TEXTBOOK OF DIAGNOSTIC RADIOLOGY

VOLUME 2:
ADVANCED APPLICATIONS AND IMAGING SPECIALTIES

Farid Ezat

ALLIED
HEALTH
PRESS

Textbook of Diagnostic Radiology

Volume 2: Advanced Applications and Imaging Specialties

Author: **Farid Ezat**

Allied Health Press
4164 Lakeshore Road
Burlington ON L7L 1A4
Canada
www.alliedhealthpress.com
Email: orders@arclereducation.com

ISBN: 978-1-77956-784-0

Allied Health Press publishes wide variety of books and eBooks. For more information about Allied Health Press and its products, visit our website at www.alliedhealthpress.com

ABOUT THE AUTHOR

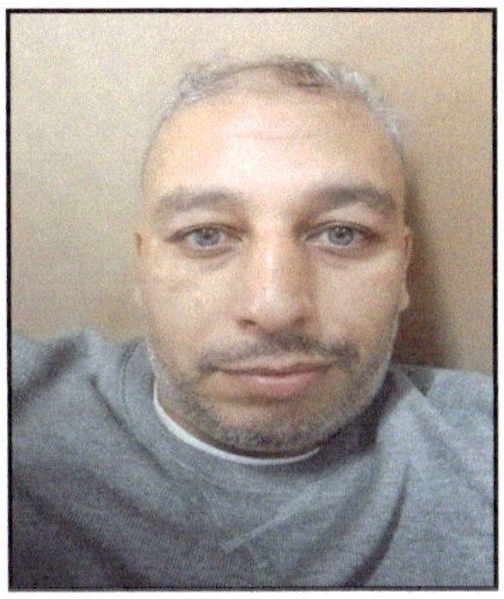

Farid ezat is a dedicated medical doctor with a diverse background in radiology, general practice, and research. Currently serving as a consultant teleradiologist for teleradiology solution , Bangaluru , India , He meticulously analyzes radiological images and engages in research. Previously, Farid honed his clinical skills as a General Practitioner in Alexandria main university hospitals. Farid's academic journey includes earning his Master degree from the Alexandria university ", Faculty of Medicine in Egypt. Committed to continuous learning, Farud actively participates in extracurricular activities and preparing for final FRCR exam.

Brief Table of Contents

Getting Started with This Book

Chapter Openers

A list of Chapter Outline is presented providing a brief Introduction to what will be covered in the chapter.

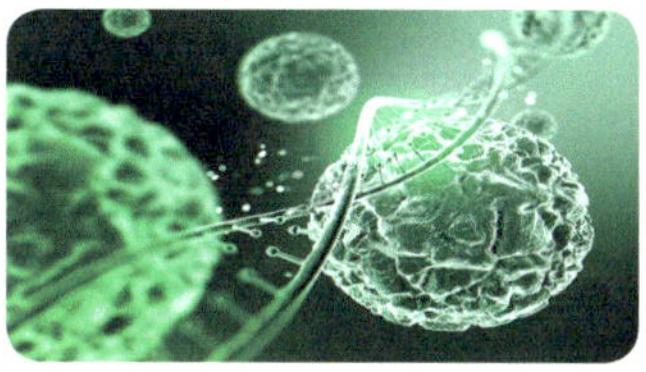

LEARNING OBJECTIVES

After studying this chapter, you will be able to:

1. Discuss the scientific method in biology;
2. Explain the cell theory;
3. Discuss the genetics and heredity;
4. Evolution and natural selection;
5. Focus on ecology and ecosystems;
6. Learn about human biology;
7. Evaluate the plant biology;
8. Explain the microbiology;
9. Focus on current trends in biology.

Introduction

Often referred to as the science of life, biology is a broad field of study aimed at comprehending the several kinds of life on Earth, from tiny creatures to sophisticated multicellular entities. Comprising several subfields, including molecular biology, ecology, and evolutionary biology, each of which advances our knowledge of living systems, this field clarifies the mechanisms controlling life events, including development, reproduction, and interaction with the surroundings, which is the central goal of biology. Moreover, biology fills in the void between the natural sciences and medicine by offering a necessary understanding of health, illness, and the interactions between organisms and their environments. Dealing with urgent global issues such as climate change, biodiversity loss, and new diseases depends on an awareness of these complex biological interactions, therefore highlighting the critical part biology plays in modern civilization. Fundamentally, biology explores and tests ideas about the living world using the scientific method. Through methodical observation and experimentation,

1.1. The Scientific Method in Biology

Learning Outcome

1. Describe the steps of the scientific method;
2. Focus on hypothesis formation;
3. Learn about experimental design.

Learning Outcomes

The beginning of each section of every chapter contains a set of Learning Outcomes that inform students of concepts they should understand. These outcomes help students understand what they should be able to do if they have mastered the material in that section.

Test Your Knowledge

Throughout each chapter, Test Your Knowledge cues you to note which topics have been covered and to self-test your understanding of the material presented.

Test Your Knowledge

1. Explain why correlation does not imply causation in scientific experiments.
2. How does the scientific method help reduce the influence of personal opinions in research?

Chapter Summary

The Summary Section appear at the end of each chapter and summarize main concepts covered throughout the chapter. These points provide key concepts in an engaging and meaningful way.

Summary

The investigation of biological principles highlights the importance of a comprehensive view of life by reflecting the intricate interactions that occur within living systems. The complexity of biology goes beyond individual species or systems, as this essay highlights; it also includes the interactions that mold ecosystems and affect biodiversity. Researchers can conduct in-depth analyses of metabolomic data using sophisticated technologies like MetaboAnalyst, which offer insights into the molecular mechanisms underlying these interactions. As demonstrated by the developments in MetaboAnalyst, for example, the integration of diverse omics data promotes a thorough understanding of metabolic pathways and helps identify important biological markers necessary for research on development and disease (Chong et al., 2018). Additionally, the phenomenon of ecological invasions is a key component of biological research and a vital field of study. The introduction of non-native species into unfamiliar habitats has significant ramifications and calls for multidisciplinary management strategies. Examining the origins and effects of these biological incursions, invasion science has become a crucial field that highlights the need to comprehend ecological dynamics and community interactions. As interest in biological invasions increases, new findings are emerging that put conventional ecological theories and practices to the test. The importance of incorporating various scientific viewpoints is shown by this developing discipline, which also highlights how invasive species shape ecosystems and advances our knowledge of ecological resilience (David et al., 2013). When taken as a whole, these discoveries from invasion science and metabolomics highlight the value of multidisciplinary biology research. Fostering cross-disciplinary collaboration and utilizing technological breakthroughs to improve our comprehension of intricate biological interactions are crucial as we look to the future of biological research. In addition to deepening our understanding of the complexities of life, this method lays the groundwork for tackling urgent environmental issues. Future studies can ensure the continued relevance of biology in a world that is constantly changing by acknowledging the interconnection of biological systems and opening the door to creative solutions that support sustainability and biodiversity conservation. We might imagine a thorough comprehension of life that serves both academia and society at large through ongoing investigation and integration of scientific knowledge.

Knowledge Assessment

The chapter includes material designed to review and reinforce each content. It includes Critical Thinking Questions to help test of your understanding of information presented in the chapter and Short answer Questions to review your understanding of the key concepts presented in the chapter.

Critical Thinking Questions

1. **Who is known as the "Father of Modern Biology"?**
   a. Aristotle
   b. Charles Darwin
   c. Gregor Mendel
   d. Louis Pasteur
2. **What is the basic unit of life?**
   a. Atom
   b. Molecule
   c. Cell
   d. Organism
3. **Which branch of biology studies the interaction of organisms with their environment?**
   a. Genetics
   b. Ecology
   c. Physiology
   d. Botany
4. **Which macromolecule is the main source of energy for living organisms?**
   a. Proteins
   b. Lipids
   c. Carbohydrates
   d. Nucleic acids
5. **DNA is primarily responsible for which function in living organisms?**
   a. Energy production
   b. Protein synthesis
   c. Storing genetic information
   d. Regulating body temperature

Short Answer Questions

1. What is biology, and why is it important to study biology?
2. What are the three main domains of life, and how are they different from one another?
3. Define homeostasis and give an example of how it works in living organisms.
4. What is the cell theory, and why is it fundamental to biology?
5. How do autotrophs and heterotrophs differ in the way they obtain energy?
6. What is the scientific method, and how is it applied in biological research?
7. Discuss how biology helps address global challenges such as climate change, disease, and food security.
8. Explain the levels of biological organization from the smallest unit to the largest. Provide examples at each level.
9. Describe the relationship between structure and function in biology, giving specific examples from cells or organs.
10. How has the discovery of genetics shaped our understanding of inheritance and variation among organisms?

Supplementary Materials

Key Terms: A list of key terms is given for quick reference

KEY TERMS FROM THIS CHAPTER

Annotation enrichment analysis	Biological structure	Cell
Cell theory	Cellular structure	Ecology
Ecosystems	Genetics	Human biology
Microbiology	Natural selection	Organism
Plant biology		

Further Resources: Recommendations for additional readings, websites, and multimedia resources.

References

1. Argelaguet, R., Velten, B., Arnol, D., Dietrich, S., Zenz, T., Marioni, J. C., Buettner, F., et al. (2018). Multi-omics factor analysis—A framework for unsupervised integration of multi-omics data sets. *Molecular Systems Biology, 14*. https://doi.org/10.15252/msb.20178124.
2. Bacher, S., Blackburn, T. M., Essl, F., & Genovesi, P. (2017). *Socio-Economic Impact Classification of Alien Taxa (SEICAT).* https://core.ac.uk/download/286567949.pdf (accessed on 8th March 2025).
3. Barnett, R., Brace, S., Cucchi, T., & Dobney, K. (2013). *Divergent Evolutionary Processes Associated with Colonization of Offshore Islands.* https://core.ac.uk/download/20664364.pdf (accessed on 8th March 2025).

Detailed Table of Contents

CHAPTER 3

Neuroradiology – Brain 65

CHAPTER 4

CHAPTER 5

CHAPTER 9

Nuclear Medicine and PET-CT 255

CHAPTER 10

Interventional Radiology 285

CHAPTER 11

Emergency and Trauma Radiology 319

CHAPTER 12

LIST OF FIGURES

PREFACE

With the growth of advanced imaging, radiology now covers dynamic procedures, detailed studies of body structures, and measurements of body functions. Volume 2 follows Volume 1 by focusing on how imaging is used for specific patient groups and body parts, and it covers the newest techniques in imaging and its analysis. The text points out how radiology is now part of team care, and it stresses the role of new technologies in making diagnoses and guiding treatment more accurately.

The second volume of Textbook of Diagnostic Radiology looks closely at advanced imaging techniques and new areas of practice. It combines knowledge about musculoskeletal, pediatric, neuro, head and neck and emergency imaging. Chapters focusing on computed tomography and magnetic resonance imaging explain how to perfect protocols and handle artifacts. It also discusses imaging methods in nuclear medicine, the practical steps of interventional radiology, and the rising impact of informatics and artificial intelligence on clinical routines.

Chapter 1 explains how to use radiographs to diagnose fractures and deformities, CT scans for complex trauma, MRI for cartilage, ligament, and marrow issues, and ultrasound for tendon and soft tissue problems, and it also explains how to tell apart degenerative, inflammatory, infectious, and neoplastic conditions.

In Chapter 2, the book gives information about pediatric radiology, including methods to keep radiation dose low, detailed sonography of neonatal organs, proper CT and MR imaging for congenital problems, and the main features of common pediatric diseases like developmental dysplasia of the hip and Wilms tumor.

Chapter 3 looks at imaging of the brain, discussing CT scans without and with contrast, MRI sequences for tumors and demyelinating diseases, advanced techniques such as diffusion and perfusion imaging, and ways to tell apart vascular malformations, infection, and metabolic disorders.

Chapter 4 focuses on the spine, explaining how CT myelography and MR help diagnose disc problems, spinal canal stenosis, and traumatic cord injury, and it reviews proper alignment measurements, signs of infection and tumors, and methods for preparing and checking treatment results.

Chapter 5 covers imaging of the head and neck, showing CT and MR scans of the sinuses, orbits, salivary glands, and pharynx; describing the common appearances of inflammation, tumors, and vascular and perineural diseases.

In Chapter 6, ultrasound and Doppler imaging are described, with high resolution techniques shown for thyroid, breast, and musculoskeletal examinations, principles of spectral and color Doppler for vascular assessment explained, protocols for abdominal and pelvic applications included, and safety and operator factors mentioned.

Chapter 7 analyzes computed tomography (CT), reviewing multi-detector and dual energy systems, image reconstruction algorithms, and dose reduction strategies; it covers protocol selection for thoracic, abdominal, and vascular studies, addresses common artifacts and troubleshooting, and discusses the role of CT in guidance for interventional procedures.

Chapter 8 describes magnetic resonance imaging (MRI), explaining fundamental pulse sequences (T1, T2, FLAIR, GRE), advanced techniques such as diffusion tensor imaging and spectroscopy, approaches to reduce scan time without compromising image quality, safety issues related to implants and contrast agents, and applications across all organ systems.

Chapter 9 looks at nuclear medicine and PET-CT, discussing the physics of radionuclide imaging, how to carry out studies for cancer, heart, and brain, choosing tracers, their uptake, and the use of PET data together with CT or MR for exact lesion detection

Chapter 10 explains interventional radiology, discussing image-guided procedures for blood vessels and other structures, the types of equipment and methods used, materials for embolization and ablation, managing patients before and after the procedure, and handling possible complications.

Chapter 11 talks about emergency and trauma radiology, explaining how to quickly image patients with polytrauma using whole body CT, use FAST ultrasound in both blunt and penetrating injuries, perform stroke code CT and MR, and communicate and interpret findings as quickly as possible in emergencies.

Chapter 12 presents a focus on radiology informatics and artificial intelligence, explaining picture archiving and communication systems (PACS), integration of electronic health records, structured reporting templates, fundamentals of machine learning and deep learning in image analysis, and examples of AI tools for lesion detection, quantification, and workflow optimization.

The book is meant for radiology residents moving into specialty training, practicing radiologists who need a reference for challenging cases, and sonographers and technologists who do advanced imaging procedures. The discussion of new technologies and procedures will be useful for clinician-investigators and educators. Along with Volume 1, this two-volume set prepares the reader to handle diagnostic radiology in general and in various specialized areas.

MUSCULOSKELETAL IMAGING

1

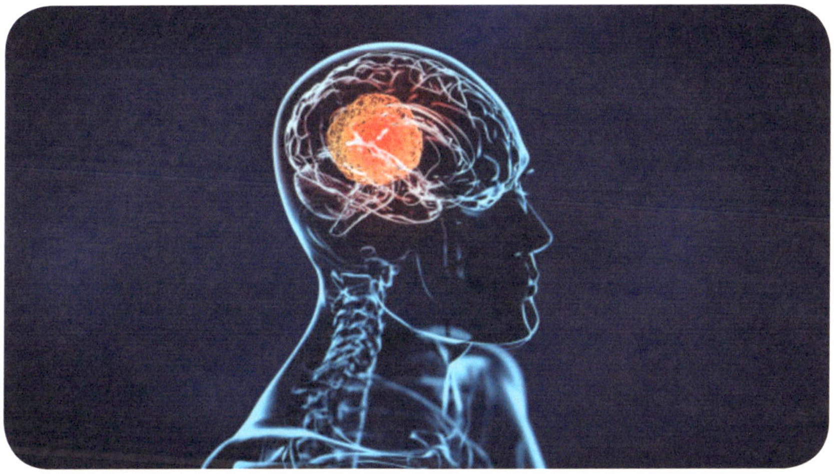

LEARNING OBJECTIVES

After studying this chapter, you will be able to:

1. Identify types of musculoskeletal imaging techniques;
2. Explain applications of musculoskeletal imaging;
3. Focus on the interpretation of musculoskeletal imaging;
4. Describe challenges and limitations in musculoskeletal imaging.

Introduction

New diagnostic tools have made it possible to see and understand many internal organs, which helps in understanding various medical problems. Musculoskeletal imaging is very important for detecting disorders of bones, joints, muscles, and soft tissues, which enables doctors to provide the best treatment possible. Using Computed Tomography, Magnetic Resonance Imaging, and high-resolution ultrasonography has made it possible to see and diagnose problems more clearly and accurately. They make it possible to clearly identify anatomical structures and diseases that were previously difficult to see. For instance, recent improvements in ultrasound technology have permitted nearly microscopic visualization of musculoskeletal anatomy, elevating diagnostic confidence and clinical decision-making (Tamborrini et al., 2024). Similarly, the development of advanced image segmentation techniques, including deep learning frameworks like U-Net and nnU-Net, has refined the interpretation of CT and MRI scans, supporting improved identification of lesions and injury patterns (Palazzo et al., 2024). All of these advances highlight the key role of musculoskeletal imaging in today's healthcare.

Definition of Musculoskeletal Imaging

Medical technology has greatly improved the way scientists and doctors look at the structures inside the body, mainly when it comes to bones and soft tissues. There are many imaging methods in musculoskeletal medicine that allow doctors to see the structure and function of muscles, bones, joints, and related tissue closely. Using computer tomography, magnetic resonance imaging, and ultrasound enables doctors to clearly see the area in three dimensions and plan proper treatment. Segmentation and geometrical description of soft tissues from detailed scans help create anatomical models that are useful in musculoskeletal biomechanics and in medical procedures (Audenaert *et al.*, 2010). Moreover, orthopedic surgery systems assisted by computers can benefit the treatment of musculoskeletal illnesses by accessing and integrating images and joint information (Kalová *et al.*, 2019). So, imaging of the musculoskeletal system benefits collaboration between surgeons and radiologists and helps improve patient results (Figure 1.1).

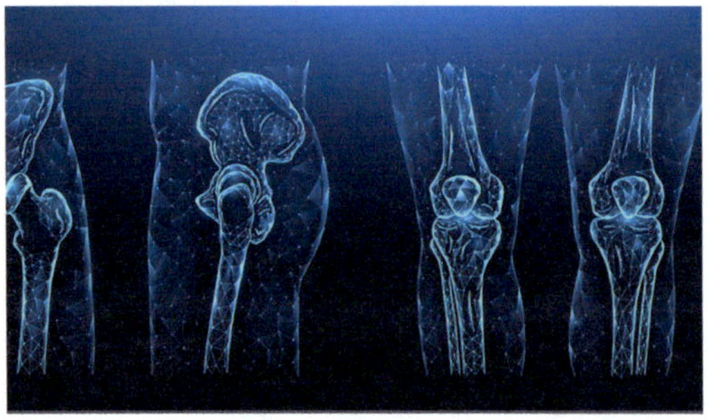

Figure 1.1. Musculoskeletal imaging.

Source: https://www.guthrie.org/sites/default/files/styles/1600x900/public/2021-09/musculoskeletal-imaging.jpg?itok=zdmpZ-6B.

Importance in Medical Diagnosis

Modern imaging changes have made diagnosing issues in musculoskeletal medicine much more precise and quicker. Thanks to magnetic resonance imaging (MRI), clinicians are now able to see small changes in bones and soft tissues, helping in the diagnosis and management of different diseases and injuries.

An example is musculoskeletal tuberculosis, which can be tough to recognize because it often shows in a variety of ways and may result in major complications if it's not addressed appropriately. Because MRI can detect tuberculous spondylitis earlier, doctors can take action quickly and help patients heal without complications (Garg *et al.*, 2024). For people involved in sports, using precise imaging methods helps correctly identify small bone injuries and fractures that are not displaced, which supports the creation of treatment plans and predicts when they can return to sports (Belair *et al.*, 2024). They demonstrate that musculoskeletal imaging is necessary to improve diagnosis and decide on the best therapies for a patient.

Historical Development of Musculoskeletal Imaging

New technology has repeatedly changed musculoskeletal imaging, going from simple X-rays to much more advanced approaches that make diagnoses more accurate. Earlier progress was mostly about X-ray imaging, allowing scientists to see inside bones without surgery. Gradually, using better imaging methods allowed doctors to recognize both clear and subtle fractures and abnormalities in joints. Nowadays, MRI is very helpful in assessing the musculoskeletal system by giving highly detailed pictures of soft tissues, cartilage, and bone marrow, while being free of ionizing radiation. Thanks to this advance, procedures such as Magnetic Resonance-guided Focused

Ultrasound Surgery (MRgFUS)can be used, which use imaging to direct ultrasound waves for treatment without removing or damaging large amounts of tissue (Albisinni *et al.*, 2015). All these advancements show a continuous improvement in the way musculoskeletal examinations are performed.

Target Audience for Musculoskeletal Imaging

Because medical imaging is always changing, it is important to thoroughly understand the people who use it the most, especially in musculoskeletal imaging. People using this technology include radiologists, rheumatologists, orthopedic surgeons, and physical therapists, all of whom need clear and appropriate data to help them make choices in clinical settings. Researchers studying rheumatoid arthritis and spondyloarthropathy look at detailed images from ultrasound to see signs of inflammation and erosion, since it offers a very clear view compared to X-ray and MRI (Bálint *et al.*, 2002).

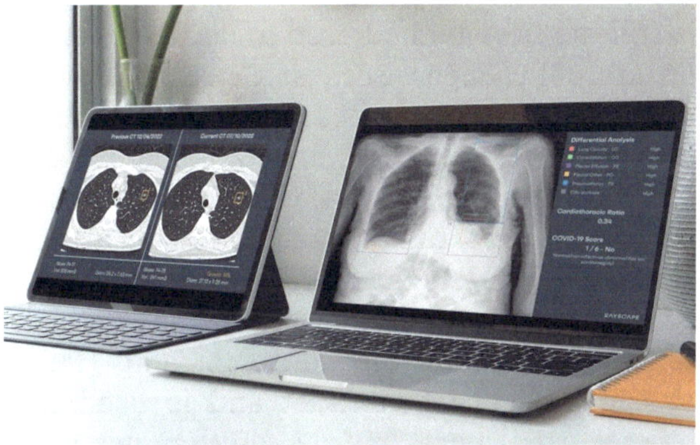

Figure 1.2. The evolving landscape of medical imaging necessitates a nuanced understanding of its primary users, particularly in musculoskeletal imaging.

Source: https://images.prismic.io/rayscape/87a4e503-ea68-4285-8044-960080bb1f27_smartmockups_lj3z7kx0%281%29.webp?auto=compress,format.

Also, understanding how images are created and understood society-wide is important, as examining the historical and social impacts sheds light on the fact that they cannot simply be seen as objective descriptions (Correll *et al.*, 2024). Therefore, these images are important for doctors, as well as for designers and other data users who need to carefully handle and apply them in different healthcare settings for better patient outcomes (Figure 1.2).

Challenges in Musculoskeletal Imaging

While diagnosing musculoskeletal problems, good visualization of bones and tissues is very important, but it is often met with several obstacles. A major difficulty arises when trying to separate muscles in the spine, since the patterns of such muscles and the image clarity vary from case to case. Automatic segmentation procedures based on artificial intelligence sometimes give inconsistent results when applied to various patient types and imaging machines, so they are not very reliable for clinical work use (Kim *et al.*, 2024).

It is also difficult to assess muscle quality using imaging among seniors, because various methods and approaches are used (Virto *et al.*, 2024). Because there are different ways to image the muscle, it can be hard to choose common evaluation standards. Getting past these difficulties will need better imaging algorithms, regularized evaluation methods, and increased access to data to help make musculoskeletal imaging more precise and reproducible.

Future Directions in the Field

New technology in imaging is changing the musculoskeletal field by making diagnoses more accurate and providing greater benefits for patients. Integrating AI with imaging will help improve interpretation, making it more reliable and efficient, which in turn simplifies medical planning. Now, with portable, high-quality, and user-friendly ultrasound tools, real-time images can be made available to many different healthcare settings, helping with early and precise actions (Chen *et al.*, 2024).

The application of 3D surface imaging, used earlier in plastic surgery, may now play a role in musculoskeletal surgery, giving surgeons access to accurate and exhaustive details before and after surgery (Kastrup *et al.*, 2024). Utilizing such technologies along with ordinary imaging can improve communication with patients, because they can use visual tools to better understand and agree to the planned treatments. Moving forward, dealing with issues related to cost, radiation doses, and consistency will be necessary to use these innovations widely in regular medical care (Figure 1.3).

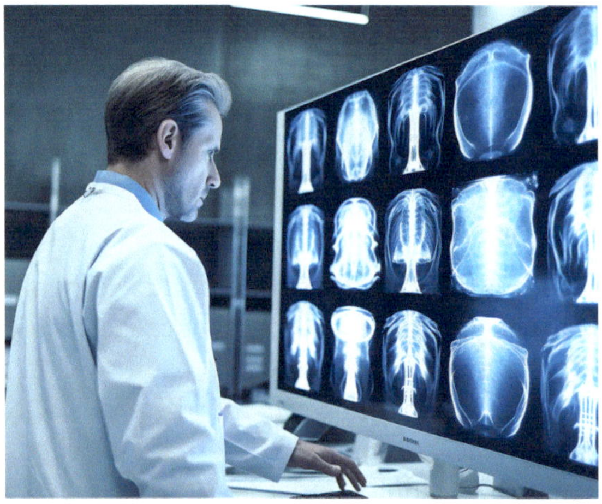

Figure 1.3. The integration of artificial intelligence into imaging modalities is poised to revolutionize interpretation by reducing variability and increasing efficiency, thereby streamlining clinical decision-making processes.

Source: https://nextgeninvent.com/wp-content/uploads/2025/02/use-of-ai-in-radiology.jpg.

1.1. Types of Musculoskeletal Imaging Techniques

Learning Outcome

1. Know how to operate an X-ray machine.
2. Discuss what magnetic resonance imaging (MRI) is.
3. Place greater emphasis on computed tomography (CT).
4. Study how ultrasound imaging works.
5. Be able to perform bone scintigraphy.
6. Describe what dual-energy x-ray absorptiometry (DEXA) is.
7. Share the information on fluoroscopy, arthrography, and fluoroscopy with the team.
8. Understand what new imaging technologies are available.

New imaging technology has improved the assessment and care of problems involving the musculoskeletal system. Because it is simple to perform and clearly shows bones, radiography is still the first method used to locate fractures or unusual changes. Because CT scans provide detailed pictures of slices through the body, they show detailed structures of the bones and any changes after surgery, which helps a lot in managing bone tumors and following up on surgery. When looking at injuries or tumors in soft tissue, including muscles, ligaments, and tendons, magnetic resonance imaging (MRI) provides the best contrast and is used the most. Furthermore, improved techniques used in MRI, like diffusion-weighted imaging and dynamic contrast-enhanced MRI, allow doctors to distinguish between what is normal after surgery and any problems or tumors that might have come back far more precisely (Lee *et al.*, 2024). Along with other imaging tests, procedures like biopsies and ablations, guided by imaging, help improve the way tumors in the musculoskeletal system are diagnosed and managed (Uldin *et al.*, 2024).

1.1.1. X-ray Imaging

The use of new technological tools has made it much easier for clinicians to accurately diagnose problems affecting the musculoskeletal system. Because of its fast and inexpensive nature, X-ray imaging continues to be relied on to assess bone and joint conditions. Still, the usual way of reading ECGs can sometimes fail to notice minor abnormalities. Recent approaches are using artificial intelligence to solve these issues, as illustrated by DeepSpine's example. This method helps both detect early symptoms of scoliosis and vertebral compression fractures and improves both treatment and recovery for patients (Degadwala *et al.*, 2024). When used with different measurements of body composition, X-ray imaging can offer additional insights into health problems that impact the musculoskeletal system, and AI is proving useful as well (Gazzotti *et al.*, 2024). As a result of these new technologies, X-ray is becoming a more important part of a complete musculoskeletal assessment (Figure 1.4).

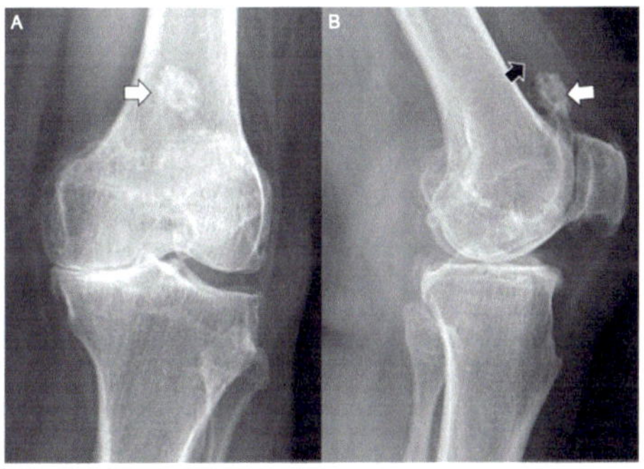

Figure 1.4. X-ray imaging remains a cornerstone in evaluating bone and joint integrity due to its rapid acquisition and cost-effectiveness.

Source: https://ars.els-cdn.com/content/image/1-s2.0-S1521694223000529-gr3.jpg.

1.1.2. Magnetic Resonance Imaging (MRI)

Thanks to new imaging techniques, we can now describe musculoskeletal tumors more accurately, and this is done without the need for invasive exams. MRI plays a pivotal role in this context, particularly through advanced techniques such as perfusion MRI and diffusion-weighted imaging (DW-MRI). Perfusion MRI quantitatively assesses tumor vascularity and permeability using parameters like K^{trans} (volume transfer constant) and K_{ep} (the rate constant of contrast transfer), which reflect increased permeability associated with malignancy, while the V_e (volume fraction of extravascular extracellular space) value indicates extracellular volume, aiding in tumor differentiation and guiding biopsy site selection (Sar *et al.*, 2024). Complementing this, DW-MRI measures the apparent diffusion coefficient (ADC), with malignant tumors generally exhibiting lower ADC values due to their dense cellularity and restricted diffusion. Studies have demonstrated high sensitivity and diagnostic accuracy of ADC measurements in distinguishing malignant from benign musculoskeletal lesions, though specificity varies, and larger cohorts are needed to validate these findings across diverse populations (Shirin *et al.*, 2024). All of these MRI advancements give clinicians important information without surgery, which helps them better treat and manage patients with musculoskeletal issues.

1.1.3. Computed Tomography (CT)

New imaging methods have greatly improved how musculoskeletal disorders are diagnosed and treated, and CT is now a key tool in this area. CT gives a clear picture of complicated bone structures and is very useful for identifying fractures, joint problems, and bone tumors that are not always visible on plain radiography. Dual-energy CT (DECT), a recent development, offers improved diagnostic capabilities by differentiating between various crystal deposits, such as uric acid and calcium, aiding in the precise identification of conditions like gout and other crystal arthropathies. Also, low-dose protocols and advanced reconstruction methods have helped to reduce radiation and keep the images clear and quickly acquired, which is safer for patients and more efficient for staff. The integration of functional postprocessing techniques further enables detailed assessment of inflammation and tissue perfusion, making CT an indispensable component in comprehensive musculoskeletal imaging strategies (Alsoliman *et al.*, 2024; Ulas *et al.*, 2024) (Figure 1.5).

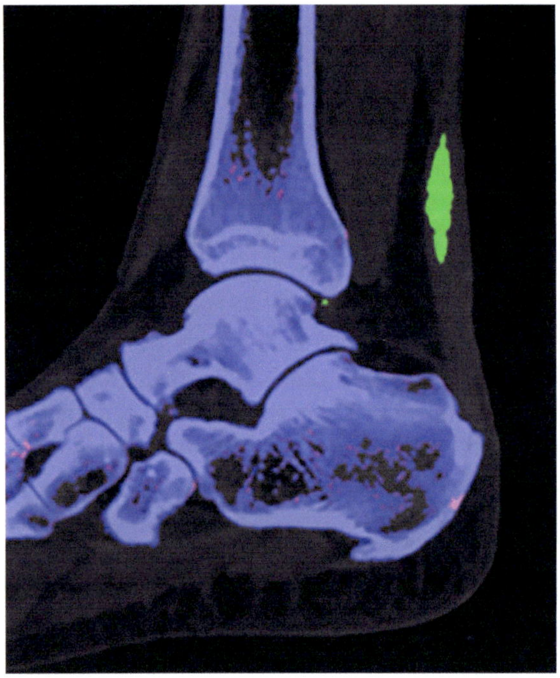

Figure 1.5. Dual-energy CT (DECT), a recent development, offers improved diagnostic capabilities by differentiating between various crystal deposits, such as uric acid and calcium, aiding in the precise identification of conditions like gout and other crystal arthropathies.

Source: https://media.springernature.com/lw685/springer-static/image/art%3A10.1007%2Fs00256-024-04856-4/MediaObjects/256_2024_4856_Fig3_HTML.jpg.

1.1.4. Ultrasound Imaging

Developments in diagnostic techniques have always improved the accuracy and care given to patients in musculoskeletal imaging. Ultrasound imaging is notable because it is both versatile and safe. It makes it possible to see soft tissues, joints, and superficial bone surfaces in great detail without using ionizing radiation on the patients. Ultrasound is also important for directing musculoskeletal procedures such as aspirations, injections, and biopsies, thereby reducing complications and improving results. Although operators' skill affects how well it works, using ultrasound skillfully has made it essential in orthopedic care. In the case of pregnant patients, ultrasound is a helpful tool because it is non-invasive and does not harm the fetus, making it safer to manage injuries of the mother's bones and joints. This synergy between diagnostic precision and safety underscores ultrasound's foundational role within musculoskeletal imaging (Tzatzairis *et al.*, 2024).

1.1.5. Bone Scintigraphy

Thanks to progress in nuclear medicine, diagnosing problems in the bones and joints has become much easier, especially with the use of bone scintigraphy. By using radiotracers, this technique can spot changes in bone metabolism and is very sensitive to detecting fractures, infections, and tumors. While bone scintigraphy can find problems early, before any changes are seen on regular X-rays, its specificity is still a concern, so it must be checked with other information and imaging tests. FDG-PET/CT has improved the way musculoskeletal infections are diagnosed, especially in cases where prosthetic joints or diabetic foot infections are involved. Nonetheless, the nonspecific uptake seen in postsurgical sites or metallic implants underscores the need for cautious interpretation (Gielen *et al.*, 2014). Combining bone scintigraphy with emerging nuclear imaging techniques fosters a more comprehensive understanding of bone pathology, thus enhancing patient management within musculoskeletal disorders (Gielen *et al.*, 2014) (Figure 1.6).

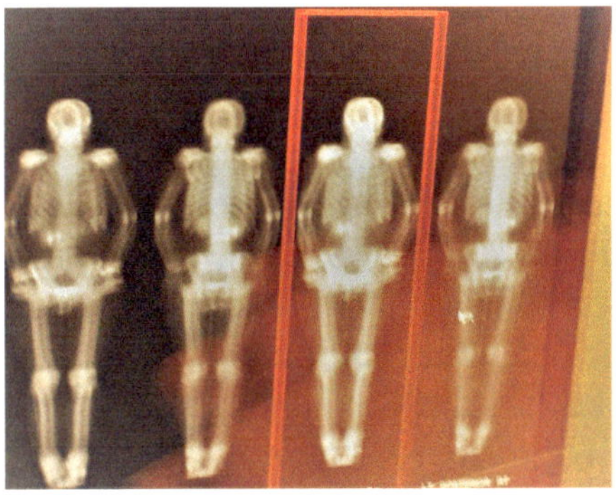

Figure 1.6. Bone scintigraphy.

Source: https://elytis-hospital.ro/wp-content/uploads/2025/02/human-skeleton-images-2025-02-22-04-54-37-utc-scaled.jpg.

1.1.6. Dual-Energy X-ray Absorptiometry (DEXA)

New imaging technology has improved the way we assess musculoskeletal health, particularly in the diagnosis and management of bone-related diseases. Among the various technologies, DEXA is now widely used to check bone mineral density with very little radiation exposure. Besides measuring, it uses advanced techniques like machine learning and deep neural networks to improve the accuracy of diagnoses and predictions of fracture risks. For example, combining fuzzy logic and artificial neural networks with features extracted from DEXA images has demonstrated impressive classification success rates in detecting osteoporosis, reaching nearly 99.4% accuracy in certain studies (Salami *et al.*, 2025). Furthermore, recent developments using deep learning architectures like vision transformers and convolutional neural networks have shown promising results in fracture risk assessment by integrating DEXA-derived imaging data with clinical information, achieving classification performance with an AUROC score of 74.3% (Senanayake *et al.*, 2023). These innovations reinforce DEXA's vital role in musculoskeletal imaging, enhancing early diagnosis and personalized treatment planning (Figure 1.7).

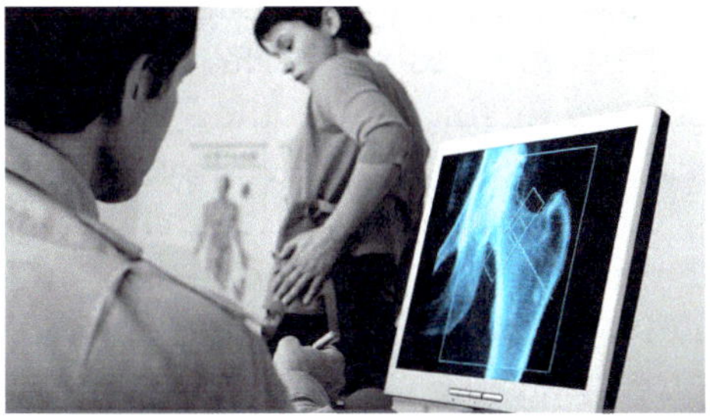

Figure 1.7. Dual-Energy X-ray Absorptiometry (DEXA) has emerged as a critical tool for evaluating bone mineral density with minimal radiation exposure.

Source: https://i0.wp.com/post.medicalnewstoday.com/wp-content/uploads/sites/3/2022/04/Dexa-scan-doctor-office-header-1024x575.jpg?w=1155&h=1528.

1.1.7. Fluoroscopy

Because of progress in musculoskeletal imaging, dynamic and real-time techniques are now used with static imaging methods. Fluoroscopy is one of these, and it offers continuous X-ray imaging to help doctors check joint movement, guide treatments, and assess the muscles and bones during surgery. The real-time movement it can show is very important for diagnosing loose ligaments, guiding arthrography, and helping to reduce fractures that must be aligned carefully. Although MRI and CT have advanced in showing bone and soft tissue, fluoroscopy is still needed for interventions that require a live view, such as manipulations and injections. While MRI advancements have improved tissue contrast without radiation exposure (Rai *et al.*, 2025), fluoroscopy's unique contribution lies in its capacity for dynamic assessment and procedural guidance. This ability often complements the strengths of MRI, CT, and ultrasound, as noted in multimodal imaging approaches that optimize diagnostic accuracy and therapeutic outcomes in musculoskeletal practice (Alsoliman *et al.*, 2024).

1.1.8. Arthrography

Thanks to new imaging methods, the way intra-articular pathologies are evaluated has greatly changed, requiring a detailed approach to diagnosing the musculoskeletal system. Among these, arthrography—particularly magnetic resonance arthrography (MRA)—has emerged as a vital tool for the detailed assessment of joint structures that are often difficult to visualize with conventional imaging. With contrast agents injected into the joint, arthrography provides a clearer view of the cartilage, ligaments, and labrum and allows the identification of small problems and instabilities. It is useful for shoulder and hip disorders, as accurately identifying capsuloligamentous and labral injuries is very important. Although arthrography involves a small procedure and requires the patient to cooperate with contrast, it is more sensitive and specific than a standard MRI for certain problems within the joints. Furthermore, the integration of imaging guidance techniques facilitates accuracy while minimizing patient discomfort, underscoring arthrography's role in contemporary musculoskeletal imaging (Fawcett *et al.*, 2022; Filho, 2018) (Figure 1.8).

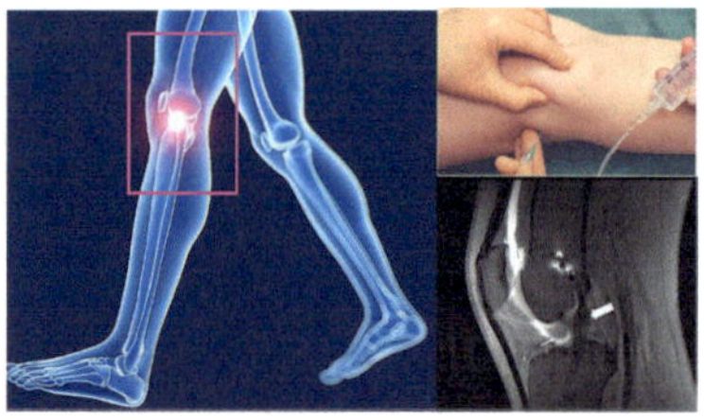

Figure 1.8. Arthrography.

Source: https://www.medifee.com/blog/wp-content/uploads/2017/06/Untitled-design-3-1.jpg.

1.1.9. Emerging Imaging Technologies

Progress in imaging has greatly improved the accuracy and safety of tests used for musculoskeletal diagnostics. With whole-body MRI and CT-like MRI sequences, radiation exposure has been reduced, and the ability to diagnose has improved in children. Photon-counting detector computed tomography and deep learning algorithms work together, bringing about improved images, faster analysis, and no risks to patients.

Artificial intelligence helps improve workflow and makes it possible to detect pathology more accurately, but there are still problems with proving its effectiveness and getting it used in many clinics. They are in line with efforts to create standard rules and encourage teamwork between different medical fields, making sure new treatments address gaps in current care. While some technological advances in dental imaging also highlight the potential of AI and molecular diagnostics to personalize treatment, their relevance underscores a broader trend toward patient-centered care across medical specialties (Kraus *et al.*, 2025; Amélia de Magalhães *et al.*, 2025). This progress could raise the standard of musculoskeletal imaging by using advanced imaging methods and smart data analysis.

Test Your Knowledge

1. How does conventional radiography (X-ray) contribute to the initial evaluation of bone and joint disorders?
2. What are the advantages of using MRI in the evaluation of soft tissue injuries and bone marrow abnormalities?

1.2. Applications of Musculoskeletal Imaging

Learning Outcome

1. Perform diagnosis of fractures;
2. Explain the evaluation of joint disorders;
3. Understand assessment of soft tissue injuries;
4. Monitor degenerative diseases;
5. Discuss preoperative planning;
6. Focus on postoperative evaluation;
7. Discuss sports medicine applications;
8. Know pediatric imaging considerations;
9. Understand oncology and tumor assessment.

Better ways to diagnose musculoskeletal problems have helped doctors detect them earlier and plan more accurate treatments. X-rays and CT scans are mainly used to check the bones and look for structural changes, but MRI and ultrasonography are better for examining soft tissues such as tendon and ligament injuries. Also, scintigraphy and fluorescence tomography allow for observing metabolic activity and inflammation, which is important for disease monitoring and predicting outcomes. When imaging is combined with biomarkers, it helps improve diagnosis, especially for osteoarthritis and osteoporosis, which supports personalized medicine. Emerging technologies, including artificial intelligence and 3D printing, promise to refine these applications by improving image interpretation and enabling customized implant designs, which can enhance surgical outcomes and patient recovery (Adamczyk *et al.*, 2025). Thus, musculoskeletal imaging remains indispensable in contemporary orthopedic practice.

1.2.1. Diagnosis of Fractures

The correct identification of fractures and related soft tissue injuries depends on choosing and interpreting the right imaging methods. Although radiography is most often used for initial fracture assessment, CT and MRI are better at finding subtle or complicated fractures, especially in areas of complex anatomy. For instance, MRI provides superior evaluation of ligamentous injuries, such as those affecting the deltoid ligament in the ankle, which often accompany fractures and influence treatment decisions (Manske *et al.*, 2025). Additionally, emerging imaging approaches facilitate the assessment of fracture risk and bone quality, as observed in metabolic bone diseases where vertebral fractures are prevalent; tools like DEXA and advanced ultrasonography techniques contribute significantly to both diagnosis and management (Bazzocchi *et al.*, 2022). Thus, integrating multiple imaging modalities optimizes diagnostic accuracy and informs comprehensive fracture care in musculoskeletal imaging (Figure 1.9).

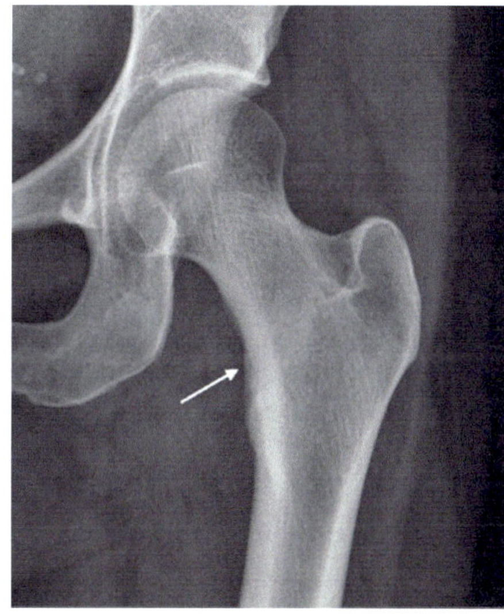

Figure 1.9. Effective diagnosis of fractures relies heavily on the appropriate selection and interpretation of imaging modalities to accurately identify bone disruptions and associated soft tissue injuries.

Source: https://onlinelibrary.wiley.com/cms/asset/89fab4a6-a52b-4487-ad7a-406e7515fe7f/rrp7412540-fig-0006a-m.jpg.

1.2.2. Evaluation of Joint Disorders

Better imaging methods have transformed how musculoskeletal conditions are diagnosed, mainly for joint disorders. Because MRI provides excellent contrast for soft tissues and can be viewed from multiple angles, it is considered essential for diagnosis. For instance, in the assessment of knee injuries, MRI not only detects anterior cruciate ligament tears but also reveals associated meniscal and collateral ligament damage, which is crucial for comprehensive treatment planning since meniscal tears frequently accompany ACL injuries (Reddy *et al.*, 2024). Similarly, ankle joint evaluation benefits significantly from MRI's ability to visualize soft tissue structures such as ligaments, tendons, and fascia, while also identifying occult bone lesions that may be missed on conventional imaging (Gebriel *et al.*, 2024). Thanks to the noninvasive and detailed imaging of MRI, diagnosing joint trauma is more accurate, which helps with quick and effective treatment of musculoskeletal disorders.

1.2.3. Assessment of Soft Tissue Injuries

Thanks to new imaging methods, it is now easier to find and treat problems in soft tissue injuries. MRI is essential because it provides excellent detail of muscles, tendons, ligaments, and cartilage, all without using ionizing radiation. MRI's efficacy in detecting subtle tissue changes, edema, and partial tears makes it indispensable in assessing sports-related injuries and degenerative conditions (Dhimar *et al.*, 2025). Complementing MRI, emerging quantitative ultrasound methods offer non-invasive assessment of tissue properties and real-time evaluation of mechanical loading during physical activity, providing critical insights into tissue health and injury mechanisms (Wearing *et al.*, 2024). These imaging advancements facilitate not only accurate diagnosis but also monitoring of healing and rehabilitation progress, underscoring the importance of integrating multiple modalities to enhance the comprehensive assessment of soft tissue injuries within musculoskeletal imaging (Figure 1.10).

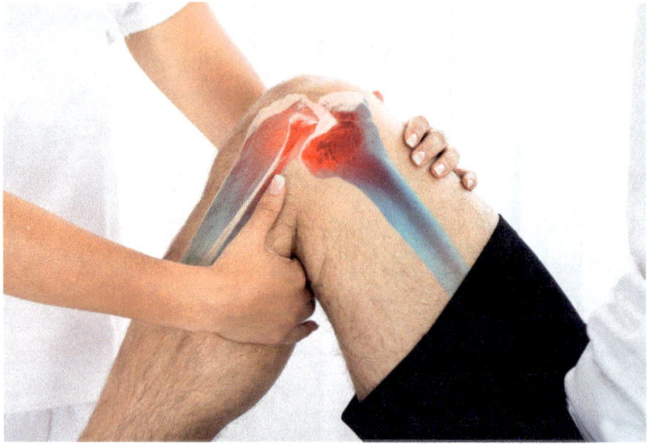

Figure 1.10. MRI's efficacy in detecting subtle tissue changes, edema, and partial tears makes it indispensable in assessing sports-related injuries and degenerative conditions.

Source: https://www.caringmedical.com/wp-content/uploads/2023/10/ACL-knee-PT.jpg.

1.2.4. Monitoring of Degenerative Diseases

New imaging techniques have made it much easier to observe degenerative musculoskeletal diseases by showing the condition of tissues and blood vessels in great detail. Ultrasonographic measurements of muscle thickness and cross-sectional area have emerged as reliable indicators of muscle degeneration, demonstrating strong correlation with histological findings and enabling effective semiquantitative scoring of muscle morphology in conditions such as sarcopenia (Blasi *et al.*, 2023). They enable doctors to closely watch how the disease develops and how well the treatment is working. Power Doppler ultrasound is also helpful in noticing increased blood flow that often happens with inflammation in degenerative tendon diseases such as rotator cuff disease. This imaging modality, combined with cytokine profiling of angiogenesis-related factors in peripheral blood, reveals the complex interaction between pro-inflammatory and anti-inflammatory mechanisms that drive tissue degeneration and repair (Badet *et al.*, 2011). Therefore, using both musculoskeletal imaging and biochemical markers provides a , and develop a comprehensive approach to monitoring the progression of degenerative diseases, informing treatment decisions, and developing personalized treatment plans.

1.2.5. Preoperative Planning

Achieving successful outcomes from musculoskeletal surgery depends on careful planning before the operation, which highlights the importance of advanced imaging. Assessing all the soft tissue and bone parts carefully helps doctors choose the right surgery for complex joints like the shoulder. Using different imaging techniques to study soft tissue injuries and bone lesions helps doctors make the right diagnosis and choose the proper treatment, which reduces risks and speeds up recovery.

For instance, preoperative imaging in shoulder arthroplasty enables surgeons to select the appropriate prosthesis and anticipate challenges, enhancing procedural success and patient outcomes (Vaswani *et al.*, 2025). Similarly, precise measurement and reporting of bone loss in cases of anterior glenohumeral instability are essential for choosing between labral repair or bone augmentation procedures, directly impacting surgical technique and prognosis (Symanski *et al.*, 2025). Thus, integration of comprehensive musculoskeletal imaging into preoperative workflows is indispensable for optimizing patient-specific interventions and advancing orthopedic care (Figure 1.11).

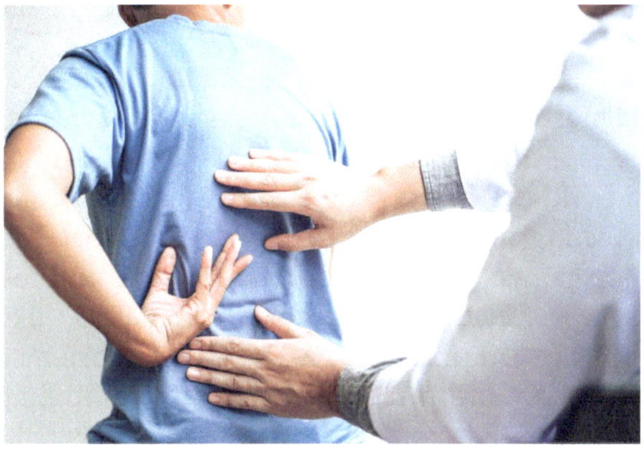

Figure 1.11. Detailed assessment of both soft tissue and bony structures facilitates appropriate surgical decision-making, especially in complex joints such as the shoulder.

Source: https://spinehealth.org/wp-content/uploads/2023/01/shutterstock_1193820529-scaled.jpg.

1.2.6. Postoperative Evaluation

Evaluating the patient after surgery is necessary in musculoskeletal imaging to help them heal well and catch any problems early. In assessing the success of rotator cuff surgeries, CT and MRI imaging are very important. Recent innovations, such as magnesium-based suture anchors, have demonstrated promising results through improved osseointegration and reduced stress shielding, which can be effectively monitored via postoperative imaging to confirm tissue healing and bone regeneration (Hsu *et al.*, 2024). When a pregnant patient is involved, the postoperative evaluation calls for extra coordination among different healthcare professionals to ensure the safety of both the mother and the fetus. For this reason, postoperative assessment includes not only checking the structure but also examining the body's function and the presence of chemicals. Using multiple approaches to evaluate patients improves outcomes in musculoskeletal surgery.

1.2.7. Sports Medicine Applications

New imaging methods have made it easier to diagnose and treat sports-related injuries to the muscles and bones. While X-rays, CT scans, and MRI are helpful, they usually have difficulty detecting minor soft tissue and early cartilage damage, as well as checking how the injured tissues function. Emerging techniques like photoacoustic imaging (PAI) have shown promise in overcoming these challenges by combining optical and ultrasound imaging to deliver high-resolution visualization of blood vessels and soft tissues, offering valuable insights into tissue oxygenation and metabolic activity essential for monitoring healing processes (Ma *et al.*, 2025). Additionally, point-of-care ultrasound (POCUS) has become increasingly integral in sports medicine due to its portability, real-time dynamic imaging, and cost-effectiveness, facilitating rapid assessment and treatment decisions for muscle, tendon, ligament, and joint injuries, thus optimizing clinical outcomes and return-to-play strategies (Koziak *et al.*, 2025). These innovations underscore the evolving role of musculoskeletal imaging in enhancing sports medicine applications (Figure 1.12).

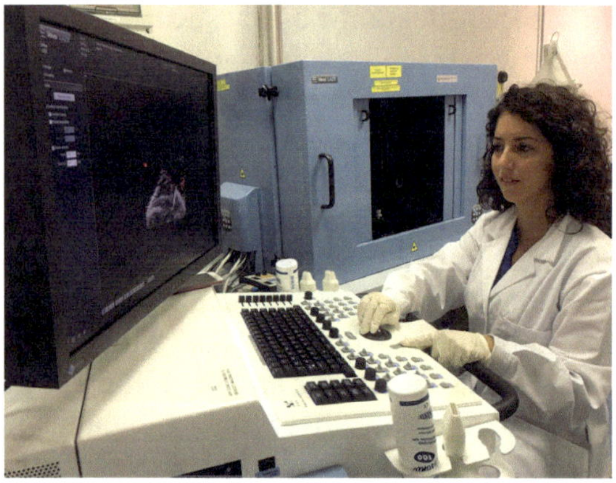

Figure 1.12. Photoacoustic imaging (PAI).

Source: https://focalplane.biologists.com/wp-content/uploads/2020/11/image001.jpg.

1.2.8. Pediatric Imaging Considerations

It is important to pay attention to certain factors when imaging the musculoskeletal system in children to ensure the results are accurate and the risks are low. Children's bones are not fully formed, so their growth plates and different levels of ossification must be interpreted differently from those of adults. Because younger patients may move during scans, it is important to use the right positioning and immobilization methods to avoid motion artifacts. Furthermore, radiation exposure is a paramount concern; thus, imaging modalities and protocols must be judiciously chosen to adhere to the ALARA (As Low As Reasonably Achievable) principle, favoring non-ionizing techniques like ultrasound or MRI when feasible. Selecting the right equipment settings and focal spot sizes made for children helps produce clear images and improves diagnostic results while keeping radiation low. Moreover, training radiologists to spot pediatric musculoskeletal problems ensures that diagnoses are accurate and the right treatment is planned.

1.2.9. Oncology and Tumor Assessment

To evaluate musculoskeletal tumors well, advanced imaging is needed to show the shape, blood supply, and the way the lesion relates to nearby tissues. To tell the difference between benign and malignant masses, MRI and CT are key tests in oncology. With these tools, clinicians can see how large the tumor is, where the margins are, and if it has spread into the bones or soft tissues, which are important for both staging and predicting the outcome. Also, imaging is essential for checking how well the therapy is working and for finding any signs of cancer returning after treatment. New developments have made it possible to see images with higher quality and better contrast, making it easier to diagnose difficult cases where the symptoms are not clear. New functional imaging techniques also give important metabolic and blood flow information that adds to what is seen in standard brain scans. Thus, comprehensive tumor assessment through musculoskeletal imaging not only facilitates diagnosis but also underpins personalized oncologic management strategies (Figure 1.13).

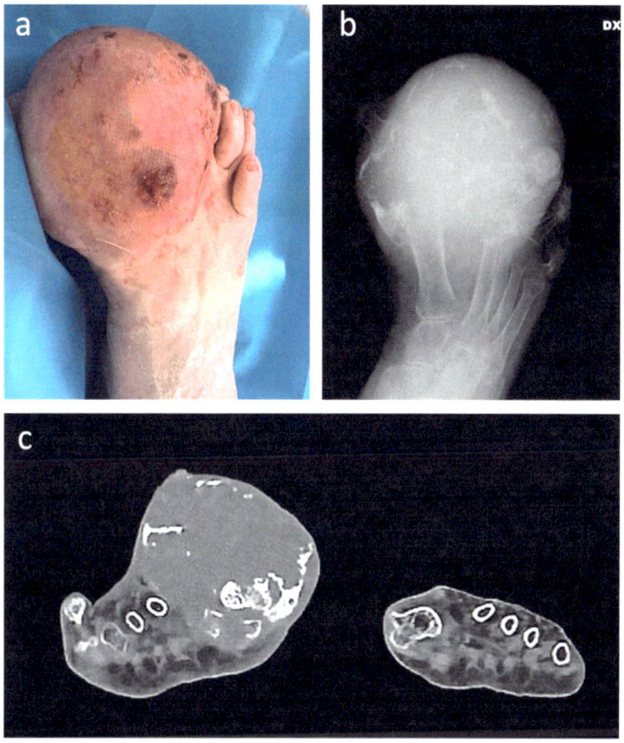

Figure 1.13. Accurate evaluation of musculoskeletal tumors necessitates advanced imaging techniques that provide detailed characterization of lesion morphology, vascularity, and relation to surrounding tissues.

Source: https://www.mdpi.com/jcm/jcm-12-03038/article_deploy/html/images/jcm-12-03038-g001.png.

Test Your Knowledge

1. In what situations is musculoskeletal ultrasound used to assess joint and soft tissue conditions?
2. What is the role of musculoskeletal imaging in the assessment of pediatric fractures or growth plate injuries?

1.3. Interpretation of Musculoskeletal Imaging

Learning Outcome

1. Know the role of radiologists;
2. Explain common imaging findings;
3. Identify differential diagnosis techniques;
4. Explain the importance of clinical correlation;
5. List limitations of imaging techniques;
6. Discuss the use of contrast agents;
7. Know reporting standards and protocols;
8. Focus on integration with other diagnostic tools;
9. Understand continuing education for practitioners.

Because of new technology, diagnostic radiology is now able to analyze musculoskeletal images more accurately and speedily. As more imaging studies are performed, it has become clear that there are not enough subspecialized musculoskeletal radiologists, which has led to the need for new approaches to keep accuracy and efficiency high. Artificial intelligence (AI) emerges as a promising adjunct, capable of assisting radiologists by triaging cases, enhancing image interpretation, and reducing reporting times, thereby improving overall patient care. Working together, AI researchers and clinical experts ensure that new tools can be trusted and easily used in the medical field. AI can also be used in education and research, which helps improve the field even further. Nevertheless, challenges such as overfitting and data imbalance must be addressed to ensure robust AI performance, paralleling strategies seen in other medical imaging domains where deep learning models are optimized through targeted augmentation and adaptive training techniques (Guermazi *et al.*, 2024; Mahesh *et al.*, 2024).

1.3.1. Role of Radiologists

New imaging methods have improved how accurately doctors can diagnose and plan treatment for musculoskeletal problems. Much of this advancement depends on radiologists who study complex images such as MRI, CT scans, and ultrasounds to spot minor problems in the bones, joints, and soft tissues. Because of their wide-ranging knowledge, radiologists can detect fractures, tumors, and inflammatory diseases and also assist doctors in selecting the right treatment. Besides, radiologists are responsible for performing image-guided procedures such as biopsies and injections, which are important for managing patients. By connecting what is seen on imaging with the patient's symptoms, they can give an accurate diagnosis and prevent unneeded treatments. The evolving landscape of musculoskeletal imaging increasingly relies on radiologists' integrated approach to technology and clinical insight, underscoring their indispensable role in modern medical practice (Figure 1.14).

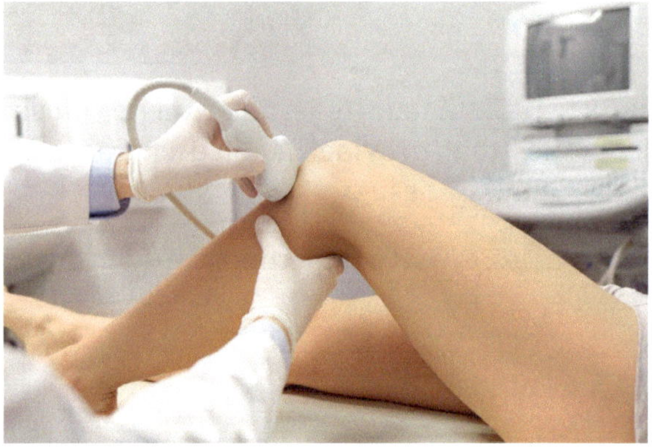

Figure 1.14. Advancements in imaging technology have significantly enhanced the diagnostic accuracy and treatment planning for musculoskeletal conditions.

Source: https://lakezurichopenmri.com/wp-content/uploads/2024/10/Ultrasound-in-musculoskeletal-diagnostics.jpeg.

1.3.2. Common Imaging Findings

Imaging is very important in finding the specific signs that help doctors diagnose and treat musculoskeletal conditions. Usually, joint effusions, increased thickness in the synovium, and bone marrow edema are seen on imaging, which may indicate either inflammation or degeneration. For instance, differentiating juvenile idiopathic arthritis from other synovial disorders can be challenging due to overlapping imaging features, such as synovial hypertrophy and joint swelling, necessitating adjunctive biomarkers to improve diagnostic accuracy, as highlighted by elevated synovial calprotectin levels in arthritis patients (Kozhevnikov *et al.*, 2025). Ultrasound and MRI are useful for finding soft tissue problems and early cartilage damage before they show up on X-rays. It is important to notice subtle signs on imaging in pediatric patients, because early care can prevent serious long-term consequences. Overall, familiarity with these common imaging findings enhances the clinician's ability to interpret musculoskeletal pathology accurately and tailor patient management effectively (Kozhevnikov *et al.*, 2025).

1.3.3. Differential Diagnosis Techniques

A good diagnosis in musculoskeletal imaging requires a well-structured process to tell apart different conditions that can have similar symptoms and images. Often, doctors need to use several imaging techniques, since each one offers its own information about the tissue, the type of lesion, and signs of inflammation. For example, the use of DECT has revolutionized the detection and distinction of crystal arthropathies by differentiating uric acid from calcium deposits, thereby refining the differential diagnosis of inflammatory joint diseases and aiding in accurate treatment planning (Ulas *et al.*, 2024). Similarly, complex cases involving masses or lesions require a multimodality strategy, combining clinical data with advanced imaging techniques to discern benign from malignant processes, particularly when standard imaging is inconclusive (Sozzi *et al.*, 2025). Employing tailored imaging algorithms and postprocessing protocols enhances diagnostic accuracy, minimizes unnecessary biopsies, and guides clinical decision-making, underscoring the essential role of differential diagnosis techniques in musculoskeletal imaging (Figure 1.15).

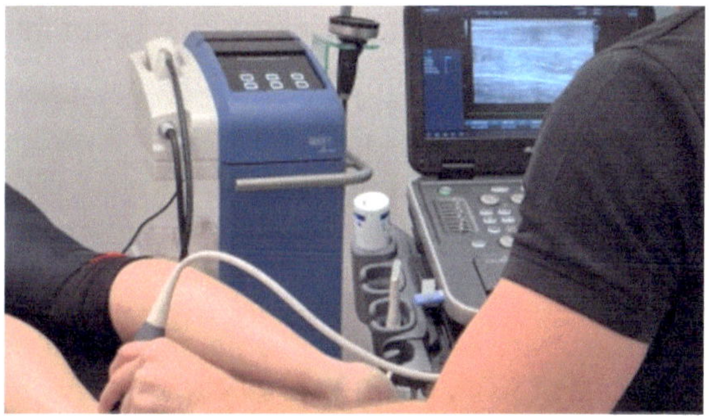

Figure 1.15. Employing tailored imaging algorithms and postprocessing protocols enhances diagnostic accuracy, minimizes unnecessary biopsies, and guides clinical decision-making, underscoring the essential role of differential diagnosis techniques in musculoskeletal imaging.

Source: https://www.sonoskills.com/clients/sonoskills/themes/uploads/crop_1719852278 UltrasoundGuidedShockwave11.png.

1.3.4. Importance of Clinical Correlation

Getting the right diagnosis in musculoskeletal imaging goes beyond reading the images; it also involves understanding how the patient's history and complaints relate to the findings on the images. For instance, low back pain in women of reproductive age presents multifactorial challenges, where imaging must be integrated with clinical factors like hormonal influences and lifestyle to identify precise etiologies effectively, as highlighted in studies exploring prevalence and causative associations (Bilkish *et al.*, 2024). Similarly, post-arthroscopy alterations in lumbopelvic mobility demonstrate that imaging changes must be correlated with functional outcomes and patient-reported pain to assess the true clinical impact (Stambaugh *et al.*, 2024). If there is no integration, images could be misunderstood, which might result in incorrect care decisions. Hence, it is essential to link clinical information with imaging in musculoskeletal care, so that the findings guide the right treatment for each patient, not just point out isolated abnormalities.

1.3.5. Limitations of Imaging Techniques

Although musculoskeletal imaging has improved a lot, there are still some problems that affect how accurate the results are and the choices doctors make. As an illustration, MRI can clearly show soft tissues, yet it may not detect cortical bone problems as well as CT, and because it is costly and takes a long time, not everyone can use it. CT imaging gives clear details of bones, but it also involves exposure to ionizing radiation, which becomes a concern when scans are done many times. Ultrasound is cost-effective and portable but is highly operator-dependent and limited in evaluating deep or complex anatomical regions (Alsoliman *et al.*, 2024). Recent innovations like the zero-echo time (ZTE) MRI sequence attempt to address some limitations by enabling imaging of short-T2 tissues with ultrafast readouts; however, practical challenges in image reconstruction and integration into routine workflows remain (Fujisaki *et al.*, 2023). Collectively, these constraints highlight the necessity for multimodal approaches to optimize musculoskeletal imaging outcomes (Figure 1.16).

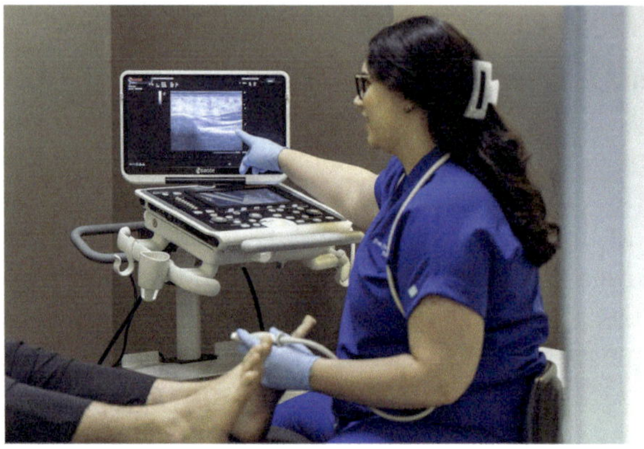

Figure 1.16. Ultrasound is cost-effective and portable, but is highly operator-dependent and limited in evaluating deep or complex anatomical regions.

Source: https://images.prismic.io/ndgpodiatry/ZtH64EaF0TcGJmfR_NDGPodiatryClinic-CliniquePodiatriqueNDG-17.jpg?auto=format%2Ccompress&w=1200.

1.3.6. Use of Contrast Agents

Contrast agents have played a key role in improving the imaging of soft tissues, blood vessels, and any disease that might be unclear without them. The most common types of these agents are gadolinium for MRI and iodine for CT, and they make it easier to see differences between inflamed, tumorous, or ischemic tissues and healthy tissues. This improvement is very important for spotting small changes in complex joints and for distinguishing between benign and malignant lesions. Moreover, contrast-enhanced imaging makes it easier to identify synovial inflammation and blood flow, which are key for diagnosing diseases such as arthritis or osteomyelitis. Even though contrast is useful, doctors should be careful when choosing it because it can cause allergic reactions and harm to the kidneys. These developments in contrast technology keep improving the accuracy of musculoskeletal imaging, which helps patients recover more effectively.

1.3.7. Reporting Standards and Protocols

It is essential to clearly explain imaging findings in musculoskeletal imaging because this helps guide doctors in their care and affects the outcomes of patients. Following standardized ways to report information helps ensure that all important details are always shared, lowers the risk of misunderstanding, and allows for quick and proper actions. For instance, the European Society of Musculoskeletal Radiology (ESSR) guidelines emphasize specific MRI sequences and detailed descriptions to distinguish malignant lesions from benign conditions. However, studies reveal frequent deviations from these standards, with incomplete imaging protocols and inaccurate diagnoses resulting in potential treatment delays and suboptimal patient care (Weiss *et al.*, 2021). Similarly, thorough reporting after procedures such as curettage for chondroblastoma must include tumor location, recurrence risk, and functional outcomes to guide effective management (Tosyal *et al.*, 2024). Thus, rigorous adherence to reporting standards not only supports diagnostic accuracy but also enhances interdisciplinary communication, ultimately improving overall patient management in musculoskeletal disorders (Figure 1.17).

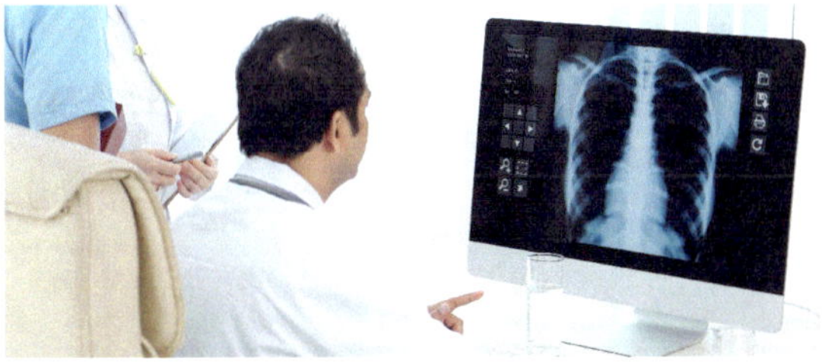

Figure 1.17. Effective communication of imaging findings is critical in musculoskeletal imaging, as the clarity and completeness of radiology reports directly influence clinical decision-making and patient outcomes.

Source: https://d35oenyzp35321.cloudfront.net/Radiology_67178ca3e8.jpg.

1.3.8. Integration with Other Diagnostic Tools

The use of a combination of diagnostic tools is now being stressed in musculoskeletal imaging to help doctors make more accurate diagnoses and improve patient outcomes. While modalities such as MRI and X-ray remain indispensable for detailed anatomic and osseous evaluation, the integration of musculoskeletal ultrasound (MSK-US) offers dynamic, high-resolution visualization of soft tissue structures that may be less apparent on traditional imaging. This way of working helps clinicians gather real-time data, plan treatments, and track the patient's progress. Physical therapists, in particular, have begun incorporating MSK-US into their diagnostic repertoire, benefiting from its portability and cost-effectiveness, as well as supportive employment environments that foster skill development and mentorship (Hayward *et al.*, 2022). Furthermore, the precise imaging of soft tissue abnormalities in conditions like lateral elbow pathologies through ultrasound enriches the interpretive context provided by other imaging forms, highlighting the value of multimodal integration in comprehensive musculoskeletal assessment (Manske *et al.*, 2025).

1.3.9. Continuing Education for Practitioners

It is important for practitioners to regularly learn new things in musculoskeletal imaging to provide accurate diagnoses and the best care for patients. Since AI-assisted imaging and three-dimensional reconstruction are now used, radiologists have to keep learning new skills. With these programs, clinicians can follow a planned path to learn about new advances, which helps them choose better diagnostic and treatment strategies. In addition, interactive and evidence-based platforms, as seen in healthcare settings, help practitioners stay involved and retain their knowledge, as they can discuss and get feedback from experts right away. Education programs like these help people become more skilled and also ensure that imaging is done the same way everywhere, benefiting patients. The commitment to lifelong learning reflects the dynamic nature of musculoskeletal imaging and supports practitioners in meeting the evolving demands of their profession (Alhejji *et al.*, 2024; Morhaim *et al.*, 2024) (Figure 1.18).

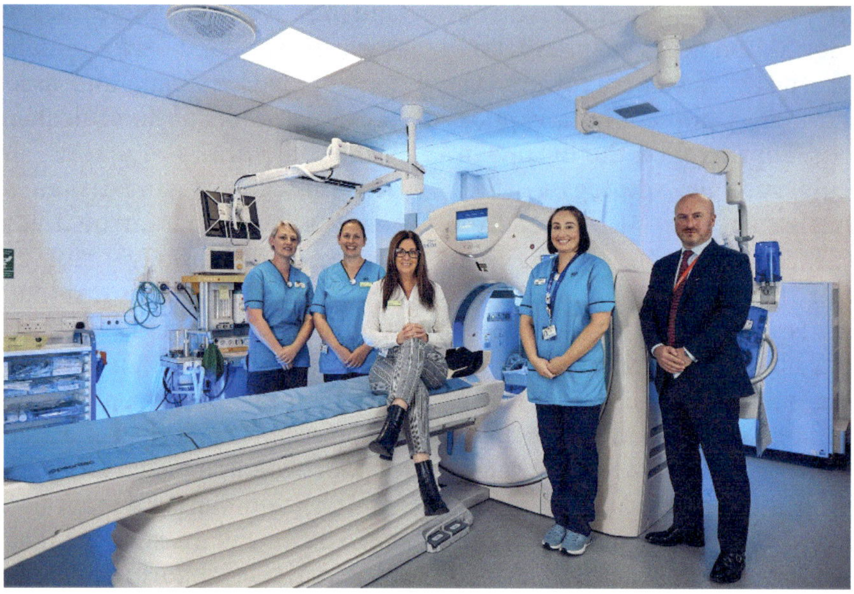

Figure 1.18. Continuing education programs provide a structured approach for clinicians to stay abreast of these innovations, facilitating the adoption of new methodologies that improve diagnostic precision and treatment planning.

Source: https://uk.medical.canon/wp-content/uploads/sites/8/2022/10/Canon-Medical-CT-Kilmarnock-26-scaled.jpg.

Test Your Knowledge

1. Which aspects should be considered when reviewing an X-ray of a long bone for a possible fracture?
2. What are the differences between a stress fracture and a pathological fracture that can be seen on X-ray or MRI?

1.4. Challenges and Limitations in Musculoskeletal Imaging

Learning Outcome

1. Understand radiation exposure concerns;
2. Define cost and accessibility issues;
3. Explain variability in imaging quality;
4. Focus on patient compliance and preparation;
5. Identify interpretation errors and misdiagnosis;
6. Know technological limitations;
7. Focus on ethical considerations in imaging;
8. Describe the impact of insurance and reimbursement policies;
9. Know future research needs.

Although musculoskeletal imaging has improved a lot, there are still some issues that prevent it from being used perfectly in diagnosis and treatment. Although X-ray and CT are good for evaluating bones, they expose patients to radiation and provide limited detail about soft tissues. MRI is better at seeing soft tissues, but it fails to clearly show bone and ligaments which have short T2 relaxation times, leading to blurry and similar-looking images. Although UTE and ZTE have improved the previous problems, their use is limited by their difficulty to perform and the lack of availability. Biomarkers used with imaging techniques allow for early detection and monitoring, though there are problems with standardization and validation. Because more people are developing musculoskeletal diseases due to their age and habits, it is important to overcome these issues to detect and treat them earlier. Future innovations such as artificial intelligence and advanced imaging technology hold promise, but their successful implementation requires addressing current limitations in access, cost, and technical expertise (Rai *et al.*, 2025; Trestka *et al.*, 2025).

1.4.1. Radiation Exposure Concerns

Although new musculoskeletal imaging tools have made it easier to diagnose, they also increase worries about radiation exposure, mainly for children. Because CT and other ionizing radiation methods are being used more, it is important to examine the health risks, such as cancer and brain problems, that can occur in children after being exposed to high doses. Even though spectral CT is safer and more accurate than regular CT scans, it is still necessary to have strict safety protocols to prevent unnecessary exposure. In places like Saudi Arabia, where there are not many detailed guidelines for radiation safety in healthcare, the risk of overexposure during musculoskeletal examinations is higher. Addressing these challenges demands policy reforms and heightened educational efforts aimed at optimizing patient safety without compromising diagnostic efficacy (Aleid *et al.*, 2024; Eibschutz *et al.*, 2024) (Figure 1.19).

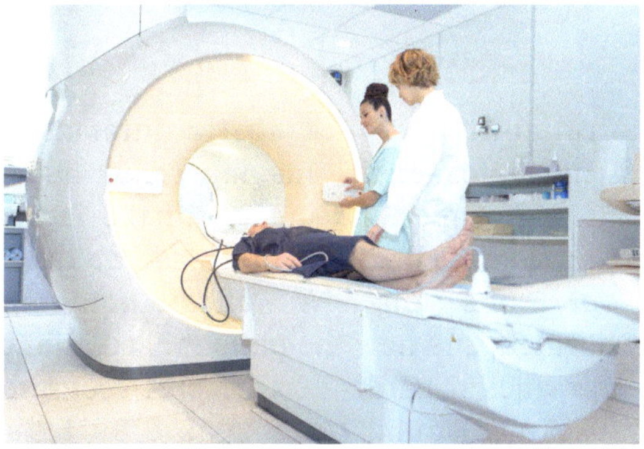

Figure 1.19. The increasing reliance on ionizing radiation-based modalities, including computed tomography (CT), necessitates a critical evaluation of associated health risks, such as carcinogenesis and neurotoxicity.

Source: https://www.simplypsychology.org/wp-content/uploads/mri-scanner.jpg.

1.4.2. Cost and Accessibility Issues

Better musculoskeletal imaging has greatly improved how conditions are diagnosed and treated, yet there are still major obstacles because of cost and availability. Because these imaging procedures are costly, they are not available as often in healthcare settings that lack resources. Besides putting pressure on patients, this burden also affects healthcare systems that are trying to carry out regular screening and early treatment. Such limitations are especially concerning given the prevalence of disorders like osteoporosis, where early detection through imaging is crucial to prevent fractures and subsequent disability (LeBoff *et al.*, 2022). Additionally, accessibility challenges hinder the effective monitoring of musculoskeletal diseases, potentially delaying timely treatment adjustments recommended in clinical guidelines (Kolasinski *et al.*, 2020). Such differences show that we need to focus on increasing insurance coverage, helping with diagnostic costs, and ensuring equal use of imaging services to improve outcomes for people from different groups.

1.4.3. Variability in Imaging Quality

The reliability of diagnostic information from musculoskeletal imaging relies heavily on the uniformity and quality of the images. Imaging quality may be inconsistent due to the operator's skill, how well the equipment is calibrated, and how the patient is positioned, which makes it harder to interpret accurately. Because ultrasound imaging is easy to use and gives instant results, it is more likely to be affected by changes in machine settings and the way the scan is performed. Recent studies have demonstrated that applying advanced image pre-processing techniques, such as adaptive contrast enhancement, can significantly improve the reproducibility of radiomic features extracted from ultrasound images, thereby enhancing diagnostic precision in musculoskeletal conditions (Triantafyllou *et al.*, 2025). Moreover, comparative analyses across imaging modalities emphasize that variability not only impacts accuracy but also influences clinical decision-making and treatment outcomes, underscoring the need for standardized protocols and technological advancements to reduce such disparities (Chen *et al.*, 2024) (Figure 1.20).

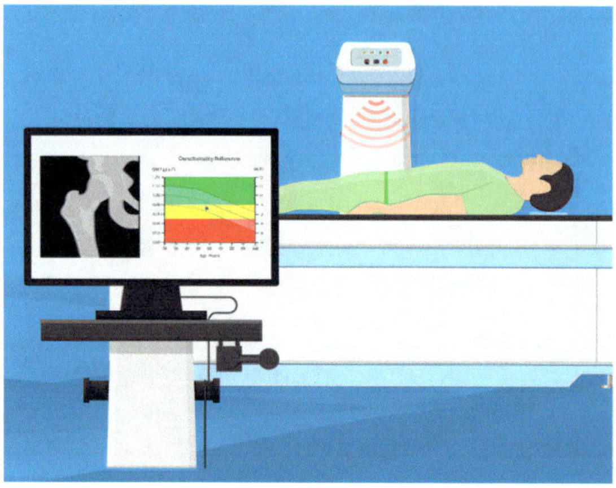

Figure 1.20. Variability in imaging quality arises from multiple factors, including operator skill, equipment calibration, and patient positioning, all of which can introduce inconsistencies that complicate accurate interpretation.

Source: https://pub.mdpi-res.com/diagnostics/diagnostics-14-01328/article_deploy/html/images/diagnostics-14-01328-g001.png?1719057491.

1.4.4. Patient Compliance and Preparation

To get good musculoskeletal images, you need advanced tools and also make sure the patient is prepared and cooperates. Following the pre-procedural guidelines, such as not eating or exercising, allows imaging modalities to give the most accurate and clear results. For example, following the right preparation steps in ultrasound and computed tomography can make the images and diagnosis more reliable. When patients are informed and follow the instructions, it reduces artifacts, makes them more comfortable, and helps avoid having to repeat scans, improving the overall efficiency of the process. Moreover, controlled and sustained drug release methods, like microsponge-based formulations, have demonstrated improved patient compliance by reducing side effects in topical treatments, highlighting the broader relevance of compliance across imaging-related interventions (Tushir *et al.*, 2025). Similarly, cross-sectional imaging in chronic conditions underscores the necessity of patient cooperation for consistent monitoring and diagnosis, further stressing that preparation protocols and compliance are indispensable elements in delivering optimal musculoskeletal imaging outcomes (Leş *et al.*, 2025).

1.4.5. Interpretation Errors and Misdiagnosis

Improvements in imaging have made it much easier to see musculoskeletal structures, but mistakes in interpretation and diagnosis are still a major problem for patients. Sometimes, not all abnormalities or similar symptoms in MRI scans are easy to spot, which can result in reading the injury as less or more severe than it actually is. For instance, differentiating between partial and complete anterior cruciate ligament injuries can be complex, as evidenced by machine learning models that, despite high overall accuracy, still face difficulties accurately identifying completely ruptured cases (Diqi *et al.*, 2024). Additionally, the integration of artificial intelligence tools into clinical workflows necessitates careful evaluation to mitigate errors caused by algorithm limitations or inappropriate application (Ducarouge *et al.*, 2021). To reduce errors, radiologists should be well-trained, AI solutions should be regularly tested, and clinicians should communicate more effectively to ensure correct diagnosis and effective patient care in musculoskeletal imaging.

1.4.6. Technological Limitations

Although musculoskeletal imaging has advanced a lot, some limitations still affect how well these tests can be used and how accurately they diagnose. For instance, while CT has expanded veterinary and human musculoskeletal examinations due to improved accessibility and cost efficiency, challenges such as radiation exposure and suboptimal soft tissue contrast remain problematic (Keane *et al.*, 2017). MRI is better than CT at seeing soft tissues, but it takes longer and can be affected by metal objects in the body, which may make evaluations more complicated. Novel technologies like photon-counting detectors (PCDs) promise enhanced spatial resolution and spectral imaging capabilities; however, their clinical integration is still in developmental stages and requires extensive validation to overcome technical and practical barriers (Becce *et al.*, 2024). These limitations highlight the necessity for ongoing research focused on optimizing existing modalities and developing hybrid techniques that balance detail, safety, and efficiency in musculoskeletal imaging (Figure 1.21).

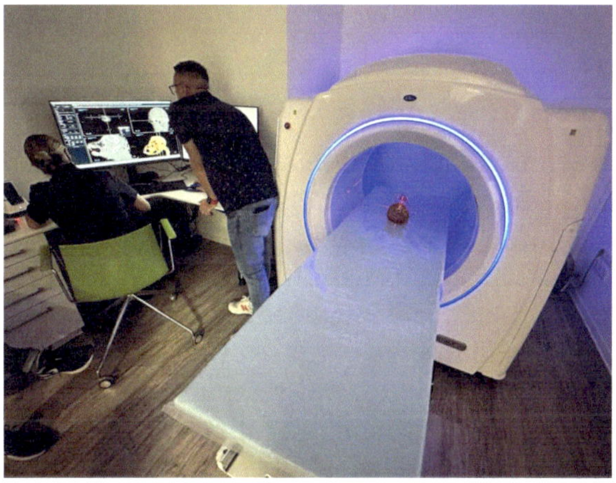

Figure 1.21. Computed Tomography (CT) has expanded veterinary and human musculoskeletal examinations due to improved accessibility and cost efficiency, challenges such as radiation exposure and suboptimal soft tissue contrast remain problematic.

Source: https://q9c5t3u9.delivery.rocketcdn.me/wp-content/uploads/2024/07/IMG_6003-1024x768.jpeg.

1.4.7. Ethical Considerations in Imaging

Better imaging techniques for muscles and bones have improved how accurately doctors diagnose, but they have also sparked ethical questions that require attention. It is very important to respect patient privacy and get consent since digital tools can easily store and move sensitive medical images. All healthcare providers and radiologists should prevent unnecessary radiation exposure by ensuring that imaging is only done when necessary. It is also difficult for all patients to use the latest imaging tools, highlighting the importance of reducing disparities that could affect their outcomes. Because incidental findings can arise, doctors must weigh the rights of patients with their professional duties. Sticking to these standards helps build trust and protects patients in musculoskeletal imaging. Following ethical rules protects patients and also ensures that the diagnostic process is done correctly.

1.4.8. Impact of Insurance and Reimbursement Policies

How musculoskeletal imaging technologies are used and improved depends greatly on the rules of health insurance and reimbursement. Innovation in imaging software, especially those based on artificial intelligence, is fast, but using them is still limited because of the long process for approval and careful reimbursement rules. For instance, although artificial intelligence-driven Software as Medical Device (SaMD) demonstrates enhanced diagnostic accuracy and cost-effectiveness, only a small fraction of these technologies have obtained separate health insurance claims, limiting broader integration into clinical practice (Kwon *et al.*, 2023). Meanwhile, policy changes and clinical guidelines can influence imaging utilization rates; however, their effect may be modest in altering established practices, as evidenced by the relatively minor reduction in spinal radiography use in Danish chiropractic clinics despite guideline dissemination and reimbursement adjustments (Reibke *et al.*, 2023). The results show that adaptable reimbursement policies are necessary to support true innovation and consider new clinical evidence, so that patients receive the best care and resources in musculoskeletal imaging.

1.4.9. Future Research Needs

While musculoskeletal imaging has improved diagnosis, more research is needed to fully help patients. Investigations into integrating AI could revolutionize image acquisition, disease detection, and clinical decision support, yet these technologies require rigorous validation for accuracy, cost-effectiveness, and ethical implementation within diverse populations (Jayakumar *et al.*, 2019). Additionally, refining bone density assessment methods and fracture risk prediction remains vital, particularly in osteoporosis management, where early detection of subclinical fractures could prevent debilitating consequences (LeBoff *et al.*, 2022). Researchers should also study how imaging-guided interventions may influence a patient's ability to function and the use of healthcare resources in the long run. It is also important to carry out prospective studies to evaluate the effects of AI-based musculoskeletal imaging on clinical routines, patient satisfaction, and health care expenses. Addressing these needs will ensure that emerging technologies translate into meaningful improvements in diagnosis, treatment, and overall musculoskeletal health (Figure 1.22).

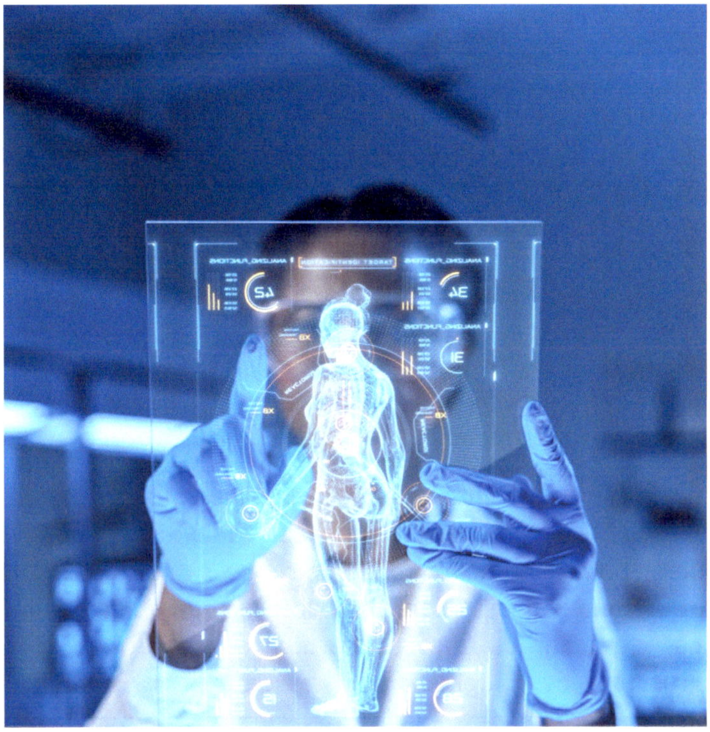

Figure 1.22. Investigations into integrating artificial intelligence (AI) could revolutionize image acquisition, disease detection, and clinical decision support.

Source: https://www.mckinsey.com/~/media/mckinsey/industries/life%20sciences/our%20insights/how%20artificial%20intelligence%20can%20power%20clinical%20development/how-advanced-analytics-can-power-clinical-development-1396801907-thumb-1536x1536.jpg.

Test Your Knowledge

1. In what ways are conventional X-rays not effective in identifying early bone problems such as bone marrow edema and microfractures?
2. How does patient body habitus (e.g., obesity) pose challenges in obtaining high-quality musculoskeletal MRI or CT images?

SUMMARY

While musculoskeletal imaging has improved both diagnosis and patient care, there are still difficulties in making the most of the information from these images. New studies highlight that a multidisciplinary approach to musculoskeletal disorders involves imaging, which helps in diagnosis, tracking the disease, and checking the effects of treatment. Persistent symptoms, such as fatigue and dyspnea observed in related systemic diseases, highlight the necessity for ongoing research into imaging biomarkers that correlate with clinical outcomes and patient quality of life (Nehme *et al.*, 2020). Moreover, adherence to established guidelines ensures standardized diagnostic protocols conducive to improving healthcare delivery (Habib *et al.*, 2015). Therefore, the future of musculoskeletal imaging involves using new technologies, thoroughly testing them in clinical settings, and working with other specialists to handle difficult conditions. Integrating advanced imaging tools with doctors' knowledge will help the field improve patient care.

mprovements in imaging for bones and muscles have helped manage patients, but some obstacles still exist in using it most effectively. Evidence suggests that direct access to physiotherapy for musculoskeletal disorders enhances referral accuracy, reduces unnecessary imaging, and promotes cost-effectiveness without compromising safety or clinical outcomes (Gallotti *et al.*, 2023). It is different from the usual physician-led approach, which often leads to more imaging and more referrals, which could result in overdiagnosis and overtreatment. Furthermore, studies highlight a global issue of low-value care in musculoskeletal conditions, particularly in low back pain, where excessive reliance on imaging frequently contributes to rising healthcare costs and patient dissatisfaction (Buchbinder *et al.*, 2020). Using imaging according to guidelines and including evidence-based pathways may address these issues. All in all, if proper imaging, clinical assessment, and conservative care are given priority, patients will benefit and the system will save resources.

KEY TERMS FROM THIS CHAPTER

- Internal organs
- Bones
- Muscles
- Magnetic Resonance Imaging
- Anatomical structures
- Visualization
- Clinical decision-making
- Musculoskeletal imaging
- Joints
- Soft tissues
- High-resolution ultrasonography
- Diseases
- Confidence
- Image segmentation techniques

CRITICAL THINKING QUESTIONS

1. **Which imaging modality is most sensitive for detecting bone marrow edema?**
   a. X-ray
   b. Ultrasound
   c. CT scan
   d. MRI
2. **What is the most appropriate initial imaging technique for evaluating a suspected bone fracture?**
   a. MRI
   b. CT
   c. X-ray
   d. PET
3. **Which modality is best for evaluating soft tissue injuries such as ligament or tendon tears?**
   a. X-ray
   b. CT scan
   c. MRI
   d. Nuclear bone scan
4. **Which of the following is most useful in detecting early osteomyelitis?**
   a. CT scan
   b. X-ray
   c. Bone scintigraphy
   d. Ultrasound
5. **Which imaging modality is preferred for evaluating a suspected rotator cuff tear?**
   a. X-ray
   b. MRI
   c. CT arthrogram
   d. Bone scan

Short Answer Questions

1. Which imaging methods are mainly used for musculoskeletal imaging, and what are the differences in their uses?
2. Under what circumstances should MRI be chosen instead of X-ray for assessing musculoskeletal problems?
3. What do X-rays usually show when there is osteoarthritis?
4. In what ways is ultrasound employed to assess soft tissue injuries such as tendonitis or bursitis?
5. How does CT contribute to evaluating complex or fractures within a joint?
6. What is the role of bone scintigraphy in finding occult fractures or metastatic disease in bones?
7. What are the pros and cons of musculoskeletal ultrasound when measured against MRI?
8. What role does MRI play in finding and classifying bone and soft tissue tumors?

Answers to Critical Thinking Questions

1. (d); 2. (c); 3. (c); 4. (c); 5. (b)

REFERENCES

1. Adamczyk, S., Domino, W., Dziewic, J., Dzwonnik, *et al.* (2025). *Imaging Diagnostics, Biomarkers, and Emerging Trends in Orthopedic Research and Treatment.* https://core.ac.uk/download/636385661.pdf (accessed on 31st May 2025).
2. Albisinni, U., Battista, G., Bazzocchi, A., Catalano, C., *et al.* (2015). *MRI-Guided Focused Ultrasound Surgery in Musculoskeletal Diseases: The Hot Topics.* https://core.ac.uk/download/98341478.pdf (accessed on 31st May 2025).
3. Aleid, A. M., Alzahrani, B., Sindi, M., Alharbi, R., Alghamdi, S., Alaradi, L., Almutairi, A., *et al.* (2024). A review of pediatric radiation exposure from diagnostic imaging in Saudi Arabia. *Journal of Advanced Trends in Medical Research.* https://www.semanticscholar.org/paper/131a06a586589262ba425e4b7db130476805b8da (accessed on 31st May 2025).
4. Alhejji, K. M., Alharbi, F. A., Faqeeh, M. A., & Alanazi, A. O. (2024). The importance of continuing education in dentistry. *International Journal of Community Medicine and Public Health.* https://www.semanticscholar.org/paper/ba0c91750e314b4181d1159e2a68ed73786726fc (accessed on 31st May 2025).
5. Alsoliman, B., Alrugebh, M., Alzahrani, A., Alshreef, N. A., & Algwiser, R. A. (2024). Advances in musculoskeletal radiology: Diagnostic techniques and clinical applications. *Journal of Advances and Scholarly Researches in Allied Education.* https://www.semanticscholar.org/paper/54e2b988afe19b56bb86b60cd00b8058d58d6ec2 (accessed on 31st May 2025).
6. Audenaert, E., Mahieu, P., Pattyn, C., Van, H., *et al.* (2010). Soft tissue structure modelling for use in orthopedic applications and musculoskeletal biomechanics. *EURASIP Journal on Advances in Signal Processing.* https://core.ac.uk/download/55761253.pdf (accessed on 31st May 2025).
7. Badet, J., Beggs, I., Candiotto, S., Cofield, R. H., Constant, C. R., Erstad, S., Gamradt, S., *et al.* (2011). Effect of angiogenesis-related cytokines on rotator cuff disease: The search for sensitive biomarkers of early tendon degeneration. *Clin. Med. Insights Arthritis Musculoskelet Disord.* https://core.ac.uk/download/pdf/8580102.pdf (accessed on 31st May 2025).
8. Bálint, P. V. (2002). *Ultrasound Imaging in Joint and Soft Tissue Inflammation.* https://core.ac.uk/download/282406.pdf (accessed on 31st May 2025).
9. Bazzocchi, A., Isaac, A., Dalili, D., Fotiadou, A., Kariki, E., Kirschke, J., Krestan, C., *et al.* (2022). Imaging of metabolic bone diseases: The spine view, Part I. *Seminars in Musculoskeletal Radiology, 26*(4), 478–490. https://www.semanticscholar.org/paper/a68dfaafea549c54aa82aa7d580f205e2e8431cc (accessed on 31st May 2025).
10. Becce, F., Booij, R., Gallego, M. L., Mourad, *et al.* (2024). *Chances and Challenges of Photon-Counting CT in Musculoskeletal Imaging.* https://core.ac.uk/download/610639100.pdf (accessed on 31st May 2025).
11. Belair, J. A., & Zoga, A. (2024). Bone bruise versus fracture on MRI and the relevance to return to play. *Seminars in Musculoskeletal Radiology, 28,* 139–145. https://www.semanticscholar.org/paper/34868403dc984ea072310e7bd268744155bf1db5 (accessed on 31st May 2025).
12. Bilkish, U. S., Hossain, M. J., Afruz, M., Rob, C. F., Mustofa, M. G., & Bodrudduza, C. A. B. (2024). Causes of low back pain (LBP) in women without pregnancy, in relation to different age groups during the reproductive period, are primarily treated as musculoskeletal disorders:

A retrospective study. *MOJ Orthopedics & Rheumatology*. https://www.semanticscholar.org/paper/74538a42be8b04e0cf700665dd32e23c1dd09fe4 (accessed on 31st May 2025).

13. Blasi, J., Hammer, H. B., Martinoli, C., Miguel, *et al.* (2023). Ultrasound assessment of degenerative muscle sarcopenia: The University of Barcelona ultrasound scoring system for sarcopenia. *RMD Open*. https://core.ac.uk/download/597057832.pdf (accessed on 31st May 2025).
14. Buchbinder, R., Underwood, M., Hartvigsen, J., & Maher, C. G. (2020). The Lancet series call to action to reduce low value care for low back pain: An update. *Pain, 161*, S57–S64. https://doi.org/10.1097/j.pain.0000000000001869 (accessed on 31st May 2025).
15. Chen, W., Zhang, Y., Wang, X., & Liu, J. (2024). Comparative analysis of imaging modalities for diagnosing musculoskeletal disorders. *Journal of Innovations in Medical Research*. https://www.semanticscholar.org/paper/b08897c482d81da296f7def6eb1fddc2d2ff9eba (accessed on 31st May 2025).
16. Correll, M., & Garrison, L. A. (2024). *When the Body Became Data: Historical Data Cultures and Anatomical Illustration.* http://arxiv.org/abs/2402.05014 (accessed on 31st May 2025).
17. De Magalhães, A. A., & Santos, A. T. (2025). Advancements in diagnostic methods and imaging technologies in dentistry: A literature review of emerging approaches. *Journal of Clinical Medicine, 14*. https://www.semanticscholar.org/paper/c0b125d5011c819fe642f05e88b36337e7d2eaf9 (accessed on 31st May 2025).
18. Degadwala, S., Krishnamurthy, V. N. D., & Vyas, D. (2024). DeepSpine: Multi-class spine X-ray conditions classification using deep learning. *2024 3rd International Conference on Sentiment Analysis and Deep Learning (ICSADL)*. https://www.semanticscholar.org/paper/da26e1f8b469d3333e236dbcaf969b7030879cb9 (accessed on 31st May 2025).
19. Dhimar, C. P., & Vaishnaw, A. (2025). Clinical applications of MRI in assessing musculoskeletal diseases and injuries. *Journal of Neonatal Surgery*. https://www.semanticscholar.org/paper/25c1e4ea7a13725eeaca5c5f4bcb3a5d7512cda1 (accessed on 31st May 2025).
20. Diqi, M., Mulyani, S. H., & Salsabil, H. A. (2024). *Generative Adversarial Networks for Anterior Cruciate Ligament Injury Detection.* https://core.ac.uk/download/604055065.pdf (accessed on 31st May 2025).
21. Ducarouge, A., Harvey, H., Kahn, C. E., Kober, T., *et al.* (2021). To buy or not to buy: Evaluating commercial AI solutions in radiology (the ECLAIR guidelines). *European Radiology*. https://core.ac.uk/download/389868724.pdf (accessed on 31st May 2025).
22. Eibschutz, L. S., Matcuk, G., Chiu, M. K. J., Lu, M. Y., & Gholamrezanezhad, A. (2024). Updates on the applications of spectral computed tomography for musculoskeletal imaging. *Diagnostics, 14*. https://www.semanticscholar.org/paper/a629dedbfeb45c014a4dba32a6a463d9a2978770 (accessed on 31st May 2025).
23. Fawcett, R., & Rowbotham, E. (2022). Interventional radiology procedures of the shoulder. *Seminars in Musculoskeletal Radiology, 26*, 611–620. https://www.semanticscholar.org/paper/d3947db838335c41a21efa6fbca5ff9722023e17 (accessed on 31st May 2025).
24. Fujisaki, A., Tsukamoto, J., Narimatsu, H., Hayashida, Y., Todoroki, Y., Hirano, N., Takeda, K., *et al.* (2023). Zero echo time magnetic resonance imaging: Techniques and clinical utility in musculoskeletal system. *Journal of Magnetic Resonance Imaging, 59*. https://www.

semanticscholar.org/paper/c17fe198e6a6a571d10d854e53acdf5272fdd145 (accessed on 31st May 2025).

25. Gallotti, M., Campagnola, B., Cocchieri, A., Mourad, F., Heick, J. D., & Maselli, F. (2023). Effectiveness and consequences of direct access in physiotherapy: A systematic review. *Journal of Clinical Medicine, 12*, 5832. https://doi.org/10.3390/jcm12185832 (accessed on 31st May 2025).

26. Garg, A., Singh, A. K., Ranjan, R. S., Yadav, A., Rajput, R. C., & Kumar, S. (2024). Reviewing imaging discoveries in tuberculosis affecting extraspinal osteoarticular regions. *MGM Journal of Medical Sciences*. https://www.semanticscholar.org/paper/43e92e685fd9a57746a30b1c7529c0899da781dd (accessed on 31st May 2025).

27. Gazzotti, S., Sassi, R., Aparisi, G. M. A., Guglielmi, R., Vasilevska, N. V., Messina, C., Guglielmi, G., *et al.* (2024). Imaging of body composition. *Seminars in Musculoskeletal Radiology, 28*(5), 594–609. https://www.semanticscholar.org/paper/1407d1d6301c7b16128b1876ac15d75986b243d9 (accessed on 31st May 2025).

28. Gebriel, M. A. O. Z., Ghieda, U., Elshafaey, K. I., & Dawoud, T. (2024). Magnetic resonance imaging in evaluation of traumatic ankle joint lesions. *SVU-International Journal of Medical Sciences*. https://www.semanticscholar.org/paper/3913ee6987285a97f2de8ae932de130780369ecb (accessed on 31st May 2025).

29. Gielen, I., & van Bree, H. (2014). *Other Imaging Techniques and Their Added Value to Diagnose Elbow Dysplasia*. https://core.ac.uk/download/55827843.pdf (accessed on 31st May 2025).

30. Glaudemans, A. W. J. M. (2022). *PET Imaging in MSK Infections*. https://core.ac.uk/download/571867327.pdf (accessed on 31st May 2025).

31. Guermazi, A., Omoumi, P., Tordjman, M., Fritz, J., Kijowski, R., Regnard, N., Carrino, J., *et al.* (2024). How AI may transform musculoskeletal imaging. *Radiology, 310*(1), e230764. https://www.semanticscholar.org/paper/077146bf368ddbe82ba7cd0933060433099e17d5 (accessed on 31st May 2025).

32. Habib, G., Lancellotti, P., Antunes, M. J., Bongiorni, M. G., Casalta, J. P., Del Zotti, F., Dulgheru, R., *et al.* (2015). 2015 ESC guidelines for the management of infective endocarditis. *European Heart Journal, 36*, 3075–3128. https://doi.org/10.1093/eurheartj/ehv319 (accessed on 31st May 2025).

33. Hayward, L., Markowski, A., Watkins, M. K., Maitland, M., Manske, R., & Beneck, G. J. (2022). Elements of learning and integration of diagnostic musculoskeletal ultrasound imaging into practice: Physical therapists' educational journeys. *Journal of Physical Therapy Education, 36*, 243–255. https://www.semanticscholar.org/paper/d1a61f6c616ea8986e4e3a4c099abf76ec96a71c (accessed on 31st May 2025).

34. Filho Hernandez, G. (2018). Magnetic resonance arthrography: What is its importance in the present day? *Radiologia Brasileira, 51*, V–V. https://www.semanticscholar.org/paper/4648f62691d8f81708ca29fcb63017f8a39b3c34 (accessed on 31st May 2025).

35. Hsu, W. C., Wu, G. L., & Yeh, M. L. (2024). Fixation technique of biodegradable magnesium alloy suture anchor in the rotator cuff repair of the shoulder in a goat model: A technical note. *BMC Musculoskeletal Disorders, 25*. https://www.semanticscholar.org/paper/490650eec60a3c59cf6525158b47f2785327e98a (accessed on 31st May 2025).

36. Jayakumar, P., Moore, M., & Bozic, K. J. (2019). Value-based healthcare: Can artificial intelligence provide value in orthopedic surgery? *Clinical Orthopedics and Related Research, 477*, 1777–1780. https://doi.org/10.1097/corr.0000000000000873 (accessed on 31st May 2025).

37. Kalová, M., Kubíček, J., Oczka, D., & Tomanec, *et al.* (2019). Recent trends, technical concepts and components of computer-assisted orthopedic surgery systems: A comprehensive review. *Sensors*. https://core.ac.uk/download/287649034.pdf (accessed on 31st May 2025).

38. Keane, M., Paul, E., Rauch, C., & Rutland, *et al.* (2017). Computed Tomography in veterinary medicine: Currently published and tomorrow's vision. *Computed Tomography – Advanced Applications*. https://core.ac.uk/download/80784172.pdf (accessed on 31st May 2025).

39. Kim, H., Kim, S., Kim, S., & Yoo, J. I. (2024). Spine muscle auto segmentation techniques in MRI imaging: A systematic review. *BMC Musculoskeletal Disorders, 25*. https://www.semanticscholar.org/paper/486fa85da189e96150d24a318bfc18c03d4fb481 (accessed on 31st May 2025).

40. Kolasinski, S. L., Neogi, T., Hochberg, M. C., Oatis, C. A., Guyatt, G., Block, J. A., Callahan, L. F., *et al.* (2020). 2019 American College of Rheumatology/Arthritis Foundation guideline for the management of osteoarthritis of the hand, hip, and knee. *Arthritis Care & Research, 72*, 149–162. https://doi.org/10.1002/acr.24131 (accessed on 31st May 2025).

41. Kozhevnikov, A. N., Derkach, E. A., Porohova, A. A., & Lukyanov, S. A. (2025). Diagnostic value of synovial calprotectin (S100A8/A9) in differential diagnosis of juvenile idiopathic arthritis and pigmented villonodular synovitis in children: Preliminary results of a single-center study. *Pediatric Traumatology, Orthopedics and Reconstructive Surgery*. https://www.semanticscholar.org/paper/7dc0109e7d854bd63ab4f88da17d2b0bf1832ef8 (accessed on 31st May 2025).

42. Koziak, W., Dudek, S., Makieła, M., Bętkowska, A., Kornacka, A., Dudek, W., Szostak, K., *et al.* (2025). The application of point-of-care ultrasound in sports medicine: A narrative review. *Quality in Sport*. https://www.semanticscholar.org/paper/c517440cb493bca3fa64412d0aa221420686c749 (accessed on 31st May 2025).

43. Kraus, M., Pertman, L., & Eshed, I. (2025). What's new in pediatric musculoskeletal imaging. *Journal of Children's Orthopedics, 19*, 109–118. https://www.semanticscholar.org/paper/8bd6dea470e372e0f20f87f2676036a47faf56eb (accessed on 31st May 2025).

44. Kwon, S., Han, S. J., & Kim, K. H. (2023). PP26 Critical review of the reimbursement process for software as a medical device and challenges in South Korea. *International Journal of Technology Assessment in Health Care, 39*, S59. https://www.semanticscholar.org/paper/dfb11cb2027f6396493e2a4232de92f58e418965 (accessed on 31st May 2025).

45. LeBoff, M. S., Greenspan, S. L., Insogna, K., Lewiecki, E. M., Saag, K. G., Singer, A., & Siris, E. S. (2022). The clinician's guide to prevention and treatment of osteoporosis. *Osteoporosis International, 33*, 2049–2102. https://doi.org/10.1007/s00198-021-05900-y (accessed on 31st May 2025).

46. Lee, S., Joo, M., Kim, J. Y., & Bernthal, N. (2024). Postoperative imaging of bone and soft tissue tumors in the extremity: A comprehensive review. *Diagnostics, 14*. https://www.semanticscholar.org/paper/869f0884bb39a1dc5d616f69715b2a669f495de8 (accessed on 31st May 2025).

47. Leş, A., Sarbu, A. M., Dumitru, R., Saizu, R., Gheorghe, L., & Gheorghe, C. (2025). P0360 Bowel ultrasonography and computed tomography tell the same story using different languages in

analyzing Crohn's disease lesions. *Journal of Crohn's and Colitis*. https://www.semanticscholar.org/paper/057dcb94f0c2218bd6b516042de911b915f6f4ea (accessed on 31st May 2025).

48. Linden, M. A., Rosenblad, T., Rosenborg, K., Hansson, S., & Brandström, P. (2024). Infant urinary tract infection in Sweden — A national study of current diagnostic procedures, imaging and treatment. *Pediatric Nephrology, 39*, 3251–3262. https://www.semanticscholar.org/paper/9744f7114f0e8d0ea253b748a023037c6a18f655 (accessed on 31st May 2025).

49. Ma, C., Chadha, A. N., Wu, C., Giannoudis, P. V., & Guo, J. J. (2025). Is there a role of photoacoustic imaging in sports medicine: Evidence today. *Orthopedic Surgery*. https://www.semanticscholar.org/paper/73ecde3b186d780ccef3deb658ed6cc5b0f803b8 (accessed on 31st May 2025).

50. Mahesh, T. R., Khan, S. B., Mishra, K. K., Alzahrani, S., & Alojail, M. (2024). Enhancing diagnostic precision in breast cancer classification through EfficientNetB7 using advanced image augmentation and interpretation techniques. *International Journal of Imaging Systems and Technology, 35*. https://www.semanticscholar.org/paper/b933d80eb98c0f6905f93ae77a8d008d76526375 (accessed on 31st May 2025).

51. Manske, R., Wolfe, C., Page, P., & Voight, M. L. (2025). Diagnostic musculoskeletal ultrasound for the evaluation of the lateral elbow: Implications for rehabilitation providers. *International Journal of Sports Physical Therapy, 20*, 137–143. https://www.semanticscholar.org/paper/aa6f2a2c204b57d047f1599da9410c440ceecd51 (accessed on 31st May 2025).

52. Morhaim, H., Rudolph, S., Davy, C. M., Wheelwright, D., & Roche, T. (2024). Abstract TP69: Development of system-wide stroke-specific nursing education for a hospital system. *Stroke*. https://www.semanticscholar.org/paper/b01c8105fef7a774ceb07965e0d97a1c2a6086b5 (accessed on 31st May 2025).

53. Nehme, M., Braillard, O., Alcoba, G., Aebischer, P. S., Courvoisier, D. S., Chappuis, F., & Guessous, I. (2020). COVID-19 symptoms: Longitudinal evolution and persistence in outpatient settings. *Annals of Internal Medicine, 174*, 723–725. https://doi.org/10.7326/m20-5926 (accessed on 31st May 2025).

54. Palazzo, S., Zambetta, G., & Calbi, R. (2024). An overview of segmentation techniques for CT and MRI images: Clinical implications and future directions in medical diagnostics. *Medical Imaging Process & Technology*. https://www.semanticscholar.org/paper/9d1721bfd41fd24c8b0cf688a7d9dc78d9447b3f (accessed on 31st May 2025).

55. Rai, P., Janu, A., Shetty, N. S., & Kulkarni, S. (2025). Current landscape of short-T2 imaging techniques in the musculoskeletal system: The past, present and future. *Journal of Magnetic Resonance Imaging*. https://www.semanticscholar.org/paper/15711c9b31cb2ea1dc7c02958d581c223eaebdf2 (accessed on 31st May 2025).

56. Reddy, M. L., Musib, J., Akshay, B., Royal, A. A., & Ramesh, V. (2024). Evaluation of ligamentous tears of the knee joint and correlation between meniscal and anterior cruciate ligament tears using magnetic resonance imaging. *IOSR Journal of Dental and Medical Sciences*. https://www.semanticscholar.org/paper/d345985e11287fc2df9d0741c72a693bf53d7645 (accessed on 31st May 2025).

57. Reibke, P. S., Godskesen, H., Jensen, R. K., French, S. D., Bussières, A., Christensen, H. W., & Jensen, T. (2023). The effect of clinical guidelines on the utilization of radiographs in chiropractic clinics in Denmark – An interrupted time series analysis. *Chiropractic & Manual Therapies, 31*. https://www.semanticscholar.org/paper/794d338cf81370788cefdcf25eef60f5

2a1a19be (accessed on 31st May 2025).

58. Salami, A. M., Salih, L. M., & Alluhaibi, O. (2025). Fuzzy logic and FFBNN-based detection of spine osteoporosis through dual energy X-ray absorptiometry (DEXA) images. *Journal of Research in Engineering and Computer Sciences*. https://www.semanticscholar.org/paper/e55269b5c40898280e81a9f6503cb604f8d33e70 (accessed on 31st May 2025).

59. Sar, S., Sar, E. A., Balcı, A., Havıtçıoğlu, H., & Tuna, B. (2024). The role of perfusion magnetic resonance imaging in discrimination of benign vs malign character of musculoskeletal tumors. *Journal of Basic and Clinical Health Sciences*. https://www.semanticscholar.org/paper/9af0df60bb2f8397eaec0cdd39d124c613dace0a (accessed on 31st May 2025).

60. Senanayake, D. A., Seneviratne, S., Imani, M., Harijanto, C., Sales, M., Lee, P., Duque, G., *et al.* (2023). Classification of fracture risk in fallers using dual-energy X-ray absorptiometry (DXA) images and deep learning-based feature extraction. *JBMR Plus, 7*. https://www.semanticscholar.org/paper/20798377a496cc87c1ad820f6f2698a1ef6f0e05 (accessed on 31st May 2025).

61. Shirin, M., Rahman, S., Chowdhury, P., Showkat, M., Paul Karki, B., & Al Azad, M. S. (2024). Accuracy of diffusion-weighted magnetic resonance imaging in diagnosing malignant musculoskeletal tumors. *Bangabandhu Sheikh Mujib Medical University Journal*. https://www.semanticscholar.org/paper/9223cf6cf55ce5c251af223ecc1edcca75b1cfff (accessed on 31st May 2025).

62. Sozzi, F. B., Gnan, E., Pandolfi, A., Iacuzio, L., Kim, J. K., Canetta, C., Rizzuto, A., *et al.* (2025). Diagnostic algorithm using multimodal imaging for the differential diagnosis of intra-cardiac masses. *Journal of Clinical Medicine, 14*. https://www.semanticscholar.org/paper/c47bcdf77d30afefb36cf8281284afacb389d81f (accessed on 31st May 2025).

63. Stambaugh, J., Morrissey, P., Hurvitz, A., Bernstein, E., & Barlow, B. (2024). Hip-spine relationship in femoroacetabular impingement: Does hip arthroscopy affect pelvic mobility? *Clinical Orthopedics and Related Research*. https://www.semanticscholar.org/paper/05c045b6bbbc999bb5821c06562569a9d9861d08 (accessed on 31st May 2025).

64. Symanski, J. S., Cooley, M., Stoeckl, E. M., Grogan, B. F., McKean, L., & Markhardt, B. (2025). Anterior shoulder instability: Pre- and postoperative imaging. *Seminars in Musculoskeletal Radiology, 29*(1), 3–16. https://www.semanticscholar.org/paper/699fcd156dc27512880431a449b8a900b8179ed7 (accessed on 31st May 2025).

65. Tamborrini, G., Micheroli, R., Ricci, V., Becciolini, M., Garcia-Pompermayer, M., Serrano, B. G. A., Müller-Gerbl, M., *et al.* (2024). Advancing high-resolution musculoskeletal ultrasound: A histology- and anatomy-driven approach for enhanced shoulder imaging. Part 2: Anterior and lateral shoulder. *Journal of Ultrasonography, 24*, 1–12. https://www.semanticscholar.org/paper/1b0b8991255752a506f1a2931584126a261b0b9a (accessed on 31st May 2025).

66. Tosyal, H. K., Kaya, H., Keçeci, B., & Sabah, D. (2024). Management of chondroblastoma in pediatric patients: 21 years of single-center experience. *Children, 11*. https://www.semanticscholar.org/paper/5063ea9acff9f2bf1e7c9aed7df5384c99dbd7bb (accessed on 31st May 2025).

67. Trestka, G., Domino, W., Zelik, U., Przygoda, M., Śnieżna, J., Stępień, K., Adamczyk, S., *et al.* (2025). Imaging diagnostics, biomarkers, and emerging trends in orthopedic research and treatment. *Quality in Sport*. https://www.semanticscholar.org/paper/17c923ae4e91ce0fd82e4b31a36fce76988ee790 (accessed on 31st May 2025).

68. Triantafyllou, M., Vassalou, E., Goulianou, A. M., Tosounidis, T. H., Marias, K., Karantanas, A., & Klontzas, M. (2025). The effect of ultrasound image pre-processing on radiomics feature quality: A study on shoulder ultrasound. *Journal of Imaging Informatics in Medicine*. https://www.semanticscholar.org/paper/ccb511461c828102f0b0760ecc1a9fc90e49dafe (accessed on 31st May 2025).

69. Tushir, R., Dhall, M., & Goel, N. (2025). Preparation and in-vitro evaluation of anti-fungal activity of clotrimazole loaded microsponge based gel. *International Journal of Pharmaceutical Sciences and Nanotechnology (IJPSN)*. https://www.semanticscholar.org/paper/fd62b8101680e69e0fcc417f099acbaf4465c40b (accessed on 31st May 2025).

70. Tzatzairis, T., Skarentzos, K., Grammatikos, C., Karamalis, C., Korakianitis, K., Kourempeles, R., & Drosos, G. (2024). Ultrasound applications in pediatric orthopedics. *Archives of Bone and Joint Surgery, 12*, 457–468. https://www.semanticscholar.org/paper/59925c2de86c06c9431d2c10ff413b9a2621bbc3 (accessed on 31st May 2025).

71. Ulas, S., & Diekhoff, T. (2024). Computed tomography—Current status and future directions for arthritis imaging. *Therapeutic Advances in Musculoskeletal Disease, 16*. https://www.semanticscholar.org/paper/400ac30dba4cbdfe4eaeb9c6c56bdece66818d81 (accessed on 31st May 2025).

72. Uldin, H., Kanbour, I., Patel, A., & Botchu, R. (2024). Image-guided musculoskeletal interventional radiology in the personalized management of musculoskeletal tumors. *Journal of Personalized Medicine, 14*. https://www.semanticscholar.org/paper/00930c713df115dd5fd1c485356e9a32a2ea5f5d (accessed on 31st May 2025).

73. Vaswani, D., Cohn, R. M., & Walsh, P. J. (2025). Shoulder arthroplasty: Preoperative evaluation and postoperative imaging. *Seminars in Musculoskeletal Radiology, 29*(1), 45–59. https://www.semanticscholar.org/paper/b2f20d9f9cf8ee2caade41037822862872723822 (accessed on 31st May 2025).

74. Virto, N., Río, X., Méndez-Zorrilla, A., & García-Zapirain, S. B. (2024). Non-invasive techniques for direct muscle quality assessment after exercise intervention in older adults: A systematic review. *BMC Geriatrics, 24*. https://www.semanticscholar.org/paper/aa5cb5fed756a139aee52e557f6d4bfea664de5e (accessed on 31st May 2025).

75. Wearing, S. C., Hooper, S. L., Langton, C. M., Keiner, M., Horstmann, T., Crevier-Denoix, N., & Pourcelot, P. (2024). The biomechanics of musculoskeletal tissues during activities of daily living: Dynamic assessment using quantitative transmission-mode ultrasound techniques. *Healthcare, 12*. https://www.semanticscholar.org/paper/fb9bababd9fc0f443e344f210921fd38b9768189 (accessed on 31st May 2025).

76. Weiss, S., Korthaus, A., Baumann, N., Yamamura, J., Spiro, A., Lübke, A., Frosch, K., *et al.* (2021). Musculoskeletal soft-tissue sarcoma: Quality assessment of initial MRI reports shows frequent deviation from ESSR guidelines. *Diagnostics, 11*. https://www.semanticscholar.org/paper/748acbb4e451dc0947a56aaf36042d93ef41786c (accessed on 31st May 2025).

PEDIATRIC RADIOLOGY

2

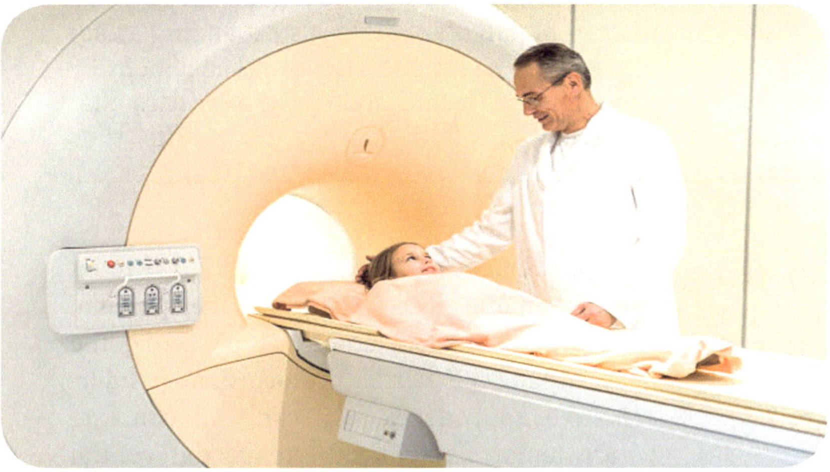

LEARNING OBJECTIVES

After studying this chapter, you will be able to:

1. Identify imaging techniques in pediatric radiology;
2. Know common pediatric conditions diagnosed with radiology;
3. Explain challenges and considerations in pediatric radiology;
4. Focus on future directions in pediatric radiology.

Introduction

Improvements in medical imaging have greatly helped with diagnoses in all groups, but using radiology for children brings specific issues and needs. Because of their growing bodies and increased sensitivity to radiation, children need special care when they are exposed to X-rays. Pediatric radiology needs to help diagnose congenital problems, injuries, infections, and cancers, which means using imaging methods that are both accurate and safe for children. This area of medicine pays special attention to reducing radiation while still producing clear images so that interpretations are accurate and patients are not harmed. Also, knowing the differences in children's and adults' bodies is important for correctly understanding radiologic images and getting better outcomes in treatment. Because of new technologies and ongoing research, pediatric imaging protocols are improved, stressing the value of having experts in this field to help with accurate diagnosis and treatment decisions.

Definition of Pediatric Radiology

Because children are not like adults, their medical images must be interpreted with knowledge of their special physiology and development. Using X-rays, ultrasound, MRI, and CT scans, pediatric radiology helps diagnose and monitor health problems in children. Unique challenges include minimizing radiation exposure and employing sedation when necessary to obtain accurate results, especially since many young patients may be unable to remain still during procedures (Kudchadkar, 2015). In addition, pediatric radiology goes beyond imaging and requires working with other specialties to help patients. For instance, accurately assessing trauma cases involves using resource utilization criteria developed through expert consensus to determine the appropriate level of pediatric trauma center care (Snyder *et al.*, 2023). This complexity underscores pediatric radiology's essential role in delivering precise, safe, and effective diagnostic services specialized for children's distinct medical needs (Figure 2.1).

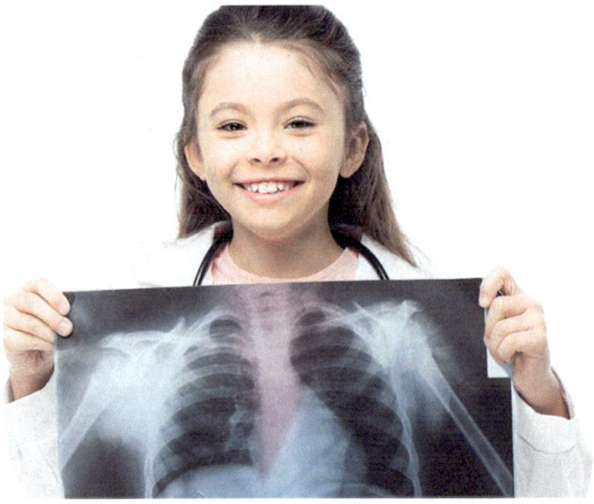

Figure 2.1. Pediatric radiology.

Source: https://www.arnoldpalmerhospital.com/-/media/images/arnold-palmer-hospital/services-and-specialties/sub-specialties/pediatric-radiology-and-diagnostic-imaging-mobile.jpg.

Importance of Radiology in Pediatric Medicine

Improvements in medical imaging have made it much easier to detect diseases in children, which is very important for proper treatment. Radiology is important for finding congenital problems, infections, and injuries in children, and it often allows for less painful tests. Additionally, the integration of artificial intelligence in radiographic analysis, as demonstrated in the rapid screening of COVID-19 through CT images, highlights radiology's expanding utility in pediatric infectious disease management by providing swift and reliable diagnostics that can anticipate pathogen testing results, thus accelerating clinical decisions (Wang *et al.*, 2021).

Furthermore, pediatric radiology must consider unique physiological and developmental factors distinct from adults, emphasizing the necessity for specialized protocols and gender-sensitive approaches, especially in contexts where females might experience differential health impacts during pandemics or treatment (Gausman *et al.*, 2020). Therefore, radiology helps detect illnesses early, provides proper treatment, and ensures fair and personalized care for children.

Historical Development of Pediatric Radiology

Pediatric radiology has advanced because of wider advancements in medical imaging and its specific use on children's systems. At first, radiographic methods were made for adults, but slowly these were modified for children to reduce the amount of radiation and improve the quality of the images. Innovations like computed tomography (CT) and positron emission tomography (PET), which later merged as PET/CT, revolutionized imaging by combining functional and anatomical data, allowing for more precise diagnosis and treatment planning, particularly in pediatric oncology (Carsrud *et al.*, 2024).

Alongside technological progress, improved understanding of embryonic vascular and craniofacial development through high-resolution imaging methods such as micro-CT enriched the capacity to visualize complex anatomical structures in early human development (Cordewener *et al.*, 2024). Because of this combination, pediatric radiology has advanced, helping doctors identify problems early and design better, customized treatments for children.

Differences Between Pediatric and Adult Radiology

Because bodies and systems change with age, healthcare imaging needs to be adapted for each age group. There are several important differences between pediatric radiology and adult radiology, mainly because children are smaller, still growing, and their tissues react differently. Children have different body structures and a faster metabolism than adults, which means the way diseases appear and progress is different, so imaging methods should be adjusted to use less radiation.

It can also be difficult to interpret symptoms since some normal changes during childhood can look like pathology, so doctors need extra training. Because children are often less cooperative, it is often necessary to sedate or immobilize them to get clear images. Also, the types and amounts of certain diseases are not the same in children and adults, which changes the way imaging is done and what is prioritized in diagnosis. These distinctions emphasize the importance of specialized training and guidelines in pediatric imaging to enhance diagnostic accuracy and patient safety (Chalasani *et al.*, 2017; Rosen *et al.*, 2018) (Figure 2.2).

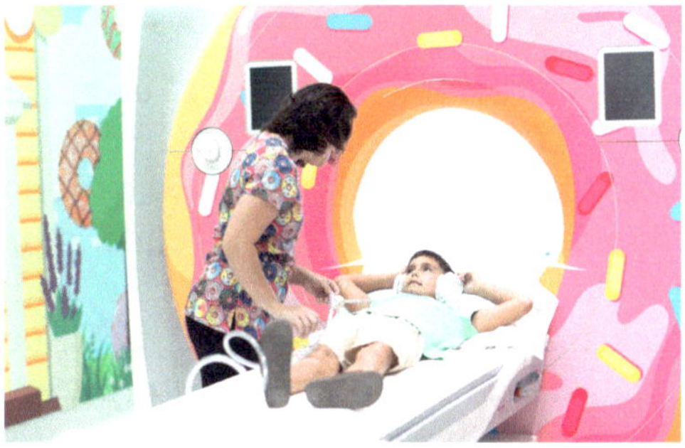

Figure 2.2. Pediatric radiology significantly differs from adult radiology in several critical aspects, primarily due to children's smaller size, ongoing growth, and differing tissue sensitivities.

Source: https://blog.erlanger.org/wp-content/uploads/2023/10/2023-10-13_15-18-09-1080x675.jpg.

Common Imaging Techniques Used in Pediatrics

Because of progress in medical imaging, diagnosing and treating children has become easier, and new techniques are needed to fit their unique bodies and growth. Many doctors use ultrasound first in children because it is safe, does not use radiation, and allows for real-time monitoring. In liver diseases, ultrasound elastography and attenuation imaging help give specific information about the condition without needing sedation or invasive methods. Magnetic resonance imaging (MRI), despite the need for sedation in younger patients, provides detailed anatomical and functional information crucial for complex diagnoses and follow-up, such as fatty liver and hepatic fibrosis (Otmane *et al.*, 2025). In oncology, specialized nuclear medicine techniques like MIBG scintigraphy play a critical role in diagnosing and staging neuroblastoma, enabling precise tumor localization and effective monitoring of treatment response (Otmane *et al.*, 2025). All these imaging methods are essential in pediatric radiology, ensuring that tests are accurate and cause as little trouble and risk to the child as possible.

Role of Pediatric Radiologists

Many times, pediatricians depend on advanced imaging to find and manage different conditions, which highlights the key role played by pediatric radiologists. They have a special understanding of the way children's bodies grow and the diseases that affect them, which are not the same as those in adults. Doctors rely on radiologists to interpret imaging results that can help decide on the right treatment for patients, such as spotting faint fractures or the first signs of diseases. For instance, in cases of acute appendicitis, pediatric radiologists contribute to precise diagnosis through tailored imaging protocols that consider the patient's age and clinical presentation, thereby improving treatment outcomes (Saverio *et al.*, 2020). Similarly, they address challenges related to pediatric musculoskeletal injuries, such as ankle and foot fractures, by applying specialized classification systems and imaging techniques to ensure accurate diagnosis and appropriate management, thus preventing complications related to growth plate injuries (Chaturvedi *et al.*, 2020). Pediatric radiologists ultimately enhance patient care through their specialized skills and collaboration with multidisciplinary teams (Figure 2.3).

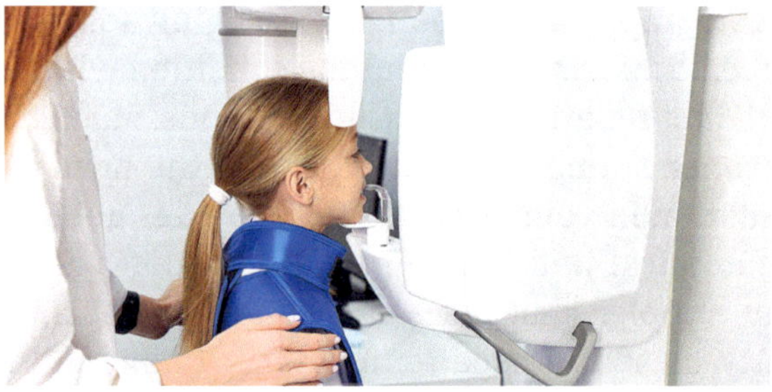

Figure 2.3. The diagnostic process in pediatric healthcare often relies heavily on specialized imaging to accurately identify and manage various conditions, emphasizing the critical role of pediatric radiologists.

Source: https://abingtonradiology.com/wp-content/uploads/2022/10/pediatric-01.jpg.

Overview of Pediatric Patient Considerations

Working with children in radiology requires knowing their specific physiological and developmental traits, which are not the same as those of adults. The variety in patient size, from premature infants weighing under 1 kg to adolescents comparable to adult body mass, demands adaptable equipment and tailored procedural approaches to ensure safety and efficacy (Young *et al.*, 2022). Also, children have unique illnesses and reactions to treatment, which means radiologists should use different imaging methods and plans. In resource-limited settings, these challenges are compounded by limited access to specialized care and diagnostic tools, increasing the complexity of managing critically ill children such as those with sepsis (Williams, 2022). Therefore, pediatric radiologists need to weigh the need for quick action with a sensitivity to the environment and the fragility of children. Using this approach is important for getting the best results and avoiding risks, which shows how vital pediatric expertise is in radiology.

Ethical Considerations in Pediatric Imaging

New tools in medical technology have made it easier to diagnose children, but they also bring up important ethical issues that require careful consideration. Because young patients are more sensitive to radiation, it is very important to use the lowest amount of radiation possible and make sure each procedure is required by their medical condition. Informed consent is hard because parents or guardians have to understand the risks and benefits for their child, who might not yet understand them. Furthermore, the integration of emerging technologies, such as generative artificial intelligence, in imaging analysis highlights the need for transparency, bias mitigation, and responsible application to protect patient privacy and data integrity

(Bahroun *et al.*, 2023). The COVID-19 pandemic exemplifies additional ethical challenges, underscoring the importance of balancing urgent clinical demands with safeguarding pediatric patients' well-being in resource-constrained environments (Fix *et al.*, 2020). Ultimately, ethical pediatric imaging requires continuous evaluation of protocols to prioritize safety, consent, and equitable access (Figure 2.4).

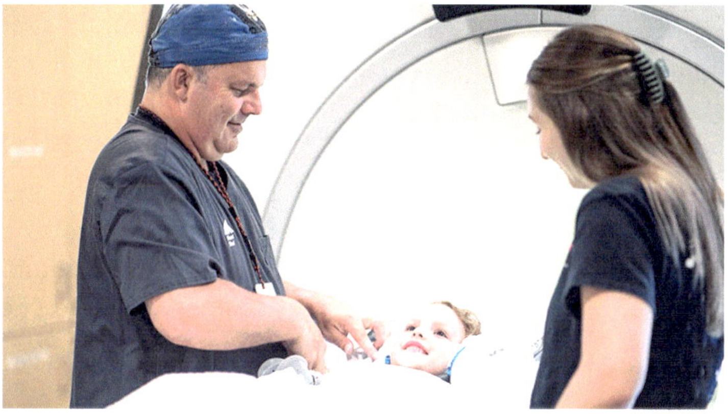

Figure 2.4. Informed consent is particularly complex, as parents or guardians must comprehend the potential risks and benefits on behalf of the child, who may not fully understand the implications.

Source: https://www.mountsinai.org/files/MSHealth/Assets/HS/Care/Pediatrics/MSHS-Pediatrics-Radiology-2col-770x420.jpg.

2.1. Imaging Techniques in Pediatric Radiology

Learning Outcome

1. Understand X-ray imaging;
2. Explain ultrasound in pediatrics;
3. Focus on computed tomography (CT) scans;
4. Define magnetic resonance imaging (MRI);
5. Explain nuclear medicine in children;
6. Describe fluoroscopy applications;
7. Know safety protocols for imaging techniques;
8. Identify contrast agents in pediatric imaging;
9. Discuss innovations in imaging technology.

Thanks to better imaging methods, pediatric radiology can now offer precise diagnosis of many conditions, always with a focus on patient safety. For instance, cone-beam computed tomography (CBCT) has revolutionized orthodontic assessments by offering detailed three-dimensional images necessary for managing craniofacial abnormalities, although its higher radiation dose necessitates stringent adherence to dose optimization guidelines and the ALARA principle (Rafighi *et al.*, 2024). Complementary modalities such as magnetic resonance imaging (MRI) and ultrasound provide valuable radiation-free alternatives, increasingly important in pediatric care. In the context of assessing pediatric renal tumors, MRI protocols refined through expert consensus enable differentiation between Wilms tumor and non-Wilms renal masses, facilitating tailored clinical management without routine biopsy (van der Pol *et al.*, 2021). Diffusion-weighted imaging helps to distinguish tissues, but there are still no common ways to interpret and report its findings. In general, using different types of imaging and new technologies like AI is gradually making it safer and more accurate to diagnose children.

2.1.1. X-ray Imaging

Thanks to new developments in medical imaging, especially X-ray, the way pediatric radiology diagnoses patients has greatly improved. This method, which quickly and clearly shows both bones and soft tissues, is still necessary to diagnose common childhood problems such as fractures, birth defects, and breathing problems. But because children are more sensitive to radiation, it is very important to limit their exposure to minimize any long-term harm. New advances in X-ray machines have made images clearer, reduced the amount of radiation used, and improved safety for children. Also, research into focal spots and imaging resolution helps doctors make more precise diagnoses for children. Ultimately, the integration of these advancements within pediatric radiology underscores the balance between diagnostic efficacy and patient safety, reflecting a critical evolution in child healthcare (Figure 2.5).

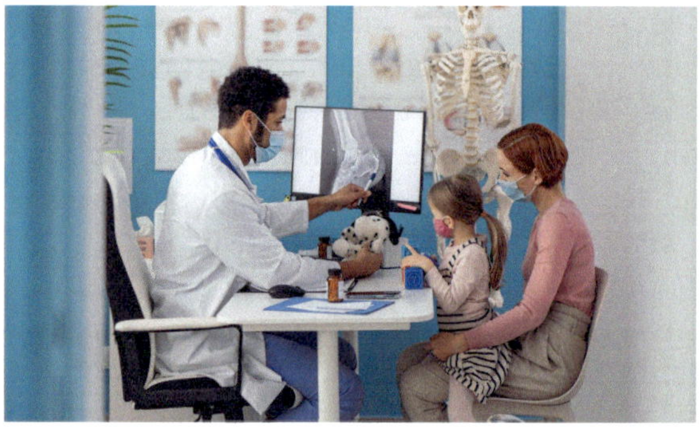

Figure 2.5. Innovations in X-ray technology, including improved detector sensitivity and tailored exposure settings, have significantly enhanced image quality while reducing radiation exposure.

Source: https://www.wmchealth.org/wp-content/uploads/2024/11/GettyImages-1368917031-sized.jpg.

2.1.2. Ultrasound in Pediatrics

The use of advanced imaging has greatly improved the ability to diagnose in pediatric medicine, and ultrasound is considered very useful. Since it does not use ionizing radiation, is portable, and provides instant images, CT is best for children and other sensitive patients. The use of contrast-enhanced ultrasound (CEUS) has expanded rapidly in pediatric care, offering dynamic evaluation of vascular structures and improving the characterization of focal liver lesions, among other applications.

This technique is increasingly recognized as a safer alternative to CT scans, particularly in cases of blunt abdominal trauma, thereby minimizing radiation exposure in young patients (Squires *et al.*, 2021). Additionally, point-of-care ultrasound (POCUS) performed by trained pediatric emergency physicians has demonstrated high diagnostic accuracy, particularly for common presentations such as neck masses, while also significantly reducing imaging delays in emergency settings (Friedman *et al.*, 2019). All of these new developments highlight that ultrasound is very important for pediatric radiology, combining accuracy, safety, and efficiency.

2.1.3. Computed Tomography (CT) Scans

When other imaging methods are not enough, CT scans are very helpful in diagnosing complex diseases in children. Because CT scans show cross-sections, they make it possible for clinicians to look at bones, soft tissues, and blood vessels with great accuracy, which helps in quick diagnosis and planning treatment. Radiation exposure concerns are higher for children because they are more sensitive and have a long life ahead, but new CT technology has made it possible to reduce radiation without compromising image quality. It is very important to keep this balance, especially when looking at metabolic bone diseases or genetic syndromes that influence several systems. For instance, the identification of sclerotic bone lesions related to certain genetic disorders benefits from CT imaging's clarity and specificity, complementing findings in other diagnostic criteria (Northrup *et al.*, 2021). Additionally, CT scans assist in the assessment of fracture risk by revealing detailed bone architecture, which informs preventative measures and treatment strategies within pediatric care contexts (LeBoff *et al.*, 2022) (Figure 2.6).

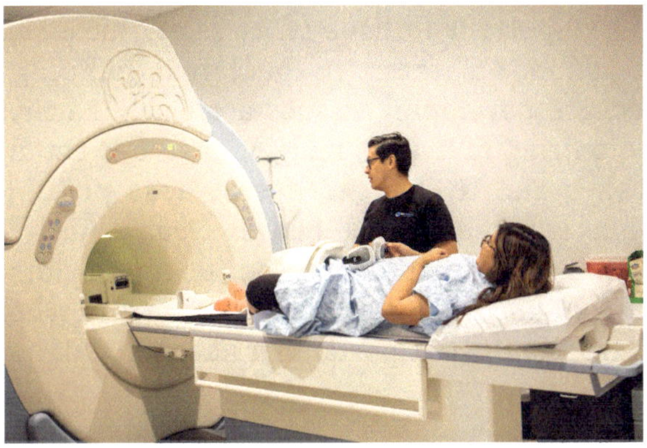

Figure 2.6. In pediatric radiology, the application of computed tomography (CT) scans plays a critical role in diagnosing complex conditions that may not be readily apparent through other imaging modalities.

Source: https://images.squarespace-cdn.com/content/v1/62cf0df2880df468dd7df097/1657828273019-5AL32CU23MUF8QV8QN1L/IMG_7967.jpg.

2.1.4. Magnetic Resonance Imaging (MRI)

New imaging technology has greatly improved how pediatricians diagnose various and complicated conditions in children. MRI is very important because it can clearly show soft tissues and does not use ionizing radiation, which is safer for children. Evaluating hepatobiliary diseases requires this modality, and various MRI techniques such as fat quantification, diffusion-weighted imaging, and elastography, help diagnose conditions such as biliary atresia and hepatic fibrosis. These approaches provide detailed functional and structural information that guides effective management without exposing young patients to harmful radiation (Yoon *et al.*, 2019).

Moreover, whole-body MRI has emerged as a powerful tool for comprehensive evaluation of pediatric oncologic and non-oncologic diseases, utilizing pulse sequences such as short tau inversion recovery and diffusion-weighted imaging to optimize detection and characterization within a timeframe tolerable for children (Goo, 2015). Using these several MRI techniques emphasizes the importance of MRI for pediatric radiology.

2.1.5. Nuclear Medicine in Children

Developments in medical imaging have made it much easier to diagnose pediatric patients, mainly with the help of nuclear medicine. Rather than the usual radiology methods, nuclear medicine uses a small quantity of radioactive substances to examine how different organs and tissues function, which is important for finding congenital and acquired diseases in children.

Since children are very sensitive to radiation, the protocols are set up to reduce their exposure and still give good results. Early and accurate diagnosis is crucial in congenital heart disease and pediatric oncology, because it can strongly affect the outcomes of treatment. Because nuclear medicine is non-invasive and offers whole-body images, it helps in thorough evaluation, aids in planning surgery, and monitors treatment effectiveness. Continued refinement in radiotracer development and imaging technology promises further to improve safety and efficacy in pediatric nuclear medicine (Figure 2.7).

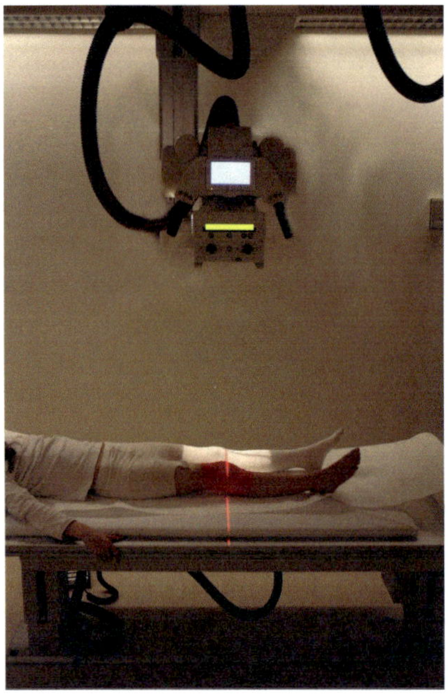

Figure 2.7. Advancements in medical imaging have significantly enhanced the diagnostic capabilities available for pediatric patients, particularly through the use of nuclear medicine.

Source: https://upload.wikimedia.org/wikipedia/commons/0/0a/Xraymachine.JPG.

2.1.6. Fluoroscopy Applications

Better imaging tools have improved the way pediatric conditions can be diagnosed and treated safely. Fluoroscopy is very important in pediatric radiology because it allows for real-time viewing of structures and their functions. It is used to guide catheter insertion, barium studies, and complicated surgeries, where seeing the procedure in real time helps ensure success and keeps risks low. Fluoroscopy is very useful for checking developmental issues and problems with the movement of food in children's digestive systems. Because children are more sensitive to radiation, it is essential to use optimized protocols and alternative imaging methods. Emerging integration with advanced guidance systems, including robotics, holds promise for improving procedural accuracy while reducing radiation doses to patients and staff alike (Kochanski *et al.*, 2018). Additionally, the incorporation of deep learning in fluoroscopic imaging advances may further refine diagnostic capabilities and workflow efficiency (Sahiner *et al.*, 2018).

2.1.7. Safety Protocols for Imaging Techniques

Since children are more sensitive to radiation, it is important to have strict safety measures designed for them in pediatric radiology. Because developing tissues are easily harmed by ionizing radiation, imaging methods should always aim to use the lowest dose possible while still keeping the images clear. Adjusting how much radiation is used, using shielding devices, and opting for ultrasound or MRI when appropriate are important for keeping radiation risks low.

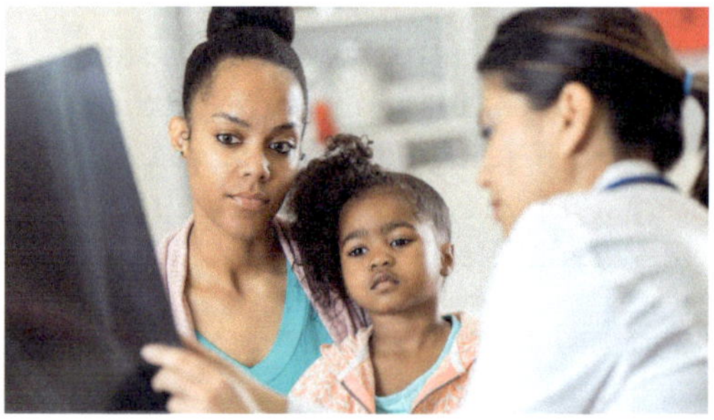

Figure 2.8. Continual monitoring and quality assurance protocols help ensure consistency in image quality and adherence to safety standards.

Source: https://www.fda.gov/files/pediatric%20xray_drupal.jpg.

Also, regularly checking and following quality assurance steps maintains the quality of images and safety standards. Giving radiologic technologists thorough training and using standard protocols for pediatric imaging makes patients safer. Digital imaging has improved, which helps to cut down on radiation because images can be acquired more efficiently. Moreover, incorporating real-time dose tracking and patient-specific adjustments reflects a commitment to optimizing safety while maintaining diagnostic efficacy in pediatric imaging (Figure 2.8).

2.1.8. Contrast Agents in Pediatric Imaging

The progress of imaging methods in pediatric radiology has been greatly helped by the use of contrast agents, which make it easier to see both normal and abnormal structures in the body. Because children have unique bodies, the main concern for contrast agents in pediatrics is safety and effectiveness. Water-soluble contrast agents, such as those used in retrograde urethrography, have demonstrated high diagnostic accuracy in evaluating urethral abnormalities with minimal complications when appropriate catheterization techniques are employed (Elsingergy *et al.*, 2023). Furthermore, ultrasound contrast agents (UCAs) offer a promising alternative, providing a non-ionizing, low-risk option for enhanced imaging across multiple organ systems. Despite their proven safety profile and potential for broader clinical applications, the limited FDA approval for UCAs in pediatrics restricts their use primarily to hepatic lesions and voiding cystourethrograms, thereby constraining optimal utilization in pediatric patients (Barr, 2022). Gaining more regulatory approval may help improve diagnostic accuracy and lower the risks linked to other imaging methods.

2.1.9. Innovations in Imaging Technology

New imaging technology has made a big difference in how pediatric radiology diagnoses are made, with a focus on safety. Especially, new types of ultrasound such as contrast-enhanced ultrasound, microvascular imaging, elastography, and fat quantification, have shown great potential for use in pediatric abdominal examinations. These innovations allow comprehensive assessments previously reliant on more invasive or radiation-heavy methods, potentially reducing the need for MRI and CT scans in children due to their non-invasiveness and absence of ionizing radiation exposure (Davis *et al.*, 2024). Also, using 3D images and AI-based tools in preoperative imaging has started to change the way surgeons plan for complicated injuries in children. This integration facilitates precise evaluation of fracture patterns and soft tissue involvement, ultimately improving surgical outcomes and recovery times (Suárez *et al.*, 2024). Collectively, these technological advancements underscore an important shift towards safer, more effective imaging strategies tailored to the unique needs of pediatric patients (Figure 2.9).

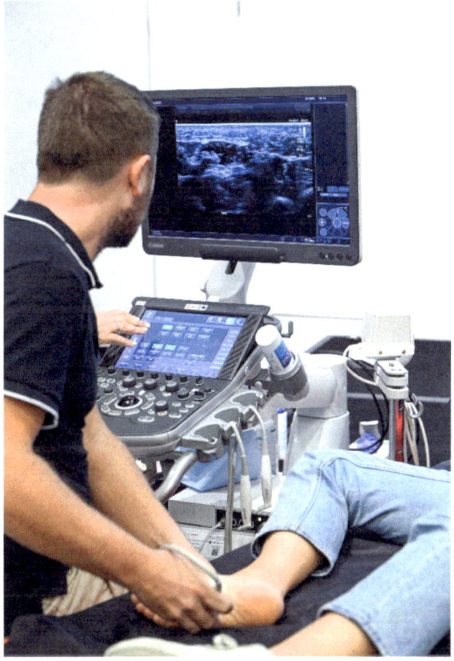

Figure 2.9. Emerging ultrasound modalities such as contrast-enhanced ultrasound, microvascular imaging, elastography, and fat quantification have demonstrated significant promise for pediatric abdominal applications.

Source: https://assets.isu.pub/document-structure/250121214143-d746303983780cb646a350c47c343540/v1/ae120d6f90fd3f7fc51a1bcf2d86a930.jpeg.

Test Your Knowledge

1. In which cases should MRI be chosen instead of CT for children, and what are the benefits?
2. What are the most important benefits of using ultrasound instead of other imaging methods for children?

2.2. Common Pediatric Conditions Diagnosed with Radiology

Learning Outcome

1. Understand congenital anomalies;
2. Identify respiratory disorders;
3. Know gastrointestinal issues;
4. Define musculoskeletal disorders;
5. Focus on neurological conditions;
6. Discuss oncological diagnoses;
7. Describe cardiovascular abnormalities;
8. Learn infectious diseases;
9. Know trauma and injury assessment.

Better imaging tools have made it much easier to diagnose conditions in children, which supports quick and proper treatment. Many common pediatric conditions like appendicitis, pneumonia, anomalies, and injuries are detected using radiology techniques. For suspected appendicitis, an abdominal ultrasound is the preferred imaging test because it is fast, requires little radiation, and gives dependable results. Moreover, the integration of oral radiocontrast material before computed tomography scans has been shown not to compromise subsequent ultrasound image quality, allowing for efficient diagnostics and management without prolonging emergency department stays (Arroyo *et al.*, 2020). X-rays are used to find musculoskeletal deformities, and MRI is important for finding brain abnormalities. Radiology in pediatrics is helpful for diagnosis and also helps choose the best treatment and monitor disease progression. Because of these capabilities, radiology is essential for caring for children with health problems.

2.2.1. Congenital Anomalies

New imaging tools have made it much easier to identify and care for complex fetal conditions, especially congenital anomalies, which are still a major concern in pediatric radiology. Though ultrasound is the main screening method, it is not always accurate in finding complex malformations, which is why other techniques are used along with it.

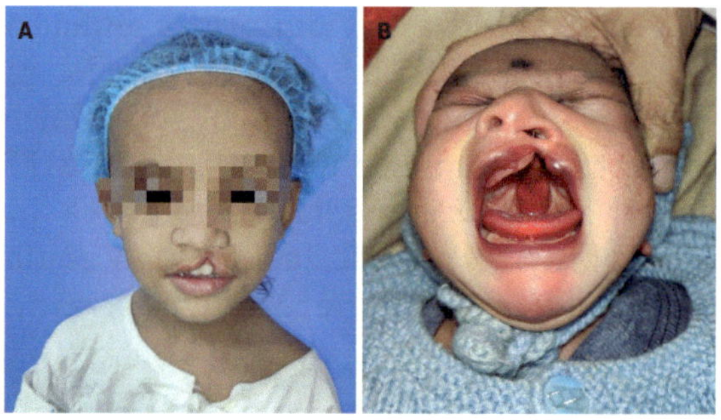

Figure 2.10. Pediatric congenital anomalies.

Source: https://f6publishing.blob.core.windows.net/8adce44e-6b86-4b8a-b5ec-c4b47b54a49d/90583-g002.png.

Fetal MRI is now used because it offers better soft tissue contrast and the ability to view images from different angles, which helps with diagnosis. Evidence shows that fetal MRI can sometimes improve or change the results found by ultrasound, which affects clinical choices, parental guidance, and evaluation of the fetus's prognosis. Earlier, the worry about fetal movement and safety meant ultrasound was not used often, but nowadays, new technology has made it easier to use more frequently. Consequently, fetal MRI serves as a problem-solving modality, particularly in cases where ultrasound findings are ambiguous or incomplete, ultimately improving patient management in the context of congenital anomalies (Baldacchino *et al.*, 2016; Stafrace *et al.*, 2008) (Figure 2.10).

2.2.2. Respiratory Disorders

Because respiratory problems in children can be complex, it is often necessary for doctors to collaborate with other specialists, mainly when there are structural issues. If the left mainstem bronchus is compressed, patients may develop frequent pneumonia, wheezing, and stridor, which can make treatment more difficult. To accurately find airway and blood vessel issues that can lead to breathing problems, advanced imaging tools like computed tomography and bronchoscopy are very important. Surgical interventions like posterior aortopexy have demonstrated efficacy in relieving compression by anchoring vascular structures away from the bronchus, thereby improving airway patency without significant mortality or need for reoperation (Arcieri *et al.*, 2016). The results point out that using both radiology and clinical knowledge helps in making the right treatment decisions. Pediatric radiology aids in making a diagnosis, assessing patients before surgery, and monitoring respiratory conditions over time, which helps provide better care for children.

2.2.3. Gastrointestinal Issues

Common gastrointestinal symptoms in children can make it hard to diagnose and may suggest that a systemic condition is present, so detailed radiology is often needed. A good example is Fabry Disease, which often starts in childhood and brings digestive issues like abdominal pain, diarrhea, and constipation, seriously affecting nutrition and growth. Radiologic imaging can help find these symptoms early, which supports prompt diagnosis and can prevent serious problems from developing. When radiologic techniques are used along with clinical and nutritional assessments, they offer a complete way to look at gastrointestinal symptoms in affected children. Also, improvements in pediatric radiology, using AI, have helped find subtle problems that might go unnoticed in regular evaluations, making diagnoses more accurate. These technological innovations complement thorough clinical assessments, facilitating early intervention and better outcomes in pediatric gastrointestinal disorders (Alrawi *et al.*, 2025; Dargenio *et al.*, 2025) (Figure 2.11).

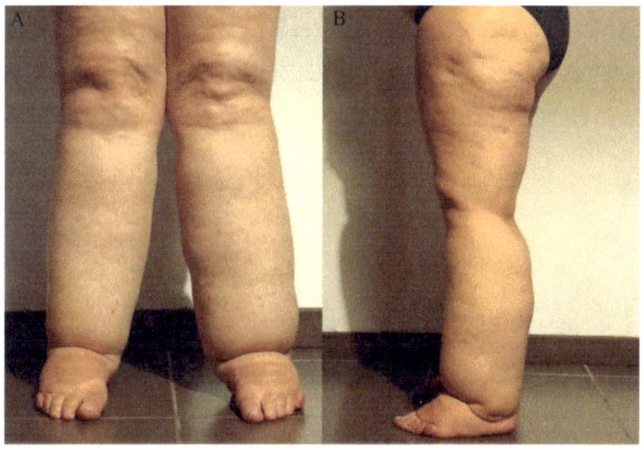

Figure 2.11. Fabry disease.

Source: https://image.oaes.cc/350e514e-769e-464c-9967-4f307fcf1aff/rdodj4061.fig.2.jpg.

2.2.4. Musculoskeletal Disorders

It is very important to diagnose musculoskeletal disorders in children accurately, because their body and growth stages can affect how the disease appears and is seen on images. Radiologic tests help discover congenital problems, injuries, and inflammation in the bones of growing children. MRI and ultrasound are used with traditional radiographs to help detect changes in soft tissue and bone marrow, which are often very hard to spot in the early stages of the disease. Radiologists working with children must make sure to examine them fully while using the least amount of radiation, because children are more sensitive to it. Interpreting what the findings mean involves looking at normal developmental variations to avoid making the wrong diagnosis. A combination of clinical history and diagnostic imaging supports fast and accurate treatment of musculoskeletal conditions, which helps patients in the long run. Better ways of imaging are helping doctors monitor disease progression, and how patients respond to treatment.

2.2.5. Neurological Conditions

Better imaging tools have made it easier to diagnose and treat different neurological problems in children. Identifying problems such as congenital malformations, brain injuries caused by accidents, and tumors early and correctly helps with better treatment and a better outlook.

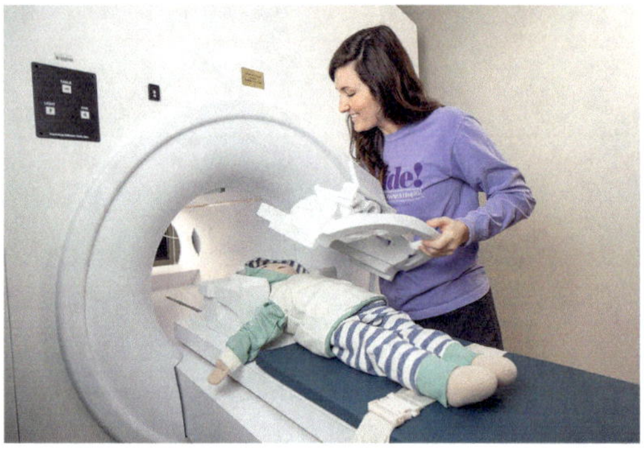

Figure 2.12. Pediatric radiology leverages modalities like magnetic resonance imaging (MRI) and computed tomography (CT) to visualize intricate neural structures with high resolution, facilitating detailed assessment of brain development and pathologies.

Source: https://media.springernature.com/lw1200/springer-static/image/art%3A10.1007%2Fs00247-021-05044-5/MediaObjects/247_2021_5044_Fig4_HTML.jpg.

Radiology in pediatrics makes use of MRI and CT to clearly see the brain's structures, which helps in studying brain development and diseases. These methods are beneficial for finding small changes in white matter and cortical formation, which are important in epilepsy and cerebral palsy. Also, using low-dose radiation and sedation techniques helps keep patients safe and makes them more likely to follow the imaging procedure. Continued refinement of pediatric neuroimaging protocols promises better diagnostic accuracy and personalized therapeutic interventions in childhood neurological disorders (Figure 2.12).

2.2.6. Oncological Diagnoses

Progress in pediatric radiology has made it much easier to find and classify oncological conditions, which has greatly helped patients recover. Using imaging tools is necessary to find the main tumor and to check for secondary cancers, which occur frequently in children with genetic conditions. Recent studies highlight that approximately 10% of children with cancer carry germline mutations that elevate the risk of both initial and secondary cancers, complicating treatment strategies due to increased toxicity from standard chemotherapy protocols (Czarny *et al.*, 2025). Additionally, accurate radiological assessment remains challenging in differentiating benign from malignant lesions, as illustrated in complex cases involving sublingual masses where imaging alone may lead to misdiagnosis, reinforcing the necessity of integrating histopathological confirmation with imaging findings (Alanazi *et al.*, 2024). This shows that pediatric radiologists play a key role in managing cancer cases by working together with other specialists, using genetic details, advanced imaging, and pathology.

2.2.7. Cardiovascular Abnormalities

Because of new developments in pediatric radiology, diagnosing and managing heart problems in children is much easier. It is crucial to detect congenital heart defects and vascular malformations early, which usually depends on using echocardiography, computed tomography, and magnetic resonance imaging. They make it possible to clearly see the heart's structures, which helps doctors make better diagnoses and treatment choices. Additionally, guidelines like the 2022 ACC/AHA provide a framework for assessing aortic diseases in pediatric populations, emphasizing the importance of genetic evaluation and continuous monitoring to prevent complications (Isselbacher *et al.*, 2022). Furthermore, the integration of artificial intelligence in radiologic practices shows promise for augmenting diagnostic precision, as demonstrated by recent innovations in deep learning algorithms applied to chest imaging (Chowdhury *et al.*, 2020). Such developments hold potential for more efficient identification of cardiovascular anomalies, ultimately improving prognostic outcomes and tailoring therapeutic approaches for young patients (Figure 2.13).

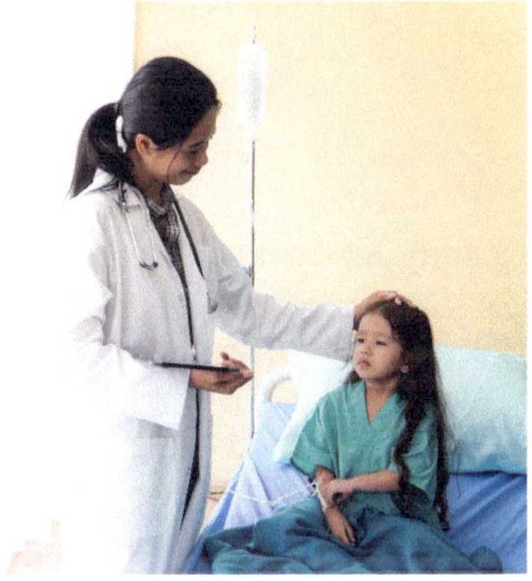

Figure 2.13. Advancements in pediatric radiology have significantly enhanced the ability to diagnose and manage cardiovascular abnormalities in children.

Source: https://medanta.s3.ap-south-1.amazonaws.com/blogs/December2024/DuBoDUM6l09JpzbJttQiXToGGzKRFc-metaUGFlZGlhdHJpYyBjYXJkaW9sb2d5LmpwZw==-.jpg.

2.2.8. Infectious Diseases

Thanks to progress in pediatric radiology, diagnosing and treating infectious diseases in children, such as those caused by SARS-CoV-2, has become much easier. Clinical presentation often varies, making imaging a critical adjunct to clinical assessment in identifying complications such as pneumonia, gastrointestinal involvement, and multisystem inflammatory syndrome in children (MIS-C). While chest CT scans can reveal subclinical lung lesions that indicate moderate COVID-19 severity, their routine use is limited by concerns over radiation exposure, sedation requirements, and healthcare costs, emphasizing the need for judicious imaging based on clinical judgment (Buonsenso *et al.*, 2020). Similarly, abdominal imaging plays a pivotal role in detecting severe gastrointestinal manifestations linked to COVID-19, including appendicitis and pancreatitis, which may require urgent surgical intervention (Vecchio *et al.*, 2021). This demonstrates that pediatric radiology is now focused on both detecting infections and helping with early treatment, which improves outcomes for children with infectious diseases.

2.2.9. Trauma and Injury Assessment

Evaluating injured pediatric patients correctly and promptly matters a lot since children have different body structures and systems than adults. In pediatric radiology, different imaging methods are important for assessing trauma and injuries by allowing a clear view of the inside without exposing the child to much radiation. The focused assessment with sonography in trauma (FAST) has gained prominence in this context, evolving to provide rapid bedside evaluation of the abdomen, chest, heart, and inferior vena cava, thus guiding clinical decision-making without the need for more invasive procedures (Richards *et al.*, 2017). Moreover, imaging is indispensable when assessing suspected child abuse cases, where subtle fracture patterns and soft tissue injuries can be indicative of maltreatment; pediatricians rely on radiologic findings to support diagnosis and subsequent intervention (Christian, 2015). Together, these advancements underscore the integral function of radiology in comprehensive trauma care, emphasizing a careful balance between diagnostic efficacy and child safety (Figure 2.14).

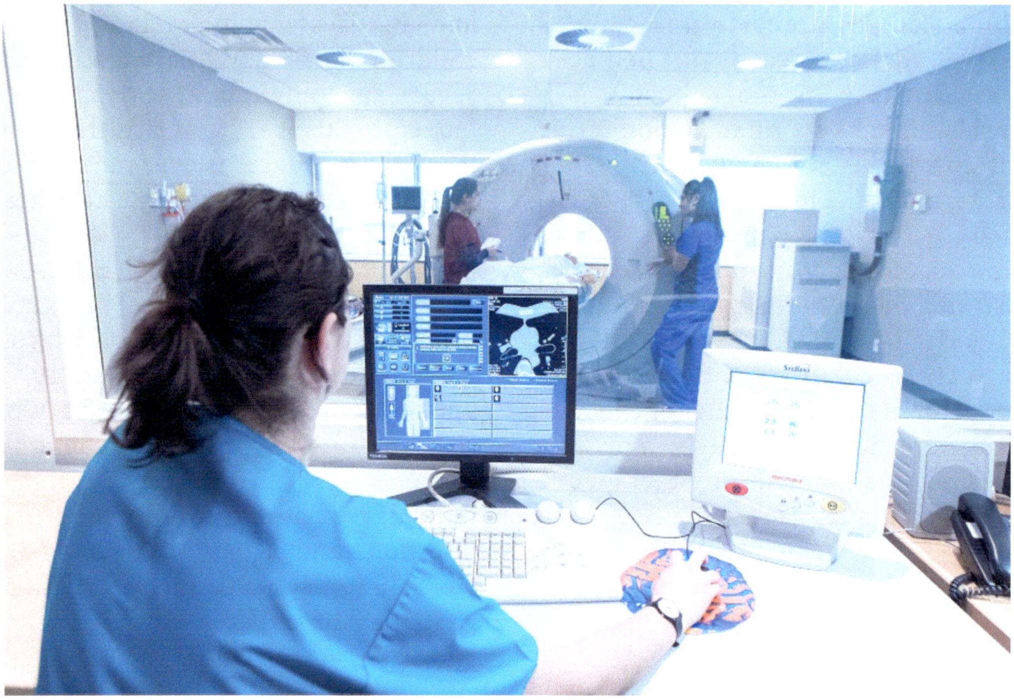

Figure 2.14. Imaging modalities in pediatric radiology play an essential role in trauma and injury assessment, enabling noninvasive visualization of internal structures while minimizing exposure to ionizing radiation.

Source: https://radonc.utoronto.ca/sites/default/files/styles/landscape_3_2_1800/public/assets/images/MRS_Radiological-Technology_21.jpg?itok=4bj2MULQ.

Test Your Knowledge

1. How is pneumonia identified in young patients by looking at their chest X-rays and what symptoms should you expect to notice?
2. For a child suspected of having congenital heart disease, which imaging technique is used first and why?

2.3. Challenges and Considerations in Pediatric Radiology

Learning Outcome

1. Know radiation exposure concerns;
2. Define sedation and anesthesia in imaging;
3. Focus on communication with pediatric patients;
4. Explain parental involvement and consent;
5. Learn developmental considerations in imaging;
6. Identify variability in pediatric anatomy;
7. Describe the psychological impact of imaging procedures;
8. Discuss access to pediatric radiology services;
9. Focus on training and education for radiologists.

Pediatric radiology requires dealing with many unique issues that are different from adult imaging, mainly regarding patient safety, accurate diagnosis, and ethical questions. Since young patients are more sensitive to radiation, it is essential to use strict dose reduction methods to avoid risks in the future while still maintaining clear images, which requires both new technology and skilled practitioners. In addition, because children grow and develop differently, it is not always easy for radiologists to correctly distinguish between normal and abnormal, so they need special training. It becomes more complicated when parents or caregivers do not communicate well, so special strategies are needed to get their cooperation and informed consent. Additionally, integrating emerging technologies such as artificial intelligence must be approached cautiously, balancing potential benefits in diagnostic precision with concerns over data security and ethical transparency in pediatric contexts (Semerci *et al.*, 2024). These multifaceted considerations underscore the critical importance of a specialized, vigilant approach in pediatric radiological practice (Chalasani *et al.*, 2017).

2.3.1. Radiation Exposure Concerns

Because medical imaging is used more often in children, there are concerns about the possible health problems caused by radiation.

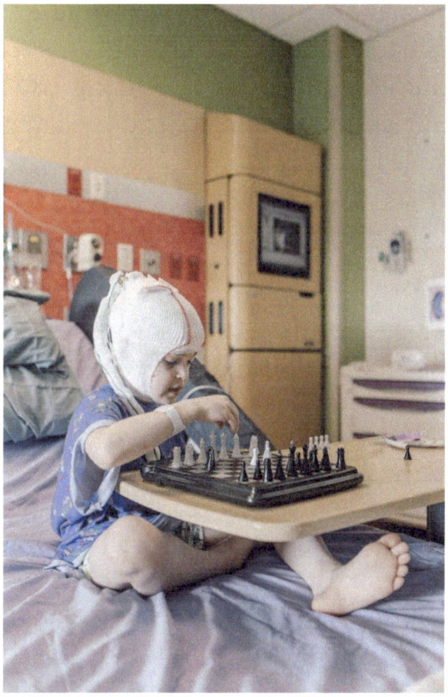

Figure 2.15. Children are more radiosensitive than adults due to their developing tissues and longer expected lifespans, which increase the cumulative risk of radiation-induced complications.

Source: https://www.itnonline.com/sites/default/files/Image1.jpg.

Children are more sensitive to radiation than adults because their tissues are still developing, and they are expected to live longer, which raises the risk of radiation-related problems. Even so, talking to caregivers about these risks is not always done well which can lead them to be reluctant or refuse important imaging tests. Studies have demonstrated that educational interventions, such as informational handouts, can effectively improve parental understanding and alleviate apprehensions without decreasing willingness to permit essential radiographic examinations (Hwang *et al.*, 2017). So, being open about information is necessary to manage the pros and cons of pediatric imaging. Also, new methods for reducing radiation doses help to make pediatric radiology safer. Thus, addressing radiation exposure concerns requires a multifaceted approach combining education, technological improvements, and vigilant clinical practice (Figure 2.15).

2.3.2. Sedation and Anesthesia in Imaging

Sedation or anesthesia is often given to pediatric patients during imaging procedures, as it is hard for them to stay still for the required time. Depending on the type of imaging, the sedation may last only a short time for a CT scan or a much longer time for MRI, which may need radiologists to be well organized. A multidisciplinary consensus highlights that such interventions are integral to resource utilization within pediatric trauma centers, recognizing anesthesia and sedation as essential components of comprehensive care in complex cases (Snyder *et al.*, 2023). However, the administration of sedation and anesthesia involves careful patient assessment to minimize risks, alongside adherence to institutional protocols that differ widely across regions and healthcare settings (Choudhary *et al.*, 2022). The purpose of using different drugs and techniques is always the same: to ensure safety, the best images, and accurate diagnoses for children.

2.3.3. Communication with Pediatric Patients

For pediatric radiology to be successful, healthcare providers must interact well with pediatric patients. Good communication that shows empathy helps children stay calm and cooperate during imaging, which may seem scary because of the equipment and the need to stay put. Additionally, involving parents or caregivers by presenting them with educational materials can significantly enhance their understanding and comfort with radiologic procedures, as demonstrated by increased parental willingness following exposure to informational handouts about radiation risks and benefits in dental radiography (Hwang *et al.*, 2017). They help the child feel better and also support getting informed consent and trust. Explaining procedures with pictures and age-appropriate language, sometimes with the help of online resources, is very important for understanding them. Altogether, tailored communication with pediatric patients and their families represents a cornerstone in optimizing outcomes and ensuring ethical practice within pediatric radiology (Figure 2.16).

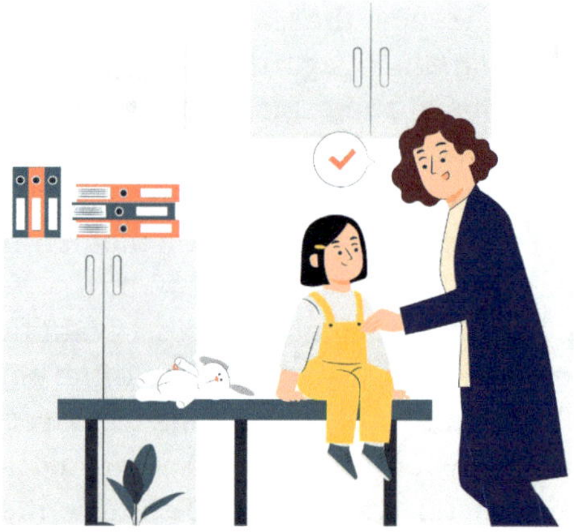

Figure 2.16. Establishing clear, empathetic communication helps alleviate children's anxiety and fosters cooperation during imaging, which can be intimidating due to unfamiliar equipment and the need to remain still.

Source: https://2af91d24.delivery.rocketcdn.me/wp-content/uploads/2024/06/Child-counsilng-350-x-250px-03-1.jpg.

2.3.4. Parental Involvement and Consent

To protect children and respect their families, those in pediatric radiology must know the rules and ethics involved in getting consent. Since minors usually depend on their parents to decide certain things, such as undergoing diagnostic imaging with radiation, parental involvement is very important in the consent process. Recent advancements in standardizing consent forms, such as those proposed in the Consent for Treatment Framework, demonstrate how formalized and digitized processes can reduce ambiguities and enhance legal compliance, fostering more transparent communication between healthcare providers and families (Voronov *et al.*, 2024). Furthermore, legislative changes removing parental involvement mandates in certain medical procedures have influenced the timing and accessibility of care for minors, underscoring the delicate balance between protecting child welfare and enabling autonomous healthcare decisions (Fulcher *et al.*, 2025). Therefore, having parents involved and giving their consent is still essential for the best results in pediatric radiology and following new rules and advances.

2.3.5. Developmental Considerations in Imaging

Improvements in imaging have made it simpler to find and follow conditions in kids, though there are still challenges because of their development. In babies, brain imaging requires techniques that are sensitive to rapid brain growth, and minimize risks from sedatives and radiation. Techniques such as MR Fingerprinting show promise by providing motion-robust, quantitative assessments of brain tissue in non-sedated infants, addressing practical obstacles linked to traditional MRI protocols, and improving image quality in younger populations (Badve *et al.*, 2023). Furthermore, the vulnerability of children necessitates ethical vigilance in employing neuroimaging, as its results may have implications beyond clinical care, including potential stigmatization and issues of confidentiality (Downie *et al.*, 2007). Thus, developmental considerations not only influence the technical selection of imaging modalities but also shape the ethical framework guiding pediatric radiology practices to ensure safety, accuracy, and respect for the child's long-term well-being (Figure 2.17).

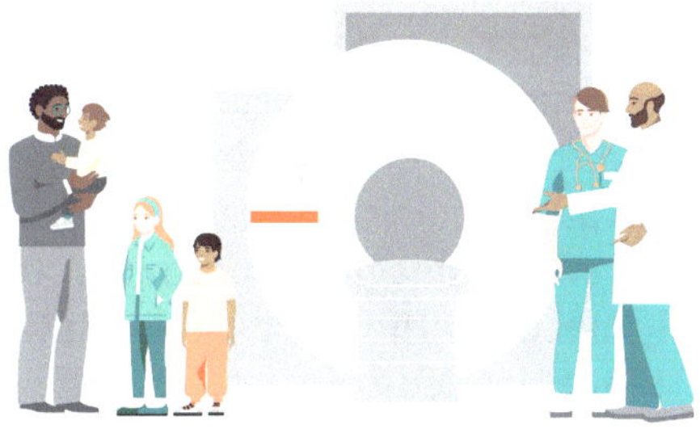

Figure 2.17. MR Fingerprinting.

Source: https://marketing.webassets.siemens-healthineers.com/fc01c286c8cf303b/3efce182a772/v/45ad7d307489/siemens-healthineers_MRI_pediatric_graphic.png?nowebp=1.

2.3.6. Variability in Pediatric Anatomy

One must understand the changes in development that can change the way organs and tissues are seen in imaging studies. Unlike adults, children's organs, their positions, and their tissues undergo significant changes as they develop and grow. Since the body changes a lot during childhood, special imaging methods are needed because standard adult methods may not be enough. For instance, the variation in vascular and cardiac anatomy among pediatric patients requires careful interpretation to avoid misdiagnoses, especially in conditions like aortic disease, where guidelines emphasize patient-specific evaluation and management (Isselbacher *et al.*, 2022). Additionally, advances in imaging technology, including deep learning applications for chest radiographs, must account for these anatomical variations to enhance diagnostic precision and clinical outcomes in children (Çall *et al.*, 2021). So, being aware of the differences in pediatric anatomy is important for using the best techniques and providing safe and effective care in pediatric radiology.

2.3.7. Psychological Impact of Imaging Procedures

Medical imaging is very important for diagnosing children in radiology, but it can also have psychological effects that must be considered. Many children find imaging procedures stressful, especially because they are in an unfamiliar setting, there are loud noises, and they must not move.

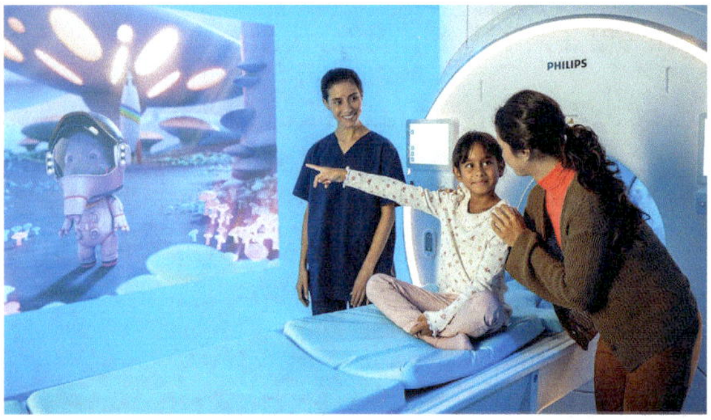

Figure 2.18. Children undergoing imaging procedures often experience anxiety and fear, exacerbated by unfamiliar environments, loud noises, and the requirement to remain still.

Source: https://www.philips.com/c-dam/corporate/newscenter/global/standard/resources/healthcare/2024/q-and-a-with-atul-gupta-md/pedatric-hero-header.jpg.

Because of this distress, patients may not cooperate well, which can lower the image quality and make it harder to diagnose accurately. Also, when a person is exposed to stressors in healthcare too often, it can lead to long-lasting negative feelings about these settings. Talking to children in a way they can understand and using distraction methods can help relieve their fears and improve their experience. Being present during procedures, caregivers can give emotional support that can ease anxiety. Addressing these psychological factors is very important for helping children follow medical advice and for improving their general well-being during radiologic exams. This holistic approach underscores the importance of empathy and psychological sensitivity alongside technical precision in pediatric radiology (Figure 2.18).

2.3.8. Access to Pediatric Radiology Services

It is still difficult for children in underserved and rural areas to get equal access to pediatric radiology services because there are not many experts in those regions. Technological advancements, such as AI-assisted interpretation of diagnostic images, offer promising avenues to augment clinician capacity and reduce wait times, yet the opacity and integration challenges of these tools can hinder their effective deployment in pediatric settings (Lebovitz *et al.*, 2022). Furthermore, the increasing reliance on telemedicine and virtual consultations during the COVID-19 pandemic has transformed healthcare delivery but also introduced new challenges related to digital fatigue and communication barriers that may affect both providers and families seeking radiologic care (Wiederhold, 2020). Investing in infrastructure, training, and technology that focuses on users is needed to handle these various challenges and give accurate, appropriate, and prompt radiologic evaluations to children. By using comprehensive strategies, pediatric radiology services can be made more available, which helps improve the outcomes and health of all children.

2.3.9. Training and Education for Radiologists

To be ready for pediatric imaging, radiologists must go through a challenging and focused educational program that covers both general radiology and things unique to children. Programs for pediatrics training are not the same everywhere, usually last several years, and include working with children to sharpen the ability to diagnose and notice the special features of their bodies. In Europe, for instance, radiology residency ranges from two to six years, often preceded by an internship, with subspecialty fellowships available in just over half of the surveyed countries, highlighting ongoing efforts to enhance subspecialized skills in pediatric radiology (Dillon *et al.*, 2017). Adding formal exams and research projects helps these programs by filling in any missing knowledge and skills. Radiologists can become familiar with pediatric diseases using detailed imaging archives, which are important visual educational tools. Thus, the continuous evolution of structured training remains essential for advancing the quality of pediatric radiologic care (Figure 2.19).

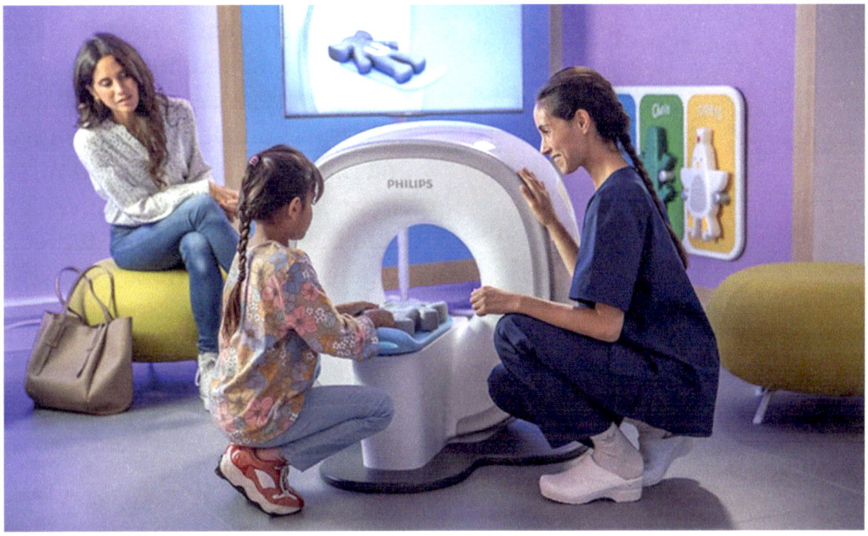

Figure 2.19. Training programs vary internationally, typically spanning several years and embedding hands-on experience with pediatric cases to sharpen diagnostic accuracy and sensitivity to the unique anatomical and physiological characteristics of children.

Source: https://www.philips.com/c-dam/corporate/newscenter/global/standard/resources/healthcare/2024/q-and-a-with-atul-gupta-md/pediatric-coaching-0272.jpg.

Test Your Knowledge

1. What are the main difficulties radiologists have when imaging babies and children, and how can these be resolved?
2. Why are children especially at risk from radiation, and what can be done to reduce this risk?

2.4. Future Directions in Pediatric Radiology

Learning Outcome

1. Learn advances in imaging technology;
2. Focus on artificial intelligence in radiology;
3. Identify personalized medicine approaches;
4. Focus on telemedicine and remote consultations;
5. Describe research and clinical trials;
6. Explain interdisciplinary collaboration;
7. Know global health perspectives;
8. Describe education and training innovations;
9. Understand policy and advocacy for pediatric radiology.

Using new technologies in radiology will likely improve how pediatric cases are diagnosed and how patients are treated. Artificial intelligence, particularly in neuro-oncology, has demonstrated superior precision compared to traditional methods, suggesting significant potential for pediatric applications where early and accurate diagnosis is critical (Khalighi *et al.*, 2024). AI can help with workflow by quickly analyzing images and identifying what is happening inside the body so that doctors may avoid invasive procedures. Moreover, the incorporation of AI into medical education ensures that future radiologists will be better equipped to interpret complex pediatric imaging and implement personalized treatment plans (Gordon *et al.*, 2024).

More research is needed to address ethical issues and guarantee that these technologies are available to all kinds of people. With the rise of more flexible and advanced AI, pediatric radiology will be able to provide tailored medicine by using information from imaging, genetics, and clinical details.

2.4.1. Advances in Imaging Technology

Lately, better imaging technology has helped pediatric radiology by making diagnoses more accurate and reducing radiation exposure to children. Digital radiography and new ultrasound methods help clinicians get images that are clearer and more suited to children's bodies. They make it easier to find and judge congenital problems and injuries, and they also decrease the number of invasive procedures. Also, using low-dose computed tomography and magnetic resonance imaging protocols created for children demonstrates a strong dedication to safety and maintaining high image quality. This progress is shown by better detectors, higher resolutions, and improved real-time imaging that allow for monitoring pediatric organ function in real-time. Collectively, these technological strides foster earlier diagnosis, targeted interventions, and better long-term outcomes in pediatric healthcare (Figure 2.20).

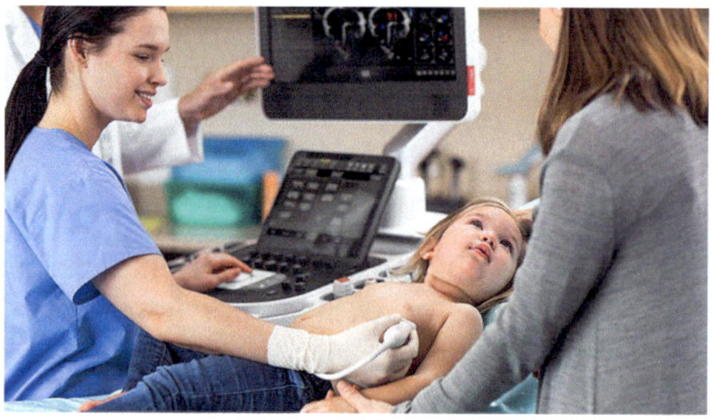

Figure 2.20. Innovations such as digital radiography and advanced ultrasound techniques have allowed clinicians to obtain clearer, more detailed images tailored to the unique anatomical considerations of children.

Source: https://www.philips.com/c-dam/corporate/innovation-and-you/global/jun-2021/teaser-child-being-scanned.jpg.

2.4.2. Artificial Intelligence (AI) in Radiology

The use of AI in radiology has created new opportunities for pediatric imaging, especially by helping to ensure that both the diagnosis and radiation levels are kept low. Because pediatric patients are more at risk from ionizing radiation, advanced techniques are needed to ensure the image is clear without using too much radiation. Using AI, such as deep learning models and convolutional neural networks, has helped to reduce noise and artifacts in low-dose imaging, increasing the accuracy of diagnoses and not endangering patients. These tools also make it easier to manage workflow and reduce the need for repeated scans, which helps clinics work more efficiently. Still, despite all these improvements, there are still major difficulties such as rules, ethics, and users' reluctance to accept AI. Overcoming these obstacles requires multifaceted strategies to ensure AI's successful integration, ultimately promising a safer, more precise pediatric radiology practice (Adeleke *et al.*, 2025; Eymann *et al.*, 2024).

2.4.3. Personalized Medicine Approaches

Because of progress in medical technology, doctors now focus on personalized treatment methods, especially in pediatrics, where children's development is very important. Using genetic, chemical, and imaging information, personalized medicine in pediatric radiology helps doctors choose the right treatment for each child. It increases the chances of accurate diagnosis and helps avoid unneeded radiation, which is very important for growing tissues. By combining advanced imaging with molecular profiling, doctors can find and identify diseases earlier and more precisely, which helps them choose the best treatment and monitor its effectiveness. Also, including artificial intelligence and machine learning in radiology helps improve image analysis and the grouping of patients by risk, which supports a better patient-centered approach. Such innovations underscore the transformative potential of personalized medicine in improving pediatric outcomes, reflecting the evolving landscape of radiological practice (Burity *et al.*, 2014) (Figure 2.21).

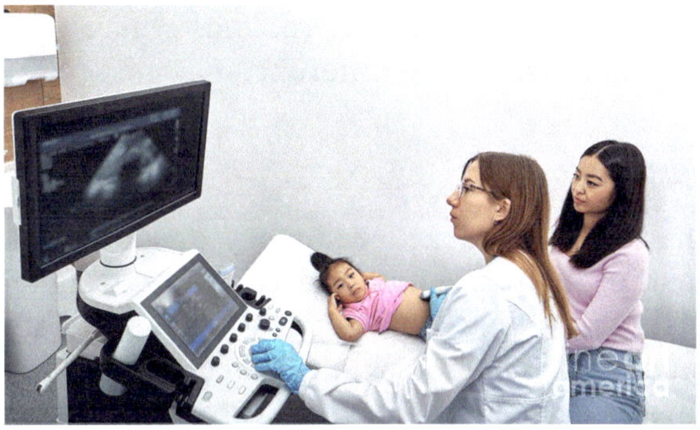

Figure 2.21. Personalized medicine approaches in pediatric radiology leverage genetic, biochemical, and imaging data to tailor interventions specifically to a child's unique physiological and pathological profile.

Source: https://lakezurichopenmri.com/wp-content/uploads/2024/06/A-high-resolution-image-of-a-child-undergoing-an-ultrasound-scan-in-a-pediatric-imaging-clinic.jpg.

2.4.4. Telemedicine and Remote Consultations

The use of new technology has helped pediatric radiology improve its diagnostic methods and better look after patients. Telemedicine and remote consultations, which used to be experimental, have now become an important part of healthcare services. Despite initial slow adoption, successful telemedicine services have demonstrated the potential to enhance access to pediatric radiological expertise, particularly for patients in remote or underserved areas (AlDossary *et al.*, 2017). Studies have shown that teleradiology maintains diagnostic accuracy comparable to conventional radiology, ensuring reliable interpretations essential for pediatric cases (Bashshur *et al.*, 2016). Besides, by using telemedicine, patients may not need to be transferred as much, can stay at home longer, and can get regular care with the help of remote consultations and image sharing. Thanks to these technologies, diagnoses are made more quickly and treatment is customized for each child, which is very important for managing serious pediatric health problems where early care can make a big difference.

2.4.5. Research and Clinical Trials

The field of pediatric radiology depends a lot on thorough research and carefully designed trials to evaluate new imaging techniques and check their safety in children. Because children have special physiology and growing tissues, special studies should be done to improve the accuracy of diagnosis and reduce the amount of radiation they receive.

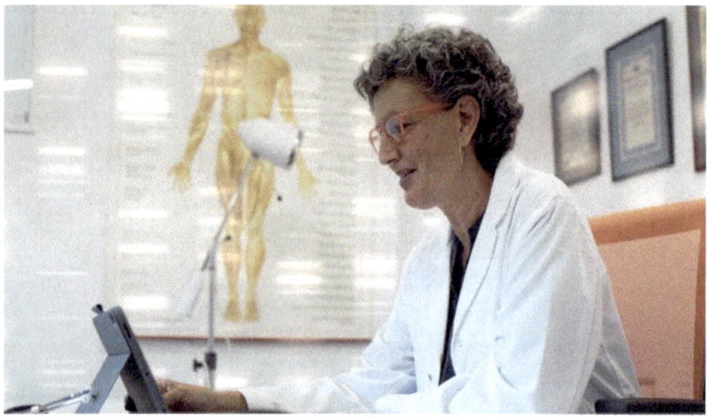

Figure 2.22. Clinical trials in this field often face challenges related to ethical considerations, informed consent, and recruitment, yet they are crucial for validating new modalities and protocols that improve patient outcomes.

Source: https://www.astrazeneca.com/content/dam/az/r-and-d/clinical-innovation/AZ2998-BioPharma.jpg/jcr:content/renditions/cq5dam.web.1200.AZ2998-BioPharma.jpg.

Ethical matters, getting informed consent, and recruiting enough participants are common challenges in this field, but clinical trials are necessary for proving the benefits of new ways and rules in medicine. Using new technologies such as artificial intelligence and telemedicine in healthcare means they should be tested thoroughly through experiments to check their usefulness and any possible side effects. Notably, the COVID-19 pandemic has heightened the importance of adapting research methodologies, underscoring the need for gender-sensitive and equitable data collection to address disparities and ensure inclusive care, as reflected in broader healthcare research contexts (Gausman *et al.*, 2020; Wiederhold, 2020). Such nuanced approaches strengthen the evidence base guiding pediatric radiology practice (Figure 2.22).

2.4.6. Interdisciplinary Collaboration

Good healthcare in pediatric radiology requires all medical specialists to communicate and cooperate well. All imaging reports must be interpreted by radiologists, pediatricians, surgeons, and technologists, who must take into account the special needs of children. Working together in this way makes it easier to diagnose correctly and gives patients the right treatment, which reduces the risks of radiation and improves the outcomes.

Also, including knowledge from nursing staff and child life specialists helps make the environment more supportive for young patients in all aspects. Such collaboration is increasingly facilitated by institutional frameworks promoting shared decision-making and continuous feedback loops, as evidenced in recent healthcare models (Artenstein *et al.*, 2016). The emphasis on teamwork not only streamlines workflow but also drives innovation in imaging protocols specifically designed for pediatric care (Artenstein *et al.*, 2020), underscoring the vital role of interdisciplinary collaboration in advancing pediatric radiology.

2.4.7. Global Health Perspectives

The availability of advanced pediatric radiology services varies significantly, which affects how childhood diseases are handled and treated. Because of a lack of specialized imaging and trained staff, early detection and treatment are limited in low- and middle-income countries, which mostly affects the most vulnerable people. For instance, children with sickle cell anemia often require transcranial Doppler screening and hydroxyurea counseling, yet adherence to these interventions remains inconsistent due to systemic barriers, including inadequate follow-up and resource shortages (Bardach *et al.*, 2019). Achieving this requires using technology, training workers, and making healthcare policies sensitive to different cultures. In addition, including global health in pediatric radiology encourages regions to cooperate, share information, and improve imaging methods to fit different health conditions. In the end, closing these gaps improves the accuracy of diagnoses and the success of treatments, which highlights the key role of equal radiologic care for children globally.

2.4.8. Education and Training Innovations

Thanks to technological progress, medical education has been dramatically changed, especially in areas like pediatric radiology. Learning traditionally is now often combined with new methods such as simulation and digital image databases, which improve both theoretical and practical knowledge. Because of these innovations, learners can examine clear pediatric images safely, which helps them make accurate diagnoses and protects patients from radiation. Also, virtual reality and augmented reality help students experience challenging medical situations, which helps them think critically and make decisions in emergencies. Online modules that people can collaborate on allow trainees from all over the world to learn about new topics and discuss cases, making education more equal for everyone. Such ways of learning help people become more skilled in reading pediatric radiology images and also make them better prepared to help patients. Consequently, these educational advancements represent a vital component in evolving pediatric radiology training paradigms (Figure 2.23).

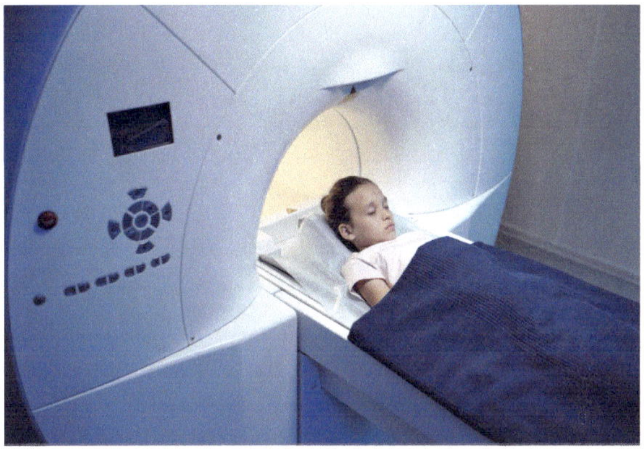

Figure 2.23. Advancements in technology have profoundly transformed the landscape of medical education, particularly within specialized fields such as pediatric radiology.

Source: https://www.itnonline.com/sites/default/files/inline-images/Screenshot%20 2024-01-15%20at%202.59.31%E2%80%AFPM.png.

2.4.9. Policy and Advocacy for Pediatric Radiology

Improving how pediatric radiology is delivered calls for strong policies and ongoing advocacy to help apply new clinical developments in practice. Advocacy is very important in bringing evidence-based changes to care that is fair and accessible, especially in places where pediatric radiology services are underdeveloped. Models such as the MAP through advocacy demonstrate how professional organizations can systematically develop and maintain public policy initiatives that support specialized fields, thereby enhancing the capacity of pediatric radiology to meet growing demands and complex clinical challenges (Boyd *et al.*, 2024). Furthermore, experiences from other pediatric healthcare domains, including tuberculosis care, illustrate the importance of clinician confidence and coordinated policies in expanding the reach of diagnostic and treatment tools, a principle readily applicable to pediatric radiology (Moore *et al.*, 2024). For this reason, a mix of clinical practices, advocacy, and policy changes is necessary to advance the field and improve health outcomes for children globally.

Test Your Knowledge

1. How might artificial intelligence (AI) and machine learning change the landscape of pediatric radiology in the coming years?
2. How do you think pediatric radiology supports precision medicine, especially for children with rare genetic problems and cancer?

SUMMARY

Although pediatric radiology has advanced a lot, there are still difficulties in finding the right balance between good diagnosis and safety. The frequent repetition of computed tomography scans in children, as documented in recent studies, highlights a pressing issue regarding radiation exposure, underscoring the urgent need for stringent dose management strategies and implementation of dose-tracking technologies to mitigate risks (Albahiti, 2023). Concurrently, magnetic resonance imaging has proven invaluable in evaluating complex pediatric conditions such as seizures, offering detailed insights into structural abnormalities without the associated radiation risks, thereby enhancing diagnostic precision in a vulnerable population (Raj *et al.*, 2021). The progress of pediatric radiology should focus on reducing the risk of harm, improving diagnosis, and making sure new technologies benefit the unique needs of children. Having this dual focus is the main idea guiding future pediatric imaging.

Better tools in pediatric radiology have improved how doctors diagnose and treat congenital and metabolic conditions in children. Tracking the progress of the disease and the effectiveness of treatment is now possible because of the latest imaging scales and methods. For example, the Radiographic Global Impression of Change (RGI-C) scale has demonstrated substantial validity and reliability in quantifying skeletal changes in children with hypophosphatasia, facilitating more precise monitoring of enzyme replacement therapy outcomes through standardized radiographic assessments (Fujita *et al.*, 2018). Additionally, diffusion imaging techniques, such as diffusion tensor imaging and high angular resolution diffusion imaging, have transformed our understanding of white matter microstructure and brain connectivity in congenital brain malformations, revealing critical insights into neurodevelopmental abnormalities and guiding both clinical and research applications (Barkovich *et al.*, 2010). All these improvements in technology and methods highlight how pediatric radiology plays a key role in accurate diagnosis, treatment planning, and caring for children with severe conditions.

KEY TERMS FROM THIS CHAPTER

- X-rays
- Congenital problems
- Infections
- Children
- Health problems
- Computed tomography (CT)
- Pediatric oncology
- Craniofacial development
- Pediatric radiology
- Injuries
- Cancers
- Imaging protocols
- Radiographic analysis
- Positron emission tomography (PET)
- Embryonic vascular
- Fatty liver

CRITICAL THINKING QUESTIONS

1. **Which type of imaging is usually chosen for examining fractures in children?**
   a. MRI
   b. X-ray
   c. CT scan
   d. Ultrasound
2. **For what medical conditions would a chest X-ray be performed on children?**
   a. To diagnose a simple cold
   b. To assess suspected pneumonia
   c. To detect a fractured rib
   d. Both B and C
3. **What is a major issue with using CT scans in pediatric radiology?**
   a. Increased exposure to radiation
   b. Poor image resolution
   c. High cost
   d. Limited accessibility
4. **Which of the following is a common feature seen in the imaging of pediatric patients with respiratory distress syndrome (RDS)?**
   a. Hyperinflation of the lungs
   b. Ground-glass appearance on chest X-ray
   c. Pulmonary edema
   d. Pneumothorax
5. **What is the main way imaging is used to assess congenital heart defects in infants?**
   a. Chest X-ray
   b. Echocardiogram
   c. CT scan
   d. MRI

Short Answer Questions

1. Why do pediatric radiology and adult radiology follow different imaging procedures and techniques?
2. What are the main problems in pediatric imaging, especially with infants and young children?
3. Which things should be considered when choosing an imaging test for children?
4. What dangers are there from radiation in pediatric radiology, and how can these dangers be reduced?
5. What types of imaging are used most often for finding fractures in children, and why?

Answers to Critical Thinking Questions

1. (b); 2. (d); 3. (a); 4. (b); 5. (b)

REFERENCES

1. Adeleke, S., Adeleke, S., Akpan, A. O., Akpan, *et al.* (2025). *AI-Driven Advances in Low-Dose Imaging and Enhancement—A Review*. https://core.ac.uk/download/647986101.pdf (accessed on 31st May 2025).
2. Alanazi, O. I., Halawani, M. S., Marhoon, S. E., Ali, A. H., & Awad, B. I. (2024). Congenital sublingual dermoid cyst mimicking a recurrent ranula in a pediatric patient: A case report. *Cureus, 16*. https://www.semanticscholar.org/paper/f723b025b026772e2b0819a49fdad44c7e8e3258 (accessed on 31st May 2025).
3. Albahiti, S. (2023). RSSA Conference: Radiation exposure from repeated CT scans in children: A quantitative analysis. *Saudi Journal of Radiology*. https://www.semanticscholar.org/paper/9480ceaed77ffafadb5695b744388480d38ce0f3 (accessed on 31st May 2025).
4. AlDossary, S., Bradford, N. K., Martin-Khan, M. G., Smith, *et al.* (2017). A systematic review of the methodologies used to evaluate telemedicine service initiatives in hospital facilities. *International Journal of Medical Informatics*. https://core.ac.uk/download/83972862.pdf (accessed on 31st May 2025).
5. Alrawi, R. M. S., & Basheer, N. M. (2025). Pediatric radiology: An analysis of AI-powered bone age determination methods. *NTU Journal of Engineering and Technology*. https://www.semanticscholar.org/paper/093a9aae8d5c79299e82ea24a4e30c89166617eb (accessed on 31st May 2025).
6. Arcieri, L., Assanta, N., Baggi, R., Di Maurizio, *et al.* (2016). The role of posterior aortopexy in the treatment of left mainstem bronchus compression. *Interactive Cardio Vascular and Thoracic Surgery*. https://core.ac.uk/download/74319435.pdf (accessed on 31st May 2025).
7. Arroyo, A., Dickman, E., Drapkin, J., Haines, *et al.* (2020). Does orally-administered radiocontrast impair ultrasound image quality in pediatric patients? *West J. Emerg. Med.* https://core.ac.uk/download/287622001.pdf (accessed on 31st May 2025).
8. Artenstein, A. (2016). *Baystate Medical Practices Annual Report – 2016*. https://core.ac.uk/download/234573495.pdf (accessed on 31st May 2025).
9. Badve, C., Chen, Y., Costello, D. W., Durieux, *et al.* (2023). *Motion Robust MR Fingerprinting Scan to Image Neonates with Prenatal Opioid Exposure*. http://arxiv.org/abs/2306.16656 (accessed on 31st May 2025).
10. Bahroun, Z., Anane, C., Ahmed, V., & Zacca, A. (2023). Transforming education: A comprehensive review of generative artificial intelligence in educational settings through bibliometric and content analysis. *Sustainability, 15*, 12983. https://doi.org/10.3390/su151712983 (accessed on 31st May 2025).
11. Baldacchino, I., Gatt, A. S., & Saliba, I. (2016). *Fetal MRI: An Essential Step in Interpreting Complex Ultrasound Findings*. https://core.ac.uk/download/46604247.pdf (accessed on 31st May 2025).
12. Bardach, N. S., Cabana, M. D., Kanter, J., Marsh, *et al.* (2019). *Barriers to Pediatric Sickle Cell Disease Guideline Recommendations*. https://core.ac.uk/download/323062997.pdf (accessed on 31st May 2025).

13. Barkovich, A. J., Mukherjee, P., & Wahl, M. (2010). *Diffusion Imaging and Tractography of Congenital Brain Malformations*. https://core.ac.uk/download/323074405.pdf (accessed on 31st May 2025).

14. Barr, R. (2022). The urgent need for FDA to approve a whole-body application of ultrasound contrast agents. *Journal of Ultrasound in Medicine, 42*. https://www.semanticscholar.org/paper/e9d50eb0a7470ca3eb67cd756baa97c2857f4fe9 (accessed on 31st May 2025).

15. Bashshur, N., Bashshur, R. L., Krupinski, E. A., Thrall, *et al.* (2016). The empirical foundations of teleradiology and related applications: A review of the evidence. *Telemed. J. E-Health*. http://deepblue.lib.umich.edu/bitstream/2027.42/140295/1/tmj.2016.0149.pdf (accessed on 31st May 2025).

16. Boyd, D. P., Nice, M. L., Hays, D. G., & Lenz, S. (2024). Best practices for associational advocacy in the counseling profession: A grounded theory investigation. *Journal of Counseling & Development*. https://www.semanticscholar.org/paper/203f9178cf13c10e2965ad744f56301d62001ac6 (accessed on 31st May 2025).

17. Buonsenso, D., Parri, N., De Rose, C., & Valentini, P. (2020). Toward a clinically based classification of disease severity for pediatric COVID-19. *The Lancet Infectious Diseases, 21*, 22. https://doi.org/10.1016/s1473-3099(20)30396-0 (accessed on 31st May 2025).

18. Burity, J., Fonte, I. B. Da., & Melo, P. B. De. (2014). Radiological Society of North America (RSNA) 3D printing Special Interest Group (SIG): Guidelines for medical 3D printing and appropriateness for clinical scenarios. *3D Printing in Medicine*. https://core.ac.uk/download/212867900.pdf (accessed on 31st May 2025).

19. Çall, E., Sogancioglu, E., van Ginneken, B., van Leeuwen, K. G., & Murphy, K. (2021). Deep learning for chest X-ray analysis: A survey. *Medical Image Analysis, 72*, 102125. https://doi.org/10.1016/j.media.2021.102125 (accessed on 31st May 2025).

20. Carsrud, N. D. V., Flores, J. V., Holets, H. M., Kadivi, *et al.* (2024). Transformative precision: Investigative summary of PET/CT-guided radiation therapy simulation in comprehensive cancer management. *European Journal of Theoretical and Applied Sciences*. https://core.ac.uk/download/603903713.pdf (accessed on 31st May 2025).

21. Chalasani, N., Younossi, Z. M., Lavine, J. E., Charlton, M., Cusi, K., Rinella, M. E., Harrison, S. A., *et al.* (2017). The diagnosis and management of nonalcoholic fatty liver disease: Practice guidance from the American Association for the Study of Liver Diseases. *Hepatology, 67*, 328–357. https://doi.org/10.1002/hep.29367 (accessed on 31st May 2025).

22. Chaturvedi, A., Mann, L., Cain, U., Chaturvedi, A., & Klionsky, N. (2020). Acute fractures and dislocations of the ankle and foot in children. *Radiographics, 40*, 754–774. https://doi.org/10.1148/rg.2020190154 (accessed on 31st May 2025).

23. Choudhary, P., & Boski, N. (2022). Sedation and general anesthesia in diagnostic pediatric imaging. *Indographics, 1*, 101–109. https://www.semanticscholar.org/paper/b7965ee8f97a5225c7ee66d492e748c5d1961833 (accessed on 31st May 2025).

24. Chowdhury, M. E. H., Rahman, T., Khandakar, A., Mazhar, R., Kadir, M. A., Mahbub, Z. B., Islam, K. R., *et al.* (2020). Can AI help in screening viral and COVID-19 pneumonia? *IEEE Access, 8*, 132665–132676. https://doi.org/10.1109/access.2020.3010287 (accessed on 31st May 2025).

25. Christian, C. W. (2015). The evaluation of suspected child physical abuse. *Pediatrics, 135*. https://doi.org/10.1542/peds.2015-0356 (accessed on 31st May 2025).

26. Cordewener, P. A. M., De Bakker, B. S., Docter, D., Hagoort, *et al.* (2024). Imaging the development of the human craniofacial arterial system – An experimental study. *Pediatric Radiology*. https://core.ac.uk/download/621203037.pdf (accessed on 31st May 2025).

27. Czarny, J., Galli, D., Wziątek, A., Pastorczak, A., Szmyd, B., Przybyszewski, B., Raciborska, A., *et al.* (2025). Hodgkin lymphoma and Ewing sarcoma in pediatric patient carrying germline *PALB2* variant: A case report and literature review. *Frontiers in Oncology, 15*. https://www.semanticscholar.org/paper/594a0114f4aedaec3c76424ee507f349f1032ed8 (accessed on 31st May 2025).

28. Dargenio, V., Natale, M., Castellaneta, S., La Grasta, G., Paulucci, L., Dargenio, C., Francavilla, R., *et al.* (2025). Unraveling the hidden burden of gastrointestinal and nutritional challenges in children with Fabry disease: A systematic review with meta-analysis. *Nutrients, 17*. https://www.semanticscholar.org/paper/a146db020f4a21770f6ee4417df3dd0ee8f5b660 (accessed on 31st May 2025).

29. Davis, L. M., Martinez-Correa, S., Freeman, C., Adams, C., Sultan, L. R., Le, D. Q., Lemessa, N. F., *et al.* (2024). Ultrasound innovations in abdominal radiology: Techniques and clinical applications in pediatric imaging. *Abdominal Radiology (New York), 50*, 1744–1762. https://www.semanticscholar.org/paper/384926c5227775a5ff44582cb2924f7566a01039 (accessed on 31st May 2025).

30. Di Saverio, S., Podda, M., De Simone, B., Ceresoli, M., Augustin, G., Tugnoli, G., Boermeester, M. A., *et al.* (2020). Diagnosis and treatment of acute appendicitis: 2020 update of the WSES Jerusalem guidelines. *World Journal of Emergency Surgery, 15*. https://doi.org/10.1186/s13017-020-00306-3 (accessed on 31st May 2025).

31. Dillon, W. P., Lau, L., Lette, M. N. M., Mikhail, P., Palkó, *et al.* (2017). *Radiology Education in Europe: Analysis of Results from 22 European Countries*. https://core.ac.uk/download/323072369.pdf (accessed on 31st May 2025).

32. Downie, J., & Marshall, J. (2007). *Pediatric Neuroimaging Ethics*. https://core.ac.uk/download/478607561.pdf (accessed on 31st May 2025).

33. Elsingergy, M., Bellah, R., Back, S. J., Weiss, D., & Darge, K. (2023). Retrograde urethrography in children: A decade of experience at a children's hospital. *Pediatric Radiology, 53*, 862–874. https://www.semanticscholar.org/paper/9c05202afcd65af41e3e262c0366ae0ad13c91c8 (accessed on 31st May 2025).

34. Eymann, T., Fuhrmann, H., & Hennrich, J. (2024). Accelerating the adoption of artificial intelligence technologies in radiology: A comprehensive overview on current obstacles. *Proceedings of the 57th Hawaii International Conference on System Sciences*. https://core.ac.uk/download/616566150.pdf (accessed on 31st May 2025).

35. Fix, O. K., Hameed, B., Fontana, R. J., Kwok, R. M., McGuire, B. M., Mulligan, D. C., Pratt, D. S., *et al.* (2020). Clinical best practice advice for hepatology and liver transplant providers during the COVID-19 pandemic: AASLD expert panel consensus statement. *Hepatology, 72*, 287–304. https://doi.org/10.1002/hep.31281 (accessed on 31st May 2025).

36. Friedman, N., Tseng, F., Savic, R., Diallo, M., Fathi, K., McLean, L., & Tessaro, M. O. (2019). Reliability of neck mass point-of-care ultrasound by pediatric emergency physicians. *Journal of Ultrasound in Medicine, 38*, 2893–2900. https://doi.org/10.1002/jum.14993 (accessed on 31st May 2025).

37. Fujita, K. P., McAlister, W. H., Moseley, S., Thompson, *et al.* (2018). Validation of a novel scoring system for changes in skeletal manifestations of hypophosphatasia in newborns, infants, and children: The Radiographic Global Impression of Change scale. *JBMR*. https://core.ac.uk/download/287888099.pdf (accessed on 31st May 2025).

38. Fulcher, I., Kimball, K., Rosen, Z., Fortin, J., Arunkumar, N., Gelfand, D., Janiak, E., *et al.* (2025). Changes to parental consent requirements for abortion in Massachusetts and impact on timeliness of care for adolescents aged 16 to 17 years. *American Journal of Public Health, 115*(3), 397–402. https://www.semanticscholar.org/paper/a83476b3eea61e188864c9f7eadea6abc8cab07e (accessed on 31st May 2025).

39. Gausman, J., & Langer, A. (2020). Sex and gender disparities in the COVID-19 pandemic. *Journal of Women's Health, 29*, 465, 466. https://doi.org/10.1089/jwh.2020.8472 (accessed on 31st May 2025).

40. Goo, H. (2015). Whole-body MRI in children: Current imaging techniques and clinical applications. *Korean Journal of Radiology, 16*, 973–985. https://www.semanticscholar.org/paper/5bd6d1c8ba2b530a6f643a01e013b1f9b6de8032 (accessed on 31st May 2025).

41. Gordon, M., Daniel, M., Ajiboye, A., Uraiby, H., Xu, N. Y., Bartlett, R., Hanson, J. L., *et al.* (2024). A scoping review of artificial intelligence in medical education: BEME Guide No. 84. *Medical Teacher, 46*, 446–470. https://doi.org/10.1080/0142159x.2024.2314198 (accessed on 31st May 2025).

42. Hwang, H. (2017). Knowledge, attitude and perception on radiation imaging among children's caregivers in the pediatric dental clinic. https://open.bu.edu/bitstream/2144/23797/5/Hwang_bu_0017N_12842.pdf (accessed on 31st May 2025).

43. Isselbacher, E. M., Preventza, O., Black, J. H., Augoustides, J., Beck, A. W., Bolen, M. A., Braverman, A. C., *et al.* (2022). 2022 ACC/AHA guideline for the diagnosis and management of aortic disease: A report of the American Heart Association/American College of Cardiology Joint Committee on Clinical Practice Guidelines. *Circulation, 146*. https://doi.org/10.1161/cir.0000000000001106 (accessed on 31st May 2025).

44. Khalighi, S., Reddy, K., Midya, A., Pandav, K., Madabhushi, A., & Abedalthagafi, M. (2024). Artificial intelligence in neuro-oncology: Advances and challenges in brain tumor diagnosis, prognosis, and precision treatment. *NPJ Precision Oncology, 8*. https://doi.org/10.1038/s41698-024-00575-0 (accessed on 31st May 2025).

45. Kochanski, R. B., Lombardi, J. M., Laratta, J. L., Lehman, R. A., & O'Toole, J. E. (2018). Image-guided navigation and robotics in spine surgery. *Neurosurgery, 84*, 1179–1189. https://doi.org/10.1093/neuros/nyy630 (accessed on 31st May 2025).

46. Kudchadkar, S. (2015). Pediatric intensivists and elective procedural sedation: Paradox or perfect pair? *Pediatric Critical Care Medicine*. https://www.semanticscholar.org/paper/456110e756eed018086099a78bdb7c51f6b10661 (accessed on 31st May 2025).

47. LeBoff, M. S., Greenspan, S. L., Insogna, K., Lewiecki, E. M., Saag, K. G., Singer, A., & Siris, E. S. (2022). The clinician's guide to prevention and treatment of osteoporosis. *Osteoporosis International, 33*, 2049–2102. https://doi.org/10.1007/s00198-021-05900-y (accessed on 31st May 2025).

48. Lebovitz, S., Lifshitz-Assaf, H., & Levina, N. (2022). To engage or not to engage with AI for critical judgments: How professionals deal with opacity when using AI for medical diagnosis.

Organization Science, 33, 126–148. https://doi.org/10.1287/orsc.2021.1549 (accessed on 31st May 2025).

49. Vecchio Lo , A., Garazzino, S., Smarrazzo, A., Venturini, E., Poeta, M., Berlese, P., Denina, M., *et al.* (2021). Factors associated with severe gastrointestinal diagnoses in children with SARS-CoV-2 infection or multisystem inflammatory syndrome. *JAMA Network Open, 4*, e2139974. https://doi.org/10.1001/jamanetworkopen.2021.39974 (accessed on 31st May 2025).
50. Miranda, S. K., Fabara, V. M. D., Arias, A. G. A., Serrano, O. E. M., & Alava, S. C. L. (2024). Preoperative imaging-guided surgical planning in complex pelvic fractures – Innovations in traumatology and radiology for enhanced clinical outcomes: A systematic review. *Arandu UTIC*. https://www.semanticscholar.org/paper/f09483b899df97a14b230b887fc0a3a6b53efb53 (accessed on 31st May 2025).
51. Moore, B. K., Graham, S. M., Nandakumar, S., Doyle, J., & Maloney, S. A. (2024). Pediatric tuberculosis: A review of evidence-based best practices for clinicians and health care providers. *Pathogens, 13*. https://www.semanticscholar.org/paper/51c93f0e21331cebcc90ecaaa4103e40dc4cfa2c (accessed on 31st May 2025).
52. Northrup, H., Aronow, M. E., Bebin, E. M., Bissler, J. J., Darling, T. N., De Vries, P. J., Frost, M., *et al.* (2021). Updated international tuberous sclerosis complex diagnostic criteria and surveillance and management recommendations. *Pediatric Neurology, 123*, 50–66. https://doi.org/10.1016/j.pediatrneurol.2021.07.011 (accessed on 31st May 2025).
53. Otmane, M., & Ismaili, N. A. (2025). The pediatric neuroblastoma: Application of MIBG scintigraphy in diagnosis, staging, and follow-up – Analysis of three cases. *Swiss Journal of Radiology and Nuclear Medicine*. https://www.semanticscholar.org/paper/100b623602f5512f1ff520b33de068cadcb9158b (accessed on 31st May 2025).
54. Rafighi, A., Jahanbani, M., & Mahmoudi, A. R. (2024). A critical review of the efficacy and safety of radiological imaging techniques in pediatric orthodontics. *Galen Medical Journal*. https://www.semanticscholar.org/paper/b3e77d846a298068efbb78ec79de8435015afe28 (accessed on 31st May 2025).
55. Raj, N., & Dhande, R. (2021). MRI evaluation of seizures in pediatric age group patients in a rural hospital of Central India. *Journal of Pharmaceutical Research International*. https://www.semanticscholar.org/paper/8eceb30c6e8c76182f34477d5f08f05061da7bac (accessed on 31st May 2025).
56. Richards, J. R., & McGahan, J. P. (2017). Focused assessment with sonography in trauma (FAST) in 2017: What radiologists can learn. *Radiology, 283*, 30–48. https://doi.org/10.1148/radiol.2017160107 (accessed on 31st May 2025).
57. Rosen, R., Vandenplas, Y., Singendonk, M., Cabana, M. D., DiLorenzo, C., Gottrand, F., Gupta, S. K., *et al.* (2018). Pediatric gastroesophageal reflux clinical practice guidelines. *Journal of Pediatric Gastroenterology and Nutrition, 66*, 516–554. https://doi.org/10.1097/mpg.0000000000001889 (accessed on 31st May 2025).
58. Sahiner, B., Pezeshk, A., Hadjiiski, L. M., Wang, X., Drukker, K., Kenny, H., Summers, R. M., *et al.* (2018). Deep learning in medical imaging and radiation therapy. *Medical Physics, 46*. https://doi.org/10.1002/mp.13264 (accessed on 31st May 2025).
59. Semerci, Z. M., & Yardımcı, S. (2024). Empowering modern dentistry: The impact of artificial intelligence on patient care and clinical decision making. *Diagnostics, 14*, 1260. https://doi.

org/10.3390/diagnostics14121260 (accessed on 31st May 2025).

60. Snyder, C. W., Kristiansen, K. O., Jensen, A. R., Sribnick, E. A., Anders, J. F., Md, C. X., Md, E. B., *et al.* (2023). Defining pediatric trauma center resource utilization: Multidisciplinary consensus-based criteria from the Pediatric Trauma Society. *Journal of Trauma and Acute Care Surgery, 96*, 799–804. https://www.semanticscholar.org/paper/68c6e1f7c7f519e624b5cdc7c760f68cc3a05d2b (accessed on 31st May 2025).

61. Squires, J., & McCarville, M. B. (2021). Contrast-enhanced ultrasound in children: Implementation and key diagnostic applications. *American Journal of Roentgenology, 217*, 1217–1231. https://doi.org/10.2214/ajr.21.25713 (accessed on 31st May 2025).

62. Stafrace, S. (2008). *Fetal MRI: Advances in the Evaluation of the Developing Fetus.* https://core.ac.uk/download/46602180.pdf (accessed on 31st May 2025).

63. Van Der, P. C. B., Yıkılmaz, A., & Schieda, N. (2021). Editorial for "MRI-characteristics of pediatric renal tumors: A SIOP-RTSG radiology panel Delphi study": Standardized assessment of pediatric renal tumors with MRI: A laudable objective that requires further investigation. *Journal of Magnetic Resonance Imaging, 55.* https://www.semanticscholar.org/paper/0ebe8b755a7814960e5cd62b670fedeada191826 (accessed on 31st May 2025).

64. Voronov, A., Jafari, M., Zhao, L., Soliz, M., Hong, Q., Pope, J., Chern, D., *et al.* (2024). Pediatric consent on FHIR. *Applied Clinical Informatics, 15*, 342–356. https://www.semanticscholar.org/paper/77be744409d06f9ec2800ebd40b1365ac0ac4c8a (accessed on 31st May 2025).

65. Wang, S., Kang, B. K., Ma, J., Zeng, X., Xiao, M., Guo, J., Cai, M., *et al.* (2021). A deep learning algorithm using CT images to screen for coronavirus disease (COVID-19). *European Radiology, 31*, 6096–6104. https://doi.org/10.1007/s00330-021-07715-1 (accessed on 31st May 2025).

66. Wiederhold, B. K. (2020). Connecting through technology during the coronavirus disease 2019 pandemic: Avoiding "Zoom fatigue." *Cyberpsychology, Behavior, and Social Networking, 23*, 437, 438. https://doi.org/10.1089/cyber.2020.29188.bkw (accessed on 31st May 2025).

67. Williams, N. C. (2022). Management of pediatric sepsis: Considerations for the austere prehospital setting. *Journal of Special Operations Medicine: A Peer Reviewed Journal for SOF Medical Professionals, 22*(2), 120–125. https://www.semanticscholar.org/paper/465c2e193b8714eb37875757d809b0d81d6f7a42 (accessed on 31st May 2025).

68. Yoon, H., Kim, J., Lim, H. J., & Lee, M. J. (2024). Quantitative liver imaging in children. *Investigative Radiology.* https://www.semanticscholar.org/paper/7c0ca221671ae2d6e3d0846e3d01b7a1705cfeb7 (accessed on 31st May 2025).

69. Yoon, H., Shin, H. J., Kim, M. J., & Lee, M. J. (2019). Quantitative imaging in pediatric hepatobiliary disease. *Korean Journal of Radiology, 20*, 1342–1357. https://www.semanticscholar.org/paper/b81f8914e4fc5f4b9d389dea4853839138fbe0ae (accessed on 31st May 2025).

70. Young, V. A., Thakor, A., & Josephs, S. (2022). Update on pediatric interventional radiology. *Radiographics, 42*(6), 1580–1597. https://www.semanticscholar.org/paper/4b0a4288b34f3a3100fedec0a2d436b471dfd5ab (accessed on 31st May 2025).

NEURORADIOLOGY – BRAIN

3

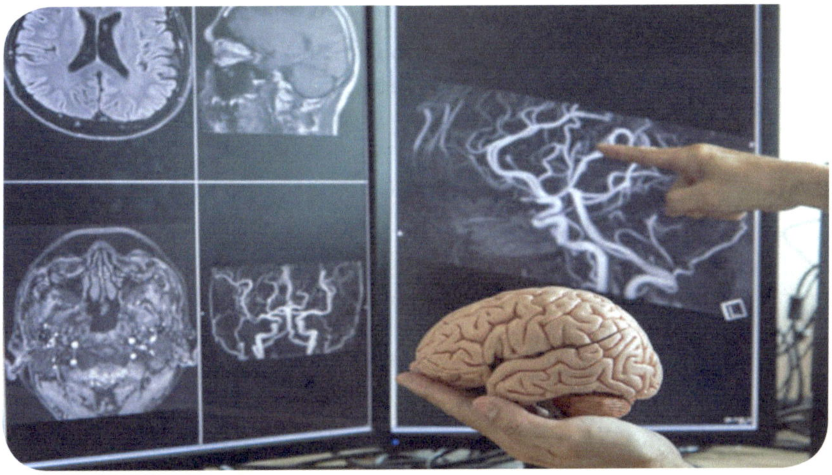

LEARNING OBJECTIVES

After studying this chapter, you will be able to:

1. Identify imaging techniques in neuroradiology;
2. Explain common neurological conditions diagnosed by neuroradiology;
3. Focus on the interpretation of neuroradiological images;
4. Know future trends in neuroradiology.

Introduction

Thanks to new medical imaging techniques, clinicians can now see the brain's structures with far greater detail, which has greatly improved the diagnosis and care of neurological disorders. Among various techniques, magnetic resonance imaging (MRI) stands out as a crucial tool, providing essential insights into brain pathology without invasive procedures. Even so, a regular MRI scan might not be sensitive enough to detect and describe brain problems such as tumors or epileptic foci. Thus, integration of specialized imaging modalities like Diffusion-Weighted Imaging (DWI) and the calculation of Apparent Diffusion Coefficient (ADC) values has become increasingly important in neuroradiology. They help doctors tell apart harmless and dangerous lesions or find the areas responsible for seizures, which directs treatment decisions. Despite these advances, some correlations, such as between MRI findings and electroencephalogram (EEG) abnormalities in epilepsy, remain inconclusive, emphasizing the need for continued research in this field (Awad *et al.*, 2025; Elmi *et al.*, 2024).

Definition of Neuroradiology

Because of new developments in medical imaging, it is now easier to detect and treat neurological conditions, stressing the role of specialized branches in radiology. Neuroradiology focuses on the visualization and interpretation of the nervous system using various imaging modalities, including MRI and computed tomography (CT). This subspecialty helps find problems with the structure and function of the brain and spinal cord, which aids in finding tumors, blood vessel diseases, and diseases that cause the brain and spinal cord to deteriorate.

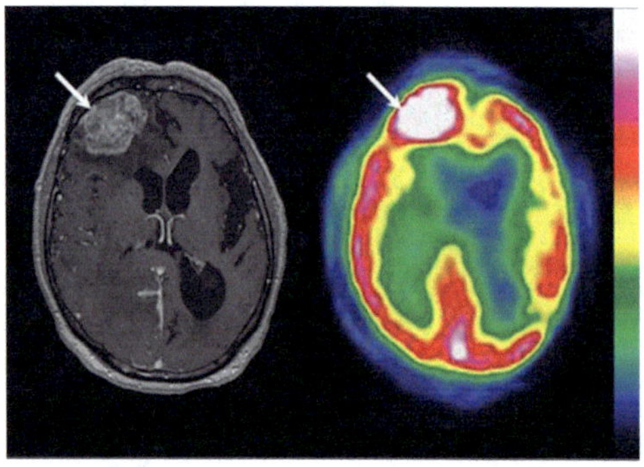

Figure 3.1. Neuroradiology focuses on the visualization and interpretation of the nervous system using various imaging modalities, including magnetic resonance imaging (MRI) and computed tomography (CT).

Source: https://cdn.technologynetworks.com/tn/images/body/neuroimaging-seo-article-fig-4_resized1657186793919.jpg.

Particularly, neuroradiology contributes to the nuanced diagnosis of brain tumors by correlating imaging features with molecular and histologic profiles, exemplified by markers such as the T2-FLAIR mismatch sign, which facilitates precise tumor classification and prognosis assessment (Dagher *et al.*, 2023). Beyond structural imaging, neuroradiological techniques also delve into dynamic brain functions, contributing to the understanding of neural circuit heterogeneity and brain activity patterns (Sharpee *et al.*, 2016). This integration of imaging technology and neuroscience underscores neuroradiology as an indispensable component of modern neurodiagnostics and treatment planning (Figure 3.1).

Importance of Brain Imaging

Thanks to new imaging techniques, neuroradiology has seen major progress in understanding the brain's structure and functions, which helps with correct diagnosis and treatment decisions. Techniques such as multiparametric MRI combined with deep learning algorithms enable precise tumor segmentation, aiding clinicians in distinguishing malignant growths from surrounding healthy tissue and monitoring therapeutic responses effectively (Ghadimi *et al.*, 2024). Moreover, innovations in diffusion-weighted imaging, functional MRI, and advanced CT modalities enhance the ability to detect subtle neurological changes associated with cerebrovascular events, neurodegenerative diseases, and traumatic injuries (Vitrio *et al.*, 2024). Such methods in imaging help doctors make accurate diagnoses and provide personalized care and predictions about the outcome. For this reason, brain imaging is now a key part of neuroradiology, helping make decisions in patient care and driving research into neurological diseases, which leads to better patient results and advances early and precise treatment.

Historical Development of Neuroradiology

As imaging technology has improved, so has neuroradiology, which in turn has helped improve the diagnosis and management of neurological problems. First discoveries, such as X-rays, helped build the foundation by showing the cranial structure without surgery.

After that, CT and MRI made it possible to see the brain from different angles, which helped doctors find abnormalities more accurately. More recent incorporation of sophisticated AI techniques has revolutionized image analysis, enabling automated detection and segmentation of brain lesions, thereby improving diagnostic accuracy and workflow efficiency in clinical settings (Najjar, 2023). These technological strides have been particularly critical in acute conditions like ischemic stroke, where advanced imaging guides interventions such as mechanical thrombectomy, optimizing patient selection and outcomes within crucial time windows (Turc *et al.*, 2019). For this reason, the history of neuroradiology shows a steady integration of new ideas, advanced technology, and practical uses which have greatly changed how neurological care is provided.

Role of Neuroradiologists

Interpreting neuroimaging correctly is essential for diagnosing brain diseases, which makes neuroradiologists key members of multidisciplinary teams. Their expertise extends beyond routine imaging to intricate analyses of pathological changes associated with diseases such as COVID-19, where neurologic involvement can be life-threatening and demands precise identification of acute encephalopathy or stroke via advanced imaging modalities (LaRovere *et al.*, 2021). In cases like primary central nervous system lymphoma, neuroradiologists play a pivotal role by confirming diagnoses through detailed MRI evaluation, guiding stereotactic biopsies, and differentiating tumor characteristics from mimicking pathologies, which impacts treatment pathways significantly (Fox *et al.*, 2018). Their skill helps them watch for changes in the patient's condition and identify relapses, which guide decisions about further therapies such as whole-brain radiotherapy or high-dose chemotherapy. Ultimately, the neuroradiologist's role is vital for integrating imaging findings with clinical data, ensuring accurate diagnosis, effective treatment planning, and improved patient outcomes in neuro-oncology and infectious neurological disorders (Figure 3.2).

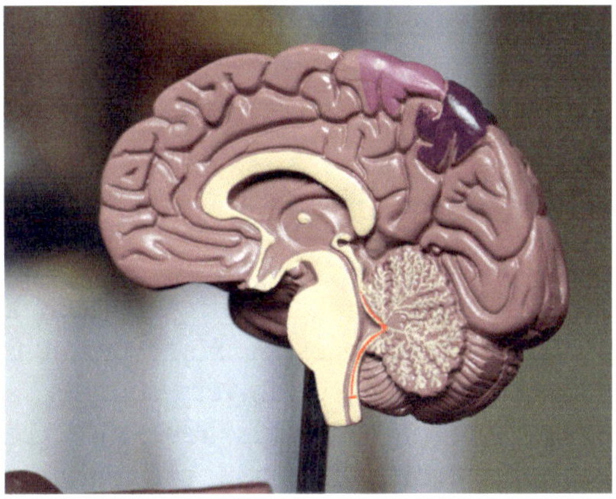

Figure 3.2. Accurate interpretation of neuroimaging is indispensable in diagnosing complex brain conditions, positioning neuroradiologists as critical figures within multidisciplinary teams.

Source: https://3dicomviewer.com/wp-content/uploads/2024/11/a-brain-diagram-showing-the-anatomy-of-the-brain-768x432.png.

Relevance to Modern Medicine

With the help of technology and new models, neuroradiology has greatly linked brain research to practical use in medicine. Using multiscale dynamic generative models helps explain how the brain works, which supports better diagnosis and better treatment options for each patient. Platforms like EBRAINS exemplify how digital neuroscience infrastructures foster collaboration between disciplines, enhancing the ability to interpret complex brain data and accelerating the translation of research findings into therapeutic interventions (Amunts *et al.*, 2022). In addition, using magnetic resonance imaging to find and classify brain tumors highlights the key role neuroradiology has in today's healthcare. Despite challenges posed by tumor heterogeneity, advancements in image processing, deep learning, and quantum machine learning techniques offer promising improvements in early and accurate tumor identification (Amin *et al.*, 2021). All these developments together demonstrate that neuroradiology is important for achieving better patient outcomes by improving diagnosis and treatment in modern medicine.

Challenges in the Field

Advances in technology have not solved all the issues that make it challenging to treat and diagnose brain diseases. A major problem is that brain tumors are often very complex, and standard imaging methods have difficulties telling apart different tumors, which can slow down diagnosis and treatment. While emerging AI and deep learning models show promise in enhancing classification accuracy, many existing approaches remain confined to binary categorization, which restricts clinical applicability and undermines comprehensive care (Tariq *et al.*, 2025).

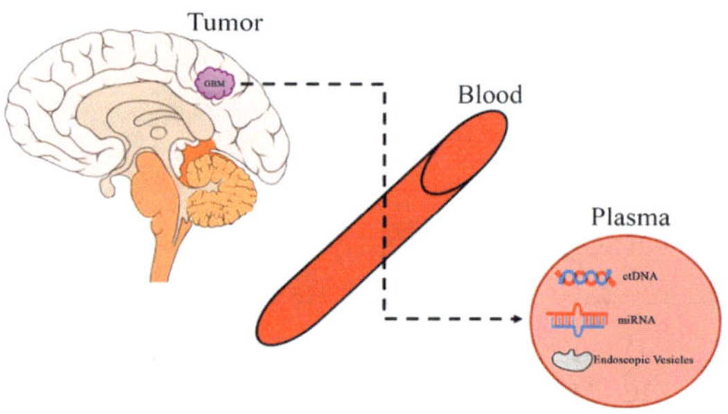

Figure 3.3. One major obstacle involves the inherent complexity of brain tumors, where conventional imaging techniques often struggle to differentiate between multiple tumor types, limiting diagnostic precision and timely intervention.

Source: https://www.frontiersin.org/files/Articles/1441460/fonc-14-1441460-HTML/image_m/fonc-14-1441460-g002.jpg.

Furthermore, even advanced imaging modalities such as diffusion-weighted imaging, perfusion MRI, and dual-energy CT, although invaluable, carry limitations related to resolution, interpretation variability, and accessibility, contributing to diagnostic uncertainty and patient management difficulties (Vitrio *et al.*, 2024). These challenges emphasize the need for continued innovation in imaging technologies and analytical methods, as well as improved integration of computational tools to support neuroradiologists in overcoming current constraints and optimizing brain disorder diagnoses (Figure 3.3).

Future Directions in Neuroradiology

New technologies are always changing medical imaging, which is likely to bring major improvements to neuroradiology. New techniques such as diffusion-weighted imaging, functional MRI, and dual-energy CT are helping doctors spot problems in the brain more precisely and with more information. These innovations are not only improving patient outcomes but also facilitating earlier detection and more personalized treatment strategies (Destefani *et al.*, 2024). Also, using artificial intelligence and machine learning is expected to change neuroradiology by automating image review, detecting small changes that humans cannot, and making work more efficient. The abundance of neuroimaging data and established public datasets creates an ideal environment for developing robust AI algorithms, although challenges remain in their full clinical adoption (Jha *et al.*, 2022). As technology improves, neuroradiology will probably depend on both advanced scans and smart computer programs to support better treatment for brain diseases.

3.1. Imaging Techniques in Neuroradiology

Learning Outcome

1. Define computed tomography (CT);
2. Explain magnetic resonance imaging (MRI);
3. Focus on positron emission tomography (PET);
4. Know single photon emission computed tomography (SPECT);
5. Learn ultrasound in brain imaging;
6. Explain advanced MRI techniques (fMRI, DTI);
7. Describe contrast agents in imaging;
8. Know radiation safety and protocols;
9. Give a comparison of imaging modalities.

Better imaging methods have improved the ability of neuroradiology to diagnose complicated brain diseases. Although MRI is still a primary tool for spotting recurrent cerebral metastases, it can be hard to tell the difference between these and changes caused by radiation, so MR perfusion is often used to help with diagnosis. However, no single imaging approach definitively differentiates these conditions, underscoring the ongoing need for histopathological confirmation to guide treatment decisions and prognostication (Schack *et al.*, 2024). Concurrently, the integration of deep learning algorithms with computed tomography (CT) has demonstrated promising results in volumetric brain analyses, especially for conditions like idiopathic normal pressure hydrocephalus. Automated CT segmentation models can reliably quantify ventricular cerebrospinal fluid, offering comparable diagnostic performance to traditional radiological assessments and enhancing accessibility due to CT's widespread availability (Srikrishna *et al.*, 2024). All these developments together demonstrate how neuroradiology is changing, as the use of multiple imaging methods and advanced technology helps doctors make more accurate diagnoses and manage patients better.

3.1.1. Computed Tomography (CT)

When the outcome for a patient depends on a quick diagnosis, easy-to-use imaging is very important in neurological emergencies. Because CT is widely available and efficient, it is the main imaging method used in these cases. CT is especially important in emergencies for spotting brain metastases and traumatic brain injuries, showing details about the lesions such as their location, size, and any edema or bleeding. While MRI has better detail and lower radiation worries, CT is still the leading choice for initial testing in pediatric trauma, since fast action is necessary. Also, using advanced CT and other imaging techniques increases the accuracy of diagnosing brain tumors and injuries. By enabling multimodal analysis, CT contributes significantly to individualized treatment planning and prognosis in neuro-oncology and neurotrauma contexts (Grazzini *et al.*, 2023; Murphy *et al.*, 2016) (Figure 3.4).

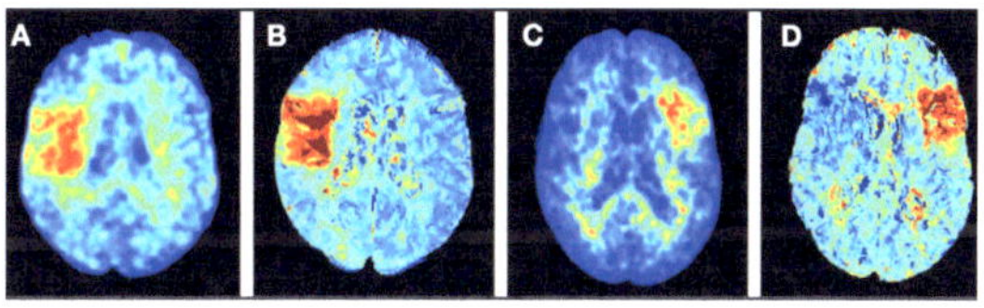

Figure 3.4. Rapid and accessible imaging techniques are crucial in acute neurological assessments, especially when timely diagnosis influences patient outcomes significantly.

Source: https://journals.sagepub.com/cms/10.1177/08465371211028823/asset/6b08c815-e367-4852-b1f0-7c06c83836cf/assets/images/large/10.1177_08465371211028823-fig4.jpg.

3.1.2. Magnetic Resonance Imaging (MRI)

New imaging technologies have greatly improved our knowledge of brain development and diseases, especially by allowing detailed study of the brain without invasive procedures. MRI is now considered very important in neuroradiology, allowing detailed images of the brain without using ionizing radiation. In addition to examining the structure, it can also show how the brain functions and its blood vessels, which helps assess both blood flow and brain tissue. In neonatal care, MRI's ability to detect subtle morphological and functional vascular differences between term and preterm infants provides valuable prognostic information critical for early intervention planning (Spampinato, 2012). Furthermore, the striking aesthetic qualities of MRI images have even fostered a unique intersection of science and art within neuroradiology, highlighting both the scientific and cultural significance of this modality (Marinković *et al.*, 2010). Because of these roles, MRI is central to both brain imaging and research.

3.1.3. Positron Emission Tomography (PET)

Having knowledge of cerebral physiology is necessary in neuroradiology for proper diagnosis and planning of treatment. PET plays a pivotal role by enabling the visualization and quantification of cerebral blood flow (CBF) and metabolic activity, critical markers of brain function. Using radiotracers, PET imaging can observe brain metabolism and give useful information about healthy and unhealthy brain states. For instance, pediatric neuroimaging studies highlight the importance of age, sedation, and other physiological factors in accurately measuring CBF using PET, underscoring its complexity and precision in a developing brain (Zhao *et al.*, 2023). While primarily utilized in brain imaging, PET's applications extend to cardiac inflammation, where its sensitivity to metabolic changes aids in diagnosing conditions such as myocarditis, illustrating its versatility (Caobelli *et al.*, 2023). Thus, PET is an indispensable tool in neuroradiology, providing crucial data for understanding brain health and disease (Figure 3.5).

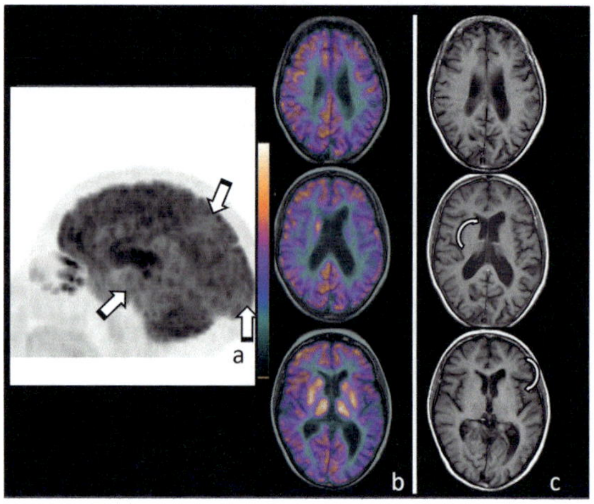

Figure 3.5. Positron Emission Tomography (PET) plays a pivotal role by enabling the visualization and quantification of cerebral blood flow (CBF) and metabolic activity, critical markers of brain function.

Source: https://article.imrpress.com/journal/JIN/22/6/10.31083/j.jin2206172/1757-448X-22-6-172/fig5.jpg.

3.1.4. Single Photon Emission Computed Tomography (SPECT)

Thanks to new imaging technologies, it is now possible to understand how the brain works in detail, which has improved the diagnosis and care of neurological disorders. One method, Single Photon Emission Computed Tomography (SPECT), creates three-dimensional images using radioactive tracers in the brain. New collimator designs, such as multi-pinhole collimators, have greatly improved both the detail and sensitivity that SPECT scans can provide, mainly in brain imaging. These improvements not only allow for more accurate localization of cerebral abnormalities but also promote broader clinical adoption (Ozsahin *et al.*, 2020). Also, new radiotracers that target signs of brain diseases, such as β-amyloid plaques, help SPECT detect these diseases and monitor their treatment. This theragnostic potential, combining diagnostic imaging with anti-amyloid therapeutic effects, underscores the expanding role of SPECT in the nuanced landscape of neuroradiology (Sagnou *et al.*, 2019).

3.1.5. Ultrasound in Brain Imaging

Because of new technology, ultrasound can now be used to view brain structures and measure blood flow inside the brain in real time. Because it is dynamic, ultrasound is important for stroke and neonatal brain injuries, which require immediate treatment. Clinicians can check the blood flow in the brain using transcranial Doppler sonography, which improves diagnosis without using ionizing radiation. Also, the use of portable ultrasound has made it possible to examine the brain at the bedside in critical care, making things easier for both doctors and patients. Because ultrasound technology keeps improving, it now helps to better identify brain tissues and blood vessel problems, which has led to more uses in neuroradiology. These advancements underscore ultrasound's evolving role, complementing more conventional imaging methods while addressing limitations related to safety, cost, and immediate diagnostic feedback within brain imaging (Figure 3.6).

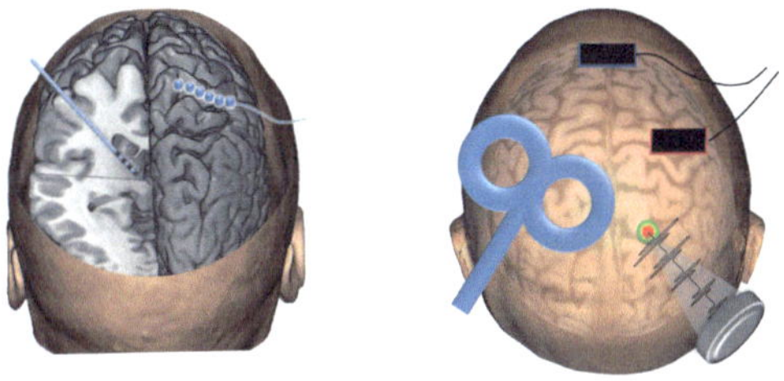

Figure 3.6. Technological advancements have significantly expanded the capabilities of ultrasound in neuroimaging, offering a non-invasive and real-time method to visualize brain structures and assess cerebral blood flow.

Source: https://www.researchgate.net/publication/283753260/figure/fig7/AS:613949519179808@1523388380728/A-summary-of-invasive-and-noninvasive-neuromodulation-technologies-Invasive-techniques.png.

3.1.6. Advanced MRI Techniques] Functional MRI (fMRI), Diffusion Tensor Imaging (DTI)]

The evolution of imaging technologies has significantly refined our understanding of brain structure and function, particularly through advanced MRI techniques that extend beyond conventional anatomical imaging. fMRI captures dynamic brain activity by detecting blood oxygen level-dependent (BOLD) signals, enabling the mapping of neural networks involved in cognitive and motor functions. At the same time, DTI provides a special view of white matter structure, making it possible to study neural connections and their integrity, which is important for understanding changes in neurological diseases. When used together, fMRI and DTI give additional details; fMRI points out how the brain functions, and DTI reveals any structural changes, which help with accurate diagnosis and selecting the best treatment. Their integration has become instrumental in clinical contexts, notably in cerebrovascular disorders, neurodegeneration, and trauma, where traditional imaging falls short (Vitrio *et al.*, 2024). Despite ongoing challenges in fully interpreting these complex data, advances in fMRI and DTI continue to bridge critical knowledge gaps in neuroradiology, advancing both research and clinical applications (Mahmoud *et al.*, 2024).

3.1.7. Contrast Agents in Imaging

Because of contrast agents, brain imaging has greatly helped improve how neurological conditions are diagnosed and managed. They make it easier to see vascular structures and diseased tissues, which helps to outline tumors, signs of inflammation, and damage to the blood-brain barrier in neuroradiology. Contrast agents such as gadolinium-based compounds in MRI help doctors to tell apart normal and abnormal brain tissue more accurately. Also, using iodine-based agents in CT scans allows for checking cerebral blood flow and finding signs of ischemia. The distribution of these agents allows doctors to see the blood vessels and integrity of the lesion, which are usually not visible on plain images. As imaging techniques continually evolve, the role of contrast agents remains pivotal in enhancing diagnostic confidence and guiding therapeutic decisions in brain pathology (Figure 3.7).

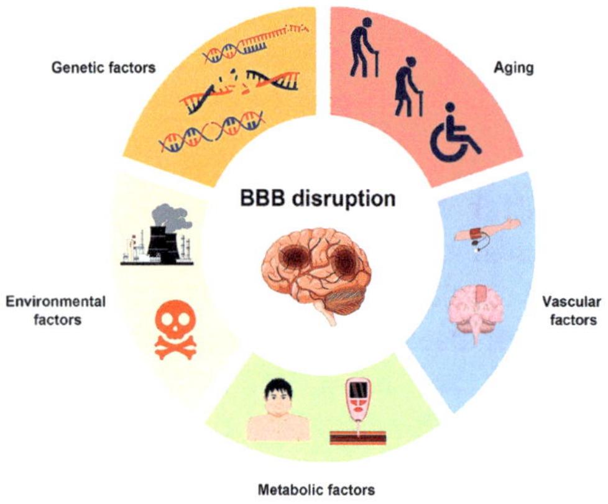

Figure 3.7. Blood-brain barrier disruptions in neuroradiology.

Source: https://media.springernature.com/lw1200/springer-static/image/art%3A10.1186%2Fs12987-024-00563-3/MediaObjects/12987_2024_563_Fig2_HTML.png.

3.1.8. Radiation Safety and Protocols

Although neuroimaging has made it much easier to find brain problems, it is important to take extra steps to protect against radiation. In particular, CT and cerebral vascular digital subtraction angiography (DSA) are prevalent modalities in neuroradiology that expose patients to ionizing radiation. Children are especially vulnerable, as radiation-induced carcinogenesis remains a significant concern, prompting careful consideration in imaging decisions, especially when alternatives like MRI can provide diagnostic value without radiation exposure (Aleid *et al.*, 2024). Studies have demonstrated that radiation dose during DSA varies significantly with factors such as the number of projections and anatomical coverage, with bilateral procedures yielding higher doses (Modlińska *et al.*, 2024). Continually optimizing the tube voltage, current, and the way scans are performed is necessary to reduce radiation and maintain clear images. Specialized radiation safety measures help protect patients and still allow for accurate diagnosis, so the need for scans is not overdone.

3.1.9. Comparison of Imaging Modalities

Neuroimaging advances have made it easier to tell apart different brain diseases, but deciding which test is best is still not simple. MRI techniques, including dynamic contrast-enhanced and susceptibility-weighted imaging, offer detailed physiological and vascular insights, crucial for distinguishing tumor recurrence from post-radiation necrosis; however, these methods can be limited by overlapping features and patient-specific factors such as radiation dose and inflammation (Arif *et al.*, 2025). Using 18F-FET PET and 11C-MET PET in nuclear medicine adds metabolic details, making the diagnosis more accurate, along with MRI. Additionally, the integration of artificial intelligence algorithms with imaging data introduces a promising frontier by enabling more objective and efficient interpretation, mitigating reliance on operator expertise while fostering early detection and treatment planning (Urooj *et al.*, 2024). So, using advanced MRI, PET imaging, and AI analysis together is the best way to make precise assessments in neuroradiology.

Test Your Knowledge:
1.

Test Your Knowledge

1. Why is Diffusion-Weighted Imaging (DWI) critical in the early detection of ischemic stroke?
2. How does functional MRI (fMRI) differ from structural MRI, and what is its role in brain mapping for pre-surgical planning?

3.2. Common Neurological Conditions Diagnosed by Neuroradiology

Learning Outcome

1. Identify stroke and its types;
2. Explain brain tumors and classifications;
3. Focus on neurodegenerative diseases;
4. Explain traumatic brain injuries;
5. Define multiple sclerosis;
6. Discuss infections affecting the brain;
7. Know vascular malformations;
8. Learn about epilepsy and seizure disorders;
9. Understand congenital brain anomalies.

With better neuroimaging, it is now much easier to detect several neurological diseases that were previously hard to find in their early stages. MRI and CT are very important for finding abnormalities linked to diseases such as cerebrovascular accidents, brain tumors, and neurodegenerative disorders. Especially, using diffusion-weighted imaging and perfusion-weighted imaging allows MRI to detect the microstructural and blood flow changes seen in stroke and multiple sclerosis. Functional MRI is used to find areas of the brain that are not working properly in epilepsy or Parkinson's disease. Using artificial intelligence with these methods helps doctors find problems earlier and with more accuracy by examining data that might be missed by humans. These innovations collectively support more precise and timely treatment plans, ultimately enhancing patient outcomes in neurological care (Kumar, 2025; Vitrio *et al.*, 2024).

3.2.1. Stroke and its Types

Because cerebrovascular events can be complicated, it is important to identify and classify them accurately to support the right treatment. Strokes are divided into ischemic and hemorrhagic types, and each type needs specific ways of diagnosis and treatment in neuroradiology. An arterial blockage in the brain causes an ischemic stroke, which leads to brain tissue damage and requires prompt imaging to check blood vessel status. Hemorrhagic strokes happen when a blood vessel bursts, and this is usually noticed on CT or MRI by the presence of bleeding inside the brain. Additionally, evolving conditions such as COVID-19 have revealed atypical neurologic presentations, including stroke in pediatric populations, highlighting the importance of recognizing life-threatening neurologic involvement linked to systemic diseases (LaRovere *et al.*, 2021). Stroke management protocols, informed by organizations like the ESC, emphasize evidence-based imaging and treatment strategies that balance urgency and accuracy, underscoring the critical role of neuroradiological assessment in tailoring patient-specific interventions (Habib *et al.*, 2015). This multidimensional understanding is essential for improving stroke outcomes through precise diagnosis and individualized care (Figure 3.8).

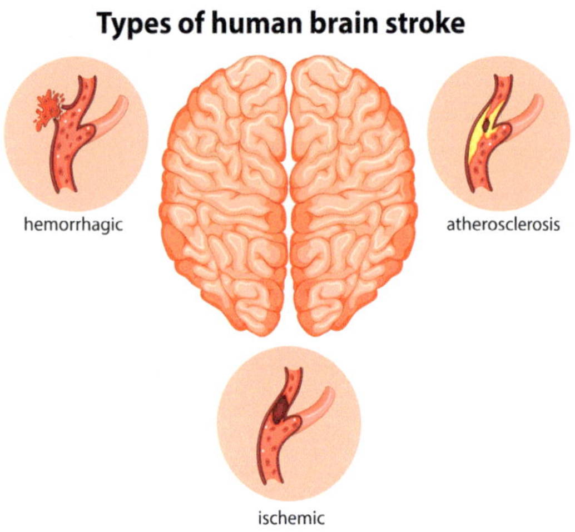

Figure 3.8. Strokes are broadly categorized into ischemic and hemorrhagic types, each requiring distinct diagnostic and therapeutic approaches within neuroradiology.

Source: https://lh7-rt.googleusercontent.com/docsz/AD_4nXd4wUbzTgD6Awfk0fmCFsKKfKGz_EKRqM-DLi-m3OWOXznnrbm7COnIPQiOLAhRMwEMIFirXWUwqIKl8Y0wNXRED1knLVROx4orXpnpN3gfYMfUER0T1lqqGkT4b0mtF2cP9ViXWiAHjrUywnXKqj7H-I4?key=xjTpeWYehELc-J-ELOX11Pw.

3.2.2. Brain Tumors and Classifications

Thanks to new developments in neuroradiology, diagnosing and classifying brain tumors is now much more accurate which is very important for choosing the right treatment. The 2021 World Health Organization's classification provides a refined framework that integrates molecular markers with traditional histopathological features, allowing differentiation among various tumor entities, including pediatric diffuse low-grade gliomas and embryonal tumors with multilayered rosettes (Rameh *et al.*, 2024). Because each type of tumor has its own biological behavior and outcome, such distinctions are necessary. Moreover, intraoperative imaging techniques like superb microvascular imaging (SMI) have proven valuable in delineating tumor boundaries more precisely than conventional ultrasound, facilitating gross-total resection and potentially improving patient outcomes (Cai *et al.*, 2024). Together, these two advances in medicine have made a big change in treating brain tumors, showing how important neuroradiology is for accurate diagnosis and safe surgery.

3.2.3. Neurodegenerative Diseases (Alzheimer's)

Better neuroimaging tools have made it much easier to learn about and diagnose brain disorders. Such diseases, for example, Alzheimer's, are hard to diagnose since their effects on the brain are gradual and not always noticeable. Neuroradiology helps in finding the typical signs of brain shrinkage, iron buildup, and small vessel changes that happen in these conditions.

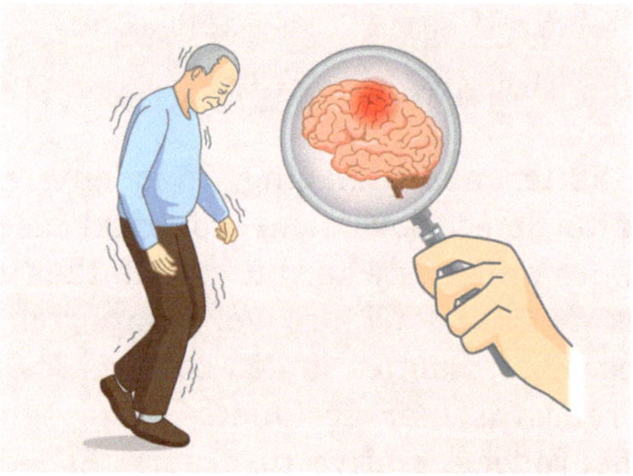

Figure 3.9. Alzheimer's disease.

Source: https://cdn.apollohospitals.com/health-library-prod/2019/06/p1.png.

Susceptibility weighted imaging (SWI), for instance, has emerged as a valuable MRI approach, enabling the detection of cerebral microbleeds and quantification of abnormal iron accumulation, which are often implicated in the pathophysiology of neurodegeneration and cognitive decline (Halefoğlu *et al.*, 2018). Moreover, integrating clinical assessments with imaging findings improves diagnostic accuracy, informing better patient management strategies (Eratne *et al.*, 2018). Thus, neuroradiological methods not only support early detection but also aid in differentiating Alzheimer's from other dementias, underscoring their essential role in advancing neurological care (Figure 3.9).

3.2.4. Traumatic Brain Injuries (TBIs)

With new techniques in neuroradiology, it is now easier to identify and diagnose TBIs, especially by spotting small changes in white matter and blood vessels. DTI has revealed that repetitive subconcussive impacts, even without clinically evident concussions, can lead to measurable alterations in white matter tracts such as the inferior fronto-occipital and superior longitudinal fasciculi, indicating microstructural brain injury (Bahrami *et al.*, 2016). Furthermore, blunt trauma to the cervical spine can induce vertebral artery injuries (VAIs), which, although rare, pose a severe risk of ischemic stroke due to vessel occlusion and thrombosis. These vascular injuries often go undetected initially, leading to catastrophic cerebellar infarctions and fatal outcomes if not promptly identified and managed (Golinvaux *et al.*, 2015). Using advanced imaging and evidence-based diagnostic methods helps find and treat TBIs and related vascular issues early, which is important for improving patient outcomes.

3.2.5. Multiple Sclerosis

For many neurological disorders, doctors depend on imaging techniques, especially when the symptoms are unusual or do not respond to the first treatments. Such conditions, for example, multiple sclerosis, which damages the central nervous system, rely heavily on neuroradiology. MRI is the main way to detect scattered lesions in the brain and spinal cord, which helps with both diagnosing and tracking changes in the disease. A young man was first thought to have cervical radiculopathy, but an MRI later showed typical multiple sclerosis plaques, which was the correct diagnosis. Because of this discovery, doctors now use corticosteroids and beta-interferon therapies, and advanced imaging is important to confirm a diagnosis when regular findings are unclear. Thus, neuroradiology is pivotal for distinguishing multiple sclerosis from other neurological conditions and guiding effective management strategies (Stafrace *et al.*, 2015) (Figure 3.10).

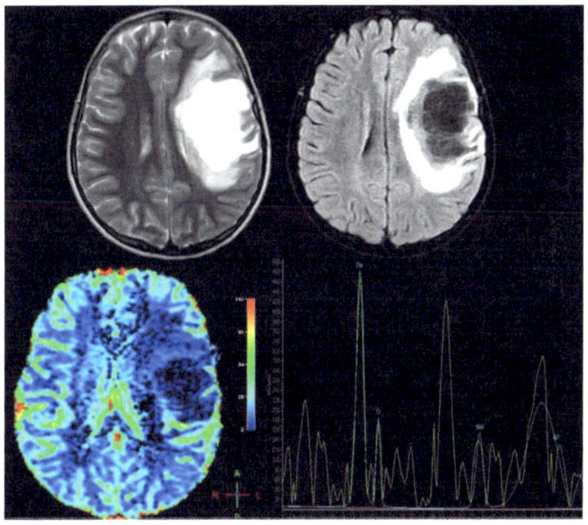

Figure 3.10. Multiple sclerosis, a demyelinating disease affecting the central nervous system, exemplifies such challenges where neuroradiological evaluation is indispensable.

Source: https://static.elsevier.es/multimedia/21735808/0000003000000002/v2_201503060225/S2173580815000024/v2_201503060225/en/main.assets/gr2.jpeg.

3.2.6. Infections Affecting the Brain

Infections in the brain can cause serious complications, and handling them requires careful use of neuroradiology to assist in treatment. Viral pathogens, such as SARS-CoV-2, have been shown to indirectly impact cerebral function and exacerbate conditions like stroke by overwhelming healthcare resources and delaying acute interventions, illustrating the broader consequences of infectious diseases on brain health (Bersano *et al.*, 2020). Besides, infections of the central nervous system can look like neoplastic diseases, which makes it difficult to distinguish between them. For example, primary central nervous system lymphoma, while not infectious itself, requires extensive imaging and tissue analysis to distinguish it from infections causing similar radiological patterns (Fox *et al.*, 2018). It is important to detect infections early, and MRI is very useful for this, since infections may show as inflammation, abscesses, or issues with blood vessels. Noticing these patterns can help doctors treat patients early, which may help reduce lasting neurological problems and improve patient outcomes.

3.2.7. Vascular Malformations

Because vascular malformations in the brain can be varied and may cause major bleeding, their management is quite complex. Particularly, hereditary hemorrhagic telangiectasia presents a unique challenge; this autosomal dominant disorder manifests with high-flow arteriovenous malformations (AVMs) and fistulas, which carry a significant rupture risk estimated at 0.7% per lesion annually. Screening with contrast-enhanced MRI is advocated at diagnosis to detect these malformations early, especially in children, to enable timely intervention and reduce morbidity (Beslow *et al.*, 2024). Surgical resection of brain AVMs, while potentially curative, carries risks such as delayed postoperative hemorrhage (DPH), which occurs more frequently with larger AVMs or those located in periventricular regions. Identifying risk factors like maximum lesion diameter and lesion location aids in stratifying patient risk and tailoring perioperative strategies to minimize adverse outcomes (Yan *et al.*, 2024). This underscores the importance of a nuanced neuroradiological approach in guiding both diagnosis and treatment planning (Figure 3.11).

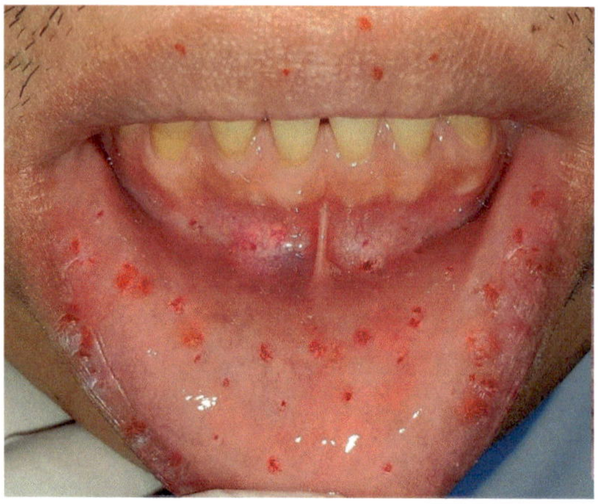

Figure 3.11. Hereditary hemorrhagic telangiectasia.

Source: https://www.bmj.com/content/bmj/376/bmj-2021-067906/F1.large.jpg.

3.2.8. Epilepsy and Seizure Disorders

New techniques in neuroimaging have greatly improved the way epilepsy and seizures are managed, especially in children, since their causes can be different and include cerebral anoxia, metabolic conditions, and brain malformations. MRI is still the primary test to find structural problems, help with pre-surgery planning, and predict outcomes, yet it may not detect small lesions such as focal cortical dysplasia, so other tests such as positron emission tomography or diffusion tensor imaging are needed. Using syndromic classification, which connects neurophysiology and neuroimaging, has helped doctors give more accurate diagnoses and better treatments. Using these categories makes it easier for clinicians to discuss cases and choose the proper treatment for the specific problem. Integrating advanced imaging techniques with detailed clinical syndromic frameworks optimizes management and assists in surgical planning, especially in refractory epilepsy cases where localization of epileptogenic foci is critical (Lin *et al.*, 2013; Morris, 2008).

3.2.9. Congenital Brain Anomalies

Using new neuroimaging techniques has made it much easier to diagnose and treat complex neurological disorders in children. Among all these, having a brain anomaly from birth is a key type of developmental disorder with major effects on health. These problems develop during pregnancy, often because of mutations in genes, harmful things in the environment, or infections in the womb, which may lead to severe brain problems such as epilepsy that does not respond to drugs. Using tools like magnetic resonance imaging and computed tomography allows doctors to clearly see these abnormalities, which helps them plan surgery if medications are ineffective. Because refractory seizures are common in these children, early and correct diagnosis is very important for the best results. Also, advanced imaging methods help determine the location and size of tumors, as well as whether surgery is an option, showing the importance of neuroradiology in managing these patients with a team approach. Despite overlaps with systemic congenital conditions, the brain's unique vulnerability necessitates specialized assessment protocols to mitigate long-term disabilities (Crișan *et al.*, 2024; Donald *et al.*, 2024) (Figure 3.12).

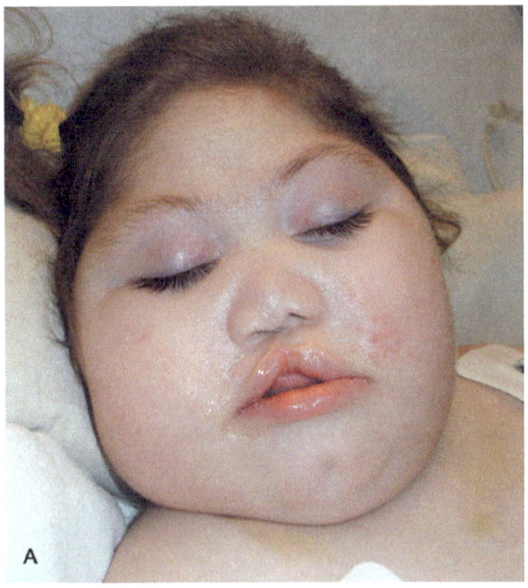

Figure 3.12. Congenital brain anomalies.

Source: https://s3.amazonaws.com/HMP/c360/imported/transfer/Screen_Shot_2013-05-23_at_9.17.57_AM_1.png.

Test Your Knowledge

1. How does brain imaging assist in finding and handling ischemic stroke?
2. What are the types of strokes?

3.3. Interpretation of Neuroradiological Images

Learning Outcome

1. Understand image artifacts;
2. Identify normal versus abnormal findings;
3. Explain the role of clinical history in interpretation;
4. Focus on a multidisciplinary approach to diagnosis;
5. Know the use of computer-aided detection systems;
6. Identify challenges in image interpretation;
7. Discuss the importance of follow-up imaging;
8. Explain reporting standards and protocols;
9. Learn case studies in image interpretation.

Interpreting neuroradiological images correctly depends on knowing both normal and abnormal changes in brain structures. Advances in MRI techniques, including susceptibility-weighted imaging and quantitative susceptibility mapping, have enhanced the detection of subtle abnormalities such as paramagnetic copper accumulation in Wilson's disease, enabling more precise diagnosis and disease severity assessment (Litwin *et al.*, 2024). Similarly, volumetric analyses in patients with systemic conditions like Type 1 diabetes reveal specific brain volume reductions, notably in the thalamus and deep gray matter, which correlate with cerebral small vessel disease indicators (Tor-Björn Claesson *et al.*, 2024). These changing imaging techniques help find important markers, showing how changes in the body are linked to symptoms and make it simpler to track the disease. So, the interpretation process should combine information from advanced imaging with what is known about the patient, using semi-quantitative scales and post-processing to better identify signs of disease in the brain. Neuroradiology can only progress by using this multidimensional approach.

3.3.1. Understanding Image Artifacts

The brain and its problems must be accurately shown in neuroradiological images, but image artifacts can make this complicated by either obscuring or mimicking disease. The sources of artifacts are patient movement, hardware limitations, and the way the imaging technique is used, which may result in distortions and signal loss. For instance, susceptibility-induced geometric distortions in diffusion-weighted MRI impact the fidelity of ischemic lesion visualization, but techniques such as field map-based correction have been demonstrated to significantly reduce these distortions, thereby enhancing diagnostic confidence and image quality across multiple brain regions (Grauhan *et al.*, 2023).

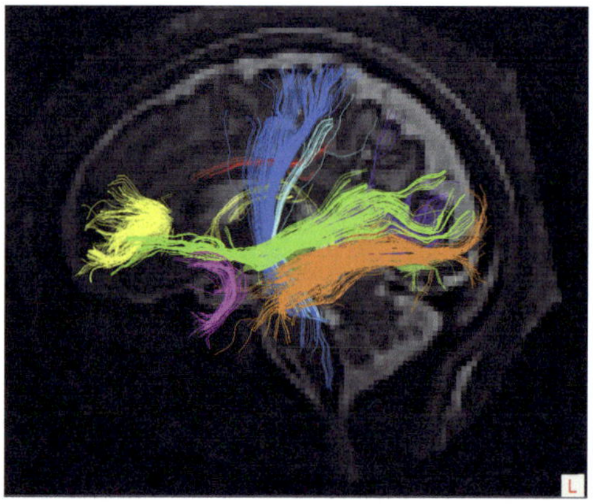

Figure 3.13. Artifacts arise from various sources, including patient movement, hardware limitations, and intrinsic imaging technique constraints, which can lead to distortions and signal loss.

Source: https://www.mri.theclinics.com/cms/10.1016/j.mric.2021.06.007/asset/4d69cedf-8755-4abd-8e18-9e21741da2c9/main.assets/gr15_lrg.jpg.

Similarly, in pediatric brain CT imaging, iterative model reconstruction methods improve signal-to-noise and contrast-to-noise ratios while minimizing artifacts compared to traditional filtered-back projection, thus maintaining diagnostic accuracy even with low-dose protocols (Rabinowich *et al.*, 2023). Understanding and addressing these artifacts is crucial for optimizing neuroradiological assessments and ensuring precise interpretation of brain imaging (Figure 3.13).

3.3.2. Identifying Normal Versus Abnormal Findings

It is very important in neuroradiology to distinguish normal from abnormal results to help with correct diagnosis and treatment decisions. Slight changes in the shape of the brain or its signals on MRI images may suggest the presence of tumors or injuries, which should be treated right away. Advanced deep learning techniques have been increasingly employed to enhance the precision of brain tumor segmentation, isolating abnormal tissues from normal structures with greater reliability despite challenges like data variability and tumor heterogeneity (Karim *et al.*, 2024). Furthermore, blood biomarker profiles complement imaging by revealing physiological abnormalities that may not be visually apparent, although factors like extracranial injuries or pre-existing conditions can produce outlier values, complicating clinical interpretation (Korhonen *et al.*, 2023). For this reason, using imaging, biochemical markers, and clinical information helps correctly identify normal and abnormal brain changes, which ultimately benefits patients in neuroradiology.

3.3.3. Role of Clinical History in Interpretation

Interpreting neuroradiological images well depends on knowing the patient's medical background which helps in finding and describing brain abnormalities. If the information is missing, radiologists could make the wrong diagnosis or not catch important changes in the body. The radiologist can use the clinical history to understand when and how the symptoms started, how they have progressed, and any related systemic problems, which helps in choosing the best diagnosis. Previous trauma, infection, or malignancy can strongly impact how doctors read and understand unclear images. In addition, clinical information aids in telling apart acute and chronic lesions, inflammatory and neoplastic conditions, and congenital from acquired abnormalities, which improves how accurately a patient is managed. As emphasized in related neuro-ophthalmic cases, integrating clinical input is critical for narrowing differential diagnoses and improving diagnostic confidence (Brennan *et al.*, 2014). Thus, the role of clinical history remains indispensable in the nuanced interpretation of brain imaging studies (Figure 3.14).

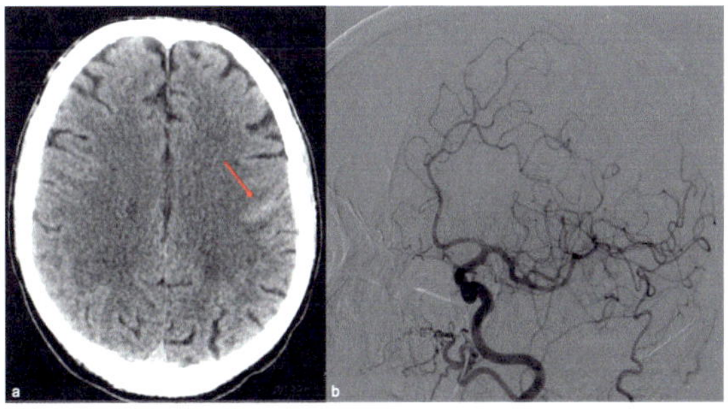

Figure 3.14. Accurate interpretation of neuroradiological imaging hinges on a comprehensive understanding of the patient's clinical history, which provides essential context for identifying and characterizing brain abnormalities.

Source: https://pub.mdpi-res.com/jcm/jcm-14-01697/article_deploy/html/images/jcm-14-01697-g001.png?1741003960.

3.3.4. Multidisciplinary Approach to Diagnosis

New brain imaging and diagnostic methods have greatly increased the speed and accuracy of finding neurological conditions. Still, because brain pathologies are so complex, it often takes the skills of several specialties to help patients recover well. A multidisciplinary approach in neuroradiology means radiological results are understood with the help of clinical, surgical, and pathological information, which leads to better patient care. This collaboration, exemplified by brain tumor centers, integrates neurosurgery, neuro-oncology, pathology, and radiology to facilitate nuanced diagnosis and tailored treatment strategies, resulting in more precise surgical planning and effective therapies (Casimiro *et al.*, 2024). Similarly, in traumatic brain injury, involving specialists such as neurologists, psychologists, and rehabilitation experts alongside radiologists enables early detection of cognitive and psychosomatic complications, promoting timely intervention and improved recovery (Yaroslavska *et al.*, 2024). Talking across different fields in neuroradiology improves the accuracy of diagnoses and raises the standard of care in the brain.

3.3.5. Use of Computer-aided Detection (CAD) Systems

Improvements in medical imaging have made it easier to diagnose brain problems in neuroradiology, but it is still difficult to find and identify brain problems early. CAD systems can be integrated to offer support to radiologists by automatically finding abnormalities that might not be noticed in regular analysis. For instance, CAD algorithms applied to hyperspectral imaging have demonstrated high precision in detecting brain cancers, although their clinical adoption is limited by a lack of external validation and small sample sizes in current studies (Leung *et al.*, 2024).

Similarly, in neurodegenerative disorders such as Alzheimer's Disease, sophisticated deep learning architectures harness multi-stage neural networks to extract and classify imaging features with remarkable accuracy, thus facilitating earlier diagnosis and better prognosis (Hassan *et al.*, 2024). These developments underscore the transformative potential of CAD systems to augment diagnostic accuracy and workflow efficiency in brain neuroradiology, though broader validation and integration into clinical practice remain critical next steps (Figure 3.15).

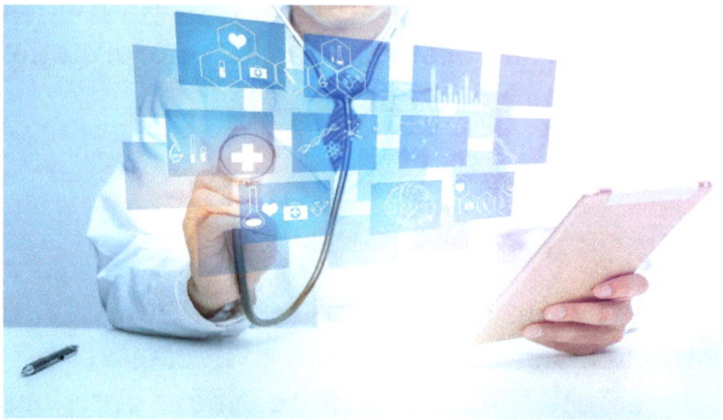

Figure 3.15. The integration of computer-aided detection (CAD) systems offers a promising solution by providing automated analysis that supports radiologists in identifying subtle abnormalities often missed in conventional assessment.

Source: https://www.market-prospects.com/storage/images/767_1200x675.jpg.

3.3.6. Challenges in Image Interpretation

Reading brain images in neuroradiology is not easy, and it affects the accuracy of disease diagnosis, and how doctors make decisions. Each type of imaging modality, such as MRI and CT, has its own contrast and resolution, which adds to the difficulty of comparing results consistently. Also, small pathological changes may be hard to detect, especially if the patient moves or if there are artifacts in the image.

Even though advanced machine learning models have been built to help with these issues, they are not widely used because they require large and varied training data and may not work well with many types of images. For example, some pretrained convolutional neural networks demonstrate high accuracy in specific modalities like MRI but perform poorly on others, indicating a challenge in creating versatile tools for broad clinical use (Fagbola *et al.*, 2024). Additionally, the high dimensionality of EEG data and the discomfort involved in acquiring multiple channels impede efficient analysis and patient compliance, necessitating novel methods for data reduction and classification (Oxenberg *et al.*, 2025). Because of these issues, it is clear that using flexible and connected strategies is necessary in neuroradiology image reading.

3.3.7. Importance of Follow-up Imaging

Monitoring how a neurological disease progresses and the effectiveness of the treatment is very important for proper diagnosis and management. Follow-up imaging is very important because it can reveal changes that the doctor may not see during the initial visit. For instance, in patients with severe COVID-19, follow-up brain MRI has revealed diverse neuroradiologic patterns associated with disease severity, underscoring its importance in detecting complications such as hemorrhagic lesions and multifocal white matter abnormalities that influence clinical outcomes (Kremer *et al.*, 2020).

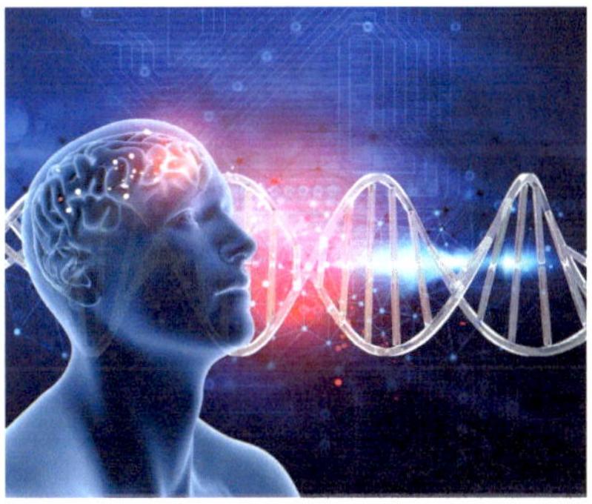

Figure 3.16. Accurate diagnosis and timely management of neurological conditions depend heavily on the ability to monitor disease progression and treatment efficacy.

Source: https://d35oenyzp35321.cloudfront.net/3d_medical_background_with_male_head_brain_dna_strands_1048_6346_650cb1a5ef.webp.

Similarly, in conditions like sickle cell disease, serial brain imaging combined with hemodynamic assessments enables the identification of cerebral infarcts and vasculopathy progression even when neurological examinations remain stable, highlighting the necessity of continuous neuroradiological evaluation for secondary stroke prevention and management after interventions such as bone marrow transplantation (Jordan *et al.*, 2019). Consequently, follow-up imaging is indispensable for optimizing patient care, guiding treatment adjustments, and improving prognostic accuracy within neuroradiology of the brain (Figure 3.16).

3.3.8. Reporting Standards and Protocols

Good and consistent reporting in neuroradiology helps move forward clinical work and research, mainly for complex brain scans. Having standard protocols guarantees that information gathered, examined, and explained can be trusted and repeated at other places. Recently, efforts have been made to develop complete frameworks, for example, for functional MRI in migraine, which stress the need to set clear guidelines for demographics, imaging, and methods to make studies more alike and easier to compare. This consensus-driven approach encompasses critical factors, including scan timing, medication status, and preprocessing documentation, thereby promoting a uniform reporting language that aids in synthesizing findings across diverse cohorts and technical setups (Schramm *et al.*, 2025). Also, because AI is being used more in neuroradiology, it is important to follow guidelines like STARD when reporting, so that AI-assisted interpretations are accurate and clear. Recognizing the variability in AI performance across different brain imaging tasks further underscores the need for precise, standardized reporting protocols to optimize diagnostic utility and patient outcomes (Gupta *et al.*, 2024).

3.3.9. Case Studies in Image Interpretation

Progress in diagnostic imaging has made it easier to study brain diseases, which underlines the need for case studies in image interpretation for neuroradiology. Detailed examinations employing multimodal approaches, such as fetal MRI following expert ultrasound, allow more precise diagnosis and inform clinical decision-making, especially in cases with incomplete or suspicious findings (Prayer *et al.*, 2023). They demonstrate that using different imaging techniques can help confirm or enhance the first diagnosis, which benefits the patient. Furthermore, the incorporation of artificial intelligence tools in real-time clinical settings demonstrates promising results in detecting critical conditions like intracranial hemorrhage, potentially reducing diagnostic errors and assisting radiologists under increasing workload pressures (Buls *et al.*, 2021). Looking at these case studies reveals the usual difficulties and challenges in interpreting brain scans, which highlights the ongoing importance of expertise in this field.

Test Your Knowledge

1. What are the usual imaging signs seen in a patient with a brain infarct on MRI?
2. How is CT angiography (CTA) used to diagnose brain aneurysms, and what are the typical imaging findings?

3.4. Future Trends in Neuroradiology

Learning Outcome

1. Understand artificial intelligence in imaging;
2. Know innovations in imaging technology;
3. Define personalized medicine and neuroradiology;
4. Focus on telemedicine and remote consultations;
5. Understand research in neuroimaging biomarkers;
6. Learn integration of imaging with genomics;
7. Discuss ethical considerations in neuroradiology;
8. Describe training and education advancements;
9. Explain the global health implications of neuroradiology.

New technologies are set to transform neuroradiology by improving how diseases are found and treated. One key development is the integration of brain-inspired computing, which offers novel computational models that mimic neural processes and could lead to more sophisticated image analysis algorithms, improving the interpretation of complex brain pathologies (Li *et al.*, 2024).

Also, new developments in deep learning and big data analytics are expected to improve the process of taking and analyzing brain images. However, these innovations also introduce challenges related to cybersecurity, as the proliferation of manipulated neuroimaging data could compromise clinical decision-making; hence, evolving detection and prevention mechanisms remain critical (Gambín *et al.*, 2024). In the future, working together, computational neuroscience, artificial intelligence, and clinical neuroradiology will help create new imaging tools, improve our knowledge of brain health and diseases, and support better patient results using personalized and precise medicine.

3.4.1. Artificial Intelligence (AI) in Imaging

AI has recently made a big difference in neuroradiology, especially in imaging needed for diagnosing urgent brain problems. AI tools in emergency neuroradiology now help doctors decide quickly about stroke, hemorrhage, and vascular problems by using deep learning on several imaging methods. These innovations not only enhance diagnostic accuracy but also support timely management strategies critical in high-stakes scenarios (Gong *et al.*, 2024). But it is still hard to confirm AI models with data from multiple institutions, as the American Society of Functional Neuroradiology's multicenter competition has shown. AI predictions differed a lot from what the experts thought, mainly when it came to judging normalcy and urgency in non-contrast CT scans. Such findings emphasize the need for rigorous external validation and cautious integration of AI tools into clinical workflows to avoid premature reliance on models that may not yet meet practical performance thresholds (Jiang *et al.*, 2024). Thus, while promising, artificial intelligence in brain imaging requires ongoing refinement to optimize its clinical utility (Figure 3.17).

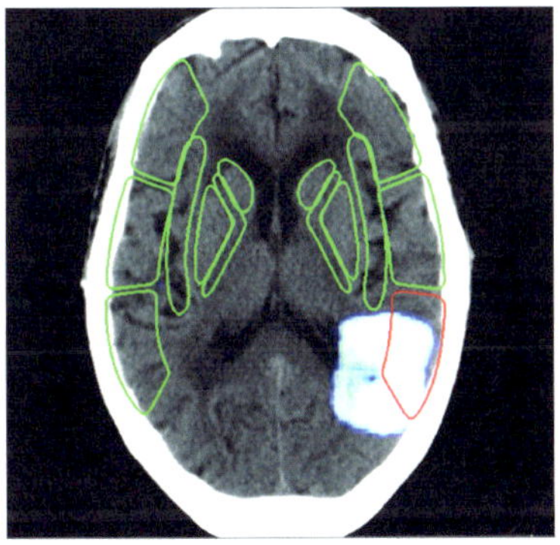

Figure 3.17. AI applications in emergency neuroradiology now aid rapid decision-making for stroke, hemorrhage, and vascular abnormalities by leveraging deep learning algorithms across various imaging modalities.

Source: https://www.ajnr.org/content/ajnr/42/1/2/F3.large.jpg.

3.4.2. Innovations in Imaging Technology

Improvements in imaging technology have made it possible to find brain problems earlier and more accurately. Thanks to high-resolution MRI and fMRI, doctors can now clearly see brain structures and how they are connected, which is very useful for diagnosing neurological disorders. Integrating artificial intelligence with these methods has made it possible to automate difficult pattern recognition tasks, which helps radiologists make more accurate diagnoses and work less. In addition, using DTI and similar techniques, doctors can precisely trace white matter tracts, which is very important for surgical planning and understanding the prognosis. AI keeps progressing, helping improve how images are taken and read, which supports the use of personalized treatments in neuro-oncology and cerebrovascular diseases. These technological strides not only improve patient outcomes but also address the increasing demand for efficient healthcare delivery, reflecting the broader impact of AI in clinical medicine (Karalis, 2024; Krishnan *et al.*, 2023).

3.4.3. Personalized Medicine and Neuroradiology

Because of technological progress, artificial intelligence and machine learning are now being used in neuroradiology, greatly affecting personalized medicine. These methods help doctors find neurological diseases by studying brain images and looking for small signs. For example, convolutional neural networks applied to structural brain scans facilitate the differentiation of dementia subtypes and provide individualized explanations for disease progression, enabling more precise prognostic evaluations tailored to patients' unique brain pathology (Leonardsen *et al.*, 2024). Furthermore, in brain tumor management, radiomic analysis coupled with AI models assists clinicians in non-invasive lesion characterization, surgical planning, and molecular target identification, optimizing treatment strategies while minimizing adverse effects on neurological function (Ce' *et al.*, 2023). With the help of detailed medical and imaging information, such protocols help predict how a patient will respond to treatment and what complications may occur. This convergence of neuroradiology and personalized medicine promises improved patient outcomes by offering targeted, data-driven care grounded in sophisticated image analysis and clinical integration (Figure 3.18).

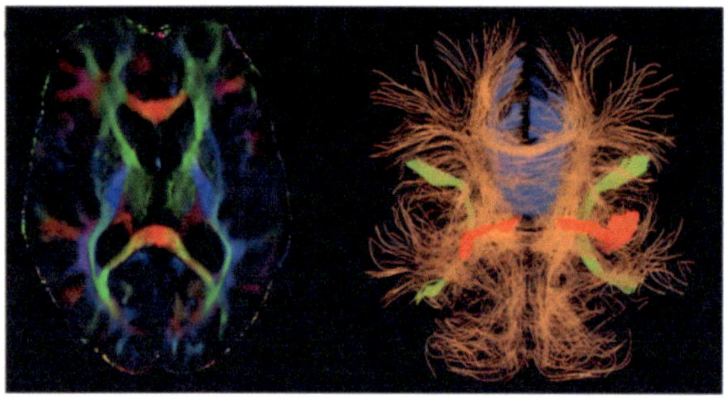

Figure 3.18. Convolutional neural networks applied to structural brain scans facilitate the differentiation of dementia subtypes and provide individualized explanations for disease progression, enabling more precise prognostic evaluations tailored to patients' unique brain pathology.

Source: https://ars.els-cdn.com/content/image/1-s2.0-S2352914824001072-gr19.jpg.

3.4.4. Telemedicine and Remote Consultations

New technologies have made a big difference in healthcare, mostly in areas like neuroradiology. Telemedicine lets patients connect with stroke specialists and have neuroradiology exams quickly, which is very important for managing brain injuries. More and more hospitals that do not have neurology departments on site are using teleneuromedical networks, as they see these networks help with better treatment, quicker access to specialists, and fewer unnecessary transfers. Despite challenges involving financing, equipment costs, and legal concerns, acceptance among collaborating institutions remains high, highlighting telemedicine's potential to enhance stroke outcomes and service competitiveness (Tenckhoff *et al.*, 2010). In addition, telemedicine platforms, which include video conferencing and messaging apps, help with postoperative checkups, educating patients, and consulting among healthcare workers in low- and middle-income countries. Such remote solutions demonstrate promise in bridging gaps in neuroradiological care access, although rigorous clinical evaluations are necessary to confirm their effectiveness (Chu *et al.*, 2022). Telemedicine is important for spreading knowledge of brain imaging over large distances.

3.4.5. Research in Neuroimaging Biomarkers

Better cognitive assessment methods have made it much easier to detect the early signs of Alzheimer's disease. Remarkably, telehealth-compatible cognitive composites have made it possible to assess people remotely with confidence in many different locations. Remote assessments have been shown to be very similar to traditional in-person tests, proving their validity. Moreover, these cognitive composites show significant associations with established neuroimaging biomarkers, including brain volume, gray matter perfusion, white matter integrity, and amyloid-β deposition, which are critical indicators of neurodegeneration and disease progression (Duran *et al.*, 2024). Also, using artificial neural networks and deep learning on neuroimaging data has made it easier to diagnose and predict the progression of Alzheimer's disease and mild cognitive impairment. The integration of multimodal neuroimaging data and advanced computational methods promises to refine biomarker discovery and enhance predictive accuracy in neuroradiology (Cabrera-León *et al.*, 2024) (Figure 3.19).

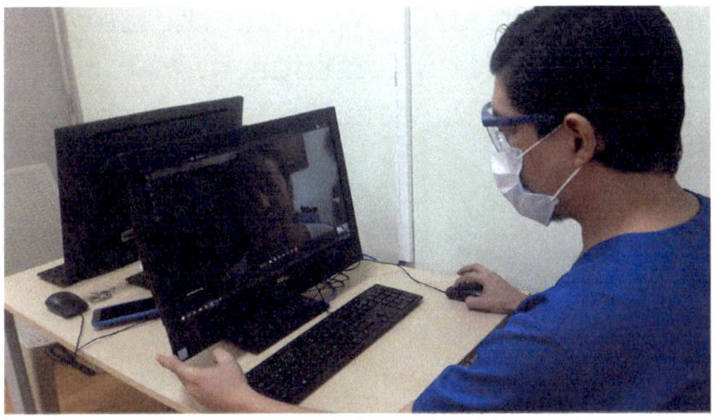

Figure 3.19. The development of telehealth-compatible cognitive composites has expanded the scope of remote evaluation, allowing for reliable measurement across diverse settings.

Source: https://upload.wikimedia.org/wikipedia/commons/thumb/f/f5/Doctor_attending_by_teleconsultation.jpg/1200px-Doctor_attending_by_teleconsultation.jpg.

3.4.6. Integration of Imaging with Genomics

Improvements in technology now allow doctors to use imaging and genomic analysis together to gain a comprehensive understanding of brain disorders. This fusion supports accurate diagnosis of complex neurological diseases by comparing imaging, structure, and genetics. Because of this integration, doctors can design treatments that fit each patient's genetic makeup and the images from radiology. Besides, using artificial intelligence helps manage and examine the large amounts of data from the multimodal approach, making diagnosis faster and more accurate, and dealing with issues related to workflow optimization. Despite obstacles such as data quality and ethical concerns, the convergence of imaging and genomics promises to revolutionize brain disorder management, fostering early detection and targeted therapies that significantly improve patient outcomes in neurological care (Krishnan *et al.*, 2023; Najjar, 2023).

3.4.7. Ethical Considerations in Neuroradiology

Thanks to progress in neuroradiology, it is now much easier to find brain problems and unexpected findings, but this also raises many ethical issues that must be carefully considered. The detection of incidental findings, such as white or grey matter abnormalities in preterm infants, raises important questions about informed consent, patient privacy, and the responsibility to communicate potentially uncertain or non-clinically significant results to families (Sullivan *et al.*, 2024). Moreover, the interdisciplinary nature of neuroradiological practice demands ongoing ethical reflection on relationships among healthcare professionals, patients, and society to maintain trust and uphold the integrity of care provision (Okoye *et al.*, 2024). Neuroradiologists have to handle matters related to using resources, respecting patient autonomy, and the possible effects of unexpected results on patients. So, encouraging openness, education, and teamwork is necessary to deal with these complex ethical issues and guarantee that the benefits of advanced imaging do not accidentally harm patients or the standards in neuroradiology.

3.4.8. Training and Education Advancements

The fast progress of technology has greatly influenced how medical education is done, especially in neuroradiology. Advances in training methods today use advanced imaging software, virtual reality, and interactive case studies, which have greatly improved the learning of brain imaging. They give trainees the opportunity to explore 3D models and live situations, which helps them understand the complex parts of the nervous system and the different diseases. In addition, workshops that bring together different fields and online platforms make it possible for professionals to learn new information about imaging and diagnosis. They help doctors make accurate diagnoses and also support critical thinking and personal care for each patient. The integration of these advanced modalities into neuroradiology training exemplifies a commitment to excellence and innovation in medical education, preparing practitioners to meet the demands of an increasingly sophisticated clinical environment (Figure 3.20).

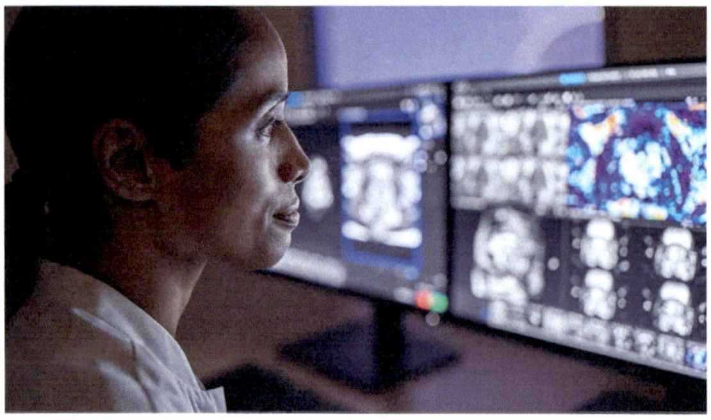

Figure 3.20. The rapid evolution of technology has profoundly influenced medical education, particularly in specialized fields such as neuroradiology.

Source: https://www.philips.com/c-dam/corporate/innovation-and-you/global/dec-2023/hero-ai-in-healthcare-realworld-examples.jpg.

3.4.9. Global Health Implications of Neuroradiology

Improvements in neuroradiology have greatly changed how neurological diseases are diagnosed, managed, and prevented, which influences health around the world. With the use of fast MRI and multi-slice CT, neuroradiology has made it easier to find and treat urgent conditions such as stroke and inflammatory diseases of the brain. Because of this, patient care improves and helps prevent health problems by catching them early and creating digital brain models for each person. Besides, reducing radiation and the use of contrast agents helps keep patients and practitioners safe and makes medical settings safer. Incorporating artificial intelligence helps improve how diseases are diagnosed and how treatment is planned everywhere. Despite this, Japan's difficulties in making extensive imaging databases available to all point out that more data democratization is needed to speed up worldwide AI progress. Addressing these issues will be crucial for neuroradiology to fulfill its potential as a cornerstone of brain health and overall global healthcare improvement (Lövblad *et al.*, 2024; Ueda *et al.*, 2024).

Test Your Knowledge

1. How will artificial intelligence (AI) revolutionize brain neuroradiology in the detection and diagnosis of neurological disorders?
2. What are the advantages and disadvantages of using AI-based algorithms to find brain tumors in MRI scans?

SUMMARY

Developments in neuroradiology have greatly improved the accuracy and efficiency of brain imaging, which has changed how diseases are diagnosed and treated. The integration of artificial intelligence into radiological practices has introduced powerful tools for image analysis, enabling more precise segmentation, diagnosis, and predictive modeling, which ultimately improve patient outcomes and clinical workflows (Najjar, 2023). Furthermore, the utilization of federated machine learning models has demonstrated substantial improvements in tumor boundary detection for complex brain pathologies such as glioblastoma, addressing challenges of data diversity and privacy while leveraging large-scale multicenter datasets (Pati *et al.*, 2022). They point to a future where technology needs to be developed by teams who care about ethics, to address the many challenges in brain imaging. To make the most of advanced imaging diagnostics in neurology, neuroradiology needs to keep collaborating with other disciplines and adopt new imaging techniques.

New methods in neuroimaging have made it possible to see the detailed structure and problems of the brain. Diffusion imaging, particularly through DTI and high angular resolution diffusion imaging (HARDI), has been instrumental in revealing white matter microstructure and aberrant connectivity associated with congenital brain malformations, enhancing both clinical and research applications in developmental disorders (Barkovich *et al.*, 2010). In addition, the use of structural MRI, functional MRI, and DTI has been very helpful for TBI research, helping to identify new biomarkers that guide treatment and prognosis. These approaches, combined with advanced volumetric analysis and connectome-based network examination, underscore a multidisciplinary effort toward refined diagnostic precision and outcome prediction in neuroradiology (Aylward *et al.*, 2012). All of these points to the important role multimodal neuroimaging plays in moving forward research and clinical practice in brain analysis.

KEY TERMS FROM THIS CHAPTER

- Neurological disorders
- Epileptic foci
- Apparent Diffusion Coefficient (ADC) values
- Lesions
- Electroencephalogram (EEG)
- Blood vessel diseases
- Deep learning algorithms
- Image processing
- Tumors
- Diffusion-Weighted Imaging (DWI)
- Neuroradiology
- Seizures
- Epilepsy
- Spinal cord
- Malignant growths
- Quantum machine learning

CRITICAL THINKING QUESTIONS

1. **Which imaging test is generally considered the best for finding acute intracranial hemorrhage?**
   a. X-ray
   b. CT Scan
   c. MRI
   d. PET Scan
2. **What is the main benefit of using an MRI instead of a CT scan for looking at the brain?**
   a. Faster scan times
   b. Superior resolution for soft tissue
   c. Lower cost
   d. Better for detecting bone fractures
3. **To find the area of ischemia in a suspected ischemic stroke patient which MRI sequence is usually used?**
   a. T1-weighted
   b. T2-weighted
   c. Diffusion-weighted Imaging (DWI)
   d. FLAIR (Fluid-Attenuated Inversion Recovery)
4. **Which of the following is a common finding on MRI in patients with multiple sclerosis (MS)?**
   a. Homogeneous white matter lesions
   b. Cortical atrophy
   c. Periventricular white matter plaques
   d. Parenchymal calcifications
5. **Which of the following conditions is most commonly diagnosed using an MR angiogram (MRA)?**
   a. Brain abscess
   b. Intracranial aneurysm
   c. Glioma
   d. Hydrocephalus

Short Answer Questions

1. What is the main way to image acute ischemic stroke?
2. How does diffusion-weighted imaging (DWI) on MRI help in the early detection of brain ischemia?
3. Why is a non-contrast CT scan usually the first test done for suspected acute intracranial hemorrhage?
4. Why is MRI better than CT for detecting brain tumors, mainly because of its superior soft tissue contrast?
5. How does functional MRI (fMRI) differ from conventional MRI, and what is its role in brain mapping?
6. What role does MR angiography (MRA) play in the assessment of cerebrovascular abnormalities, such as aneurysms or stenosis?
7. How does MRI help in detecting multiple sclerosis (MS) lesions, and what MRI sequence is typically used for this purpose?

Answers to Critical Thinking Questions

1. (b); 2. (b); 3. (c); 4. (c); 5. (b)

REFERENCES

1. Aleid, A. M., Al Omireen, R. M., Enani, M. J., Alharbi, R., Alsubaie, O. F., Aljibreen, A. F., Aldehailan, M. S., *et al.* (2024). A review of imaging modalities in pediatric traumatic brain injury: Evaluating diagnostic accuracy and clinical outcomes: Cross-sectional study. *Journal of Advanced Trends in Medical Research*. https://www.semanticscholar.org/paper/dcdebc46b9344dd18f98a485a51f76758dd18cb7 (accessed on 31st May 2025).
2. Aloumba-Gilius, D., Aloumba-Gilius, D. W., El, S., Himri, H., Oudrhiri, D., Laoudiyi, K., Siham, C., *et al.* (2024). Imaging congenital brain malformations: A cause of drug-resistant epilepsy in children. *World Journal of Advanced Research and Reviews*. https://www.semanticscholar.org/paper/b342cf4e697d78f605db19d559b5419f57dad277 (accessed on 31st May 2025).
3. Amin, J., Sharif, M., Haldorai, A., Yasmin, M., & Nayak, R. S. (2021). Brain tumor detection and classification using machine learning: A comprehensive survey. *Complex & Intelligent Systems, 8*, 3161–3183. https://doi.org/10.1007/s40747-021-00563-y (accessed on 31st May 2025).
4. Amunts, K., DeFelipe, J., Pennartz, C. M. A., Destexhe, A., Migliore, M., Ryvlin, P., Furber, S., *et al.* (2022). Linking brain structure, activity, and cognitive function through computation. *eNeuro, 9*, ENEURO.0316-21.2022. https://doi.org/10.1523/eneuro.0316-21.2022 (accessed on 31st May 2025).
5. Arif, S., Varma, R. C., Thaiparambil, S., Ahuja, A., & Nair, A. (2025). Comparison of imaging modalities in differentiating cerebral neoplastic lesions and post-radiation necrosis. *Cureus, 17*. https://www.semanticscholar.org/paper/bbdb24d33477ad9734de723ee097d7c6172387e0 (accessed on 31st May 2025).
6. Awad, N. S., Hassan, H. A., Hasan, A. A., & Elbadawi, Y. O. (2025). Assessing brain tumors through diffusion-weighted imaging techniques. *Saudi Journal of Medical and Pharmaceutical Sciences*. https://www.semanticscholar.org/paper/54f7ddf973835e7f374ff91f1ded2037e0a93d8c (accessed on 31st May 2025).
7. Aylward, S. R., Gerig, G., Hovda, D. A., & Irimia, A. (2012). Neuroimaging of structural pathology and connectomics in traumatic brain injury: Toward personalized outcome prediction. *NeuroImage: Clinical*. https://core.ac.uk/download/323078685.pdf (accessed on 31st May 2025).
8. Bahrami, N., Sharma, D., Rosenthal, S. L., Davenport, E. M., Urban, J. E., Wagner, B., Jung, Y., *et al.* (2016). Subconcussive head impact exposure and white matter tract changes over a single season of youth football. *Radiology, 281*, 919–926. https://doi.org/10.1148/radiol.2016160564 (accessed on 31st May 2025).
9. Barkovich, A. J., Mukherjee, P., & Wahl, M. (2010). *Diffusion Imaging and Tractography of Congenital Brain Malformations.* https://core.ac.uk/download/323074405.pdf (accessed on 31st May 2025).
10. Bersano, A., Kraemer, M., Touzé, E., Weber, R., Alamowitch, S., Sibon, I., & Pantoni, L. (2020). Stroke care during the COVID-19 pandemic: Experience from three large European countries. *European Journal of Neurology, 27*, 1794–1800. https://doi.org/10.1111/ene.14375 (accessed on 31st May 2025).
11. Beslow, L., White, A. J., Krings, T., Hammill, A. M., Lang, S., Baba, A., Clancy, M., *et al.* (2024). Current practice: Rationale for screening children with hereditary hemorrhagic telangiectasia

for brain vascular malformations. *AJNR. American Journal of Neuroradiology*. https://www.semanticscholar.org/paper/b4388033a5b8af199be9a4faf3f3aeaae5c2678e (accessed on 31st May 2025).

12. Brennan, P., Galvin, P. L., Grech, R., & Grech, A. (2014). *Imaging of Adult Ocular and Orbital Pathology – a Pictorial Review*. https://core.ac.uk/download/323186424.pdf (accessed on 31st May 2025).

13. Buls, N., Watté, N., Nieboer, K., Ilsen, B., & De Mey, J. (2021). Performance of an artificial intelligence tool with real-time clinical workflow integration – Detection of intracranial hemorrhage and pulmonary embolism. *Physica Medica, 83*, 154–160. https://doi.org/10.1016/j.ejmp.2021.03.015 (accessed on 31st May 2025).

14. Cabrera-León, Y., Báez, P. G., Fernández-López, P., & Suárez-Araujo, C. P. (2024). Neural computation-based methods for the early diagnosis and prognosis of Alzheimer's disease not using neuroimaging biomarkers: A systematic review. *Journal of Alzheimer's Disease, 98*, 793–823. https://www.semanticscholar.org/paper/854f96eda5da7e8d73c224de0c1f676b0f850b78 (accessed on 31st May 2025).

15. Cai, S., Xing, H., Wang, Y., Wang, Y., Ma, W., Jiang, Y., Li, J., *et al.* (2024). Clinical application of intraoperative ultrasound superb microvascular imaging in brain tumors resections: Contributing to the achievement of total tumoral resection. *BMC Medical Imaging, 24*. https://www.semanticscholar.org/paper/dbe444514cb8d392220a07e6bbf22d3facd5c974 (accessed on 31st May 2025).

16. Caobelli, F., Broncano, C. J., Galea, N., Haaf, P., Loewe, C., Luetkens, J. A., Muscogiuri, G., *et al.* (2023). Cardiovascular magnetic resonance (CMR) and positron emission tomography (PET) imaging in the diagnosis and follow-up of patients with acute myocarditis and chronic inflammatory cardiomyopathy. *The International Journal of Cardiovascular Imaging, 39*, 2221–2235. https://www.semanticscholar.org/paper/4492b2f656ac1d733929f562a91900b3362a67bc (accessed on 31st May 2025).

17. Casimiro, C., Silva, M., Monteiro, J., Viegas, C., & Cunha e Sá, M. (2024). P25.04.B ten years experience of the "Brain Tumor Center" of Almada. *Neuro-Oncology*. https://www.semanticscholar.org/paper/e9e00fa00f47e35376a32f38198cd106d87e1e3b (accessed on 31st May 2025).

18. Ce,' M., Irmici, G., Foschini, C., Danesini, G., Falsitta, L. V., Serio, M. L., Fontana, A., *et al.* (2023). Artificial intelligence in brain tumor imaging: A step toward personalized medicine. *Current Oncology, 30*, 2673–2701. https://www.semanticscholar.org/paper/dfca6c5efacb8dcea956040dac6f146f9ef4bf87 (accessed on 31st May 2025).

19. Chu, K. M., Davies, J., Louw, J., & Mac Quene, P. (2022). *Telemedicine in Surgical Care in Low- and Middle-Income Countries: A Scoping Review*. https://core.ac.uk/download/552232691.pdf (accessed on 31st May 2025).

20. Claesson, T. B., Putaala, J., Shams, S., Salli, E., Gordin, D., Mutter, S., Tatlisumak, T., *et al.* (2024). Cerebral small vessel disease is associated with smaller brain volumes in adults with type 1 diabetes. *Journal of Diabetes Research, 2024*. https://www.semanticscholar.org/paper/9ea700f97b8b473a18ec70ad894aefe5b6486d70 (accessed on 31st May 2025).

21. Crișan, S., Băghină, R. M., Luca, S. A., Pătru, O., Lazăr, M., Văcărescu, C., Rus, M., *et al.* (2024). From ECG to imaging: Challenges in the diagnosis of adult congenital heart

diseases. *Journal of Clinical Medicine, 13.* https://www.semanticscholar.org/paper/bf13fe1ce4fd24d8fb16f91604368853a69d85b4 (accessed on 31st May 2025).

22. Dagher, S. A., Lochner, R. H., Ozkara, B., Schomer, D. F., Wintermark, M., Fuller, G. N., & Ucisik, F. E. (2023). The T2-FLAIR mismatch sign in oncologic neuroradiology: History, current use, emerging data, and future directions. *The Neuroradiology Journal, 37*, 441–453. https://www.semanticscholar.org/paper/03e61697e963ee3553bd5b7204c0160a957ed6de (accessed on 31st May 2025).

23. Destefani, V. C., Destefani, A. C., & Vitrio, B. (2024). Advancing neuroimaging frontiers: A comprehensive review of novel diagnostic techniques in neuroradiology and their clinical applications. *Brazilian Journal of Implantology and Health Sciences.* https://core.ac.uk/download/617924644.pdf (accessed on 31st May 2025).

24. Duran, T., Gaussoin, S., Latham, L. A., Rundle, M. M., Espeland, M., Williams, B. J., Hughes, T. M., *et al.* (2024). Examining a preclinical Alzheimer's cognitive composite for telehealth administration for reliability between in-person and remote cognitive testing with neuroimaging biomarkers. *Journal of Alzheimer's Disease: JAD.* https://www.semanticscholar.org/paper/f28e832cb71c7225441dbb91ef4c4a23a3355a05 (accessed on 31st May 2025).

25. Elmi, A. A. I., Hassan, M., Osman, F., Çelik, C., Dirie, A. M., & Ibrahim, I. (2024). Magnetic resonance imaging findings and their association with electroencephalographic data in children with epilepsy at tertiary care hospital in Mogadishu, Somalia. *International Journal of General Medicine, 17*, 253–261. https://www.semanticscholar.org/paper/8e7ac0f17c328bc49496bca0e263a8e9866cd0cc (accessed on 31st May 2025).

26. Eratne, D., Loi, S. M., Farrand, S., Kelso, W., Velakoulis, D., & Looi, J. C. L. (2018). Alzheimer's disease: Clinical update on epidemiology, pathophysiology and diagnosis. *Australasian Psychiatry, 26*, 347–357. https://doi.org/10.1177/1039856218762308 (accessed on 31st May 2025).

27. Fagbola, T., & Success, I. (2024). Leveraging pretrained models for multimodal medical image interpretation: An exhaustive experimental analysis. https://www.semanticscholar.org/paper/a672ef0b860b3b065c66377d115fa7e73199e93f (accessed on 31st May 2025).

28. Fox, C. P., Phillips, E. H., Smith, J., Linton, K., Gallop-Evans, E., Hemmaway, C., Auer, D. P., *et al.* (2018). Guidelines for the diagnosis and management of primary central nervous system diffuse large B-cell lymphoma. *British Journal of Hematology, 184*, 348–363. https://doi.org/10.1111/bjh.15661 (accessed on 31st May 2025).

29. Gambín, Á. F., Yazidi, A., Vasilakos, A., Haugerud, H., & Djenouri, Y. (2024). Deepfakes: Current and future trends. *Artificial Intelligence Review, 57*, 64. https://www.semanticscholar.org/paper/f8c523a69250296becba5ce0850292ea114bd36c (accessed on 31st May 2025).

30. Ghadimi, D. J., Vahdani, A. M., Karimi, H., Ebrahimi, P., Fathi, M., Moodi, F., Habibzadeh, A., *et al.* (2024). Deep learning-based techniques in glioma brain tumor segmentation using multi-parametric MRI: A review on clinical applications and future outlooks. *Journal of Magnetic Resonance Imaging: JMRI.* https://www.semanticscholar.org/paper/415619acd84773a7d8313e80b2b7699d34d49d52 (accessed on 31st May 2025).

31. Golinvaux, N. S., Basques, B. A., Bohl, D. D., Laurans, M., & Grauer, J. N. (2015). Bilateral vertebral artery injury in a patient with upper cervical spine fractures leading to fatal vertebrobasilar infarction: A case report. *Orthopedic Surgery, 7*, 281–285. https://doi.org/10.1111/os.12187

(accessed on 31st May 2025).

32. Gong, B., Khalvati, F., Ertl-Wagner, B., & Patlas, M. N. (2024). Artificial intelligence in emergency neuroradiology: Current applications and perspectives. *Diagnostic and Interventional Imaging*. https://doi.org/10.1016/j.diii.2024.11.002 (accessed on 31st May 2025).

33. Grauhan, N. F., Grünebach, N., Brockstedt, L., Sanner, A. P., Feiweier, T., Schöffling, V., Brockmann, M., *et al.* (2023). Reduction of distortion artifacts in brain MRI using a field map-based correction technique in diffusion-weighted imaging. *Clinical Neuroradiology, 34*, 85–91. https://www.semanticscholar.org/paper/afbc0c4cd4f28342b0623c7b60eeb76bb93471e2 (accessed on 31st May 2025).

34. Grazzini, I., Venezia, D., Del Roscio, D., Chiarotti, I., Mazzei, M., & Cerase, A. (2023). Morphological and functional neuroradiology of brain metastases. *Seminars in Ultrasound, CT, and MR, 44*(3), 170–193. https://www.semanticscholar.org/paper/186ae990d1ace08aeee19cd0c2a0899438f80e06 (accessed on 31st May 2025).

35. Gupta, R., Hamid, A. M., Jhaveri, M., Patel, N., & Suthar, P. (2024). Comparative evaluation of AI models such as ChatGPT 3.5, ChatGPT 4.0, and Google Gemini in neuroradiology diagnostics. *Cureus, 16*. https://www.semanticscholar.org/paper/f9d6e02ea4dafbc73e81cf6a3d8397c88f81bef2 (accessed on 31st May 2025).

36. Habib, G., Lancellotti, P., Antunes, M. J., Bongiorni, M. G., Casalta, J. P., Del Zotti, F., Dulgheru, R., *et al.* (2015). 2015 ESC Guidelines for the management of infective endocarditis. *European Heart Journal, 36*, 3075–3128. https://doi.org/10.1093/eurheartj/ehv319 (accessed on 31st May 2025).

37. Halefoğlu, A. M., & Yousem, D. M. (2018). Susceptibility weighted imaging: Clinical applications and future directions. *World Journal of Radiology, 10*, 30–45. https://doi.org/10.4329/wjr.v10.i4.30 (accessed on 31st May 2025).

38. Hassan, N., Miah, A. S. M., & Shin, J. (2024). Residual-based multi-stage deep learning framework for computer-aided Alzheimer's disease detection. *Journal of Imaging, 10*. https://www.semanticscholar.org/paper/938d17e9ffb55dbb397b87215929691bf38351c1 (accessed on 31st May 2025).

39. Jha, M., & Tripathi, S. (2022). *Advancements in Neuroradiology Via Artificial Intelligence and Machine Learning*. https://core.ac.uk/download/595875554.pdf (accessed on 31st May 2025).

40. Jiang, B., Ozkara, B. B., Zhu, G., Boothroyd, D., Allen, J. W., Barboriak, D. P., Chang, P., *et al.* (2024). Assessing the performance of artificial intelligence models: Insights from the American Society of Functional Neuroradiology Artificial Intelligence Competition. *American Journal of Neuroradiology, 45*, 1276–1283. https://doi.org/10.3174/ajnr.a8317 (accessed on 31st May 2025).

41. Jordan, L. C., Juttukonda, M. R., Kassim, A. A., DeBaun, M. R., Davis, L. T., Pruthi, S., Patel, N., *et al.* (2019). Haploidentical bone marrow transplantation improves cerebral hemodynamics in adults with sickle cell disease. *American Journal of Hematology, 94*. https://doi.org/10.1002/ajh.25455 (accessed on 31st May 2025).

42. Karalis, V. (2024). The integration of artificial intelligence into clinical practice. *Applied Biosciences, 3*, 14–44. https://doi.org/10.3390/applbiosci3010002 (accessed on 31st May 2025).

43. Karim, S., Tong, G., Yu, Y., Laghari, A. A., Khan, A., Ibrar, M., & Mehmood, F. (2024). Developments in brain tumor segmentation using MRI: Deep learning insights and future perspectives. *IEEE Access, 12*, 26875–26896. https://www.semanticscholar.org/paper/c5539e51c9f362f94895bef46e89b204e51ef913 (accessed on 31st May 2025).

44. Korhonen, O., Mononen, M., Mohammadian, M., Tenovuo, O., Blennow, K., Hossain, I., Hutchinson, P. J., *et al.* (2023). An outlier analysis for acute blood biomarkers of moderate and severe traumatic brain injury. *Journal of Neurotrauma*. https://www.semanticscholar.org/paper/945eda0eb186685ebcd6aecfc00bf2c47dd36939 (accessed on 31st May 2025).

45. Kremer, S., Lersy, F., De Sèze, J. C., Ferré, J. C., Maamar, A., Carsin-Nicol, B., Collange, O., *et al.* (2020). Brain MRI findings in severe COVID-19: A retrospective observational study. *Radiology, 297*, E242–E251. https://doi.org/10.1148/radiol.2020202222 (accessed on 31st May 2025).

46. Krishnan, G., Singh, S., Pathania, M., Gosavi, S., Abhishek, S., Parchani, A., & Dhar, M. (2023). Artificial intelligence in clinical medicine: Catalyzing a sustainable global healthcare paradigm. *Frontiers in Artificial Intelligence, 6*. https://doi.org/10.3389/frai.2023.1227091 (accessed on 31st May 2025).

47. Kumar, T. A. (2025). Using artificial intelligence, the early detection of neurological disorders through brain imaging and neural data. *International Journal for Research in Applied Science and Engineering Technology*. https://www.semanticscholar.org/paper/a800cb59732693077872f2e948013eb954c4ead9 (accessed on 31st May 2025).

48. LaRovere, K. L., Riggs, B. J., Poussaint, T. Y., Young, C. C., Newhams, M. M., Maamari, M., Walker, T. C., *et al.* (2021). Neurologic involvement in children and adolescents hospitalized in the United States for COVID-19 or multisystem inflammatory syndrome. *JAMA Neurology, 78*, 536. https://doi.org/10.1001/jamaneurol.2021.0504 (accessed on 31st May 2025).

49. Leonardsen, E., Persson, K., Grødem, E., Dinsdale, N., Schellhorn, T., Roe, J. M., Vidal-Piñeiro, D., *et al.* (2024). Constructing personalized characterizations of structural brain aberrations in patients with dementia using explainable artificial intelligence. *NPJ Digital Medicine, 7*. https://www.semanticscholar.org/paper/b88392ffdd5a12849d08d77e782aab92b2747e6f (accessed on 31st May 2025).

50. Leung, J. H., Karmakar, R., Mukundan, A., Lin, W. S., Anwar, F., & Wang, H. C. (2024). Technological frontiers in brain cancer: A systematic review and meta-analysis of hyperspectral imaging in computer-aided diagnosis systems. *Diagnostics, 14*. https://www.semanticscholar.org/paper/e55607a5c8f6781511746f178540fa005690cd3b (accessed on 31st May 2025).

51. Li, G., Deng, L., Tang, H., Pan, G., Tian, Y., Roy, K., & Maass, W. (2024). Brain-inspired computing: A systematic survey and future trends. *Proceedings of the IEEE, 112*, 544–584. https://www.semanticscholar.org/paper/6392c0cd2a9dd6b43ab16d99c58c7796e8242e8f (accessed on 31st May 2025).

52. Lin, D., & Gallagher, A. (2013). Advances in pediatric epilepsy neuroimaging. *Journal of Pediatric Epilepsy, 2*, 1, 2. https://www.semanticscholar.org/paper/4b5ba807daff8ec3186f7847f88b0669a09d4f23 (accessed on 31st May 2025).

53. Litwin, T., Rędzia-Ogrodnik, B., Antos, A., Przybyłkowski, A., Członkowska, A., & Bembenek, J. (2024). Brain magnetic resonance imaging in Wilson's disease—Significance and practical aspects—A narrative review. *Brain Sciences, 14*. https://www.semanticscholar.org/paper/211775197799a10276f4bbd34f31975f08c78fdc (accessed on 31st May 2025).

54. Lövblad, K., Wanke, I., Botta, D., Kurz, F. T., Wiest, R., Rüfenacht, D., & Remonda, L. (2024). Brain health in neuroradiology. *Clinical and Translational Neuroscience*. https://www.semanticscholar.org/paper/85bf58ed5efba80c730bc41b406a6a1bb7f6621b (accessed on 31st May 2025).

55. Mahmoud, A. A. Y., Ahmed, M. K. I., Mohammed, T. H. J., Hani, A. M. M., & Mahmoud, H. M. (2024). Development of magnetic resonance imaging (MRI) techniques for studying neurological changes associated with brain diseases. *European Journal of Medical Genetics and Clinical Biology*. https://www.semanticscholar.org/paper/1ee07ff84f66364da01eacab42e84a71e4aaf697 (accessed on 31st May 2025).

56. Marinković, S., Stošić-Opinćal, T., Štrbac, M., Tomić, I., Tomić, O., & Djordjević, D. M. (2010). Neuroradiology and art: A review and personal contribution. *The Tohoku Journal of Experimental Medicine, 222*(4), 297–302. https://www.semanticscholar.org/paper/055545c6322fd7380da290cfde86b649b4672812 (accessed on 31st May 2025).

57. Modlińska, S., Kufel, J., Janik, M., Czogalik, Ł., Dudek, P., Rojek, M., & Zbroszczyk, M. (2024). Radiation dose during digital subtraction angiography of the brain—The influence of examination parameters and patient factors on the dose. *Brain Sciences, 14*. https://www.semanticscholar.org/paper/7c442b35b6ddf1f7479f8d0086e71e7fa4a62c2d (accessed on 31st May 2025).

58. Morris, G. L. (2008). A clinical guide to epileptic syndromes and their treatment (2nd ed.). *American Journal of Neuroradiology, 29*, e86–e86. https://www.semanticscholar.org/paper/7f088dcb3137e05d822190e5daf6820b060d948d (accessed on 31st May 2025).

59. Murphy, S., & Duhaime, A. (2016). The role of neuroimaging in the diagnosis, treatment, and prognosis of traumatic brain injury in children. *Journal of Pediatric Neuroradiology, 5*, 2–6. https://www.semanticscholar.org/paper/5bc824d9ef5c54c4a58e81eee452215628cf9394 (accessed on 31st May 2025).

60. Najjar, R. (2023). Redefining radiology: A review of artificial intelligence integration in medical imaging. *Diagnostics, 13*, 2760. https://doi.org/10.3390/diagnostics13172760 (accessed on 31st May 2025).

61. Okoye, O., Uche, N., Nwachukwu, N. Z., Udeh, N., & Umeh, R. (2024). Random reflections on medical professionalism: Ethical concerns for the contemporary ophthalmologist in Nigeria. *Nigerian Journal of Ophthalmology*. https://www.semanticscholar.org/paper/25cc5c72eb6db8178a140ff185a8b979053aa9e1 (accessed on 31st May 2025).

62. Oxenberg, O., Fuhrmann, A. G., & Fire, M. (2025). Automatic classification of EEG signals, based on image interpretation of spatio-temporal information. https://www.semanticscholar.org/paper/439ce7064a40bebecfa3397f0d8f0c5f11015a1b (accessed on 31st May 2025).

63. Ozsahin, I., Chen, L., Könik, A., King, M., Beekman, F., & Mok, G. (2020). The clinical utilities of multi-pinhole single photon emission computed tomography. *Quantitative Imaging in Medicine and Surgery, 10*(10), 2006–2029. https://www.semanticscholar.org/paper/61ad8d3997735391faa56551f7f71beb3289f03e (accessed on 31st May 2025).

64. Pati, S., Baid, U., Edwards, B., Sheller, M., Wang, S. H., Reina, G. A., Foley, P., *et al.* (2022). Federated learning enables big data for rare cancer boundary detection. *Nature Communications, 13*. https://doi.org/10.1038/s41467-022-33407-5 (accessed on 31st May 2025).

65. Prayer, D., Malinger, G., De Catte, L., De Keersmaecker, B., Gonçalves, L. F., Kasprian, G., Laifer-Narin, S., *et al.* (2023). ISUOG practice guidelines (updated): Performance of fetal

magnetic resonance imaging. *Ultrasound in Obstetrics and Gynecology, 61*, 278–287. https://doi.org/10.1002/uog.26129 (accessed on 31st May 2025).

66. Rabinowich, A., Shendler, G., Ben-Sira, L., & Shiran, S. (2023). Pediatric low-dose head CT: Image quality improvement using iterative model reconstruction. *The Neuroradiology Journal, 36*, 555–562. https://www.semanticscholar.org/paper/25507befd14e9441cb7f1ae20f5dd82cdd23619a (accessed on 31st May 2025).
67. Rameh, V., Löbel, U., D'Arco, F., Bhatia, A., Mankad, K., Poussaint, T., & Alves, C. A. P. (2024). Cortically-based brain tumors in children: A decision-tree approach in the radiology reading room. *AJNR. American Journal of Neuroradiology*. https://www.semanticscholar.org/paper/0111a15a417ed0c59dc02c693dc5599d5cab142e (accessed on 31st May 2025).
68. Sagnou, M., Mavroidi, B., Shegani, A., Paravatou-Petsotas, M., Raptopoulou, C., Psycharis, V., Pirmettis, I., *et al.* (2019). Remarkable brain penetration of cyclopentadienyl $M(CO)_3^+$ (M = ^{99m}Tc, Re) derivatives of benzothiazole and benzimidazole paves the way for their application as diagnostic, with single-photon-emission computed tomography (SPECT), and therapeutic agents for Alzheimer's disease. *Journal of Medicinal Chemistry, 62*(5), 2638–2650. https://www.semanticscholar.org/paper/9536955071396f0b30e9b169d0104876a4d7b8bb (accessed on 31st May 2025).
69. Schack, A., Aunan-Diop, J. S., Gerhardt, F. A., Pedersen, C. B., Halle, B., Kofoed, M. S., Markovic, L., *et al.* (2024). Evaluating the efficacy of perfusion MRI and conventional MRI in distinguishing recurrent cerebral metastasis from brain radiation necrosis. *Brain Sciences, 14*. https://www.semanticscholar.org/paper/1979dd076cc0ac85a2d505caf2f3a8d0fa80850b (accessed on 31st May 2025).
70. Schramm, S., Börner-Schröder, C., Reichert, M., Ramschütz, C., Androulakis, X., Ashina, M., Coppola, G., *et al.* (2025). Consensus recommendations to establish reporting standards in fMRI of migraine: A Delphi study. *Neurology, 104*(5), e210235. https://www.semanticscholar.org/paper/7a751e34becb6380615633 25fb7fe2fea1b4f814 (accessed on 31st May 2025).
71. Sharpee, T., Destexhe, A., Kawato, M., Sekulić, V., Skinner, F., Wójcik, D., Chintaluri, C., *et al.* (2016). 25th Annual Computational Neuroscience Meeting: CNS-2016. *BMC Neuroscience, 17*. https://www.semanticscholar.org/paper/23a30ca55aef3e307c9e761b22a34080ebf6985f (accessed on 31st May 2025).
72. Spampinato, M. (2012). Neuroimaging and the preterm infant brain. *Journal of Pediatric Neuroradiology, 1*, 69, 70. https://www.semanticscholar.org/paper/e4b2d707aa651b377198cfd5655a6c993986800e (accessed on 31st May 2025).
73. Srikrishna, M., Seo, W., Zettergren, A., Kern, S., Cantré, D., Gessler, F., Sotoudeh, H., *et al.* (2024). Assessing CT-based volumetric analysis via transfer learning with MRI and manual labels for idiopathic normal pressure hydrocephalus. *medRxiv*. https://www.semanticscholar.org/paper/aae3d095788249e12a09a2f27945c1823d5bc7bf (accessed on 31st May 2025).
74. Stafrace, M. M., Psaila, K., & Matthew, M. (2015). *An Unexpected Cause of Palmar Paraesthesia in a Soldier: A Case Report*. https://core.ac.uk/download/46603556.pdf (accessed on 31st May 2025).
75. Sullivan, G., Quigley, A., Choi, S., Teed, R., Blesa, C. M., Vaher, K., Corrigan, A., *et al.* (2024). Brain 3T magnetic resonance imaging in neonates: Features and incidental findings from a research cohort enriched for preterm birth. *Archives of Disease in Childhood. Fetal and Neonatal Edition,*

110. https://www.semanticscholar.org/paper/ab478e0fef07f9ceac2b6088ca1cf748baab4124 (accessed on 31st May 2025).

76. Tariq, A., Iqbal, M. M., Iqbal, M. J., & Ahmad, I. (2025). Transforming brain tumor detection empowering multi-class classification with vision transformers and EfficientNetV2. *IEEE Access, 13*, 63857–63876. https://www.semanticscholar.org/paper/59eb7d91e9a07125154 4b009f89f258bc4ba837c (accessed on 31st May 2025).

77. Tenckhoff, D., Ickenstein, G. W., Klisch, J., Hausn, P., Groß, S., Isenmann, S., & Becker, U. (2010). An empirical analysis of the current need for teleneuromedical care in German hospitals without neurology departments. *International Journal of Telemedicine and Applications.* https://core.ac.uk/download/208292561.pdf (accessed on 31st May 2025).

78. Turc, G., Bhogal, P., Fischer, U., Khatri, P., Lobotesis, K., Mazighi, M., Schellinger, P. D., *et al.* (2019). European Stroke Organization (ESO) – European Society for Minimally Invasive Neurological Therapy (ESMINT) guidelines on mechanical thrombectomy in acute ischemic stroke. *Journal of NeuroInterventional Surgery, 15*, e8–e8. https://doi.org/10.1136/neurintsurg-2018-014569 (accessed on 31st May 2025).

79. Ueda, D., Walston, S., Takita, H., Mitsuyama, Y., & Miki, Y. (2024). The critical need for an open medical imaging database in Japan: Implications for global health and AI development. *Japanese Journal of Radiology, 43*, 537–541. https://www.semanticscholar.org/paper/e8121553c846d27de7b638580d4c662cd755ef61 (accessed on 31st May 2025).

80. Urooj, F., Tameezuddin, A., Khalid, Z., Aftab, K., Bajwa, M. H., Siddiqui, K., Bakhshi, S., *et al.* (2024). Use of artificial intelligence and radiogenomics in neuroradiology and the future of brain tumor imaging and surgical planning in low- and middle-income countries. *JPMA. The Journal of the Pakistan Medical Association, 74*(3, Suppl. 3), S51–S63. https://www.semanticscholar.org/paper/9a06610ae172160af5a183647adff1bc9b5c0bf3 (accessed on 31st May 2025).

81. Vitrio, B., Destefani, V. C., & Destefani, A. C. (2024). Advancing neuroimaging frontiers: A comprehensive review of novel diagnostic techniques in neuroradiology and their clinical applications. *Brazilian Journal of Implantology and Health Sciences*. https://www.semanticscholar.org/paper/355651ac57197a8c833308567db32cf7d9023b86 (accessed on 31st May 2025).

82. Yan, D., Yuan, K., Chen, Y., Zheng, K., Han, H., Li, Z., Zhang, H., *et al.* (2024). Risk factors for delayed postoperative hemorrhage in patients with brain arteriovenous malformations: An analysis of the nationwide multicenter prospective registry MATCH study. *Journal of Neurosurgery*. https://www.semanticscholar.org/paper/be07c8deb7bde2d620e716be2e9ccfa1f2574602 (accessed on 31st May 2025).

83. Yaroslavska, S., Korsak, A. V., & Litvynova, L. V. (2024). Multidisciplinary approach to the treatment of traumatic brain injury in children and rehabilitation. *Ukrainian Interventional Neuroradiology and Surgery*. https://www.semanticscholar.org/paper/9c3b5742580fd1dfca 9ae69a4af333a85011c945 (accessed on 31st May 2025).

NEURORADIOLOGY–SPINE

4

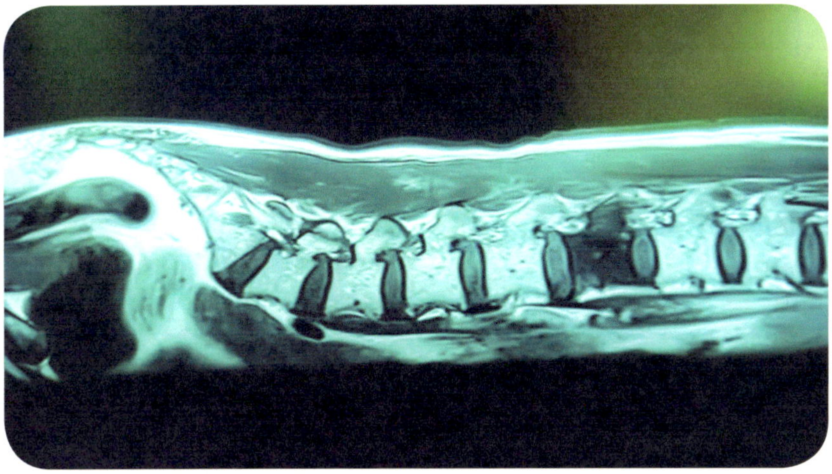

LEARNING OBJECTIVES

After studying this chapter, you will be able to:

1. Identify common spinal disorders diagnosed by neuroradiology;
2. Explain the interpretation of spinal imaging;
3. Focus on advances and innovations in neuroradiology.

Introduction

New medical imaging and surgery methods have greatly changed how spinal problems are handled. Being a complex structure, the spine has special difficulties because its nerves and bones are so detailed, and these need to be seen clearly for proper treatment. In this situation, neuroradiology is very important because it offers detailed imaging that helps find and assess different spinal issues such as trauma, degenerative diseases, and tumors like Ewing sarcoma. This malignant tumor, predominantly affecting younger populations, underscores the necessity of accurate imaging for early diagnosis and optimal treatment planning, including surgery, chemotherapy, and radiotherapy (Sakhrekar *et al.*, 2024). Additionally, recent technological advancements like robot-assisted spine surgery have enhanced the precision of interventions, reducing operative risks and improving patient outcomes through superior imaging integration and surgical navigation (Qi *et al.*, 2025). All of these changes underline the role neuroradiology plays in improving spine care.

Better medical imaging has greatly helped in finding and treating spinal issues, which has led to the development of specialized areas focusing on the complex anatomy of the spine. Neuroradiology is focused on radiology imaging and the interpretation of the brain, spine, and other parts of the nervous system. Its scope extends beyond traditional radiography to employ sophisticated techniques such as magnetic resonance imaging (MRI), computed tomography (CT), and digital subtraction angiography, enabling detailed visualization of spinal pathologies. It is important in this field to find structural issues and plan minimally invasive surgeries, which highlights the value of precise images in managing patients. The practical application of neuroradiology requires stringent attention to radiation safety and procedural protocols to mitigate risks, as highlighted by guidelines addressing radiation exposure incidents in diagnostic and interventional settings (Damilakis *et al.*, 2017). Neuroradiology today uses advanced technology and puts safety first, which strengthens its role in caring for the spine.

Importance of Spinal Imaging

Good diagnosis and treatment of spine problems depend greatly on detailed spinal imaging methods. Dynamic radiographs, CT, and MRI are radiologic tests that each provide important and different information needed to assess lumbar spinal stenosis and guide the decision on whether to perform open surgery or less invasive procedures. The ability to visualize canal dimensions, spinal deformities, and facet joint conditions across multiple planes enables clinicians to tailor interventions precisely, minimizing unnecessary tissue disruption and improving patient outcomes (Hartman *et al.*, 2019). Furthermore, advanced imaging plays a crucial role in differentiating complex inflammatory myelopathies, such as myelin oligodendrocyte glycoprotein antibody (MOG-IgG) myelitis, from other similar disorders like aquaporin-4-IgG myelitis and multiple sclerosis. Detailed MRI characteristics, including lesion location, signal abnormalities, and enhancement patterns, provide critical diagnostic clues, influencing both prognosis and treatment strategies (Dubey *et al.*, 2018). Thus, spinal imaging remains indispensable in neuroradiology, facilitating early detection, accurate diagnosis, and personalized management of spinal diseases (Figure 4.1).

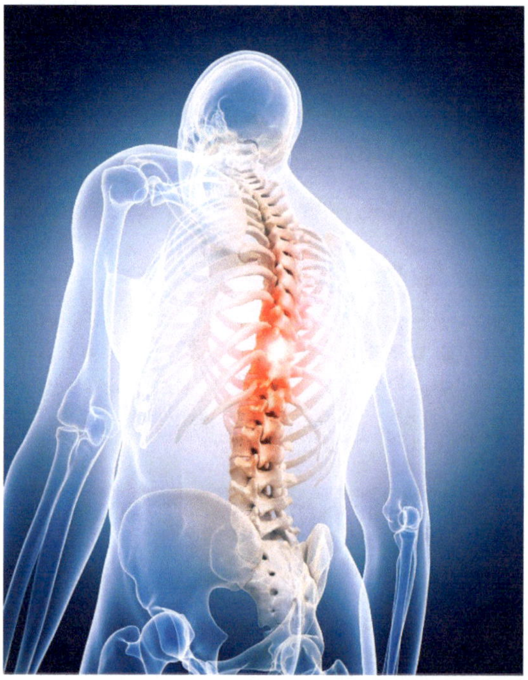

Figure 4.1. Accurate diagnosis and effective treatment of spinal pathologies rely heavily on comprehensive spinal imaging techniques.

Source: https://neurosurgeonindore.in/wp-content/uploads/2024/07/Spine-1-1160x1450-1.jpg.

Overview of Spinal Anatomy

Knowing how the spine is built helps with interpreting images taken for neuroradiological assessment. There are vertebrae, intervertebral discs, ligaments, and neural elements in the spine, and each one helps support and function the spine. The spinal cord is protected by the vertebrae, which form a canal, and the intervertebral discs allow the spine to bend and absorb shocks. Detailed knowledge of these components enhances the ability to detect pathological changes such as disc herniations or Modic changes—vertebral endplate and bone marrow alterations visible on MRI—that are linked to clinical symptoms like low back pain (Andersen *et al.*, 2022). Additionally, the lumbar spine's susceptibility to degenerative conditions, including disc herniation with radiculopathy, emphasizes the importance of correlating clinical evaluation with imaging findings for effective management strategies (Kalantaite *et al.*, 2024). So, knowing spinal anatomy well is necessary for the accurate reading and use of neuroradiologic tests.

Common Spinal Disorders

Spinal disorders are usually hard to diagnose because they have many causes and similar symptoms. Pain in the facet joints is very common and makes up a large portion of chronic back pain in the cervical, thoracic, and lumbar areas. In many cases, these syndromes are caused by degenerative changes such as osteoarthritis and hypertrophied joint processes, and sometimes these are made worse by infections or inflammation, like septic arthritis.

Patients may have local pain or radicular symptoms if joint cysts or enlarged joints put pressure on the nerves. Even with obvious changes in the structure, pain may not always match the findings on images, which often means nerve blocks or joint injections are needed to diagnose and treat the condition properly. Behçet's syndrome and similar inflammatory disorders can lead to problems in the spinal cord, such as meningoencephalitis and vascular inflammation, which can create neurological problems and other symptoms. Understanding the pathophysiology, guided by neuroradiological assessment, is crucial for tailored therapeutic strategies and improved patient outcomes (Kidd, 2023; Yoo *et al.*, 2023) (Figure 4.2).

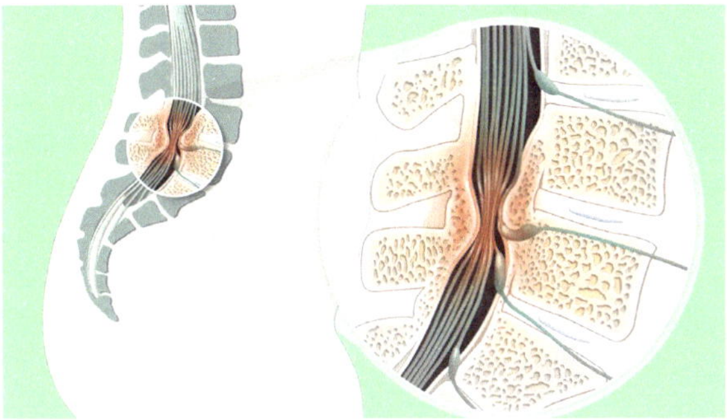

Figure 4.2. Spinal disorders often present a complex diagnostic challenge due to their diverse etiologies and overlapping clinical manifestations.

Source: https://osteomag.ca/wp-content/uploads/2019/12/for-baby-boomer-back-surgery-is-often-good-news-1440x810-1.webp.

Role of Neuroradiology in Diagnosis

Using advanced imaging methods has made it possible for clinicians to spot and describe many spinal problems with exceptional accuracy. Neuroradiology helps a lot by clearly showing images of the vertebrae, intervertebral discs, spinal cord and nerve roots in the spine. Finding out about herniated discs, spinal stenosis, tumors and inflammatory diseases is possible with the help of MRI and CT scans. They help in early detection and also show doctors the extent and type of lesions which guides their choice of treatment. Neuroradiology is also important for telling apart the causes of spinal symptoms, whether they are from degeneration or injury, which improves the accuracy of the diagnosis. Thanks to these contributions, neuroradiology greatly helps manage patients and achieve better results, proving its essential part in modern spinal care.

Advancements in Imaging Technology

Advances in medical technology have boosted the ability of neuroradiology, especially in examining the spine. Because of MRI and CT, doctors can now see deeper into the spine, which helps with accurate diagnosis and treatment decisions. Moreover, the integration of artificial intelligence (AI) into imaging technology has revolutionized the field by automating image segmentation, enhancing computer-aided diagnosis, and optimizing workflow efficiency. AI-driven tools contribute to reducing interpretation times and improving diagnostic accuracy, addressing the increasing demand for quality healthcare amidst clinician workload challenges (Krishnan *et al.*, 2023). Additionally, machine learning and deep learning algorithms enable predictive analytics that personalize patient management and improve outcomes in spinal disorders (Najjar, 2023b). These advancements underscore a paradigm shift where technological innovation and interdisciplinary collaboration are essential in advancing spinal neuroradiology and improving patient care (Figure 4.3).

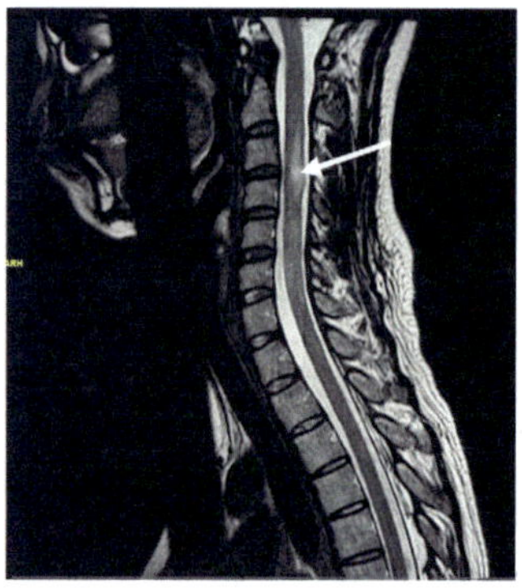

Figure 4.3. Recent developments in medical technology have significantly enhanced the capabilities of neuroradiology, particularly in spinal imaging.

Source: https://pub.mdpi-res.com/neurosci/neurosci-05-00006/article_deploy/html/images/neurosci-05-00006-g001.png?1710299546.

4.1. Common Spinal Disorders Diagnosed by Neuroradiology

Learning Outcome

1. Understand herniated discs;
2. Explain spinal stenosis;
3. Focus on spondylolisthesis and spinal tumors;
4. Know degenerative disc disease;
5. Identify infections of the spine;
6. Focus on spinal cord injuries;
7. Understand congenital spinal abnormalities;
8. Learn post-surgical complications.

Because symptoms of spinal disorders are often confused, advanced imaging is usually needed to make a correct diagnosis. Neuroradiology is important for finding conditions such as spinal cord ischemia and facet joint pathologies, which may be missed with regular examinations. For example, problems in the blood vessels of the neck can be hard to find because the symptoms and usual images are often similar to those of inflammatory or compressed disorders. In such cases, digital subtraction angiography proves indispensable when computed tomography angiography and magnetic resonance angiography fail to yield definitive results, thereby preventing misdiagnosis and guiding timely treatment (Intikhab *et al.*, 2024). Just like in the discs, degeneration in the facet joints is a major cause of ongoing back pain, especially when osteoarthritis grows in the articular processes or forms cysts, which can compress nerves and lead to radiating pain. Neuroradiological assessment assists in differentiating these disorders and informing therapeutic interventions such as joint injections or surgical decompression (Yoo *et al.*, 2023).

4.1.1. Herniated Discs

Better neuroradiological imaging has made it easier to diagnose and treat spinal problems, especially herniated discs. Such disc herniations can pinch nearby nerves, which is often seen as pain in the affected area or as radiculopathy. Magnetic resonance imaging (MRI) remains the gold standard for visualizing disc morphology and neural involvement due to its superior soft tissue contrast. Recent studies employing high-resolution MRI techniques, including magnetic resonance neurography, have demonstrated increased signal intensity in compressed cervical spinal nerves, correlating with radicular symptoms and aiding in the assessment of multilevel disc disease (Dailey *et al.*, 1996). Also, procedures like nucleoplasty have demonstrated good results in patients who used to be treated surgically for large disc extrusions. Post-treatment MRI evaluations indicate a reduction in disc expulsion and significant pain relief, supporting less invasive approaches in selected cases (Borelli *et al.*, 2018). These findings underscore the critical role of advanced imaging in guiding both diagnosis and treatment strategies for herniated discs (Figure 4.4).

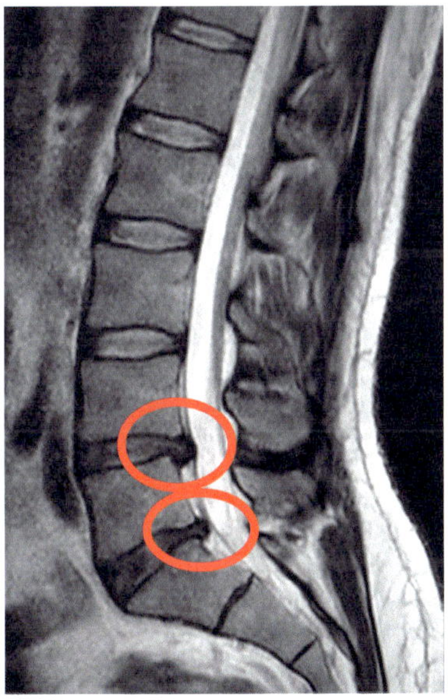

Figure 4.4. Herniated discs.

Source: https://upload.wikimedia.org/wikipedia/commons/8/84/Hernie_discale_L4_L5.png.

4.1.2. Spinal Stenosis

Many times, degenerative changes in the spine result in health problems that affect the nerves, and spinal stenosis is a common and important example. A narrowed spinal canal or neural foramina may happen because of hypertrophic ligamentum flavum, facet joint arthropathy, or disc herniation, which can put pressure on the spinal cord or nerve roots. MRI and CT myelography are important tools for identifying and describing stenotic areas, allowing doctors to distinguish between central, lateral recess, and foraminal stenosis. The results from imaging help decide the treatment approach, which can be conservative or involve surgery. Also, small signs on imaging, such as missing epidural fat and less cerebrospinal fluid, help determine the extent of nerve damage. Contemporary neuroradiology thus plays a pivotal role in spinal stenosis evaluation, guiding clinical decision-making while improving patient outcomes through precise anatomical delineation (Figure 4.5).

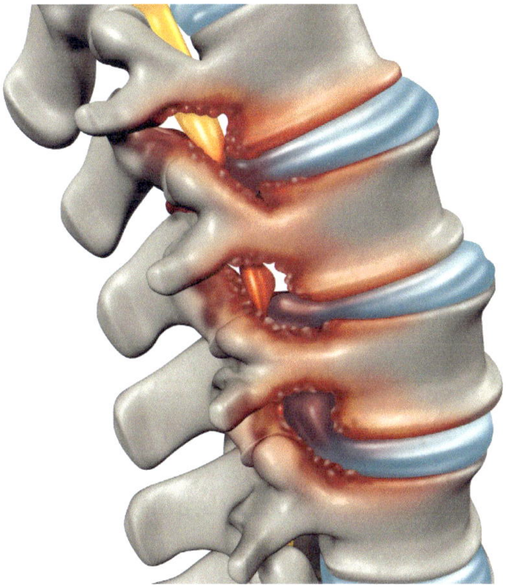

Figure 4.5. Spinal stenosis.

Source: https://deintegrativehealthcare.com/wp-content/uploads/2021/01/Spinal-stenosis.jpg.

4.1.3. Spondylolisthesis

When the spine has structural problems that affect nerves, accurate imaging is very important for diagnosis. For example, spondylolisthesis, which is when one vertebra slides forward relative to the one below, might result in serious instability of the spine and pressure on the nerves. Advanced neuroradiological techniques such as MRI and computed tomography (CT) are indispensable for identifying the degree of vertebral slippage and assessing associated degenerative changes, including osteophyte formation and canal stenosis, which frequently coexist with spondylolisthesis.

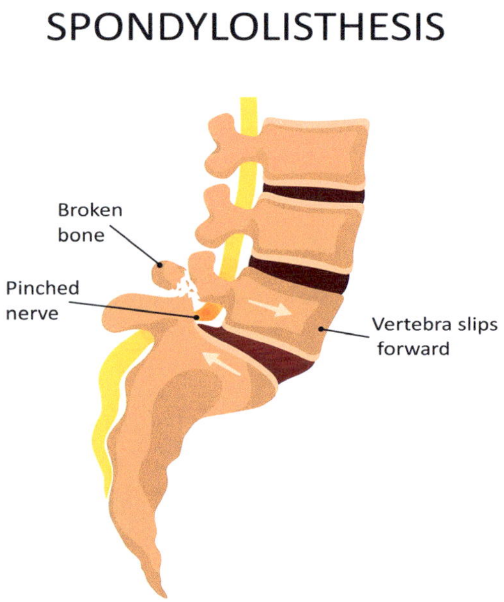

Figure 4.6. Spondylolisthesis.

Source: https://wexnermedical.osu.edu/-/media/images/wexnermedical/pages/patient-care/healthcare-services/brain-spine-neuro/spine/spondylolisthesis.jpg.

They help to show not only the position of bones but also any damage to soft tissues or nerves, which helps choose the best treatment. With increasing age, degenerative processes including spondylolisthesis become more prevalent, often correlating with adjacent disc disease and neurogenic symptoms, as observed in clinical and electromyographic evaluations (Armesto Pérez *et al.*, 2020). The integration of imaging findings with clinical symptoms facilitates a comprehensive approach to spinal disorders, underscoring the importance of CT and MRI as complementary tools in neuroradiology (García Espinosa *et al.*, 2022) (Figure 4.6).

4.1.4. Spinal Tumors

Better imaging methods have improved the way doctors diagnose and manage serious problems of the spine. Spinal tumors are different from others because they have many possible origins, can be located anywhere along the spine, and may harm neural structures. It is important to use neuroradiology to distinguish between intradural and extradural lesions and also to identify primary tumors from metastatic tumors. MRI is the best method for seeing soft tissue clearly, which helps identify the edges of tumors, involvement of the spinal cord, and surrounding swelling. Also, contrast-enhanced sequences help doctors understand the blood vessels in tumors and their aggressiveness, which influences treatment plans. CT is useful for showing bone destruction and calcifications more clearly, which are often found in vertebral metastases or primary bone tumors. A thorough examination of imaging helps both in understanding the stage of the tumor and in planning minimally invasive treatments and surgeries, which benefits the patient's outcome.

4.1.5. Degenerative Disc Disease

New imaging methods have helped a lot in understanding and treating spine problems, mainly in those where the structure worsens over time. Among these, degenerative disc disease (DDD) represents a prevalent cause of chronic low back pain, necessitating thorough neuroradiological evaluation. Magnetic resonance imaging remains the cornerstone for assessing disc integrity, yet emerging techniques such as PET/CT with 18F-fluorodeoxyglucose and 18F-sodium fluoride provide valuable metabolic insights into early disc degeneration, potentially improving diagnostic accuracy before gross morphological changes become evident (Teichner *et al.*, 2025). Clinically, patient history and physical examination are paramount in guiding diagnosis and treatment, as imaging findings often do not directly correlate with symptom severity (Beyer *et al.*, 2025). Conservative approaches are usually tried first, but surgery, such as decompression or fusion, may be needed for severe cases, although there is not much scientific proof backing up the many surgical procedures. Thus, integrating advanced imaging with clinical assessment is essential for optimizing individualized care in DDD within neuroradiological practice (Beyer *et al.*, 2025; Teichner *et al.*, 2025) (Figure 4.7).

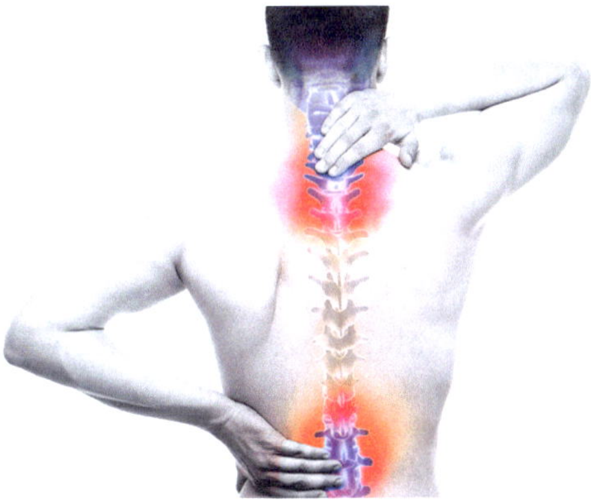

Figure 4.7. Degenerative disc disease.

Source: https://complete-physio.co.uk/wp-content/uploads/2023/04/image-2-1.png.

4.1.6. Infections of the Spine

Due to their ability to result in major neurological problems and a long treatment period, spinal infections are a serious clinical challenge. Neuroradiological methods are used to diagnose these infections and show how much the vertebrae and discs are affected, which guides the selection of treatment. MRI images are important for checking inflammation, abscess formation, and damage to the structure, which are all necessary for planning the best treatment. Patients are usually treated with antibiotics for a long time, often given through central catheters placed in a vein in the arm, which allows them to stay at home and visit the hospital less. Studies have demonstrated the safety and efficacy of such outpatient intravenous regimens, particularly for elderly populations infected with common pathogens like Staphylococcus species, resulting in favorable clinical and radiographic outcomes without catheter-related complications (Berlis *et al.*, 2024). In addition, progress in neuroradiology, such as three-dimensional augmented reality and better imaging techniques, keeps helping to diagnose and understand spinal infections related to cerebrovascular and neuroinflammatory disorders.

4.1.7. Spinal Cord Injuries (SCI)

Improvements in imaging have made it much easier to diagnose and treat SCI, especially in children, since clinical exams can be tough. High-resolution 3T MRI and advanced deep learning methods have made it possible for recent studies to discover structural changes in the spinal cord, such as differences in its cross-sectional area and dimensions, very accurately. They make it possible to tell apart ordinary development from long-term injury and to assess the severity of any injury, which supports proper treatment and forecasting of outcomes. Besides SCI from trauma, neuroradiology also covers serious conditions like metastatic epidural spinal cord compression. Using MRI and new methods such as diffusion-weighted imaging and PET-MRI helps detect problems early, which is key to preventing major damage to the brain from tumor pressure. Collectively, these innovations underscore the central role of advanced imaging in improving patient outcomes in diverse spinal cord pathologies (Kasat *et al.*, 2024; Sadeghi-Adl *et al.*, 2025) (Figure 4.8).

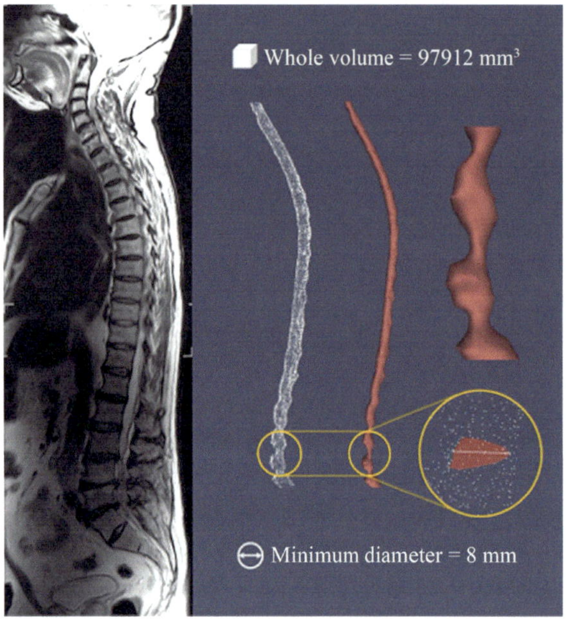

Figure 4.8. Utilizing high-resolution 3T MRI and sophisticated deep learning algorithms, recent studies have demonstrated the capacity to detect structural changes in the spinal cord, such as alterations in cross-sectional area and dimensions, with remarkable accuracy.

Source: https://www.ejradiology.com/cms/10.1016/j.ejrad.2023.110726/asset/0f3d4610-e289-4560-b9b8-04e988bca2cf/main.assets/gr4_lrg.jpg.

4.1.8. Congenital Spinal Abnormalities

Better imaging techniques have made it easier to find and evaluate congenital spinal problems early on, which helps doctors manage them more accurately. A lot of these malformations affect the lower part of the spine and may result in various neurological, orthopedic, and urologic problems. Nevertheless, differences in the way diseases are described and in the technology used have made it harder to diagnose and treat patients in the past. Using standardized procedures with plain radiography, sonography, computed tomography, and magnetic resonance imaging helps improve the accuracy of diagnosis and supports the right treatment decisions. Also, following specialized training and guidelines for pediatric neuroradiology helps ensure that imaging for congenital spinal malformations in children is done safely and effectively. Such structured approaches foster multidisciplinary collaboration and support consistent, evidence-based decision-making in clinical care, thereby minimizing morbidity associated with these complex abnormalities (Adamsbaum *et al.*, 2022; Balani *et al.*, 2024).

4.1.9. Post-surgical Complications

Since spinal surgeries for tumors or abnormalities are very complex, they can lead to a number of post-surgical problems that must be closely watched. A major issue is neurological deterioration, which can happen because of spinal cord swelling, decreased blood flow, or accidental injury during the procedure. In disorders such as Mucopolysaccharidosis IVA, where spinal instability and cord compression are prevalent, post-operative management involves careful imaging surveillance to detect early signs of deterioration and prevent irreversible deficits (Goel *et al.*, 2013). Additionally, intraoperative techniques like preoperative embolization are employed to mitigate complications such as excessive bleeding, which can complicate recovery and prolong hospitalization (Ashour *et al.*, 2013). Even with these steps, infections, hardware problems, and cerebrospinal fluid leaks are still big issues. Radiological modalities, including MRI and CT, play indispensable roles in the timely identification of these complications, facilitating prompt intervention and improving patient outcomes in spinal neuroradiology (Figure 4.9).

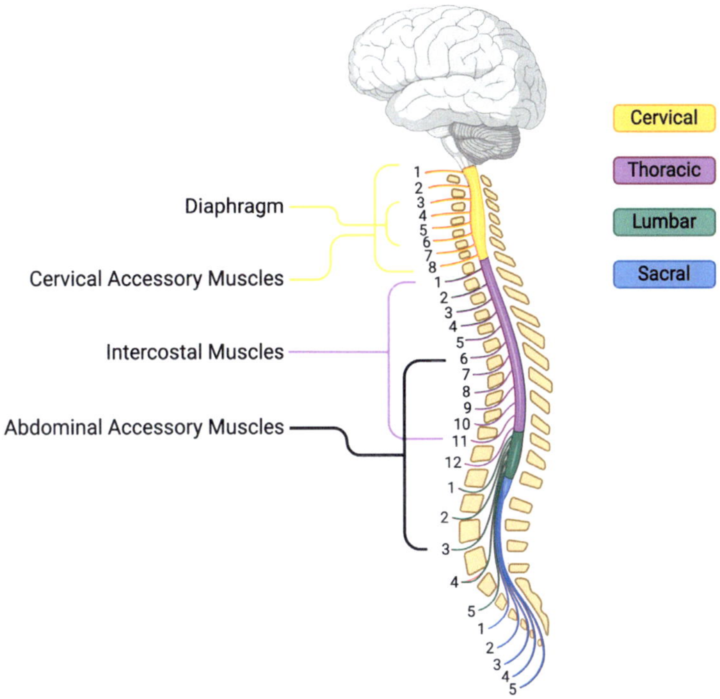

Figure 4.9. Neurological deterioration is a prominent concern, often arising from spinal cord edema, ischemia, or inadvertent injury during the procedure.

Source: https://www.mdpi.com/cells/cells-14-00288/article_deploy/html/images/cells-14-00288-g001.png.

Test Your Knowledge

1. What is the condition called spondylolisthesis, and how can it be found on imaging?
2. What can an MRI show about spinal stenosis, and what are the usual symptoms it causes?

4.2. Interpretation of Spinal Imaging

Learning Outcome

1. Understand the radiologist's role in diagnosis;
2. Identify key imaging features;
3. Know the differential diagnosis process;
4. Write the importance of clinical correlation;
5. Report findings effectively;
6. Focus on the use of imaging in treatment planning;
7. Understand a multidisciplinary approach to care;
8. Identify challenges in interpretation;
9. Learn case studies in spinal imaging.

Accurately diagnosing problems of the spine and spinal cord depends on knowing the anatomy and common diseases of the spinal column. Radiologists have to distinguish between normal variations and diseases, like lesions, degenerative problems, or injuries. Because MRI and CT give detailed images of soft tissues and bones, they help find small problems that may not be seen in regular X-rays. Also, linking what is seen on imaging with the patient's symptoms helps doctors choose the best treatment and management strategies. Because of high-resolution imaging, recent neuroradiological studies can clearly show spinal cord lesions and vertebral abnormalities, which help in deciding how to treat patients. Also, as imaging technology keeps advancing, it becomes easier to identify early signs of degeneration and problems in the blood vessels of the spinal canal, showing how spinal imaging interpretation is changing in healthcare.

4.2.1. Radiologist's Role in Diagnosis

To properly diagnose issues of the spine, imaging techniques are needed, and radiologists are key to the process of managing patients in neuroradiology. Their expertise enables differentiation among complex conditions such as chronic nonbacterial osteomyelitis, where vertebral and mandibular manifestations require careful assessment to prevent diagnostic delays and facilitate timely treatment (Silva *et al.*, 2024). Radiologists rely on modalities such as MRI and CT to assess the form of lesions and any inflammation, which is important for knowing how far and how fast the disease is spreading. Furthermore, the integration of functional imaging approaches like FDG PET-CT enhances diagnostic precision in infections such as spondylodiscitis, allowing for metabolic evaluation alongside anatomical visualization, which aids in targeted interventions and monitoring therapeutic response (Diana Páez *et al.*, 2024). Thus, the radiologist's interpretative skills ensure the synthesis of diverse imaging data, guiding clinicians toward accurate diagnosis and personalized care strategies in spinal neuroradiology (Figure 4.10).

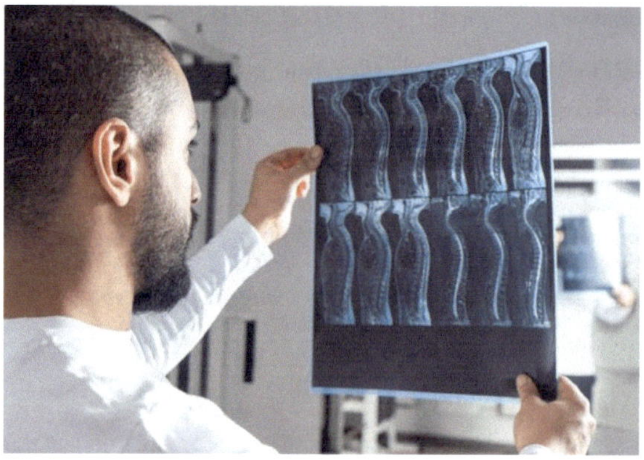

Figure 4.10. Accurate diagnosis of spinal pathologies often hinges on advanced imaging techniques interpreted by radiologists, who play a critical role in patient management within neuroradiology.

Source: https://www.chennaispinecare.com/wp-content/uploads/2024/05/Role-of-Imaging-in-Spinal-Conditions.jpg.

4.2.2. Identifying Key Imaging Features

The accurate diagnosis and prognosis in neuroradiology depend on finding important imaging features that show the underlying disease. MRI allows clinicians to clearly see the spinal structures and find small changes in the tissues and diseases. For instance, radiomic analysis from T2-weighted imaging has been shown to emphasize the significance of peritumoral edematous regions in differentiating tumor characteristics, demonstrating the potential of integrating quantitative imaging biomarkers to enhance predictive accuracy (Usuzaki *et al.*, 2024). Similarly, assessing specific imaging features such as intralesional hemorrhage and tumor morphology can provide critical prognostic information, as evidenced in studies of pineal region tumors where hemorrhage strongly correlates with poorer outcomes (Peng *et al.*, 2024). Such cases prove that the best way to read imaging data in spinal neuroradiology is to combine examining the spine's structure with radiomic and clinical information to improve diagnosis and treatment decisions.

4.2.3. Differential Diagnosis Process

Managing spinal problems in the clinic requires precise differential diagnosis, which depends on getting a good patient history, conducting a physical exam, and using advanced imaging. It is very important in neuroradiology of the spine to tell apart infectious, traumatic, neoplastic, and degenerative conditions, since they can all have similar symptoms. For instance, spinal tuberculosis, a frequently overlooked etiology in endemic areas, may mimic malignancy or degenerative changes on imaging; thus, careful assessment of characteristic radiologic findings, such as vertebral body involvement and epidural abscess formation, is essential to avoid misdiagnosis and delayed treatment (Sunwar *et al.*, 2025). Additionally, innovative computational tools like DEEP-Spine facilitate more accurate classification and localization of vertebral fractures, addressing current challenges in manual image interpretation by reducing subjectivity and improving diagnostic accuracy through automation (Li *et al.*, 2024). These advancements collectively enhance the differential diagnosis process, supporting timely and targeted therapeutic strategies in spinal neuroradiology (Figure 4.11).

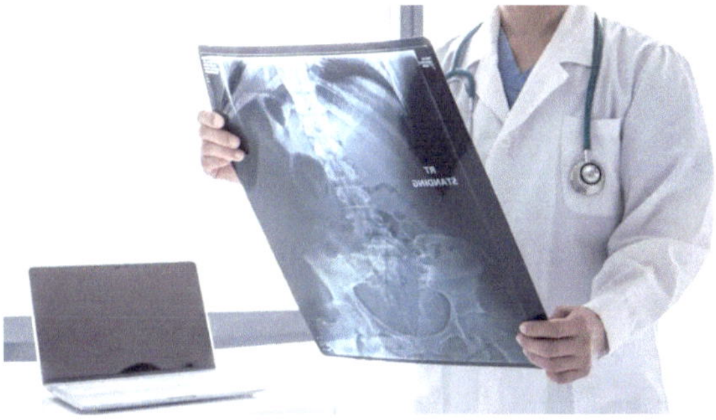

Figure 4.11. Effective clinical management of spinal pathologies relies heavily on a precise differential diagnosis process, which necessitates a thorough integration of patient history, physical examination, and advanced imaging techniques.

Source: https://chblob.icloudhospital.com/thumbnails/2-eb00ba04-a6cb-4744-8019-807c2d04bf3f.webp.

4.2.4. Importance of Clinical Correlation

It is very important in spinal imaging in neuroradiology to combine advanced imaging with what is found in clinical exams to avoid errors and provide the best care for patients. Radiological images can show many changes in the body, but without connecting them with the patient's symptoms, the results might not be interpreted correctly, which could result in ineffective care. For instance, the utilization of artificial intelligence in image analysis enhances detection accuracy and workflow efficiency, but it remains crucial to interpret these results within the patient's clinical context to ensure relevance and individualized care (Najjar, 2023a). Similarly, while deep learning tools demonstrate impressive accuracy in identifying hemorrhages or other abnormalities, the ultimate value of neuroradiological findings depends on their alignment with clinical symptoms and physical examination (Chang *et al.*, 2018). Because of this, clinical correlation connects what is seen in images to what needs to be done in patient care, ensuring effective management of spinal neuroradiology.

4.2.5. Reporting Findings Effectively

Clear communication of neuroradiological results is very important for the correct diagnosis and best treatment of patients with spine problems. If reports are well-organized, clear, and meet the needs of referring clinicians, it becomes easier for everyone to work together.

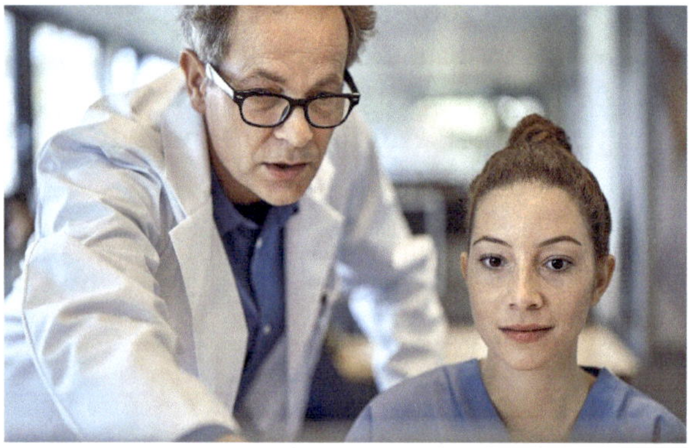

Figure 4.12. Effective communication of neuroradiological findings is crucial for accurate diagnosis and optimal patient management, particularly in spine imaging.

Source: https://www.philips.co.in/c-dam/b2bhc/master/Specialties/oncology-specialty-page/challenge-pages/orchestrating-clear-pathways/oncology-header-image.jpg.

Recent studies indicate a preference among healthcare providers for structured reporting formats over traditional free-text narratives, as they enhance readability and make critical information more accessible by reducing ambiguity and unnecessary sections (Lee *et al.*, 2025). In complex spine cases, this method is very important to clearly describe the abnormalities found and the results after surgery. Additionally, integrating quantitative data such as pain scores or postoperative assessments derived from clinical studies can further contextualize imaging findings, aiding in comprehensive patient care planning (Guan *et al.*, 2024). Thus, standardizing report structures and emphasizing clarity not only streamlines clinical workflows but also improves the practical utility of neuroradiological evaluations in spine pathology (Figure 4.12).

4.2.6. Use of Imaging in Treatment Planning

Better imaging tools have greatly improved how treatment is planned in spinal neuroradiology. By using MRI and CT scans, clinicians can clearly see the spinal anatomy and detect disc herniations, tumors, and vascular issues, which are necessary for planning the proper treatment. They help doctors make a clear diagnosis and also guide surgeons in less invasive procedures, which lowers patient risk and results in better outcomes. Also, using images during surgery allows doctors to see the brain and nearby tissues in real time, making sure the treatment is delivered correctly. Using advanced imaging in spinal care shows a move towards personalized medicine, focusing on the unique aspects of each patient's condition. New, high-quality imaging methods are being developed, which are needed for more advanced treatments in spinal neuroradiology.

4.2.7. Multidisciplinary Approach to Care

Optimizing patient outcomes from spinal pathologies now depends on involving several medical specialties. Because spinal disorders can be complex, neuroradiologists often work with neurologists, neurosurgeons, physiatrists, rehabilitation specialists, and radiologists to give patients the best possible care. Using this approach, the findings from imaging are related to the patient's overall health, which helps with choosing and monitoring the right treatments. Also, having teams with different but complementary skills helps ensure safety and success in advanced procedures, which is important in modern neuroradiology. In pediatric cases, the necessity for coordinated care is even more pronounced, with recommendations underscoring the need for well-organized teams proficient in pediatric neuroradiology's unique imaging protocols and safety considerations (Adamsbaum *et al.*, 2022). By fostering collaborative decision-making, this integrated model ultimately elevates the standard of care in spinal neuroradiology (Figure 4.13).

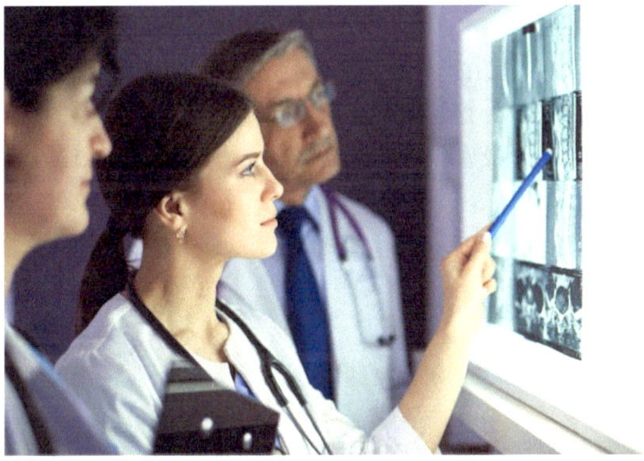

Figure 4.13. Within neuroradiology, the complexity of spinal disorders demands collaboration among radiologists, neurologists, neurosurgeons, physiatrists, and rehabilitation specialists to provide comprehensive diagnosis and tailored treatment plans.

Source: https://cdn.prod.website-files.com/652e8c998f656fbf00cb7c99/666642fcd6d5a0d4203cc5a8_group-doctors-hospital-xray-diagnostics_358354-8670.jpeg.

4.2.8. Challenges in Interpretation

Reading spinal neuroradiological images correctly is often difficult, which can affect the accuracy of the diagnosis, and how patients are treated. Because of many similarities in anatomy, subtle signs of disease, and overlapping images, it can be difficult to distinguish between normal variants and diseases. For instance, distinguishing ligament ruptures, syringomyelia, or minor vertebral fractures requires a nuanced understanding and experience, as misinterpretation can lead to diagnostic errors, as highlighted by common mistakes in these areas reported during radiographer evaluations (Piper *et al.*, 2018). Also, using different imaging techniques, settings, and ways patients are placed can change the appearance and quality of the images, making things more difficult. Because of advanced imaging, it is important that radiologists get thorough training to avoid errors and improve their accuracy. Despite high sensitivity and specificity achieved through specialized education, ongoing efforts remain essential to refine expertise in spinal neuroradiology interpretation to ensure reliable clinical application (Piper *et al.*, 2018).

4.2.9. Case Studies in Spinal Imaging

Better spinal imaging techniques have made it easier to diagnose and treat complicated spine problems, as shown by different case studies. A clinical study looking back at canine degenerative lumbosacral stenosis showed that detailed imaging helped surgeons decide on dorsal laminectomy, annulectomy, and distraction stabilization. This procedure significantly increased foraminal width and improved clinical outcomes, underscoring the importance of precise imaging metrics in pre- and post-operative assessment (Inness *et al.*, 2021). Similarly, in the context of spinal metastases, case series utilizing advanced imaging modalities have been crucial in evaluating the efficacy of separation surgery followed by stereotactic radiosurgery (SRS). Despite challenges such as imaging artifacts and variability in technique, these studies demonstrated promising local tumor control rates and emphasized the utility of neuroradiological evaluation in tailoring minimally invasive yet effective treatment protocols (Fisher *et al.*, 2013). All of these case studies highlight how spinal imaging supports better decisions for patients in neuroradiology.

Test Your Knowledge

1. What part does imaging play in both diagnosing and monitoring syringomyelia?
2. How does spondylosis (degenerative disc disease) manifest on MRI or CT scans?

4.3. Advances and Innovations in Neuroradiology

Learning Outcome

1. Understand artificial intelligence in imaging;
2. Explain 3D imaging techniques;
3. Focus on enhanced imaging resolution;
4. Learn tele-radiology applications;
5. Discuss integration of imaging with other modalities;
6. Focus on personalized medicine in spinal disorders;
7. Discuss research in spinal imaging;
8. Know the impact of technology on patient outcomes;
9. Describe ethical considerations in neuroradiology.

New developments in medical imaging have greatly changed neuroradiology, especially for spinal problems and treatments. Thanks to better MRI and CT scans, doctors can now see the spine and its problems more clearly, which helps with early diagnosis and better treatment. Innovations like diffusion tensor imaging (DTI) and functional MRI further augment the ability to assess neural integrity and functional status, critical for complex spinal cases. Also, using artificial intelligence and machine learning has made it possible to analyze images automatically and group patients by risk, which leads to , more accurate, and efficient diagnosis. Thanks to these progresses, both the effectiveness of treatment and the number of invasive procedures are improving. The current trend is to use less invasive procedures guided by images, which allows for safer procedures. These transformative technologies exemplify the dynamic evolution in spine neuroradiology, reinforcing its pivotal role in comprehensive spinal care (Figure 4.14).

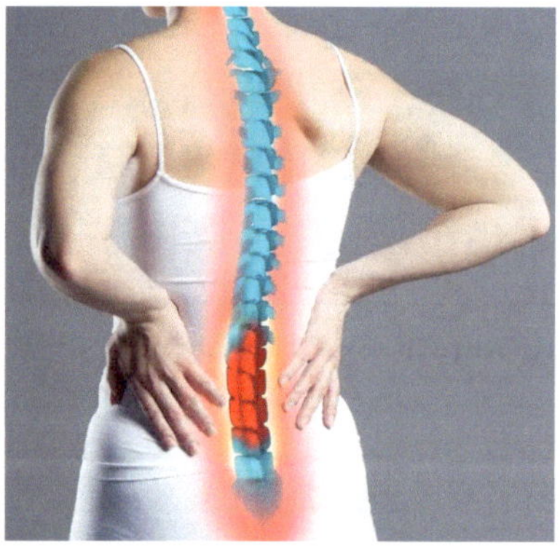

Figure 4.14. Diffusion tensor imaging (DTI) of the spine.

Source: https://spinecenteratlanta.com/wp-content/uploads/2022/10/f8c6ccd05dc702d8f07f5a4307165613.png.

4.3.1. Artificial Intelligence (AI) in Imaging

Neuroradiology, which deals with images of the spine, has been greatly influenced by recent technological changes. AI is changing the way images are taken, improved, and interpreted, which leads to better diagnoses and more efficient care. AI helps analyze detailed imaging data, which makes it easier to find issues and decide on the best approach for each patient before surgery. AI also helps during surgery by guiding surgeons and offering assistance with decisions, and it is used postoperatively to monitor outcomes and help with patient care. Yet, issues still exist in making AI algorithms clear and in the ethics of the industry using data. Increasing accessibility and openness of AI databases could mitigate biases and foster trust between surgeons and technology developers, ultimately advancing patient care in neuroradiology of the spine (Fortuni *et al.*, 2024; Yahanda *et al.*, 2024).

4.3.2 3D Imaging Techniques

New technologies in medical imaging have greatly improved the care of people with spinal problems, and three-dimensional imaging is very important in neuroradiology. These methods allow for clear pictures of the spine's small structures by using information from both CT and MRI to make detailed 3D models. Integration needs to occur for a full assessment and planning of surgery, especially when spinal tumors are involved, since the type of tissue involvement affects the surgical approach. Preparing for surgery with 3D rendering and printing enables surgeons to practice and improve their techniques, which helps patients by making the surgery safer and more accurate. The combination of MRI and CT information is also advancing, which should enhance how doctors make diagnoses and carry out interventions. Despite these advancements, ongoing research is necessary to fully harness the potential of 3D imaging, advancing its application in neuroradiology to address complex spinal pathologies more effectively (Nowak *et al.*, 2023; Tappa *et al.*, 2024) (Figure 4.15).

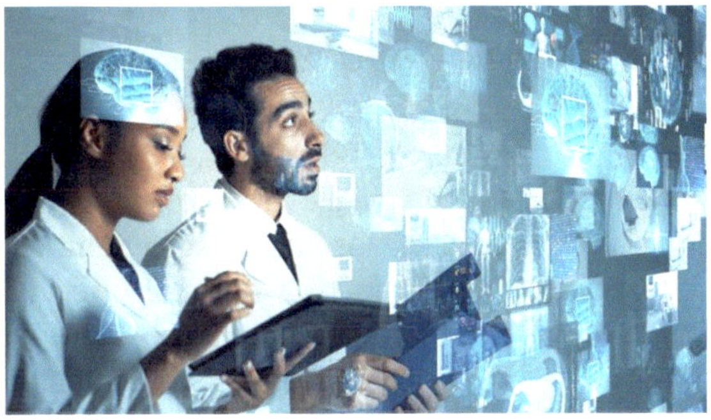

Figure 4.15. Advancements in medical imaging have profoundly enhanced the diagnosis and treatment of complex spinal conditions, with three-dimensional imaging techniques playing a pivotal role in neuroradiology.

Source: https://www.itnonline.com/sites/default/files/styles/content_large/public/GettyImages-1333328712.jpg?itok=gryN5ppe.

4.3.3. Enhanced Imaging Resolution

Improvements in imaging have made it easier to see detailed images of the spine and its problems. Better imaging resolution allows doctors to tell apart soft tissue, nerve roots, and vertebrae, which is important for accurate diagnosis and planning treatment. Better resolution in images allows doctors to spot small and delicate lesions such as demyelinating plaques or tiny tumors that might be hidden by other imaging methods. In addition, finer spatial resolution helps surgeons perform less invasive operations by providing clear images of the patient's anatomy, which reduces risks. Using advanced imaging methods helps manage patients better by allowing doctors to choose the right treatment and track the disease. Integrating these advances aligns with the recommendations for pediatric and adult neuroradiology practice, highlighting the importance of high-quality imaging in specialized clinical contexts (Adamsbaum *et al.*, 2022). In the end, better imaging resolution is a major step forward in spine neuroradiology, improving diagnostic accuracy, and patient outcomes.

4.3.4. Tele-radiology Applications

Better medical imaging technology has greatly improved how neuroradiology diagnoses spinal problems. Tele-radiology allows doctors to review and interpret complex spinal images remotely, which is very helpful in this situation. Because of these applications, neuroradiologists can view high-quality MRI and CT scans from a distance and quickly spot abnormalities in the spine such as herniated discs, spinal cord lesions, and degenerative diseases. Because of tele-radiology, patients receive faster and more accurate expert analysis, and it also helps specialists from different fields cooperate across different regions. Additionally, using digital methods to send imaging data makes communication safe and efficient, as evidenced by recent cases. Continued innovations in tele-radiology platforms promise to further enhance spine-focused neuroradiology by increasing diagnostic accessibility and workflow efficiency (Figure 4.16).

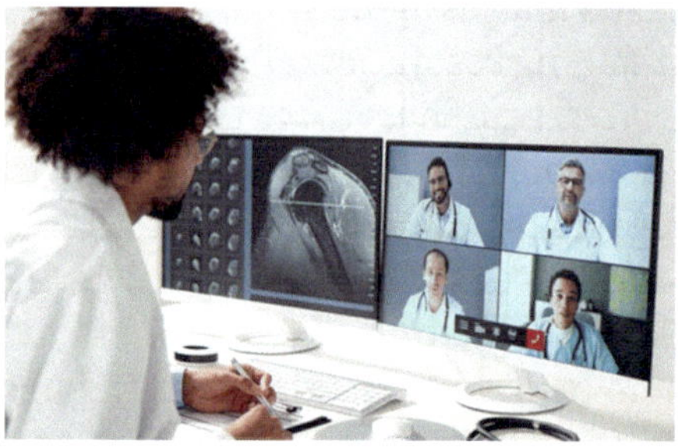

Figure 4.16. Tele-radiology applications have emerged as pivotal tools by facilitating remote interpretation and consultation of complex spinal imaging studies.

Source: https://dcmsys.com/wp-content/uploads/2023/06/Dicom_Systems_Teleradiology_Telehealth_2023_Second_Opinions.png.

4.3.5. Integration of Imaging with Other Modalities

The use of multiple imaging techniques together has greatly improved the application of spine neuroradiology in clinical practice. Combining MRI with electrophysiological studies, such as electromyography (EMG) and nerve conduction studies, provides a more comprehensive assessment of neural function alongside structural abnormalities. Also, using CT data and three-dimensional imaging makes it easier for surgeons to guide their tools during surgery for complex spine problems or injuries. The use of various methods allows doctors to tailor treatment and see how the body works and is built. Innovations in software and peer review systems, as discussed in recent frameworks, underscore the importance of optimizing image interpretation through mathematical models that consider error frequency and clinical impact, thus improving diagnostic reliability in neuroradiology (Balsim *et al.*, 2010). Seeing these relationships in images or diagrams helps people understand how imaging and other tools are now used together in spinal care.

4.3.6. Personalized Medicine in Spinal Disorders

With better diagnostic tools, doctors can now give more personalized treatment for spinal problems. Neuroradiology helps a lot in this change by making it possible to accurately see and measure problems in the spine. Quantitative MRI lets doctors view the structure of tissues in the spine, which helps them understand the extent and differences in the damage in spinal lesions.

This level of detailed imaging aids in stratifying patients for tailored interventions, optimizing outcomes, and monitoring disease progression or treatment response over time (Barkhof *et al.*, 2021). Moreover, integrating artificial intelligence with neuroradiological data holds promise in refining personalized treatment plans by simulating and predicting patient-specific responses, particularly in complex neurological conditions affecting the spine (Rajhans *et al.*, 2024). Such an interdisciplinary strategy underscores the shift from one-size-fits-all treatment paradigms toward precision medicine, ultimately improving diagnostic accuracy and enhancing individualized care in spinal disorders within a neuroradiological framework (Figure 4.17).

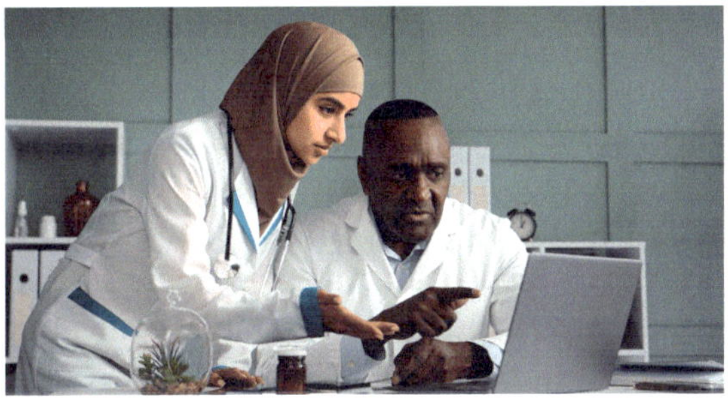

Figure 4.17. Neuroradiology plays a pivotal role in this transformation, enabling precise visualization and quantitative assessment of spinal pathology.

Source: https://dcmsys.com/wp-content/uploads/2023/06/Dicom_Systems_Teleradiology_Telehealth_2023_Provider_Collaboration.png.

4.3.7. Research in Spinal Imaging

New imaging techniques have greatly improved the ability to diagnose and treat spine-related issues, which shows the wider growth in neuroradiology. Even though traditional techniques are key, they do not always assess the biomechanical qualities of the spine well, which is why new techniques such as shear wave elastography are being used. This method offers a novel perspective by sensitively capturing tissue elasticity, which is crucial for understanding conditions like disc herniations and various degenerative disorders, thereby expanding diagnostic precision and therapeutic planning (Zhang *et al.*, 2025). At the same time, research into spinal cerebrospinal fluid leaks demonstrates how spinal imaging is always progressing, introducing new, non-invasive methods and image-guided treatments that have improved patient care. Such developments underscore the neuroradiologist's critical role in advancing spinal imaging capabilities, particularly through sophisticated myelographic techniques and enhanced imaging resolution, which contribute to more effective and targeted treatments (Mamlouk *et al.*, 2024). All of these efforts together are moving the field toward better-tailored and more accurate care for the spine.

4.3.8. Impact of Technology on Patient Outcomes

Thanks to new imaging tools, diagnosing and treating spinal problems has become much easier, improving the outcomes for patients in neuroradiology. CT and MRI allow for a clear view of the spine and its problems, which helps find and describe conditions like cervical spine instability and cord compression at an early stage.

They are important for planning surgery and also help ensure that surgery is safe and effective by giving information on the degree of spinal involvement. Also, using intraoperative neurophysiological monitoring and advanced imaging helps surgeons avoid neurological complications during surgery. Frequent imaging of the brain together with neurological checks helps doctors act quickly and prevent permanent brain damage. The integration of these technologies has thus played a crucial role in transforming spinal care, promoting better functional recovery and quality of life in affected patients (Goel *et al.*, 2013) (Figure 4.18).

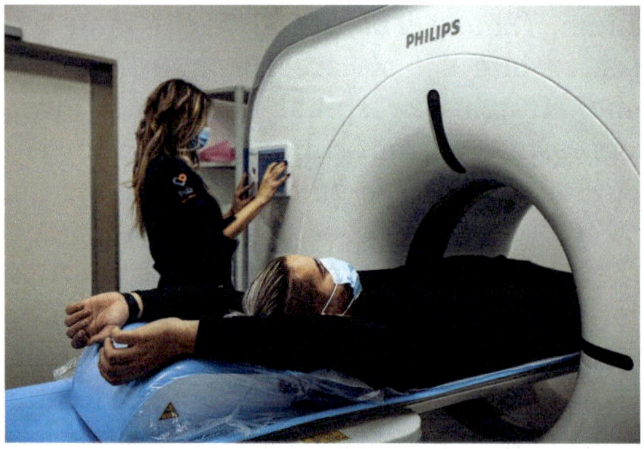

Figure 4.18. High-resolution modalities such as computed tomography (CT) and magnetic resonance imaging (MRI) enable detailed visualization of spinal anatomy and pathology, facilitating early detection and precise characterization of conditions like cervical spine instability and cord compression.

Source: https://pulskardioloskicentar.rs/wp-content/uploads/2021/02/How-Does-a-Cervical-Spine-CT-Scan-Work.jpg.

4.3.9. Ethical Considerations in Neuroradiology

Because of new techniques in neuroradiology, especially in spinal imaging, the accuracy of diagnosis and treatment planning has improved. At the same time, these advances introduce important ethical issues that should be handled to keep patients safe and protect the reputation of healthcare workers. AI being used in image interpretation adds new challenges about privacy, informed consent, and the transparency of algorithms. AI-based decisions need to be clear and without bias to keep clinicians and patients trusting each other. Also, the chance of discovering unexpected issues during spinal imaging means it is important to explain the results clearly to avoid unnecessary worry in patients. It is also an ethical issue to consider the positives of advanced images and the negatives, such as radiation and the use of resources. Addressing these issues requires continuous collaboration between neuroradiologists, AI developers, and ethicists, fostering responsible innovation anchored in patient-centered care and transparency (Najjar, 2023a; Najjar, 2023b).

Test Your Knowledge

1. How has 3D imaging and visualization changed the way surgeons plan spinal procedures such as spinal decompression and fusion?
2. How do artificial intelligence (AI) and machine learning technologies contribute to improving the diagnosis and interpretation of spine MRI and CT scans?

SUMMARY

Thanks to developments in neuroradiology, diagnosing and treating spinal disorders has become much better, though there are still issues in getting the best outcomes and avoiding complications. The integration of minimally invasive techniques such as uniportal spine endoscopy has introduced unique risks, including neurological deterioration associated with fluid insufflation, underscoring the need for precise intraoperative monitoring and standardized irrigation parameters to mitigate adverse events (Liu *et al.*, 2025). At the same time, collecting detailed information and using multiple registries helps surgeons understand risks and predict results better. The amalgamation of data from the American Spine Registry with Medicare records provides a more accurate reflection of complication rates and readmissions following lumbar fusion procedures, facilitating improved clinical decision-making and quality enhancement initiatives (Glassman *et al.*, 2025). All of these points show that research, new technology, and combining data are key to improving neuroradiological spine care for patients.

Thanks to new neuroradiology technologies, we now have a much better understanding and way to examine the spinal column. Recent research underscores the strong correlation between the C6 slope (C6S) and C7 slope (C7S), revealing that C6S can serve as a reliable surrogate when C7S visibility is compromised, which is crucial for assessing cervical alignment and balance (Sha *et al.*, 2025). Machine learning models increase the accuracy of predicting spinal parameters, which may be useful in clinical practice. Additionally, long-term outcome measurements in spinal surgery demonstrate variability in minimal important change (MIC) values, especially for disability indices, while patient-acceptable symptom state (PASS) values remain comparatively stable over time. This variability necessitates careful interpretation of patient-reported outcome measures in extended follow-up studies to ensure accurate clinical assessments (Toivonen *et al.*, 2024). All these findings point to how accurate and detailed neuroradiological exams and follow-up have become for spinal conditions.

KEY TERMS FROM THIS CHAPTER

- Trauma
- Malignant tumor
- Chemotherapy
- Nervous system
- Radiation safety
- Spine
- Spinal deformities
- Multiple sclerosis
- Degenerative diseases
- Surgery
- Radiotherapy
- Minimally invasive surgeries
- Radiation exposure
- Canal dimensions
- Aquaporin-4-IgG myelitis

CRITICAL THINKING QUESTIONS

1. **Which type of imaging is most often used to check spinal cord injuries?**
   a. X-ray
   b. CT scan
   c. MRI
   d. Ultrasound
2. **Why is MRI generally preferred over CT for looking at the spine?**
   a. MRI provides better visualization of bone fractures.
   b. MRI gives the best view of soft tissues, so it is perfect for looking at the spinal cord, nerves, and discs between the vertebrae.
   c. MRI is less expensive than CT.
   d. MRI is quicker than CT in emergency settings.
3. **MRI of the spine is NOT usually used to detect what?**
   a. Spinal cord tumors
   b. Disc herniation
   c. Spinal fractures
   d. Spinal cord inflammation
4. **For what main reason is CT myelography used in spine imaging?**
   a. Evaluation of bone tumors
   b. Radiology of the spinal cord, nerve roots, and surrounding tissues for patients who cannot have an MRI
   c. Detection of muscle spasms
   d. Routine screening for spinal degeneration
5. **A spine MRI is often done when a doctor suspects what condition?**
   a. Detection of fractures in the cervical spine
   b. Investigation of lower back pain with possible nerve involvement
   c. Evaluation of soft tissue injuries in the knee
   d. Screening for lung cancer metastasis to the spine

Short Answer Questions

1. What is the best imaging method for assessing soft tissues such as the spinal cord and nerve roots in the spine?
2. In what cases is CT myelography used for spinal imaging, and what makes it better than MRI?
3. How are CT and MRI different when used to image the spine?
4. How does an X-ray scan assist in finding out about fractures and alignment problems in the spine?
5. What is the role of dynamic radiography (flexion-extension X-rays) in evaluating spinal pathologies?

Answers to Critical Thinking Questions

1. (c); 2. (b); 3. (c); 4. (b); 5. (b)

REFERENCES

1. Adamsbaum, C., Altmann-Schneider, I., Argyropoulou, M., Boulouis, G., *et al.* (2022). European recommendations on practices in pediatric neuroradiology: Consensus document from the European Society of Neuroradiology (ESNR), European Society of Pediatric Radiology (ESPR) and European Union of Medical Specialists Division of Neuroradiology (UEMS). Pediatric Radiology. https://core.ac.uk/download/549582974.pdf (accessed on 31st May 2025).
2. Andersen, M. Ø., Carreon, L. Y., Karppinen, J., Modic, M., *et al.* (2022). *A Definition and Clinical Grading of Modic Changes.* https://core.ac.uk/download/628859523.pdf (accessed on 31st May 2025).
3. Armesto, P. V., González, U. P., & Suárez, Q. J. A. (2020). *Clinical Anatomy of Cervical Spondylosis.* https://core.ac.uk/download/389284308.pdf (accessed on 31st May 2025).
4. Ashour, R., Berkefeld, J., Bilsky, M., Chalouhi, N., Choi, I. S., Hasan, D., Deshmukh, V., *et al.* (2013). *Preoperative Spinal Tumor Embolization: An Institutional Experience with Onyx.* https://core.ac.uk/download/46972854.pdf (accessed on 31st May 2025).
5. Balani, A., Biswas, A., Capra, V., Catala, M., *et al.* (2024). International consensus statement on the radiological evaluation of dysraphic malformations of the spine and spinal cord. https://core.ac.uk/download/603247275.pdf (accessed on 31st May 2025).
6. Balsim, I., Bleicher, A. G., & Branstetter, B. F. IV. (2010). Optimizing radiology peer review: A mathematical model for selecting future cases based on prior errors. *Journal of the American College of Radiology.* https://academicworks.cuny.edu/cgi/viewcontent.cgi?article=1064&context=kb_pubs (accessed on 31st May 2025).
7. Barkhof, F., Calabrese, M., De Stefano, N., Enzinger, C., *et al.* (2021). Quantitative magnetic resonance imaging towards clinical application in multiple sclerosis. *Brain.* https://core.ac.uk/download/427084118.pdf (accessed on 31st May 2025).
8. Berlis, A., Bonk, M. N., Hofmann, R., Krauß, T., *et al.* (2024). Peripherally inserted central venous catheter in outpatient antibiotic spinal infection treatment is safe, effective and leads to significant reduction in healthcare expenses. *Neurosurgical Review.* https://core.ac.uk/download/643181514.pdf (accessed on 31st May 2025).
9. Beyer, F., Eysel, P., & Bredow, J. (2025). The diagnosis and treatment of degenerative changes of the lumbar spine. *Deutsches Ärzteblatt International (Forthcoming).* https://www.semanticscholar.org/paper/16c8c4aa9bc756a3ccda838eeda5e7523b433a0d (accessed on 31st May 2025).
10. Borelli, A., Liguori, A., Magenta, B. A. M., Masciocchi, C., Piccolo, C. L., Caranci, F., Galli, F., *et al.* (2018). Clinical and instrumental assessment of herniated discs after nucleoplasty: A preliminary study. Acta Biomed. https://core.ac.uk/download/225134303.pdf (accessed on 31st May 2025).
11. Chang, P., Kuoy, E., Grinband, J., Weinberg, B. D., Thompson, M., Homo, R. L., Chen, J. W., *et al.* (2018). Hybrid 3D/2D convolutional neural network for hemorrhage evaluation on head CT. *American Journal of Neuroradiology, 39*, 1609–1616. https://doi.org/10.3174/ajnr.a5742 (accessed on 31st May 2025).

12. Dailey, A. T., & Tsuruda, J. S. (1996). *Magnetic Resonance Neurography for Cervical Radiculopathy: A Preliminary Report.* https://core.ac.uk/download/276284998.pdf (accessed on 31st May 2025).
13. Damilakis, J., Ebdon-Jackson, S., Frush, D. P., Loose, R., *et al.* (2017). Unintended and accidental medical radiation exposures in radiology: Guidelines on investigation and prevention. *Journal of Radiological Protection.* https://core.ac.uk/download/96883276.pdf (accessed on 31st May 2025).
14. Dubey, D., Pittock, S. J., Krecke, K. N., Morris, P. P., Sechi, E., Zalewski, N. L., Weinshenker, B. G., *et al.* (2018). Clinical, radiologic, and prognostic features of myelitis associated with myelin oligodendrocyte glycoprotein autoantibody. *JAMA Neurology, 76*, 301. https://doi.org/10.1001/jamaneurol.2018.4053 (accessed on 31st May 2025).
15. Fisher, C., & Batke, J. (2013). Editorial: Separation surgery. *Journal of Neurosurgery: Spine, 18*(3), 205, 206. https://www.semanticscholar.org/paper/5608846712338b0ba5b58da34964afe745b1f6ea (accessed on 31st May 2025).
16. Fortuni, F., Ciliberti, G., De Chiara, B., Conte, E., Franchin, L., Musella, F., Vitale, E., *et al.* (2024). Advancements and applications of artificial intelligence in cardiovascular imaging: A comprehensive review. *European Heart Journal. Imaging Methods and Practice, 2.* https://www.semanticscholar.org/paper/69a618ef1cafa26e26a7e8251039302dd9ed59c3 (accessed on 31st May 2025).
17. García, E. J., Láinez, R. A. J., Martínez, B. J. P., & Martínez, M. A., *et al.* (2022). The value of magnetic resonance imaging and computed tomography in the study of spinal disorders. *Quant. Imaging Med. Surg.* https://core.ac.uk/download/527689191.pdf (accessed on 31st May 2025).
18. Glassman, S. D., Djurasovic, M., Asher, A., De, A., Murray, J., Safdar, A., Porter, K. R., *et al.* (2025). Linking American Spine Registry (ASR) and Medicare data: An analysis of 8,755 lumbar fusion cases. *Spine.* https://www.semanticscholar.org/paper/2e53150e3fe73f31552baf68f72ac003eb8a30e6 (accessed on 31st May 2025).
19. Goel, A., McDonald, A., Madawi, A. A., Brooks, A. L., McLaughlin, A. M., Montano, A. M., Ransford, A. O., *et al.* (2013). Spinal involvement in mucopolysaccharidosis IVA (Morquio-Brailsford or Morquio A syndrome): Presentation, diagnosis and management. *Journal of Inherited Metabolic Disease.* https://core.ac.uk/download/323073297.pdf (accessed on 31st May 2025).
20. Guan, J., Feng, N., Yang, K., Abudouaini, H., & Liu, P. (2024). The efficacy and safety of ketorolac for postoperative pain management in lumbar spine surgery: A meta-analysis of randomized controlled trials. *Systematic Reviews, 13.* https://www.semanticscholar.org/paper/80d6280b29c17888918f40f0cd3dccd535bbb6b8 (accessed on 31st May 2025).
21. Hartman, J., Granville, M., & Jacobson, R. E. (2019). Radiologic evaluation of lumbar spinal stenosis: The integration of sagittal and axial views in decision making for minimally invasive surgical procedures. *Cureus.* https://doi.org/10.7759/cureus.4268 (accessed on 31st May 2025).
22. Inness, P. R., Kimbrell, T. L., Nemanic, S., & Baltzer, W. (2021). Distraction stabilization of degenerative lumbosacral stenosis: Technique and mid- to long-term outcome in 30 cases. *Veterinary and Comparative Orthopedics and Traumatology: V.C.O.T.* https://www.semanticscholar.org/paper/5e08e9dc5411989e06f56429f3563015647857b0 (accessed on 31st May 2025).

23. Intikhab, O., Cristiano, B. C., Tehrani, A., Zeiler, S., Felling, R. J., & Gailloud, P. (2024). Role of digital subtraction angiography in acute cervical spinal cord ischemia. *Interventional Neuroradiology: Journal of Peritherapeutic Neuroradiology, Surgical Procedures and Related Neurosciences*. https://www.semanticscholar.org/paper/0ec2c8abd01b9d9d4b12ac58d92dbaa784317617 (accessed on 31st May 2025).

24. Kalantaite, I. (2024). Physiotherapy assessment and intervention for patients with lumbar disc herniation with radiculopathy: A self-study material for physiotherapy students. https://core.ac.uk/download/638723763.pdf (accessed on 31st May 2025).

25. Kasat, P. R., Kashikar, S., Parihar, P., Sachani, P., Shrivastava, P., Mapari, S. A., Pradeep, U., *et al.* (2024). Advances in imaging for metastatic epidural spinal cord compression: A comprehensive review of detection, diagnosis, and treatment planning. *Cureus, 16*. https://www.semanticscholar.org/paper/0aed072a7910bef0ab2b0162e37cbcabd02b3ed1 (accessed on 31st May 2025).

26. Kidd, D. (2023). Neurological involvement by Behçet's syndrome: Clinical features, diagnosis, treatment and outcome. *Practical Neurology, 23*, 386–400. https://www.semanticscholar.org/paper/95562a307a0981ee127ef065bc7168f2cab39da0 (accessed on 31st May 2025).

27. Krishnan, G., Singh, S., Pathania, M., Gosavi, S., Abhishek, S., Parchani, A., & Dhar, M. (2023). Artificial intelligence in clinical medicine: Catalyzing a sustainable global healthcare paradigm. *Frontiers in Artificial Intelligence, 6*. https://doi.org/10.3389/frai.2023.1227091 (accessed on 31st May 2025).

28. Lee, J., & Alcaide-Leon, P. (2025). Characterizing the preferred reporting methods in neuroradiology: A multispecialty survey. *Canadian Association of Radiologists Journal = Journal l'Association Canadienne des Radiologistes*. https://www.semanticscholar.org/paper/c64d83ab8f480c67a7770dc4cae784eb9866e042 (accessed on 31st May 2025).

29. Li, S., Ma, L., Li, D., Deng, Y., Yang, Y., & Xu, L. (2024). A robust detection network utilizing neural memory ordinary differential equations for vertebral fractures diagnosis. *2024 International Annual Conference on Complex Systems and Intelligent Science (CSIS-IAC)*. https://www.semanticscholar.org/paper/497ed69f603c8a64ff2f02c2fd3a3fa2059f760d (accessed on 31st May 2025).

30. Liu, D., & Mobbs, R. (2025). Risk analysis of neurological deterioration associated with fluid insufflation in uniportal spine endoscopy: A case series and literature review. *International Journal of Spine Surgery*. https://www.semanticscholar.org/paper/fe08c6a5c2ab3c0f1cfa8a27500452b6c8a62cb7 (accessed on 31st May 2025).

31. Mamlouk, M., Callen, A. L., Madhavan, A., Lützen, N., Jones, L. C., Mark, I., Brinjikji, W., *et al.* (2024). Spinal CSF leaks: The neuroradiologist transforming care. *AJNR. American Journal of Neuroradiology*. https://www.semanticscholar.org/paper/c923d7e90c7a68311ec6714e28f4abc32ca8d114 (accessed on 31st May 2025).

32. Najjar, R. (2023a). Redefining radiology: A review of artificial intelligence integration in medical imaging. *Diagnostics, 13*, 2760. https://doi.org/10.3390/diagnostics13172760 (accessed on 31st May 2025).

33. Najjar, R. (2023b). *Redefining Radiology: A Review of Artificial Intelligence Integration in Medical Imaging*. https://doi.org/10.20944/preprints202306.1124.v1 (accessed on 31st May 2025).

34. Nowak, P., Dąbrowski, M., & Kubaszewski, Ł. (2023). Current techniques of 3D reconstruction

in computed tomography and magnetic resonance in diagnostic imaging of the spine. *Chirurgia Narządów Ruchu i Ortopedia Polska*. https://www.semanticscholar.org/paper/c447f13ff9d324b503d055dad5f2c6f3f6728f37 (accessed on 31st May 2025).

35. Páez, D., Giammarile, F., Brink, A., García-Pérez, O., & Estrada-Lobato, E. (2024). The role of 18-fluorodeoxyglucose positron emission tomography/computed tomography (18F-FDG PET/CT) in the diagnosis and evaluation of spondylodiscitis. *Seminars in Nuclear Medicine*. https://www.semanticscholar.org/paper/bb06a5c656990f1af92073f1d3da19d9aa7ee86b (accessed on 31st May 2025).

36. Peng, Y., Chen, S., Li, J., Wang, Y., & Wu, B. (2024). Pineal region tumors: Prognostic stratification based on magnetic resonance imaging features—A retrospective cohort study. *Quantitative Imaging in Medicine and Surgery, 15*, 177–188. https://www.semanticscholar.org/paper/a9d74f8b9775ff5e4b9ac2e26c460c32233f131d (accessed on 31st May 2025).

37. Piper, K., Pittock, L., *et al.* (2018). Radiographer reporting of neurological magnetic resonance imaging examinations of the head and cervical spine: Findings of an accredited postgraduate program. *Radiography*. https://core.ac.uk/download/287635771.pdf (accessed on 31st May 2025).

38. Qi, Z., Da, H., Fang, Y., & Fan, M. (2025). Current status and prospects of robot-assisted spine surgery. *Expert Review of Medical Devices*. https://www.semanticscholar.org/paper/e4f5dde580c43203a665223bdf27ef8d112f57b7 (accessed on 31st May 2025).

39. Rajhans, S., Jha, S., & Singh, P. (2024). Yoga and artificial intelligence: A review of the potential applications of AI in yoga research and practice for neurological disorders. *International Journal on Recent and Innovation Trends in Computing and Communication*. https://core.ac.uk/download/603899088.pdf (accessed on 31st May 2025).

40. Sadeghi-Adl, Z., Naghizadehkashani, S., Middleton, D., Krisa, L., Alizadeh, M., Flanders, A. E., Faro, S. H., *et al.* (2025). Severity classification of pediatric spinal cord injuries using structural MRI measures and deep learning: A comprehensive analysis across all vertebral levels. *AJNR. American Journal of Neuroradiology*. https://www.semanticscholar.org/paper/a4991d50168a8cc6710c10a1042d06111c399ff9 (accessed on 31st May 2025).

41. Sakhrekar, R., Iorio, C., Yoon, S., Monjardino, M. P., Lewis, S., & Gray, R. (2024). Philosophies and surgical techniques for Ewing's sarcoma of spine with review of literature. *Journal of Orthopedic Case Reports, 14*, 168–175. https://www.semanticscholar.org/paper/99e7c63f55137b2a681a5837e00c13c0bc713199 (accessed on 31st May 2025).

42. Sha, Z., Yang, X., Ran, Y., Liu, Y., Qin, Z., Xu, L., Mu, X., *et al.* (2025). The correlation between gender, age, curvature, and symptom-related changes in C6 and C7 slope in 10,000 subjects. *Spine*. https://www.semanticscholar.org/paper/b59e29f94f34c92ad53c68513cf05b623b256e31 (accessed on 31st May 2025).

43. Silva, J. S., Bettencourt, S., Madureira, I., Conde, M., & Conceição, C. (2024). Chronic nonbacterial osteomyelitis in neuroradiology – Behavior and evolution of vertebral and mandibular lesions on imaging. *Pediatric Radiology, 54*, 2046–2059. https://www.semanticscholar.org/paper/1f5ddc148409baf6b4db752bdd8aa5e1689c0d6f (accessed on 31st May 2025).

44. Sunwar, S., & Saiyed, A. (2025). Delayed diagnosis of thoracic spine tuberculosis: A learning objective in primary care. *International Journal of Clinical Trials*. https://www.semanticscholar.org/paper/444ff12483116d11353a53be9d011e3d5b78e12d (accessed on 31st May 2025).

45. Tappa, K. K., Bird, J. E., Arribas, E. M., & Santiago, L. (2024). Multimodality imaging for 3D printing and surgical rehearsal in complex spine surgery. *Radiographics: A Review Publication of the Radiological Society of North America, Inc., 44*(3), e230116. https://www.semanticscholar.org/paper/87ae913c479fa155027e8267adeefee76d42a27f (accessed on 31st May 2025).

46. Teichner, E. M., Subtirelu, R. C., Crutchfield, C. R., Parikh, C., Ashok, A. B., Talasila, S., Anderson, V. A., *et al.* (2025). The advancement and utility of multimodal imaging in the diagnosis of degenerative disc disease. *Frontiers in Radiology, 5*. https://www.semanticscholar.org/paper/57163a28fbdb1db3ea2226b1784e4b09f158686d (accessed on 31st May 2025).

47. Toivonen, L., Laurén, J. L. C., Kautiainen, H., Häkkinen, A., & Neva, M. (2024). Ten-year heterogeneity of minimal important change and patient acceptable symptom state after lumbar fusions. *Spine, 50*, 46–52. https://www.semanticscholar.org/paper/05c18f1c5561aa7d2ff3b0c22b02b5287b65b862 (accessed on 31st May 2025).

48. Usuzaki, T., Takahashi, K., Inamori, R., Morishita, Y., Shizukuishi, T., Takagi, H., Ishikuro, M., *et al.* (2024). Identifying key factors for predicting O6-methylguanine-DNA methyltransferase status in adult patients with diffuse glioma: A multimodal analysis of demographics, radiomics, and MRI by variable Vision Transformer. *Neuroradiology, 66*, 761–773. https://www.semanticscholar.org/paper/b084f687667ede807cb76c2a8cec0a3c763213ee (accessed on 31st May 2025).

49. Yahanda, A. T., Joseph, K., Bui, T., Greenberg, J. K., Ray, W. Z., Ogunlade, J. I., Hafez, D., *et al.* (2024). Current applications and future implications of artificial intelligence in spine surgery and research: A narrative review and commentary. *Global Spine Journal, 15*, 1445–1454. https://www.semanticscholar.org/paper/9ed3b38c0de172bf5a401aaa564983b3985d4018 (accessed on 31st May 2025).

50. Yoo, Y., & Kim, K. H. (2023). Facet joint disorders: From diagnosis to treatment. *The Korean Journal of Pain, 37*, 3–12. https://www.semanticscholar.org/paper/af202a95a997f052d946ad576e80837524468d60 (accessed on 31st May 2025).

51. Zhang, Y., Luo, Y., & Wang, G. (2025). Application and research progress of SWE technology in spinal diseases. *Advances in Clinical Medicine*. https://www.semanticscholar.org/paper/c4dc96f871ea842fe33ba16a45710009751e3d8a (accessed on 31st May 2025).5811111111111111111111112

HEAD AND NECK IMAGING

5

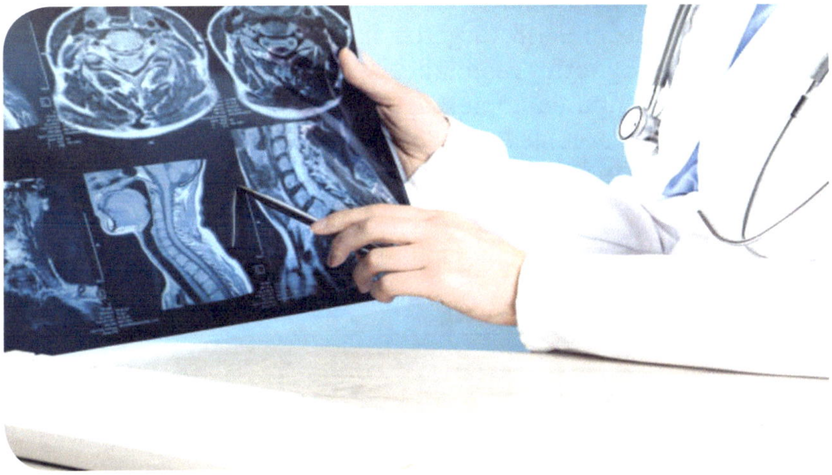

LEARNING OBJECTIVES

After studying this chapter, you will be able to:

1. Understand imaging modalities;
2. Explain clinical applications;
3. Focus on interpretation and analysis;
4. Discuss patient considerations.

Introduction

Medical imaging has greatly improved how doctors diagnose complex anatomy, mainly in the head and neck. Since this region contains many vital structures, finding and diagnosing pathological changes is very important for proper treatment. Radiographic techniques allow doctors to find diseases early and help them decide between different diagnoses, which benefits the patient's care. In dental and medical practice alike, the capability to discern abnormalities within the maxillofacial and cervical regions is essential, underscoring the interdisciplinary nature of head and neck imaging (Cardoso *et al.*, 2019). Furthermore, innovative modalities like sentinel node mapping and SPECT/CT have emerged to overcome anatomical challenges in lymph node localization, further improving diagnostic precision in oncology staging (Balm *et al.*, 2009). All of these advances in imaging underline the importance of radiography in finding and treating problems in the head and neck, which helps patients and improves their overall prognosis.

Definition of Head and Neck Imaging

Medical technology has greatly improved the ways doctors diagnose problems in the head and neck. A variety of imaging techniques are used in the head and neck area to find tumors, infections, or blood vessel problems. This specialized imaging is vital for identifying cancers of unknown primary origin, where a neck mass is the initial presentation but the primary tumor site remains elusive, necessitating precise and individualized diagnostic pathways to guide treatment effectively (Messineo *et al.*, 2025). Because MRI provides clear images of soft tissues and can measure their functions, it is now used more often in medical imaging. This comprehensive imaging approach supports adaptive treatment strategies by facilitating accurate target delineation and response monitoring during interventions like radiotherapy, thereby improving patient outcomes while minimizing damage to surrounding tissues (Ridder *et al.*, 2022). Thus, head and neck imaging serves as a cornerstone for diagnosis and treatment planning in this anatomically complex region (Figure 5.1).

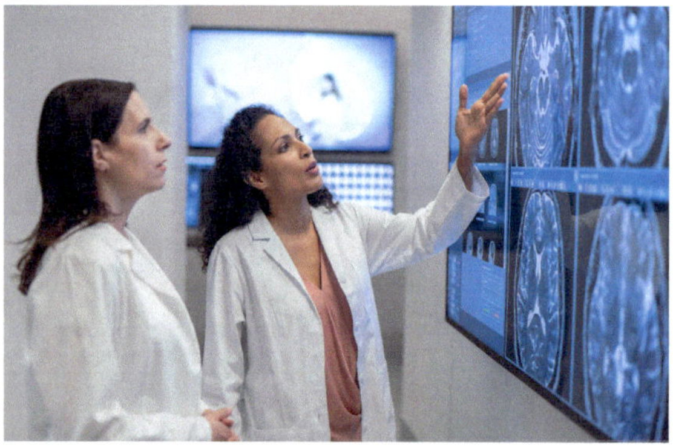

Figure 5.1. Head and neck imaging encompasses a range of techniques aimed at visualizing intricate structures to detect abnormalities such as tumors, infections, or vascular issues.

Source: https://wp04-media.cdn.ihealthspot.com/wp-content/uploads/sites/91/2022/04/iStock-1310711930.jpg.

Importance of Imaging in Medical Diagnosis

Getting an accurate diagnosis is very important for treating patients, especially in areas such as the head and neck. Imaging tests help doctors tell apart conditions that have similar symptoms and plan the correct, and timely interventions. For instance, distinguishing sensorineural hearing loss from conductive hearing loss at the initial clinical encounter is imperative, as emphasized by the clinical guidelines that recommend targeted imaging techniques like magnetic resonance imaging over routine computed tomography to identify underlying retrocochlear pathology (Chandrasekhar *et al.*, 2019a; Chandrasekhar *et al.*, 2019b).

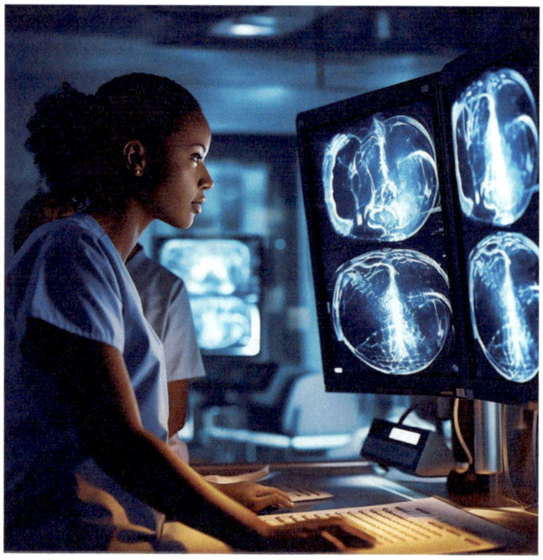

Figure 5.2. Imaging modalities play a critical role in differentiating conditions that present with overlapping symptoms, guiding clinicians toward appropriate and timely interventions.

Source: https://oncologycompass.com/digest/issue7/images/cover.png.

Thanks to these precise ways of diagnosing, patients do not have to undergo unnecessary tests, delays in treatment are avoided, and their quality of life is improved by providing the right therapy and steroid treatment. Furthermore, imaging not only facilitates immediate diagnostic clarity but also supports ongoing management through follow-up evaluations, underscoring its indispensable value in modern medical practice, especially in head and neck disorders with intricate presentations (Figure 5.2).

Historical Context of Head and Neck Imaging

The way medical imaging has advanced is closely tied to improvements in surgical techniques and technology, which have greatly improved the accuracy and speed of diagnoses. The first head and neck X-rays were difficult to take because the area is complex and the structures are easily damaged, so inventions in radiology and image reading were required. Advances in surgery led surgeons to request better imaging tools, which in turn made it possible to perform procedures with less damage to the body. This historical trajectory mirrors developments seen in other surgical fields, such as vascular surgery, where the shift from open surgeries to minimally invasive techniques was enabled by improved imaging and instrumentation (Bhogal *et al.*, 2011). In addition, combining aerospace medicine and life support systems with imaging research has contributed innovative materials and computer-aided ways to acquire and analyze images. All of these elements highlight the ongoing relationship between the needs of doctors and technological progress in the history of head and neck imaging.

Current Trends in Imaging Technology

Better diagnostic tools have made a big difference in how head and neck pathologies, including differentiated thyroid cancers, are managed. These tumors have increasingly been identified at smaller, localized stages, necessitating highly sensitive imaging modalities that can guide more conservative treatment strategies while ensuring accurate surveillance (Deandreis *et al.*, 2016). In addition to traditional ultrasonography and Doppler analysis, there is now a greater use of advanced cross-sectional and functional imaging, which helps find out if the disease has spread to other parts of the body. Furthermore, molecular image-guided surgery represents a cutting-edge trend, integrating real-time biological data to refine surgical precision and outcomes (Achilefu *et al.*, 2018). These technologies are expected to greatly improve the way surgeons make decisions during surgery and monitor patients afterward, despite some issues like dealing with tiny variations in diseases and finding suitable imaging agents for different tumors. The integration of multimodal imaging with molecular probes underscores an era where personalized, risk-adapted care in head and neck oncology is becoming increasingly feasible (Achilefu *et al.*, 2018; Deandreis *et al.*, 2016).

Scope of Head and Neck Imaging

New imaging methods have greatly increased what can be seen in head and neck imaging and helped doctors make better decisions. This domain encompasses various modalities, including ultrasound, computed tomography (CT), magnetic resonance imaging (MRI), and emerging deep learning techniques, each contributing unique strengths. Ultrasound remains crucial for real-time soft tissue evaluation and vascular assessment, while CT provides detailed bony and air-filled structure visualization, and MRI excels in soft tissue contrast resolution (Salomon *et al.*, 2022). Moreover, the integration of sophisticated segmentation methods such as U-net has revolutionized image analysis by enabling automated, accurate delineation of complex anatomical regions, thereby improving workflow efficiency and diagnostic accuracy (Siddique *et al.*, 2021). They make it easier to assess congenital problems, tumors, conditions of the immune system, and diseases of the blood vessels. Consequently, the expanding technological landscape continues to broaden the clinical applications and diagnostic capabilities of head and neck imaging, underscoring its indispensable role in multidisciplinary patient care (Figure 5.3).

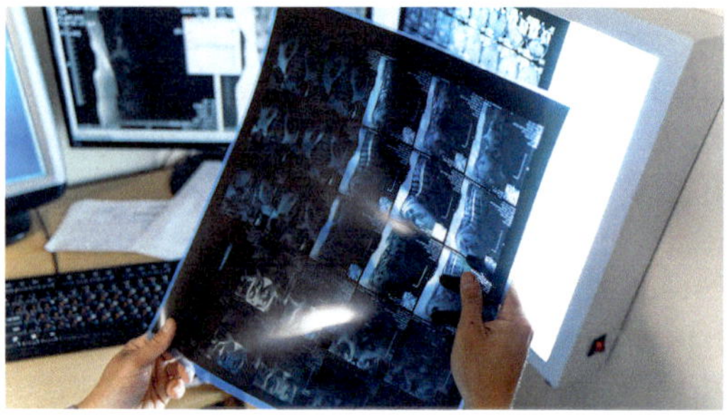

Figure 5.3. Advancements in imaging technology have significantly expanded the scope of head and neck imaging, enhancing diagnostic precision and clinical management.

Source: https://medicalbuyer.co.in/wp-content/uploads/2023/07/870X470-1.png.

Challenges in Head and Neck Imaging

Better imaging techniques have helped doctors diagnose and plan treatment for head and neck problems; still, it remains challenging to clearly outline tumors and the areas to be removed during surgery. Since the anatomy in this area is very complex and accurate tumor segmentation is required on PET and CT scans, it becomes a major challenge. Older ways of segmenting tumors are time-consuming and do not always show the precise boundaries of the tumor, which can result in less effective treatments. Recently, innovative approaches such as cross-modal attention mechanisms in transformer-based models have shown promise in enhancing inter-modality feature representation, thereby improving segmentation accuracy (Li *et al.*, 2023). Additionally, the identification of surgical margins during procedures continues to be hindered by limitations in existing intraoperative imaging modalities, which, despite demonstrating high sensitivity and specificity, require further validation in larger patient cohorts to ensure reliability and consistency (Young *et al.*, 2022). Overcoming these problems is important for making head and neck cancer management better by improving how images are used.

5.1. Imaging Modalities

Learning Outcome

1. Understand x-ray imaging techniques;
2. Define computed tomography (CT);
3. Describe magnetic resonance imaging (MRI);
4. Focus on ultrasound in head and neck imaging;
5. Learn positron emission tomography (PET);
6. Identify fluoroscopy applications;
7. Know digital imaging advancements;
8. Give a comparison of imaging modalities;
9. Focus on future directions in imaging technology.

Better imaging methods have improved both the detection and the management of diseases in the head and neck region. Of these, 18F-FDG PET/CT is most useful, mainly for finding distant metastases, other tumors at the same time, and for examining disease that returns or remains after treatment in head and neck squamous cell carcinoma. Combining metabolic and anatomical details gives it an edge in difficult anatomical areas where other imaging methods might not work well. However, while PET/CT has limitations in regional lymph node staging, modalities such as MRI and multi-slice spiral CT continue to provide complementary data for precise tumor characterization and local staging (Al-Ibraheem *et al.*, 2009). Also, fluorescence-guided imaging is a new intraoperative method that gives surgeons real-time optical information, allowing them to see the tumor borders more clearly and perform radical resection. This technique holds promising potential to improve surgical outcomes and patient survival when integrated thoughtfully into clinical practice (Keereweer *et al.*, 2014).

5.1.1. X-ray Imaging Techniques

The accuracy of diagnosing complex areas of the head and neck has improved a lot with the help of advanced imaging methods. Among these, X-ray imaging is still basic because it is accessible and can clearly show any structural problems in the body. Conventional radiography is particularly effective for assessing bony structures and detecting calcifications, while specialized techniques like computed tomography (CT) provide cross-sectional images that facilitate detailed visualization of both osseous and soft tissue components. The integration of digital enhancements and segmentation algorithms, notably those derived from deep learning architectures like U-net, further improves image interpretation by enabling precise delineation of anatomical boundaries even with limited training data, thus streamlining diagnosis and treatment planning (Siddique *et al.*, 2021). Moreover, in the context of soft tissue sarcomas and other head and neck malignancies, X-ray imaging plays a crucial role in initial assessment and staging, complementing other modalities such as MRI and PET to inform multidisciplinary management approaches (Casali *et al.*, 2018) (Figure 5.4).

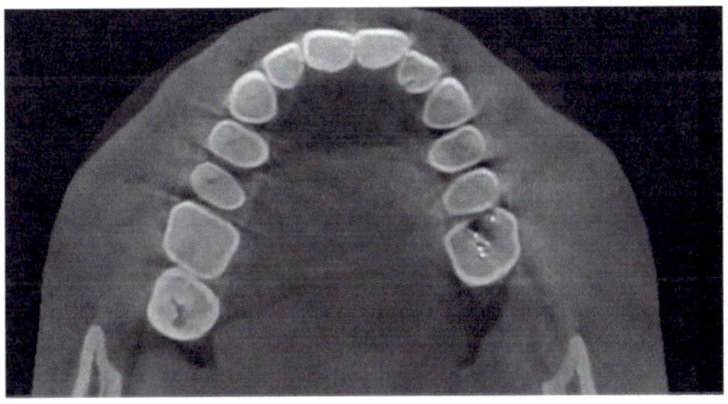

Figure 5.4. Advanced imaging modalities have significantly enhanced the diagnostic accuracy in the evaluation of complex anatomical regions such as the head and neck.

Source: https://pub.mdpi-res.com/engproc/engproc-34-00001/article_deploy/html/images/engproc-34-00001-g001.png?1684832151.

5.1.2. Computed Tomography (CT)

New imaging techniques have made it much easier to diagnose and treat problems in the head and neck. CT is especially important here because it gives very clear images and can capture them quickly, which is crucial for examining bones, soft tissues, and blood vessels in this region. CT makes it possible to see the exact size and location of the tumor, check nearby lymph nodes, and check for any invasion of neighboring tissues, which are all important for both staging and planning the treatment. Besides, using contrast-enhanced protocols helps doctors more clearly distinguish between pathological and normal tissues, which improves how accurately they can diagnose. Due to the detailed anatomy and many possible diseases in the head and neck, CT helps by providing detailed images that support both surgical and non-surgical treatments. Its role aligns with the multidisciplinary approach advocated in sarcoma management and hepatocellular carcinoma surveillance protocols, underscoring its clinical importance (Casali *et al.*, 2018; Vogel *et al.*, 2018).

5.1.3. Magnetic Resonance Imaging (MRI)

Because the head and neck region is so detailed, it is difficult to image, so advanced tools are required for proper diagnosis and treatment planning. MRI is beneficial for looking at soft tissues and complex areas because it gives clear images from all directions. Particularly in oncology, MRIs' advanced techniques, such as permeability imaging, enhance differentiation between benign and malignant tumors, including salivary gland neoplasms and squamous cell carcinomas, improving clinical decision-making and prognosis assessment (Nagano *et al.*, 2025). MRI is also important for checking if lymph nodes are involved, which is important for making a diagnosis and choosing treatment. Beyond oncology, prenatal MRI advances have expanded diagnostic precision for fetal tumors in the brain, face, and neck, guiding management strategies to mitigate severe complications associated with tumor location and metabolic demands (Feygin *et al.*, 2020). So, MRI is a primary tool in head and neck imaging because it is versatile and keeps improving with new technology.

5.1.4. Ultrasound in Head and Neck Imaging

New imaging technology has greatly improved how doctors diagnose head and neck problems, particularly in detecting cervical lymph nodes. Even though clinical examination is very important, it does not always find subclinical metastatic disease, so other methods are needed. Using high-frequency small-parts transducers, ultrasound gives a safe, inexpensive, and easy-to-access way to improve how anatomy is seen and how accurate diagnoses are made.

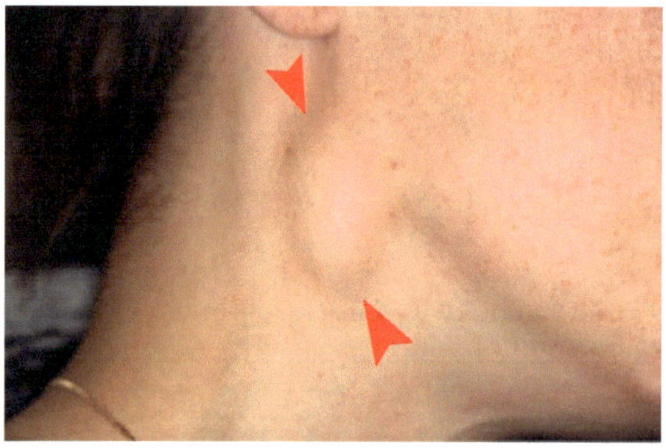

Figure 5.5. Cervical lymph nodes.

Source: https://i0.wp.com/post.medicalnewstoday.com/wp-content/uploads/sites/3/2023/01/Cervical_lymphadenopathy_right_neck_1296x728_slide-1024x575.jpg?w=1155&h=1528.

It is more detailed than palpation because it allows doctors to tell if a lymph node is solid or cystic, which helps avoid unnecessary surgery. Also, using ultrasound to guide a fine needle aspiration biopsy allows doctors to see the area and examine the cells, which helps with diagnosis and deciding on treatment. Although CT and MRI can detect cancer better, their specificity for finding metastasis is not very high, which shows why ultrasounds are still important for screening and monitoring. Given its safety profile and real-time capabilities, ultrasound remains indispensable for evaluating head and neck masses and nodal metastases, directly impacting therapeutic decisions and prognostic assessments (Baatenburg de Jong *et al.*, 1990; Dudea *et al.*, 2013) (Figure 5.5).

5.1.5. Positron Emission Tomography (PET)

Improvements in imaging methods have made it easier to diagnose problems of the head and neck. PET is now recognized as a useful method for studying metabolism and function, which adds to the findings of anatomical studies. For oncologic assessment, the use of 18F-Fluorodeoxyglucose (18F-FDG) enables the identification of primary tumors and metastatic lymph nodes with high sensitivity, particularly in vascularized regions like the lingual and laryngeal areas, where it delineates tumor margins more accurately (Culp *et al.*, 2019). Beyond conventional tracers, PET imaging with 18F-DOPA is considered the gold standard for hereditary head and neck paragangliomas, facilitating detailed tumor characterization and staging (Cantisani *et al.*, 2020). While 18F-FDG PET also contributes prognostic information by detecting aggressive disease phenotypes, newer tracers such as 68Ga-peptides hold promise for improving diagnostic accuracy further (Cantisani *et al.*, 2020). Consequently, PET plays a pivotal role not only in cancer staging but also in monitoring treatment response and detecting inflammation within head and neck structures (Culp *et al.*, 2019).

5.1.6. Fluoroscopy Applications

New medical imaging techniques have greatly improved how Otolaryngology-Head and Neck Surgery deals with diagnosis and treatment, especially by using fluoroscopy. This method gives doctors the ability to see the movement of foreign bodies in real time, which improves the accuracy of finding them in the head and neck area. For example, fluoroscopic guidance facilitates minimally invasive removal of radiopaque metallic objects lodged in the upper aerodigestive tract, reducing the need for extensive surgical exploration and enabling prompt patient recovery (Albilasi *et al.*, 2023). Historically, the development of fluoroscopy is rooted in pioneering radiographic techniques that emerged shortly after the discovery of X-rays in the late 19th century, where continuous imaging methods evolved to improve procedural precision and safety (Mould, 2018). In contemporary clinical practice, fluoroscopy has become an invaluable tool not only for diagnostic assessments but also for intraoperative guidance, ensuring that interventions are safer and more efficient by minimizing tissue trauma while simultaneously providing immediate feedback to clinicians (Figure 5.6).

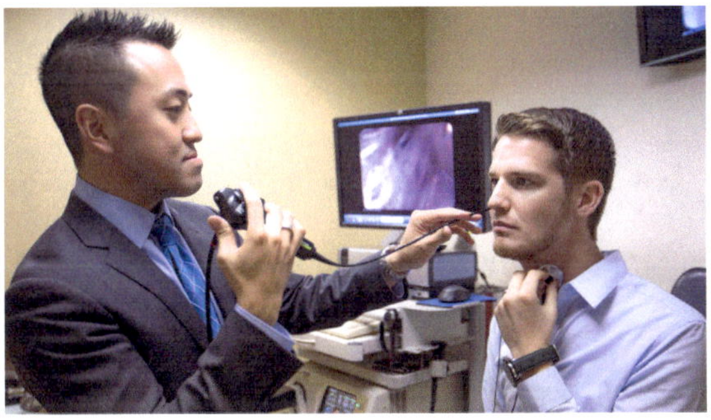

Figure 5.6. Otolaryngology-head and neck surgery.

Source: https://nyulangone.org/files/otolaryngologist-treats-a-patient.jpg.

5.1.7. Digital Imaging Advancements

Using digital imaging tools has greatly improved how head and neck oncology diagnoses are made by providing a clearer view of tumor areas. Improvements in artificial intelligence and machine learning have helped a lot in interpreting immunohistochemical tests, such as those for PD-L1, which are key for choosing immune checkpoint inhibitor treatments. These tools address the usual issues pathologists have, such as different staining patterns and subjective scoring, by ensuring the same analysis every time and improving the accuracy of diagnosis. Also, digital pathology platforms make it possible to view whole slides at high resolution, which supports thorough assessment and remote help. They help move from a simple visual review of images to using data, which improves the efficiency and quality of care for patients. Importantly, these developments position radiologists and pathologists to leverage enhanced digital workflows, ultimately improving outcomes in head and neck cancer care (Inge *et al.*, 2020; Pesapane *et al.*, 2018).

5.1.8. Comparison of Imaging Modalities

The right imaging techniques are very important for accurate diagnosis of head and neck lesions, and these depend on the specific lesion and the circumstances of the patient. Functional imaging techniques like 68 Ga-DOTATATE PET/CT have demonstrated superior sensitivity in detecting head and neck paragangliomas and related metastatic lesions, outperforming traditional anatomical methods such as contrast-enhanced CT and MRI, as well as 18 F-FDG PET/CT and 131 I-MIBG scintigraphy (Dodamani *et al.*, 2022). Conversely, when managing squamous cell carcinoma of the head and neck, ultrasound offers the highest sensitivity and diagnostic accuracy for identifying lymph node metastases, surpassing clinical examination and CT/MRI, despite operator dependency challenges (Schneider *et al.*, 2020). It points out that using both functional and anatomical imaging improves the accuracy of diagnosis. Ultimately, tailoring imaging choices to tumor characteristics and clinical objectives remains crucial in optimizing outcomes in head and neck oncology (Figure 5.7).

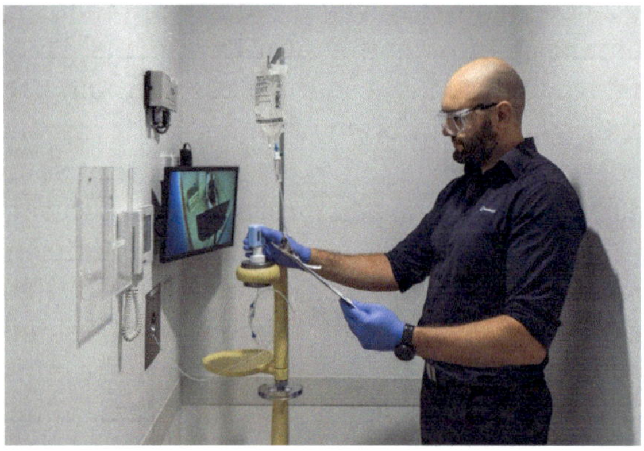

Figure 5.7. 68 Ga-DOTATATE PET/CT.

Source: https://www.qldxray.com.au/media/ohfmfkxw/image-modality-petct-psma.jpg?width=1280&height=855&quality=90&v=1d7cc14a5ba9640.

5.1.9. Future Directions in Imaging Technology

Innovations in imaging are about to significantly improve how the field of head and neck imaging works by making diagnoses and treatment planning more accurate. Emerging modalities that combine anatomical and functional imaging promise improved tumor characterization and delineation, critical for tailoring interventions such as intensity-modulated radiotherapy (IMRT). IMRT can give precise doses to the tumor while protecting healthy organs, which has led to better treatment results and lower side effects, but it is still difficult to treat resistant cancer cells. In the future, biologically guided dose escalation could be used, relying on imaging biomarkers to spot parts of a tumor that are hard to treat, which may improve the success of local control. Additionally, innovations such as intensity-modulated arc therapy (IMAT) expand on IMRT by offering enhanced delivery flexibility and precision, particularly in complex geometries (Stewart *et al.*, 2004). These technological evolutions, supported by ongoing peer-reviewed research, underscore the dynamic trajectory of head and neck imaging toward more personalized and effective care paradigms (Stewart *et al.*, 2004).

Test Your Knowledge

1. Which imaging method is most often used for looking at the nasal cavity and paranasal sinuses?
2. In what ways does MRI assist in diagnosing laryngeal tumors?

5.2. Clinical Applications

Learning Outcome

1. Understand the diagnosis of tumors and cancers;
2. Explain the evaluation of traumatic injuries;
3. Focus on assessment of congenital anomalies;
4. Learn imaging for inflammatory diseases;
5. Explain preoperative planning and guidance;
6. Describe postoperative imaging and follow-up;
7. Discuss the role in dental imaging;
8. Identify imaging for vascular conditions;
9. Known use in functional imaging studies.

The use of advanced technology has expanded both the ways to diagnose and treat diseases in the head and neck area. With artificial intelligence and radiomics working together, it is now possible to use digital images to obtain a lot of data for precise tumor analysis and monitoring. Radiomics, which collects many imaging biomarkers, helps doctors improve their understanding of head and neck cancer behavior and treatment results. Using several methods allows personalized medicine by helping doctors choose treatments that suit a patient's disease development. AI tools help radiologists find subtle changes in images, which improves how efficiently and accurately they work and manage patients. These technologies may also be used in clinical settings to help predict the success of treatments and better group patients by risk, which is important for a better outcome. Together, these innovations demonstrate a transformative impact on head and neck imaging practices, offering improved clinical utility and patient care (Peng *et al.*, 2021; Viswanathan *et al.*, 2022).

5.2.1. Diagnosis of Tumors and Cancers

To diagnose tumors and cancers correctly, imaging, histopathology, and molecular techniques are all used together. MRI and CT are major tools for assessing the extent of a lesion's impact on the body and for planning biopsies. It is important to get biopsy samples carefully to ensure sufficient tissue for microscopic examination and advanced molecular tests, which help decide the right therapy for each patient. For lung cancers, for example, techniques like endobronchial ultrasound-guided transbronchial needle aspiration allow for precise sampling of central lesions, facilitating not only diagnosis but also molecular profiling critical for targeted treatments (Planchard *et al.*, 2018). Soft tissue sarcomas, on the other hand, require a similarly rigorous protocol including core needle biopsies planned within multidisciplinary teams at specialized centers, as these tumors exhibit considerable histological heterogeneity demanding comprehensive pathological assessment (Casali *et al.*, 2018). Ultimately, a multidisciplinary approach combining high-quality imaging, expert pathology, and genomic insights is indispensable for accurate diagnosis and optimal management of tumors in the head and neck region (Figure 5.8).

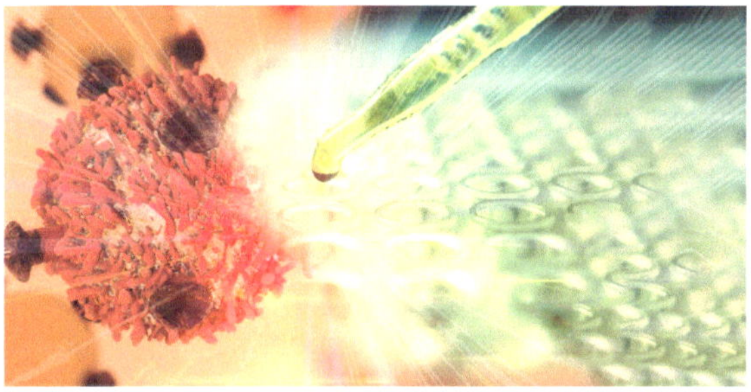

Figure 5.8. Accurate diagnosis of tumors and cancers involves a multifaceted approach that integrates imaging, histopathology, and molecular analyses.

Source: https://www.netscribes.com/wp-content/uploads/2023/08/cancer-research.webp.

5.2.2. Evaluation of Traumatic Injuries

To assess traumatic injuries in the head and neck region correctly, it is important to know how the tissues are doing and what impact they might have on nearby structures. Emerging evidence underscores the importance of evaluating cellular integrity within affected tissues to guide optimal treatment strategies, as demonstrated by studies on cartilage flaps showing high chondrocyte viability despite trauma, which may inform repair approaches in other anatomical areas (Wright *et al.*, 2017). Furthermore, the evolving landscape of concussion research emphasizes the need for refined clinical protocols to evaluate subtle neurological deficits resulting from traumatic insults, acknowledging that management must be tailored to individual injury patterns and recovery trajectories (McCrory *et al.*, 2017). Using imaging, doctors can find fractures, soft tissue issues, and blood vessel problems quickly, which helps them treat the patient properly and promptly. So, using both biological viability information and advanced imaging results helps doctors make better diagnoses and leads to improved results for patients with head and neck trauma.

5.2.3. Assessment of Congenital Anomalies

Thorough scans and the expertise of specialists are important for finding congenital issues in the head and neck region before birth. More advanced ultrasound techniques, such as examining the heart of the fetus, are now part of the usual congenital anomaly screening to improve how accurately diagnoses are made. This involves a comprehensive evaluation of the fetal situs, ventricular structures, outflow tracts, and great vessels, ensuring early identification of structural defects that could affect postnatal function and prognosis (Carvalho *et al.*, 2023). Moreover, first-trimester ultrasound screening complements this by enabling early detection of major malformations and nuchal translucency measurements predictive of chromosomal abnormalities, thus guiding further genetic counseling and management strategies (Bilardo *et al.*, 2023). Using color Doppler imaging helps see the fetus's blood vessels, which improves the detection of abnormalities. Such multidisciplinary, evidence-based approaches underscore the critical role of head and neck imaging in the timely assessment and management of congenital anomalies, ultimately supporting informed parental counseling and clinical decision-making (Figure 5.9).

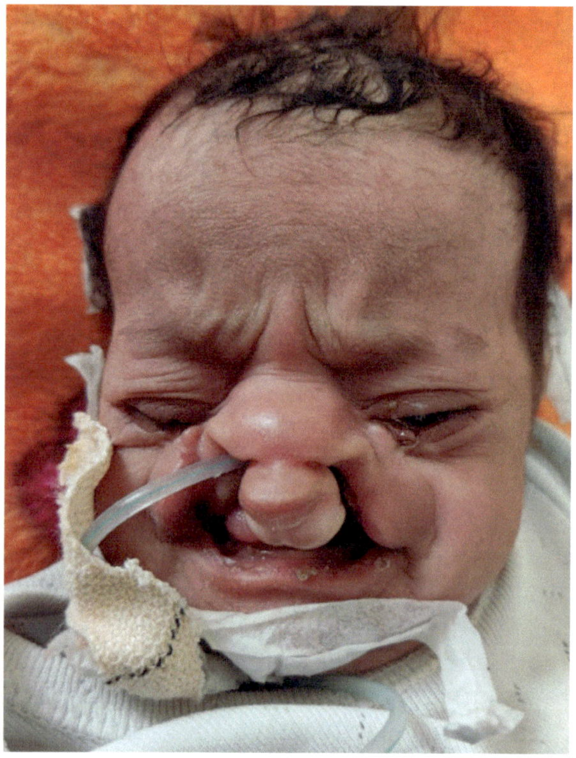

Figure 5.9. Accurate prenatal detection of congenital anomalies in the head and neck region relies on systematic imaging protocols and expert evaluation to optimize clinical outcomes.

Source: https://f6publishing.blob.core.windows.net/8adce44e-6b86-4b8a-b5ec-c4b47b54a49d/90583-g003.png.

5.2.4. Imaging for Inflammatory Diseases

The correct diagnosis and proper management of inflammatory diseases in the head and neck area rely on advanced imaging to show the extent of inflammation and related problems. MRI and CT imaging make it possible to see soft tissue swelling, abscesses, and changes in bones, which helps with quick action. Imaging helps to distinguish inflammatory lesions from cancer and also supports planning how to treat them in complicated body areas. For example, in patients with chronic inflammatory conditions or suspected neoplastic transformation, imaging complements clinical and histopathological evaluations, enhancing diagnostic accuracy (Johnson *et al.*, 2020). Additionally, standardized imaging protocols integrated within multidisciplinary approaches contribute to tailored treatment strategies, optimizing patient outcomes and monitoring response to therapy (Keohane *et al.*, 2020). For this reason, imaging is essential in the complete evaluation of inflammatory diseases in the head and neck, connecting the findings from the examination with the decisions about treatment.

5.2.5. Preoperative Planning and Guidance

Better imaging technologies have strongly improved surgery in head and neck oncology by making preoperative planning and in-surgery guidance easier. Adaptive radiation therapy models that are tailored to each patient use old images to help decide when to change the treatment plan, which results in better protection of healthy tissues and a better balance between expenses and the benefits of treatment. Such models have demonstrated significant reductions in treatment toxicity by enabling dynamic decision-making based on real-time anatomical changes, thus optimizing radiation delivery to organs at risk (Hosseinian *et al.*, 2024). At the same time, near-infrared fluorescence imaging lets surgeons see the sentinel lymph node and the tumor in real time, which is especially helpful when the area is hard to access. This fluorescence-guided approach has shown promise in enhancing the accuracy of sentinel node biopsies and improving detection rates in transoral robotic surgery, which is crucial for identifying occult primary tumors (Buchwald *et al.*, 2017). Integrating these imaging modalities into preoperative workflows exemplifies a sophisticated, evidence-based strategy that refines both surgical precision and therapeutic outcomes in head and neck cancer management (Figure 5.10).

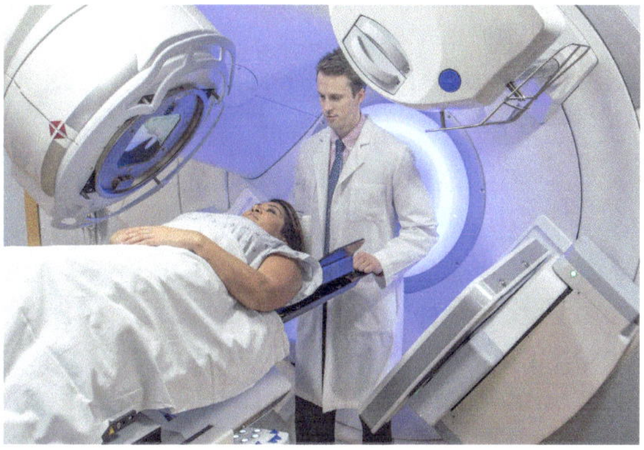

Figure 5.10. Personalized adaptive radiation therapy.

Source: https://www.oncologynurseadvisor.com/wp-content/uploads/sites/13/2020/11/radiation_G_1069315710.jpg.

5.2.6. Postoperative Imaging and Follow-up

Thorough imaging and regular check-ups are important after head and neck surgery to find any remaining disease and watch for recurrence. Modern imaging tools such as CT, MRI, and PET help surgeons see the surgical area in detail, so they can judge the success of treatment and spot any problems early. Using such imaging and careful clinical evaluation helps direct further care and improve patient results. The adaptation of auto-segmentation software in radiotherapy planning enhances the accuracy and consistency of postoperative target delineation, reducing interobserver variability and improving treatment conformity (Valentini *et al.*, 2014).

Also, having follow-up plans that match each patient's risk helps detect local recurrence quickly, which is necessary because head and neck cancers are aggressive. Moreover, understanding the patterns of tumor recurrence and integrating comprehensive imaging strategies contributes substantially to improving long-term survival rates (Sankaranarayanan *et al.*, 2015). So, checking with imaging and watching the patient closely after surgery are crucial parts of managing head and neck cancer.

5.2.7. Role in Dental Imaging

Better imaging tools have greatly improved how head and neck specialists diagnose and plan treatments, mainly in dentistry. Dental imaging helps a lot by giving clear pictures of the bones, teeth, and soft tissues, which is important for finding diseases, guiding surgery, and planning radiotherapy. For instance, the incorporation of 3D printed, tooth-borne tissue retraction devices have demonstrated potential in sparing healthy tissues during radiotherapy for head and neck cancers, thereby reducing treatment-related toxicity and improving patient outcomes (Held *et al.*, 2021). The main purpose of these developments is to use accurate imaging to help avoid harming healthy tissues during treatment. Additionally, with the rise of telehealth and remote consultations influenced by recent societal shifts, imaging has become pivotal in enhancing virtual assessments of facial and dental aesthetics, facilitating more comprehensive care beyond traditional clinical settings (Cristel *et al.*, 2020). Thus, dental imaging is indispensable for accurate diagnosis, effective treatment, and improved quality of life within head and neck imaging protocols (Figure 5.11).

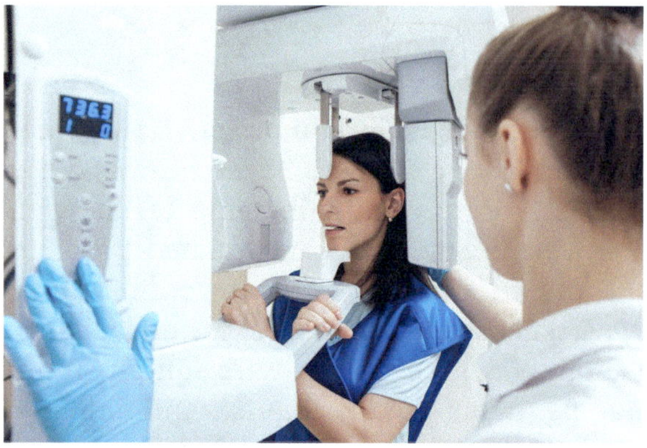

Figure 5.11. Dental imaging plays a critical role by providing detailed visualization of osseous structures, teeth, and surrounding soft tissues, which is essential for detecting pathologies, guiding surgical interventions, and planning radiotherapy.

Source: https://conescan.com/wordpress/wp-content/uploads/2022/10/Scan-Image-Left-min-scaled.jpg.

5.2.8. Imaging for Vascular Conditions

Because the head and neck region have a complex structure and serious complications can occur, advanced imaging is often needed to diagnose complex vascular lesions. A regular clinical examination might not detect all these vascular anomalies, which can result in anything from facial changes to severe bleeding. Modalities such as ultrasonography with color Doppler, magnetic resonance angiography, and cone-beam computed tomography enhance the visualization of vascular flow dynamics and lesion morphology, enabling precise characterization and differentiation of slow-flow venous malformations from other pathologies (Bonthagarla *et al.*, 2023). They help doctors make a correct diagnosis and also plan the best treatment, which reduces the risks during any intervention. Furthermore, advances in scintigraphic techniques, although more commonly applied in orthopedic vascular studies, offer insight into vascularity and tissue metabolism, suggesting a potential complementary role in assessing post-treatment vascular health (Amarasekera *et al.*, 2012). All these imaging methods are used together to handle vascular problems in the head and neck.

5.2.9. Use in Functional Imaging Studies

The use of advanced imaging has improved our ability to diagnose head and neck diseases, beyond just visual inspection. In this area, MRI has become very important because it can give detailed information about tissue metabolism, blood flow, and cell density. With these images, radiotherapy can be designed to hit the tumor precisely and save healthy tissues. For instance, functional MRI methods offer superior soft tissue contrast and non-ionizing properties, meeting the escalating demands of IMRT in head and neck cancer management (Yuan *et al.*, 2016). Radiomic approaches also make it possible to find measurable features in images, which improves the accuracy of diagnosis and tracking treatment with noninvasive markers. Platforms like PyRadiomics exemplify how standardized image processing algorithms can augment reproducibility and comparability in functional imaging studies, thereby advancing personalized treatment strategies in head and neck oncology (van Griethuysen *et al.*, 2017) (Figure 5.12).

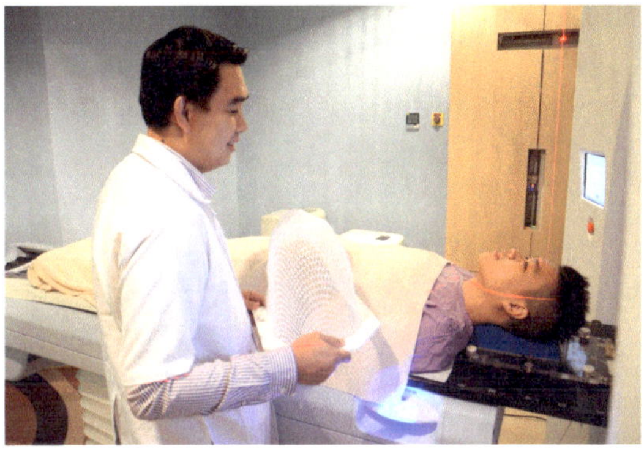

Figure 5.12. Intensity-modulated radiation therapy (IMRT) in head and neck cancer management.

Source: https://mountmiriam.com/wp-content/uploads/2017/02/tomotherapy2.jpg.

Test Your Knowledge

1. Which imaging method is most suitable for checking the cervical spine in trauma patients?
2. What is the role of CT angiography in checking for carotid artery disease?

5.3. Interpretation and Analysis

Learning Outcome

1. Identify radiological signs and symptoms;
2. Know the importance of radiologist expertise;
3. Explain common pitfalls in interpretation;
4. Understand a multidisciplinary approach to analysis;
5. Discuss the use of artificial intelligence in interpretation;
6. Learn case studies in head and neck imaging;
7. Know reporting standards and protocols;
8. Explain ethical considerations in imaging;
9. Understand continuing education for imaging professionals.

Interpreting and analyzing images is key to finding and managing problems of the head and neck. Advanced instruments like confocal laser endomicroscopy and FDG PET/CT allow doctors to see important details for their decisions. For instance, the development of deep learning algorithms applied to confocal laser endomicroscopy has significantly enhanced early detection of oral squamous cell carcinoma by accurately distinguishing malignant from healthy tissue, leading to improved treatment outcomes (Aubreville *et al.*, 2017). Similarly, FDG PET/CT plays an essential role in identifying and monitoring sarcoidosis within head and neck regions, demonstrating utility in both disease localization and therapeutic response assessment, which traditional laboratory tests fail to achieve adequately (Artiko *et al.*, 2019). These technologies prove that combining advanced analysis with imaging interpretation is vital for improving diagnosis and patient treatment, which underlines the main role of imaging in the field of head and neck pathology.

5.3.1. Radiological Signs and Symptoms

Spotting radiological signs and symptoms is very important for diagnosing many head and neck diseases and choosing the right treatment. CT and MRI scans can show mass lesions, unusual blood vessels, and signs of inflammation, which often match the symptoms seen in patients. For instance, acute cerebrovascular events associated with head and neck vasculature can manifest through ischemic changes observed on imaging, coinciding with neurological symptoms that may complicate infectious or neoplastic processes (Ellul *et al.*, 2020). Furthermore, radiological evaluation is integral in assessing tumor extent, nodal involvement, and potential perineural spread in head and neck cancers, providing essential information that influences treatment planning and prognosis (Pfister *et al.*, 2020). A proper understanding of the images helps find out sooner if the disease is progressing or causing complications, which supports better multidisciplinary care. Hence, understanding radiological signs within the clinical context remains indispensable in advanced head and neck imaging practices (Figure 5.13).

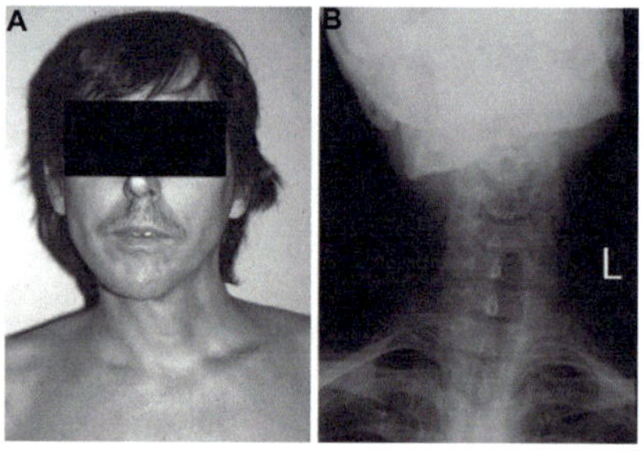

Figure 5.13. The identification of radiological signs and symptoms plays a crucial role in diagnosing a wide spectrum of head and neck pathologies, guiding appropriate clinical management.

Source: https://www.orthopedic.theclinics.com/cms/10.1016/j.ocl.2021.05.013/asset/8fd4a802-d342-4f91-9bbd-dbdb8b327be0/main.assets/gr3_lrg.jpg.

5.3.2. Importance of Radiologist Expertise

Interpreting the complex anatomy seen in head and neck imaging requires a great deal of skill from radiologists, which helps ensure the right diagnosis and treatment. Because there are many overlapping tissues and because normal and abnormal findings can be similar, it takes special training and experience to tell apart small abnormalities from benign variants. Experienced radiologists in this field help find malignancies, vascular issues, and musculoskeletal disorders early, which benefits patients. Also, using clinical data along with imaging results helps doctors make better diagnoses and prevent unneeded procedures. As new imaging techniques are introduced, such as MRI and CT angiography, radiologists must keep up with them to use them effectively. This expertise aligns with broader clinical guidelines emphasizing precision and individualized management, underlining the importance of expert interpretation akin to established recommendations in other medical imaging domains (Isselbacher *et al.*, 2022; LeBoff *et al.*, 2022).

5.3.3. Common Pitfalls in Interpretation

Interpreting head and neck images can be difficult because there are many things that can lead to mistakes in diagnosis. Because healthy structures and variations can appear similar to pathology, a good knowledge of the area and common harmless conditions is important to avoid misdiagnosis. Radiotracer uptake may also change because of inflammation or infection, which could be misinterpreted as cancer, and some tumors do not take up much radiotracer, which may result in false negatives. Problems like the patient moving, poor preparation, or artifacts in the images make it more difficult to interpret the images. Using PET metabolic data along with CT or MRI anatomy images helps confirm a diagnosis, but it is important to compare them to distinguish malignant from benign or accidental findings. Awareness of these pitfalls and appropriate use of complementary modalities are essential to improve diagnostic accuracy and optimize patient management in head and neck oncology (Mihailović *et al.*, 2021; Wiggins *et al.*, 2022).

5.3.4. Multidisciplinary Approach to Analysis

Getting the best results for head and neck cancer patients depends on bringing together different clinical viewpoints. Imaging helps both in identifying the cause and in planning the best treatment approach with a team. Imaging, pathology, and clinical details are used together to guide doctors in choosing the best surgical approach, radiation therapy, and chemotherapy for a patient.

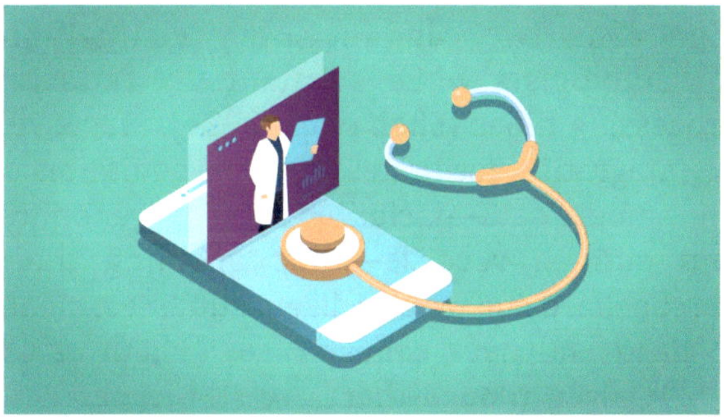

Figure 5.14. Imaging plays a crucial role not only in diagnosis but also in guiding treatment planning within a multidisciplinary framework.

Source: https://cipherhealth.com/wp-content/uploads/2019/08/CH-Communication-Blog.jpg.

Because of this teamwork, each treatment is designed to fit the patient's condition and the disease's severity, which keeps side effects low and increases the chances of controlling the disease. For instance, narrow or positive surgical margins identified through integrated imaging and pathology reports necessitate careful radiotherapy dose adjustments to avoid unnecessary tissue damage (Biedka-Paluch *et al.*, 2024). Moreover, combining advanced imaging with systemic therapies such as immunotherapy and metastasis-directed radiotherapy enhances survival rates in metastatic cases, underscoring the vital role of multidisciplinary evaluation in complex treatment scenarios (Xu *et al.*, 2025) (Figure 5.14).

5.3.5. Use of Artificial Intelligence (AI) in Interpretation

New technology has greatly improved how head and neck imaging is done, and AI has been key in making the process more accurate and efficient. AI algorithms based on deep learning have proven to be good at finding small changes in the brain that might go unnoticed by standard analysis. For instance, AI-assisted tools have been developed to identify and measure vascular abnormalities such as aneurysms, offering high sensitivity and accuracy comparable to radiologists while substantially reducing processing times (Shen *et al.*, 2024). Moreover, AI integration facilitates the amalgamation of multimodal data—including imaging, genomics, and clinical records—thus enabling more personalized and precise diagnostic assessments in head and neck cancer cases (Pham *et al.*, 2024). Even though there are still issues with data quality and the transparency of algorithms, the use of explainable AI and more teamwork between doctors and data scientists is set to enhance how diseases are diagnosed, which should lead to better patient outcomes.

5.3.6. Case Studies in Head and Neck Imaging

Improvements in artificial intelligence and imaging have greatly improved how head and neck pathologies are diagnosed. Case studies have shown significant progress, mainly in using automated segmentation and classification of lesions with both FDG-PET and CT images. For example, the HECKTOR challenge showcased how convolutional neural networks (CNNs) could accurately delineate gross tumor volumes in oropharyngeal cancers, outperforming both baseline methods and human inter-observer agreement, thus indicating a promising future for radiomics studies and reducing reliance on time-consuming manual delineation (Oreiller *et al.*, 2021). Similarly, another study employing a ResNet-based CNN for whole-body FDG PET/CT images achieved high accuracy in classifying benign, malignant, and equivocal lesions, with impressive region-specific reliability in the head and neck area (Kawauchi *et al.*, 2020). The case studies show that AI-powered tools can greatly improve both the accuracy of diagnoses and the way clinical work is done in head and neck imaging.

5.3.7. Reporting Standards and Protocols

Consistent use of reporting standards and protocols makes sure that imaging studies in head and neck oncology are interpreted accurately and patients are treated properly. Since head and neck anatomy is complicated and some inflammatory or infectious diseases can appear like cancer, using standard ways to measure metabolism is very important. For instance, distinguishing between FDG-avid lymph nodes due to malignancy versus those related to inflammatory conditions such as HIV infection requires careful consideration of nodal size, symmetry, and standardized uptake values (SUV), as noted in studies comparing these factors across patient populations (Ayeni *et al.*, 2019). Furthermore, the use of normalization techniques, such as referencing liver SUVmean, has been proposed to enhance consistency across PET/CT scans, reducing variability introduced by patient or technical factors and thereby facilitating more accurate staging and monitoring (Wilson *et al.*, 2011). Overall, adherence to rigorous reporting protocols promotes clarity, comparability, and ultimately better clinical outcomes in head and neck imaging (Figure 5.15).

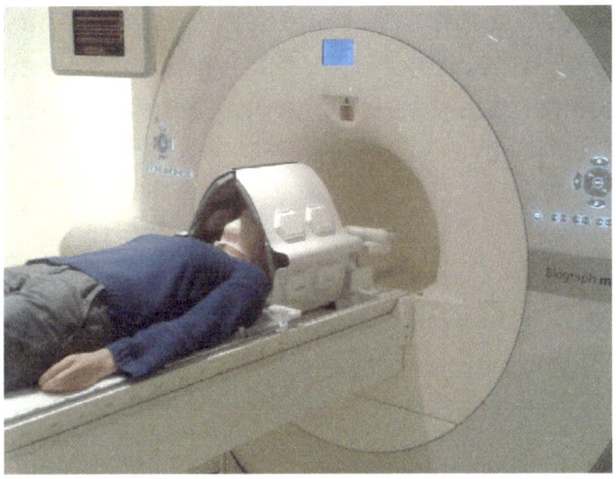

Figure 5.15. Accurate interpretation of imaging studies in head and neck oncology relies heavily on consistent reporting standards and protocols to ensure diagnostic reliability and optimal patient management.

Source: https://www.researchgate.net/publication/327772129/figure/fig1/AS:679625546014720@1539046765139/Dedicated-positioning-solution-for-MR-imaging-of-head-and-neck-cancer-patients-in-RT.png.

5.3.8. Ethical Considerations in Imaging

New imaging methods have greatly improved the process of diagnosing head and neck diseases, but they also bring up complicated ethical problems. There is a big issue with patient privacy, mainly because images that can be traced back to patients may be used or shared. Although there are clear ethical rules, many healthcare professionals and patients do not realize the consequences of uploading patient pictures online and in science. Ensuring fully informed consent before publishing any identifiable images is critical to maintaining trust and confidentiality in clinical practice and academic dissemination (Roguljić *et al.*, 2025). Also, deciding how to use adaptive imaging techniques and their costs can create ethical dilemmas about using resources and caring for patients. Implementing decision-making models that optimize radiation therapy while considering financial and quality-of-life impacts exemplifies an ethical commitment to both efficacy and equity in patient care (Hosseinian *et al.*, 2024). So, it is important to use strong privacy measures and consider the benefits and costs when performing ethical head and neck imaging.

5.3.9. Continuing Education for Imaging Professionals

Because imaging advances and new diagnostic standards keep appearing, experts in head and neck imaging should keep learning to maintain their skills and provide the best care for patients.

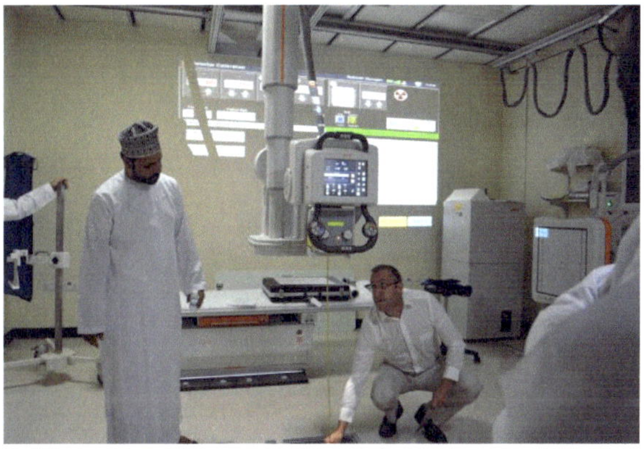

Figure 5.16. Continuing education for imaging professionals.

Source: https://www.carestream.com/blog/wp-content/uploads/2018/12/Oman_DR_Workshop_3_Carestream.jpg.

ducational courses help doctors learn about the latest techniques, such as high-resolution MRI and PET/CT, which are key for correctly identifying anatomical and pathological problems in the head and neck. Also, having access to structured learning helps imaging specialists improve their ability to distinguish between benign and malignant findings. Because of the complex anatomy and many diseases in head and neck imaging, using updated evidence-based protocols improves diagnosis and encourages teamwork. Recent educational resources, workshops, and seminars, together with case-based learning modules, play a key role in helping professionals continue their development. Consequently, continuing education ensures that imaging professionals remain adept at leveraging cutting-edge technologies and methodologies in their clinical practice (Figure 5.16).

Test Your Knowledge

1. What part does imaging have in finding and classifying head and neck cancers?
2. In what ways can imaging be applied to check for metastasis in head and neck cancers?

5.4. Patient Considerations

Learning Outcome

1. Understand patient preparation for imaging;
2. Know safety protocols and radiation exposure;
3. Identify contrast agents and their implications;
4. Manage patient anxiety during procedures;
5. Focus on informed consent processes;
6. Know special considerations for pediatric patients;
7. Address cultural sensitivities in imaging;
8. Describe follow-up care and patient education;
9. Learn the impact of imaging on patient outcomes.

Developments in treating head and neck cancers require doctors to look at each patient's situation to achieve the best results and avoid harm. Using neoadjuvant immunotherapy can lessen the tumor before surgery, which may make surgeries less invasive and help maintain organ function. Nevertheless, this method requires constant observation for any negative effects and careful evaluation of how well the treatment is working, due to differences between what is seen on images and what is found in the tissue. Concurrently, imaging modalities used for treatment planning must balance accuracy with patient safety; recent developments in magnetic resonance imaging sequences, such as optimized fat-suppressed 3D T2-weighted scans, enhance tumor and lymph node delineation while limiting radiation exposure to surrounding tissues (Joint Head and Neck Radiotherapy-MRI Development Cooperative *et al.*, 2023). For this reason, it is important to use personalized imaging and for teams from different specialties to collaborate in treating head and neck cancers, so the care is effective and causes the least harm.

5.4.1. Patient Preparation for Imaging

Good imaging of the head and neck area depends on both advanced equipment and thorough patient preparation. Before imaging, patients should be placed correctly and told to stay still to avoid motion artifacts that may affect the imaging of delicate structures and diseases. The administration of specific contrast agents, such as ultrasmall superparamagnetic iron oxide (USPIO), enhances the detection of lymph node metastases, necessitating careful scheduling and assessment protocols to ensure optimal uptake and clear differentiation between benign and malignant tissues (Driessen *et al.*, 2022). Additionally, the selection of appropriate imaging sequences, like the optimized T2-weighted fat-suppressed sequence developed for MR-Linac systems, is contingent upon preparatory steps that include patient hydration status and contraindications to imaging agents, thereby improving the segmentation accuracy and overall image quality vital for precise treatment planning (Joint Head and Neck Radiotherapy-MRI Development Cooperative *et al.*, 2023). This comprehensive preparation ultimately facilitates improved diagnostic yields and patient outcomes in head and neck imaging (Figure 5.17).

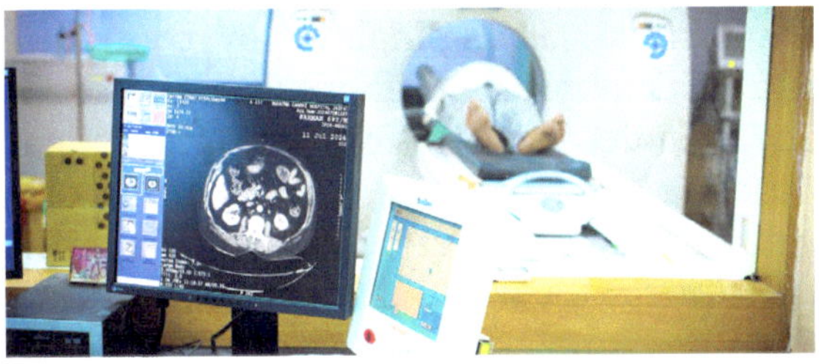

Figure 5.17. Effective imaging of the head and neck region hinges not only on advanced technology but also on meticulous patient preparation to optimize image quality and diagnostic accuracy.

Source: https://www.mgmch.org/uploads/LargeImages/24pg_radio-diagnosis.jpg.

5.4.2. Safety Protocols and Radiation Exposure

Because new imaging techniques produce more radiation, it is now very important to follow strict safety procedures, especially when scanning the head and neck. The integration of hybrid imaging technologies, such as the 1.5T MR-Linac, enables precise tumor delineation while optimizing radiation dosing to minimize collateral damage to adjacent organs at risk, thus potentially reducing toxicity and improving patient outcomes (Joint Head and Neck Radiotherapy-MRI Development Cooperative *et al.*, 2023). Similarly, the advent of PET/MRI offers improved soft tissue characterization and functional imaging with inherently lower radiation doses compared to conventional PET/CT, enhancing safety profiles especially for pediatric populations (Lyons *et al.*, 2018). Still, these advantages rely on proper handling of workflow, radiation safety, and sedation methods to ensure patient comfort and adherence to established protocols. Trying to optimize imaging settings and using dose modulation algorithms plays a big role in balancing the effectiveness of imaging with the risk of radiation exposure, highlighting the strong connection between advanced technology and safety measures in head and neck imaging.

5.4.3. Contrast Agents and Their Implications

It is very important to use contrast agents in head and neck imaging to clearly show both normal and abnormal parts of the body. Agents like these, which are often given through a vein, help CT and MRI scans by making it easier to distinguish normal tissue from lesions. Even so, the use of contrast in imaging can cause allergic reactions, harm the kidneys, and interact with any existing medical conditions, so it must be managed properly.

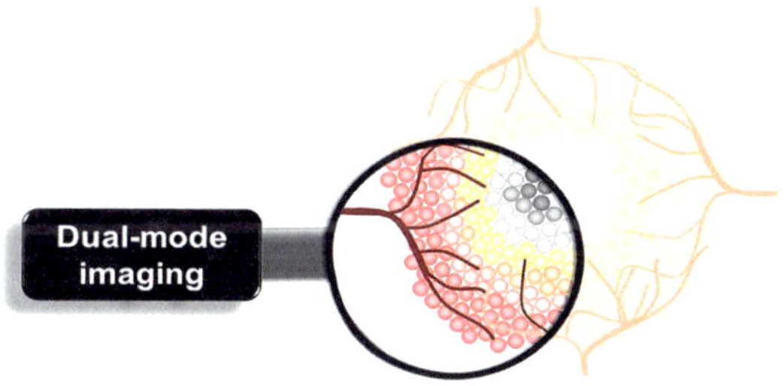

Figure 5.18. Dual mode imaging.

Source: https://pub.mdpi-res.com/biosensors/biosensors-12-00478/article_deploy/html/images/biosensors-12-00478-ag-550.jpg?1656595815.

Also, differences in the way drugs are handled by the body can affect the assessment of tumor size and the response to treatment, which can impact both medical decisions and predicting outcomes. For head and neck cancer patients undergoing radiation or proton therapy, precise delineation of organs at risk through contrast-enhanced imaging is essential to optimize treatment planning and minimize toxicities, as effective dose-sparing relies on accurately defined anatomical boundaries (Stieb *et al.*, 2021). While contrast agents present certain risks, their judicious application greatly facilitates diagnostic accuracy and therapeutic outcomes (McMullin *et al.*, 2018) (Figure 5.18).

5.4.4. Managing Patient Anxiety During Procedures

Talking clearly and focusing on the patient's needs helps to ease anxiety during head and neck imaging procedures. Many patients feel more stressed because they are afraid of the pain, do not know what to expect, or are in unfamiliar surroundings. When healthcare providers explain the procedure, what the patient will feel, and the reason for imaging, it helps the patient feel more in charge and less afraid. Relaxation methods and a supportive atmosphere can encourage patients to cooperate more, which helps produce better images for diagnosis.

Clinicians ought to take into account personal factors in patients, such as other health problems or previous unpleasant experiences, to adjust their approach and help patients tolerate and follow the treatment. Engaging patients in shared decision-making not only enhances their comfort but also aligns care with their values and preferences, thereby improving procedural outcomes and satisfaction in line with best clinical practices (Stout *et al.*, 2018). This holistic strategy reflects the broader imperative within imaging and medical care to address psychological as well as physical patient needs (LeBoff *et al.*, 2022).

5.4.5. Informed Consent Processes

Good communication between healthcare providers and patients is very important for meeting ethical and legal standards, especially in head and neck imaging, because the results can guide treatment decisions. Patients should be told in detail about what imaging means, its advantages, possible risks, and the other options available, so they can make an informed decision. This process is especially important given the complex treatment options and potential toxicities associated with head and neck cancers, as highlighted by contrasting therapeutic approaches that demand thorough patient understanding for consent adequacy (Mehanna *et al.*, 2018). Moreover, standardized guidelines and expert consensus emphasize the need for clear, transparent disclosure in emerging interventions, underscoring the broader applicability of rigorous informed consent beyond imaging to encompass novel treatments (McClintock *et al.*, 2017). Ultimately, ensuring comprehensive informed consent within head and neck imaging not only respects patient autonomy but also enhances trust and compliance in clinical care pathways (Figure 5.19).

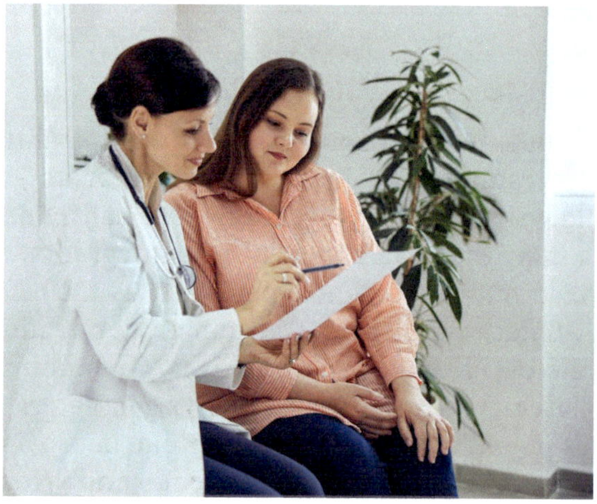

Figure 5.19. Effective communication between healthcare providers and patients is crucial to ensuring ethical and legal standards are met, particularly in the context of head and neck imaging where diagnostic procedures can have significant implications for treatment planning.

Source: https://publichealth.tulane.edu/wp-content/uploads/sites/3/2021/09/Strategies-for-Effective-Communication-in-Health-Care.jpg.

5.4.6. Special Considerations for Pediatric Patients

Because head and neck imaging in children are different, it requires special methods to get the right results and avoid risks. Because children's anatomy is not the same as adults' and keeps changing, radiologists must use appropriate imaging techniques and protocols, since congenital anomalies and rare malignancies are more frequent in this group. For example, children with chromosomal disorders like Down syndrome may exhibit characteristic craniofacial features and associated conditions that demand specialized imaging assessments and frequent monitoring (Bull *et al.*, 2022). Radiation exposure should be kept low in children by choosing the right imaging techniques when possible. When assessing rare neoplasms such as nasopharyngeal carcinoma, which is less common in children but demonstrates distinct epidemiologic and biological behaviors, understanding the underlying viral associations and histopathology can guide imaging strategies for staging and therapeutic response evaluation (Chua *et al.*, 2019). In general, imaging for children in the head and neck area should be done in a way that combines accurate diagnosis, safety, and attention to development.

5.4.7. Addressing Cultural Sensitivities in Imaging

For healthcare professionals, being able to communicate well and respect what matters to patients is very important for giving the best care. In head and neck imaging, cultural factors can play a big role in how well patients cooperate and how accurate the diagnosis is. Because people's thoughts on medical procedures, privacy, and modesty differ greatly across cultures, healthcare providers should use approaches that fit each group's beliefs. Ethical considerations such as autonomy and informed consent become particularly relevant when addressing these factors, ensuring that patients feel respected and empowered throughout the imaging process (Varkey, 2020). Furthermore, psychosocial distress linked to cultural misunderstandings or discomfort during imaging may hinder effective diagnosis and treatment, emphasizing the need for culturally competent care protocols (Riba *et al.*, 2019). By integrating cultural awareness into head and neck imaging procedures, healthcare providers can foster trust, reduce patient anxiety, and enhance diagnostic outcomes, aligning technical expertise with compassionate, patient-centered care (Figure 5.20).

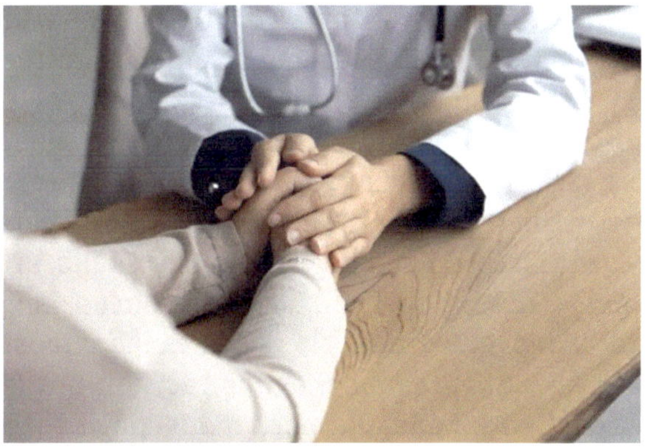

Figure 5.20. Patients' beliefs and attitudes toward medical procedures, privacy, and modesty vary widely across cultures, necessitating tailored approaches that honor these differences.

Source: https://www.thehastingscenter.org/wp-content/smush-webp/shutterstock_2093260780-doctor-patient-hands.jpg--866x573.jpg.webp.

5.4.8. Follow-up Care and Patient Education

Good follow-up care and complete education of patients play an important role in achieving the best outcomes for people having head and neck imaging. As well as working with images, clinicians should help patients understand what the results mean, what the possible diagnosis is, and what will be done next. It requires explaining that ongoing monitoring, possible interventions, and changes in lifestyle can help stop or reduce the effects of the disease. For example, patients with conditions such as obstructive sleep apnea (OSA) may benefit from understanding the importance of continuous positive airway pressure adherence, which significantly reduces mortality and cardiovascular risks associated with untreated disease (Pépin *et al.*, 2022). Similarly, in metabolic bone diseases like osteoporosis, timely follow-up and patient education about medication adherence and preventive measures are imperative to avoid recurrent fractures and associated morbidity (LeBoff *et al.*, 2022). So, when patient-centered education is included in follow-up, patients are more likely to comply, make better decisions, and enjoy better long-term health in head and neck disease.

5.4.9. Impact of Imaging on Patient Outcomes

Better imaging techniques have greatly improved how head and neck cancers are diagnosed and treated, which has a positive effect on patients. The use of MRI, CT, and FDG-PET improves the identification of tumor borders, shows signs of perineural invasion, and detects lymph node metastases, helping surgeons remove the tumor completely and save important structures. This way of treating cancer reduces the risk of cancer coming back in the same area and improves the chance of survival. In addition, using radiomics helps to quantify imaging features that can be used as noninvasive biomarkers to predict how a tumor will behave and how it will respond to treatment, making patient care more personal. But it is still challenging to standardize how algorithms are used so that their results are the same and useful in different medical centers. When different specialists use advanced imaging and molecular diagnostics, it is easier to stage and group these tumors, which helps choose the best therapy for each patient. Hence, imaging not only enhances diagnostic precision but also directly impacts prognosis and quality of life for patients with head and neck malignancies (van Griethuysen *et al.*, 2017; van Herpen *et al.*, 2022).

Test Your Knowledge

1. Why is MRI generally preferred over CT for looking at the brain and brainstem in the head and neck area?
2. What new developments have occurred in imaging during head and neck surgery?

SUMMARY

Better imaging techniques for head and neck cancers have made it easier to diagnose, plan treatment, and look after patients. Being able to see detailed changes in the body has allowed doctors to find tumors early and assess the effectiveness of treatments, and their side effects. For instance, the integration of imaging findings with clinical endpoints has allowed for better assessment of therapeutic efficacy, as highlighted by recent studies utilizing immune checkpoint inhibitors in recurrent cases demonstrating meaningful antitumor activity confirmed through imaging metrics (Bauml *et al.*, 2017). Additionally, the development of standardized imaging-based grading systems, such as DIGEST, enhances the objectivity and reliability of toxicity evaluation, contributing to more tailored therapeutic approaches and improved quality of life for patients (Hutcheson *et al.*, 2016). All in all, imaging of the head and neck is vital for oncology, helping to bring together different specialists and lead to better patient results.

The use of new imaging methods has made it much easier to diagnose and treat complex problems of the head and neck, proving that radiological evaluation is very important in making clinical decisions. Accurate imaging facilitates the detection of subtle pathological changes, such as perineural spread along cranial nerves, which significantly alter prognosis and treatment strategies for head and neck tumors (Ciurea *et al.*, 2021). Additionally, hybrid molecular imaging modalities, including FDG PET/CT, have enhanced the identification and monitoring of inflammatory disorders like head and neck sarcoidosis, enabling tailored therapeutic interventions and improved patient outcomes (Artiko *et al.*, 2019). Seeing anatomical and functional problems clearly with imaging makes it important to include complete imaging protocols in regular assessments. So, imaging of the head and neck confirms what doctors suspect and supports the use of various treatments. The use of advanced imaging is still necessary for better diagnosis, staging, and care after treatment in otolaryngology and oncology.

KEY TERMS FROM THIS CHAPTER

- Dental
- Cervical
- Lymph node localization
- Blood vessel
- Conductive hearing loss
- Doppler analysis
- U-net
- Calcifications
- Maxillofacial
- Sentinel node
- Diagnostic precision
- Sensorineural hearing loss
- Retrocochlear pathology
- Air-filled structure visualization
- Lymph node staging

CRITICAL THINKING QUESTIONS

1. **When it comes to soft tissue lesions in the head and neck, which method is considered the best?**
    a. X-ray
    b. Ultrasound
    c. MRI
    d. CT
2. **For what purpose is contrast-enhanced CT most often used in head and neck imaging?**
    a. To detect bone fractures in the skull
    b. To look at the blood vessels and find any tumors or infections in the soft tissues
    c. To evaluate brain function during surgery
    d. To diagnose hearing loss
3. **What imaging approach should be used to check the nasal cavity and paranasal sinuses for illnesses such as sinusitis or tumors?**
    a. MRI
    b. X-ray
    c. CT
    d. Ultrasound
4. **Ultrasound is often used in imaging the head and neck to examine:**
    a. Intracranial hemorrhage
    b. Salivary gland diseases, such as sialolithiasis
    c. Skull fractures
    d. Nasopharyngeal tumors
5. **What does gadolinium contrast usually help to evaluate in a contrast-enhanced MRI of the head and neck?**
    a. Bone fractures
    b. Soft tissue tumors and vascular malformations
    c. Calcifications in the skull
    d. Intracranial pressure

Short Answer Questions

1. Which imaging tests are most often used to assess head and neck conditions?
2. In what ways is MRI different from CT when looking at the head and neck area?
3. What part does X-ray play in examining the head and neck?
4. When assessing soft tissue masses in the head and neck, which imaging method is usually preferred?
5. Why do head and neck CT or MRI scans usually need contrast-enhanced imaging?
6. What are the uses of ultrasound in checking head and neck conditions?
7. In what cases is CT imaging chosen instead of MRI for head and neck evaluations?
8. What benefits come from using high-resolution CT when viewing the temporal bone and middle ear?

Answers to Critical Thinking Questions

1. (c); 2. (b); 3. (c); 4. (b); 5. (b)

REFERENCES

1. Achilefu, S., Pogue, B. W., Rosenthal, E. L., Van, D., *et al.* (2018). *Perspective Review of What is Needed for Molecular-Specific Fluorescence-Guided Surgery.* https://core.ac.uk/download/212867593.pdf (accessed on 31st May 2025).
2. Albilasi, T., AlDhawi, L. F., Alolaywi, A. N., Al Mutairy, A. S., Alghamdi, F. R., Alamry, S., & Alzhrani, H. (2023). Fluoroscopy-guided metallic foreign body removal: A report of three cases and literature review. *Cureus.* https://doi.org/10.7759/cureus.40462 (accessed on 1st June 2025).
3. Alfaro-Almagro, F., Jenkinson, M., Bangerter, N. K., Andersson, J., Griffanti, L., Douaud, G., Sotiropoulos, S. N., *et al.* (2017). Image processing and quality control for the first 10,000 brain imaging datasets from UK Biobank. *NeuroImage, 166*, 400–424. https://doi.org/10.1016/j.neuroimage.2017.10.034 (accessed on 31st May 2025).
4. Al-Ibraheem, A., Buck, A., Krause, B. J., Scheidhauer, *et al.* (2009). *Clinical Applications of FDG PET and PET/CT in Head and Neck Cancer.* https://core.ac.uk/download/pdf/8320635.pdf (accessed on 31st May 2025).
5. Amarasekera, H. W., Amarasekera, H. W., Beaulé, P. E., Beaulé, P. E., Bolland, B. J., Calder, S. J., Carrothers, A. D., *et al.* (2012). Scintigraphic assessment of bone status at one year following hip resurfacing: Comparison of two surgical approaches using SPECT-CT scan. *Bone & Joint Research.* https://core.ac.uk/download/16662900.pdf (accessed on 31st May 2025).
6. Anand, U., Dey, A., Singh, C. A. K., Sanyal, R., Mishra, A., Pandey, D. K., De Falco, V., *et al.* (2022). Cancer chemotherapy and beyond: Current status, drug candidates, associated risks and progress in targeted therapeutics. *Genes & Diseases, 10*, 1367–1401. https://doi.org/10.1016/j.gendis.2022.02.007 (accessed on 1st June 2025).
7. Artiko, V. M., Grozdic, M. I., Saponjski, J., Sobic-Saranovic, *et al.* (2019). *Hybrid Imaging in Head and Neck Sarcoidosis.* https://core.ac.uk/download/288114268.pdf (accessed on 31st May 2025).
8. Attia, A. B. E., Balasundaram, G., Moothanchery, M., Dinish, U. S., Bi, R., Ntziachristos, V., & Olivo, M. (2019). A review of clinical photoacoustic imaging: Current and future trends. *Photoacoustics, 16*, 100144. https://doi.org/10.1016/j.pacs.2019.100144 (accessed on 31st May 2025).
9. Aubreville, M., Bohr, C., Denzler, J., Jaremenko, *et al.* (2017). Automatic classification of cancerous tissue in laserendomicroscopy images of the oral cavity using deep learning. *Scientific Reports.* https://core.ac.uk/download/618224174.pdf (accessed on 31st May 2025).
10. Ayeni, O. A., Baeyens, A., Kotzen, J. A., Minnaar, *et al.* (2019). Defining characteristics of nodal disease on PET/CT scans in patients with HIV-positive and -negative locally advanced cervical cancer in South Africa. *Tomography.* https://core.ac.uk/download/322827598.pdf (accessed on 31st May 2025).
11. Ayers, M., Lunceford, J., Nebozhyn, M., Murphy, E., Loboda, A., Kaufman, D. R., Albright, A., *et al.* (2017). IFN-γ–related mRNA profile predicts clinical response to PD-1 blockade. *Journal of Clinical Investigation, 127*, 2930–2940. https://doi.org/10.1172/jci91190 (accessed on 1st June 2025).

12. Baatenburg, De. J. R. J., & Rongen, R. J. (1990). *Ultrasound Examination of the Head and Neck*. https://core.ac.uk/download/18513420.pdf (accessed on 31st May 2025).

13. Balm, A. J. M., Klop, W. M. C., Nieweg, O. E., Valdés, O., *et al.* (2009). Sentinel node detection in head and neck malignancies: Innovations in radioguided surgery. *J. Oncol.* https://core.ac.uk/download/pdf/8358696.pdf (accessed on 31st May 2025).

14. Bauml, J., Seiwert, T. Y., Pfister, D. G., Worden, F. P., Liu, S. V., Gilbert, J., Saba, N. F., *et al.* (2017). Pembrolizumab for platinum- and cetuximab-refractory head and neck cancer: Results from a single-arm, phase II study. *Journal of Clinical Oncology, 35*, 1542–1549. https://doi.org/10.1200/jco.2016.70.1524 (accessed on 31st May 2025).

15. Bhogal, R. H., & Downing, R. (2011). *The Evolution of Aortic Aneurysm Repair: Past Lessons and Future Directions*. https://core.ac.uk/download/pdf/1631327.pdf (accessed on 31st May 2025).

16. Biedka-Paluch, M., Biedka, P., & Winiecki, J. (2024). Therapeutic implications of narrow or positive surgical margins in head and neck tumors. *Acta Elbingensia*. https://www.semanticscholar.org/paper/bd03d7cf10e44be3bed992a38a0770f37c59dd90 (accessed on 1st June 2025).

17. Bilardo, C. M., Chaoui, R., Hyett, J., Kagan, K. O., Karim, J., Papageorghiou, A. T., Poon, L. C., *et al.* (2023). *ISUOG* Practice Guidelines (updated): Performance of 11–14-week ultrasound scan. *Ultrasound in Obstetrics and Gynecology, 61*, 127–143. https://doi.org/10.1002/uog.26106 (accessed on 31st May 2025).

18. Bonthagarla, K. S., Buduru, K., Deepika, A. D. N., Mounika, *et al.* (2023). *Vascular Malformation Involving the Maxillofacial Region: A Case Report*. https://core.ac.uk/download/591773001.pdf (accessed on 31st May 2025).

19. Buchwald, C., Christensen, A., Rubek, N., Juhl, K., Charabi, B., Mortensen, J., Kiss, K., *et al.* (2017). Abstract IA13: Real-time near-infrared fluorescence tracer imaging to guide sentinel node biopsy and tumor detection in head and neck cancer. *Clinical Cancer Research, 23*. https://www.semanticscholar.org/paper/d34e7be67ce76077d6ba24523db098d0bd9c5f01 (accessed on 31st May 2025).

20. Bull, M. J., Trotter, T. L., Santoro, S. L., Christensen, C. K., & Grout, R. W. (2022). Health supervision for children and adolescents with Down syndrome. *Pediatrics, 149*. https://doi.org/10.1542/peds.2022-057010 (accessed on 1st June 2025).

21. Cantisani, V., Colao, A., Di Leo, N., Faggiano, *et al.* (2020). Natural history and management of familial paraganglioma syndrome type 1: Long-term data from a large family. *J. Clin. Med.* https://core.ac.uk/download/296244529.pdf (accessed on 31st May 2025).

22. Cardoso, L. G., Lessa, A. M. G., Maia, J. P. C., Sampaio, *et al.* (2019). The importance of immunological findings in the identification of head and neck pathological changes: A literature review. *Journal of Research in Dentistry*. https://core.ac.uk/download/300482777.pdf (accessed on 31st May 2025).

23. Carvalho, J. S., Axt-Fliedner, R., Chaoui, R., Copel, J. A., Cuneo, B. F., Goff, D. A., Gordin, K. L., *et al.* (2023). ISUOG practice guidelines (updated): Fetal cardiac screening. *Ultrasound in Obstetrics and Gynecology, 61*, 788–803. https://doi.org/10.1002/uog.26224 (accessed on 31st May 2025).

24. Casali, P. G., Abecassis, N., Bauer, S., Biagini, R., Bielack, S., Bonvalot, S., Boukovinas, I., *et al.* (2018). Soft tissue and visceral sarcomas: ESMO–EURACAN Clinical Practice Guidelines for diagnosis, treatment and follow-up. *Annals of Oncology, 29*, iv51–iv67. https://doi.org/10.1093/annonc/mdy096 (accessed on 1st June 2025).

25. Chandrasekhar, S. S., Tsai, S. B., Schwartz, S., Bontempo, L., Faucett, E. A., Finestone, S. A., Hollingsworth, D. B., *et al.* (2019a). Clinical practice guideline: Sudden hearing loss (update). *Otolaryngology, 161*. https://doi.org/10.1177/0194599819859885 (accessed on 1st June 2025).

26. Chandrasekhar, S. S., Tsai, S. B., Schwartz, S., Bontempo, L., Faucett, E. A., Finestone, S. A., Hollingsworth, D. B., *et al.* (2019b). Clinical practice guideline: Sudden hearing loss (update) executive summary. *Otolaryngology, 161*, 195–210. https://doi.org/10.1177/0194599819859883 (accessed on 1st June 2025).

27. Chua, M. L. K., Sun, Y., & Supiot, S. (2019). Advances in nasopharyngeal carcinoma—"West meets East." *British Journal of Radiology, 92*. https://doi.org/10.1259/bjr.20199004 (accessed on 1st June 2025).

28. Ciurea, A., Csutak, C., Dinu, C., Hedesiu, *et al.* (2021). *Perineural Spread in Head and Neck Malignancies: Imaging Findings – an Updated Literature Review*. https://core.ac.uk/download/644449258.pdf (accessed on 31st May 2025).

29. Cristel, R. T., Demesh, D., & Dayan, S. (2020). Video conferencing impact on facial appearance: Looking beyond the COVID-19 pandemic. *Facial Plastic Surgery & Aesthetic Medicine, 22*, 238, 239. https://doi.org/10.1089/fpsam.2020.0279 (accessed on 1st June 2025).

30. Culp, W. T. N., Spriet, M., & Willcox, J. L. (2019). Role of positron emission tomography in imaging of non-neurologic disorders of the head, neck, and teeth in veterinary medicine. *Front Vet. Sci.* https://core.ac.uk/download/323070037.pdf (accessed on 31st May 2025).

31. Deandreis, D., Durante, C., Filetti, S., Lamartina, *et al.* (2016). Endocrine tumors: Imaging in the follow-up of differentiated thyroid cancer: Current evidence and future perspectives for a risk-adapted approach. *European Journal of Endocrinology*. https://core.ac.uk/download/74318453.pdf (accessed on 31st May 2025).

32. Dodamani, M. H., Jaiswal, S. K., Sarathi, V., Marfatia, H., D'Cruz, A., Malhotra, G., Hira, P., *et al.* (2022). Comparison of the sensitivity of 68Ga-DOTATATE PET/CT with other imaging modalities in detecting head and neck paraganglioma: Experience from western India. *World Journal of Nuclear Medicine, 21*, 184–191. https://doi.org/10.1055/s-0042-1751030 (accessed on 1st June 2025).

33. Driessen, D., De Gouw, D. D., Stijns, R. C. H., Litjens, G., Israël, B., Philips, B. W. J., Hermans, J., *et al.* (2022). Validation of *in vivo* nodal assessment of solid malignancies with USPIO-enhanced MRI: A workflow protocol. *Methods and Protocols, 5*. https://www.semanticscholar.org/paper/ff03230686a60e55153b625117169fba7033f0eb (accessed on 31st May 2025).

34. Dudea, Petrovic, Sham, & Torabi. (2013). Application of imaging methods in the diagnostics of malignant neck lymph nodes. *Acta Medica Mediane*. https://core.ac.uk/download/pdf/26978184.pdf (accessed on 31st May 2025).

35. Duthoy, W. (2006). Intensity modulated radiation therapy and arc therapy: Validation and evolution as applied to tumors of the head and neck, abdominal and pelvic regions. https://core.ac.uk/download/55748558.pdf (accessed on 31st May 2025).

36. Działach, E., Simlot, M., Osowiecka, K., Nowara, E., Markowski, J., & Grajek, M. (2025). Metastasis of squamous cell carcinoma of the larynx to the right adrenal gland—A case report. *Clinics and Practice, 15.* https://www.semanticscholar.org/paper/370fbccf01570e1843397c42da57318b15140fa7 (accessed on 31st May 2025).

37. Ellul, M., Benjamin, L., Singh, B., Lant, S., Michael, B., Easton, A., Kneen, R., *et al.* (2020). Neurological associations of COVID-19. *The Lancet Neurology, 19,* 767–783. https://doi.org/10.1016/s1474-4422(20)30221-0 (accessed on 1st June 2025).

38. Feygin, T., Khalek, N., & Moldenhauer, J. (2020). Fetal brain, head, and neck tumors: Prenatal imaging and management. *Prenatal Diagnosis, 40,* 1203–1219. https://www.semanticscholar.org/paper/150406043868e0ad23af745469d1133be669ea25 (accessed on 1st June 2025).

39. Gaddikeri, R. S., Gaddikeri, S., Tailor, T., & Anzai, Y. (2020). Dynamic contrast-enhanced MR imaging in head and neck cancer: Techniques and clinical applications. https://core.ac.uk/download/357585896.pdf (accessed on 1st June 2025).

40. Guk, K., Han, G., Lim, J., Jeong, K., Kang, T., Lim, E. K., & Jung, J. (2019). Evolution of wearable devices with real-time disease monitoring for personalized healthcare. *Nanomaterials, 9,* 813. https://doi.org/10.3390/nano9060813 (accessed on 1st June 2025).

41. Held, T., Herpel, C., Schwindling, F. S., Christ, L., Lang, K., Regnery, S., Eichkorn, T., *et al.* (2021). 3D-printed individualized tooth-borne tissue retraction devices compared to conventional dental splints for head and neck cancer radiotherapy: A randomized controlled trial. *Radiation Oncology, 16.* https://doi.org/10.1186/s13014-021-01803-8 (accessed on 1st June 2025).

42. Hosseinian, S., Suarez-Aguirre, D., Dede, C., Garcia, R., McCullum, L., Hemmati, M., Karagoz, A., *et al.* (2024). Cost-effectiveness of personalized policies for implementing organ-at-risk sparing adaptive radiation therapy in head and neck cancer: A Markov decision process approach. https://www.semanticscholar.org/paper/a8e315eddcca01b779789767a6ccd5ef86e4c09b (accessed on 1st June 2025).

43. Hutcheson, K. A., Barrow, M. P., Barringer, D. A., Knott, J. K., Lin, H., Weber, R. S., Fuller, C. D., *et al.* (2016). Dynamic Imaging Grade of Swallowing Toxicity (DIGEST): Scale development and validation. *Cancer, 123,* 62–70. https://doi.org/10.1002/cncr.30283 (accessed on 1st June 2025).

44. Inge, L. J., & Dennis, E. (2020). Development and applications of computer image analysis algorithms for scoring of PD-L1 immunohistochemistry. *Immuno-Oncology Technology, 6,* 2–8. https://doi.org/10.1016/j.iotech.2020.04.001 (accessed on 1st June 2025).

45. Isselbacher, E. M., Preventza, O., Black, J. H., Augoustides, J., Beck, A. W., Bolen, M. A., Braverman, A. C., *et al.* (2022). 2022 ACC/AHA guideline for the diagnosis and management of aortic disease: A report of the American Heart Association/American College of Cardiology Joint Committee on Clinical Practice Guidelines. *Circulation, 146.* https://doi.org/10.1161/cir.0000000000001106 (accessed on 31st May 2025).

46. Johnson, D. E., Burtness, B., Leemans, C. R., Lui, V. W. Y., Bauman, J. E., & Grandis, J. R. (2020). Head and neck squamous cell carcinoma. *Nature Reviews Disease Primers, 6.* https://doi.org/10.1038/s41572-020-00224-3 (accessed on 31st May 2025).

47. Joint Head and Neck Radiotherapy-MRI Development Cooperative, Salzillo, T., Dresner, M. A., Way, A., Wahid, K., McDonald, B., Mulder, S., *et al.* (2023). Development and implementation of optimized endogenous contrast sequences for delineation in adaptive radiotherapy on

a 1.5T MR-linear-accelerator: A prospective R-IDEAL stage 0-2a quantitative/qualitative evaluation of *in vivo* site-specific quality-assurance using a 3D T2 fat-suppressed platform. *Journal of Medical Imaging, 10.* https://www.semanticscholar.org/paper/b2c38d8c553adadc1fc2712f22d68551df9ecec9 (accessed on 31st May 2025).

48. Kawauchi, K., Furuya, S., Hirata, K., Katoh, C., Manabe, O., Kobayashi, K., Watanabe, S., *et al.* (2020). A convolutional neural network-based system to classify patients using FDG PET/CT examinations. *BMC Cancer, 20.* https://doi.org/10.1186/s12885-020-6694-x (accessed on 1st June 2025).

49. Keereweer, S. (2014). *Towards Fluorescence-Guided Head and Neck Cancer Surgery.* https://core.ac.uk/download/19747817.pdf (accessed on 1st June 2025).

50. LeBoff, M. S., Greenspan, S. L., Insogna, K., Lewiecki, E. M., Saag, K. G., Singer, A., & Siris, E. S. (2022). The clinician's guide to prevention and treatment of osteoporosis. *Osteoporosis International, 33*, 2049–2102. https://doi.org/10.1007/s00198-021-05900-y (accessed on 1st June 2025).

51. Li, G. Y., Chen, J., Jang, S. I., Gong, K., & Li, Q. (2023). SwinCross: Cross-modal Swin transformer for head-and-neck tumor segmentation in PET/CT images. *Medical Physics, 51*, 2096–2107. https://doi.org/10.1002/mp.16703 (accessed on 31st May 2025).

52. Lyons, K., Sher, A., Orth, R., & Seghers, V. (2018). The utility of PET/MRI in pediatric malignancies. *Applied Radiology.* https://www.semanticscholar.org/paper/885340e2107698048ccedce72ce8448255359ca2 (accessed on 1st June 2025).

53. McClintock, S. M., Reti, I. M., Carpenter, L. L., McDonald, W. M., Dubin, M. J., Taylor, S. F., Cook, I. A., *et al.* (2017). Consensus recommendations for the clinical application of repetitive transcranial magnetic stimulation (rTMS) in the treatment of depression. *The Journal of Clinical Psychiatry, 79*, 35–48. https://doi.org/10.4088/jcp.16cs10905 (accessed on 1st June 2025).

54. McCrory, P., Meeuwisse, W., Dvořák, J., Aubry, M., Bailes, J. E., Broglio, S. P., Cantu, R. C., *et al.* (2017). Consensus statement on concussion in sport—the 5th international conference on concussion in sport held in Berlin, October 2016. *British Journal of Sports Medicine, 51*, 838–847. https://doi.org/10.1136/bjsports-2017-097699 (accessed on 1st June 2025).

55. McMullin, M. F., Harrison, C., Ali, S., Cargo, C., Chen, F., Ewing, J., Garg, M., *et al.* (2018). A guideline for the diagnosis and management of polycythemia vera: A British Society for Hematology guideline. *British Journal of Hematology, 184*, 176–191. https://doi.org/10.1111/bjh.15648 (accessed on 1st June 2025).

56. Mehanna, H., Robinson, M., Hartley, A., Kong, A., Foran, B., Fulton-Lieuw, T., Dalby, M. J., *et al.* (2018). Radiotherapy plus cisplatin or cetuximab in low-risk human papillomavirus-positive oropharyngeal cancer (De-ESCALaTE HPV): An open-label randomized controlled phase 3 trial. *The Lancet, 393*, 51–60. https://doi.org/10.1016/s0140-6736(18)32752-1 (accessed on 31st May 2025).

57. Messineo, D., Valentini, F., Niccolini, G. F., Zoccali, F., Ripari, F., Marotta, E., Caratozzolo, M., *et al.* (2025). Unlocking the hidden: Advancing imaging techniques in diagnosing cancers of unknown primary in the head and neck region. *Applied Sciences.* https://www.semanticscholar.org/paper/f990c6f025f726eaef7c6885af3653aae1aed3c8 (accessed on 31st May 2025).

58. Mihailović, J., Killeen, R., & Duignan, J. (2021). PET/CT variants and pitfalls in head and neck cancers including thyroid cancer. *Seminars in Nuclear Medicine.* https://www.semanticscholar.

org/paper/b7e6cddf7dab3ae23661977c837dfe0efe79eda4 (accessed on 31st May 2025).

59. Mould, R. F. (2018). *A Century of X-rays and Radioactivity in Medicine*. CRC Press eBooks. https://doi.org/10.1201/9781315136271 (accessed on 1st June 2025).

60. Nagano, S. Y. M., Chojniak, R., & Porto, G. (2025). Magnetic resonance permeability for the evaluation of head and neck tumors: Parotid and beyond. *Journal of Clinical Imaging Science, 15*. https://www.semanticscholar.org/paper/53859f39d71839e621be6875302548e9f482e9ee (accessed on 1st June 2025).

61. Oreiller, V., Andrearczyk, V., Jreige, M., Boughdad, S., Elhalawani, H., Castelli, J., Vallières, M., *et al.* (2021). Head and neck tumor segmentation in PET/CT: The HECKTOR challenge. *Medical Image Analysis, 77*, 102336–102336. https://doi.org/10.1016/j.media.2021.102336 (accessed on 1st June 2025).

62. Park, S., & Kim, Y. G. (2022). A metaverse: Taxonomy, components, applications, and open challenges. *IEEE Access, 10*, 4209–4251. https://doi.org/10.1109/access.2021.3140175 (accessed on 1st June 2025).

63. Peng, Z., Wang, Y., Wang, Y., Jiang, S., Fan, R., Zhang, H., & Jiang, W. (2021). Application of radiomics and machine learning in head and neck cancers. *International Journal of Biological Sciences, 17*, 475–486. https://doi.org/10.7150/ijbs.55716 (accessed on 1st June 2025).

64. Pépin, J. L., Bailly, S., Rinder, P., Adler, D., Benjafield, A., Lavergne, F., Josseran, A., *et al.* (2022). Relationship between CPAP termination and all-cause mortality. *CHEST Journal, 161*, 1657–1665. https://doi.org/10.1016/j.chest.2022.02.013 (accessed on 31st May 2025).

65. Pesapane, F., Codari, M., & Sardanelli, F. (2018). Artificial intelligence in medical imaging: Threat or opportunity? Radiologists again at the forefront of innovation in medicine. *European Radiology Experimental, 2*. https://doi.org/10.1186/s41747-018-0061-6 (accessed on 31st May 2025).

66. Pfister, D. G., Spencer, S., Adelstein, D. J., Adkins, D. R., Anzai, Y., Brizel, D. M., Bruce, J. Y., *et al.* (2020). Head and neck cancers, version 2.2020, NCCN Clinical Practice Guidelines in Oncology. *Journal of the National Comprehensive Cancer Network, 18*, 873–898. https://doi.org/10.6004/jnccn.2020.0031 (accessed on 31st May 2025).

67. Pham, T. D., Teh, M., Chatzopoulou, D., Holmes, S., & Coulthard, P. (2024). Artificial intelligence in head and neck cancer: Innovations, applications, and future directions. *Current Oncology, 31*, 5255–5290. https://www.semanticscholar.org/paper/79301386f2ef45ba2dd9501c0b1a9799343a9ada (accessed on 1st June 2025).

68. Planchard, D., Popat, S., Kerr, K. M., Novello, S., Smit, E. F., Faivre-Finn, C., Mok, T., *et al.* (2018). Metastatic non-small cell lung cancer: ESMO Clinical Practice Guidelines for diagnosis, treatment and follow-up. *Annals of Oncology, 29*, iv192–iv237. https://doi.org/10.1093/annonc/mdy275 (accessed on 31st May 2025).

69. Riba, M. B., Donovan, K. A., Andersen, B. L., Braun, I., Breitbart, W., Brewer, B. W., Buchmann, L., *et al.* (2019). Distress management, version 3.2019, NCCN Clinical Practice Guidelines in Oncology. *Journal of the National Comprehensive Cancer Network, 17*, 1229–1249. https://doi.org/10.6004/jnccn.2019.0048 (accessed on 1st June 2025).

70. Ridder, M., Raaijmakers, C., Pameijer, F., Bree, R., Reinders, F. J., Doornaert, P., Terhaard, C., *et al.* (2022). Target definition in MR-guided adaptive radiotherapy for head and neck cancer.

Cancers, 14. https://www.semanticscholar.org/paper/28e2e87902f5de6f447d8a133acbd80 9c088fce0 (accessed on 1st June 2025).

71. Roguljić, M., Šimunović, D., Buljan, I., Žuljević, M. F., Turić, A., & Marušić, A. (2025). Publishing identifiable patient photographs in the digital age: Focus group study of patients, doctors, and medical students. *Journal of Medical Internet Research, 27.* https://www.semanticscholar.org/paper/967cce37d2457cf40aefe05370cc2e4818d2cc41 (accessed on 1st June 2025).

72. Salomon, L., Alfirević, Ž., Berghella, V., Bilardo, C. M., Chalouhi, G. E., Da Silva, C. F., Hernández-Andrade, E., *et al.* (2022). ISUOG practice guidelines (updated): Performance of the routine mid-trimester fetal ultrasound scan. *Ultrasound in Obstetrics and Gynecology, 59*, 840–856. https://doi.org/10.1002/uog.24888 (accessed on 1st June 2025).

73. Sankaranarayanan, R., Ramadas, K., Amarasinghe, H., Subramanian, S., & Johnson, N. W. (2015). *Oral CANCer: Prevention, Early Detection, and Treatment.* The World Bank eBooks. https://doi.org/10.1596/978-1-4648-0349-9_ch5 (accessed on 1st June 2025).

74. Schache, A., Kerawala, C., Ahmed, O. A., Brennan, P. A., Cook, F., Garrett, M., Homer, J. J., *et al.* (2021). British Association of Head and Neck Oncologists (BAHNO) standards 2020. *Journal of Oral Pathology and Medicine, 50*, 262–273. https://doi.org/10.1111/jop.13161 (accessed on 31st May 2025).

75. Schneider, U., Graß, I., Laudien, M., Quetz, J., Graefe, H., Wollenberg, B., & Meyer, J. E. (2020). Comparison of clinical examination and various imaging modalities in the diagnosis of head and neck cancer. *International Archives of Otorhinolaryngology, 25*, e179–e184. https://doi.org/10.1055/s-0039-3402435 (accessed on 1st June 2025).

76. Shen, Y., Zhu, C., Chu, B., Song, J., Geng, Y., Li, J., Liu, B., *et al.* (2024). Evaluation of the clinical application value of artificial intelligence in diagnosing head and neck aneurysms. *BMC Medical Imaging, 24.* https://www.semanticscholar.org/paper/0d76d202107161991e4d8049c068fecf7ecd7783 (accessed on 1st June 2025).

77. Siddique, N., Paheding, S., Elkin, C., & Devabhaktuni, V. (2021). U-Net and its variants for medical image segmentation: A review of theory and applications. *IEEE Access, 9*, 82031–82057. https://doi.org/10.1109/access.2021.3086020 (accessed on 1st June 2025).

78. Stewart, A., Stewart, A., Buck, A. M., Pentland, A. P., Cortet, B., Cortet, B., Snyder, B. D., *et al.* (2004). Identification of hip fracture patients from radiographs using Fourier analysis of the trabecular structure: A cross-sectional study. *BMC Med. Imaging.* https://core.ac.uk/download/pdf/3544344.pdf (accessed on 31st May 2025).

79. Stieb, S., Lee, A., Van Dijk, L. V., Frank, S. J., Fuller, C. D., & Blanchard, P. (2021). NTCP modeling of late effects for head and neck cancer: A systematic review. *International Journal of Particle Therapy, 8*, 95–107. https://doi.org/10.14338/20-00092 (accessed on 1st June 2025).

80. Stout, K., Daniels, C. J., Aboulhosn, J., Bozkurt, B., Broberg, C. S., Colman, J. M., Crumb, S. R., *et al.* (2018). 2018 AHA/ACC guideline for the management of adults with congenital heart disease: A report of the American College of Cardiology/American Heart Association Task Force on Clinical Practice Guidelines. *Circulation, 139.* https://doi.org/10.1161/cir.0000000000000603 (accessed on 1st June 2025).

81. Valentini, V., Boldrini, L., Damiani, A., & Muren, L. P. (2014). Recommendations on how to establish evidence from auto-segmentation software in radiotherapy. *Radiotherapy and*

Oncology, 112, 317–320. https://doi.org/10.1016/j.radonc.2014.09.014 (accessed on 1st June 2025).

82. Van Griethuysen, J. J. M., Fedorov, A., Parmar, C., Hosny, A., Aucoin, N., Narayan, V., Beets-Tan, R. G. H., *et al.* (2017). Computational radiomics system to decode the radiographic phenotype. *Cancer Research, 77*, e104–e107. https://doi.org/10.1158/0008-5472.can-17-0339 (accessed on 31st May 2025).

83. Van Herpen, C., Vander, P. V., Skálová, A., Terhaard, C. H. J., Maroldi, R., Van Engen, A., Baujat, B., *et al.* (2022). Salivary gland cancer: ESMO–European Reference Network on Rare Adult Solid Cancers (EURACAN) clinical practice guideline for diagnosis, treatment and follow-up. *ESMO Open, 7*, 100602–100602. https://doi.org/10.1016/j.esmoop.2022.100602 (accessed on 31st May 2025).

84. Varkey, B. (2020). Principles of clinical ethics and their application to practice. *Medical Principles and Practice, 30*, 17–28. https://doi.org/10.1159/000509119 (accessed on 31st May 2025).

85. Viswanathan, V. S., Toro, P., Corredor, G., Mukhopadhyay, S., & Madabhushi, A. (2022). The state of the art for artificial intelligence in lung digital pathology. *The Journal of Pathology, 257*, 413–429. https://doi.org/10.1002/path.5966 (accessed on 1st June 2025).

86. Vogel, A., Cervantes, A., Chau, I., Daniele, B., Llovet, J. M., Meyer, T., Nault, J. C., *et al.* (2018). Hepatocellular carcinoma: ESMO Clinical Practice Guidelines for diagnosis, treatment and follow-up. *Annals of Oncology, 29*, iv238–iv255. https://doi.org/10.1093/annonc/mdy308 (accessed on 31st May 2025).

87. Wiggins, R., Hoffman, J., Fine, G., Covington, M. F., Salem, A. E., Koppula, B., Morton, K. A. (2022). PET-CT in clinical adult oncology—V. Head and neck and neuro oncology. *Cancers, 14*. https://www.semanticscholar.org/paper/518dba54b98e93572eb336faee2b17051b01ee19 (accessed on 1st June 2025).

88. Wilson, C. M. (2011). *Value of Using Liver FDG Uptake as Background Activity in Standardizing FDG PET/CT Studies*. https://open.bu.edu/bitstream/2144/33592/1/Wilson_Colin_2011_web.pdf (accessed on 1st June 2025).

89. Wright, V. J., McCrum, C. L., Li, H., Tranovich, M. J., & Huard, J. (2017). Significant chondrocyte viability is present in acetabular chondral flaps associated with femoroacetabular impingement. *The American Journal of Sports Medicine, 46*, 149–152. https://doi.org/10.1177/0363546517732751 (accessed on 1st June 2025).

90. Xu, P., Liu, D., Zhou, J., Tang, Z., Wang, S., Huang, Y., Feng, M., *et al.* (2025). Survival analysis of patients with metastatic head and neck squamous cell carcinoma treated with metastasis-directed radiotherapy and immunotherapy. *Radiation Oncology (London, England), 20*. https://www.semanticscholar.org/paper/57bd085bc7fe82fa6708c10a6358e1d817f5cf52 (accessed on 1st June 2025).

91. Young, K., Ma, E., Kejriwal, S., Nielsen, T., Aulakh, S. S., & Birkeland, A. C. (2022). Intraoperative *in vivo* imaging modalities in head and neck cancer surgical margin delineation: A systematic review. *Cancers, 14*, 3416. https://doi.org/10.3390/cancers14143416 (accessed on 1st June 2025).

ULTRASOUND AND DOPPLER IMAGING

6

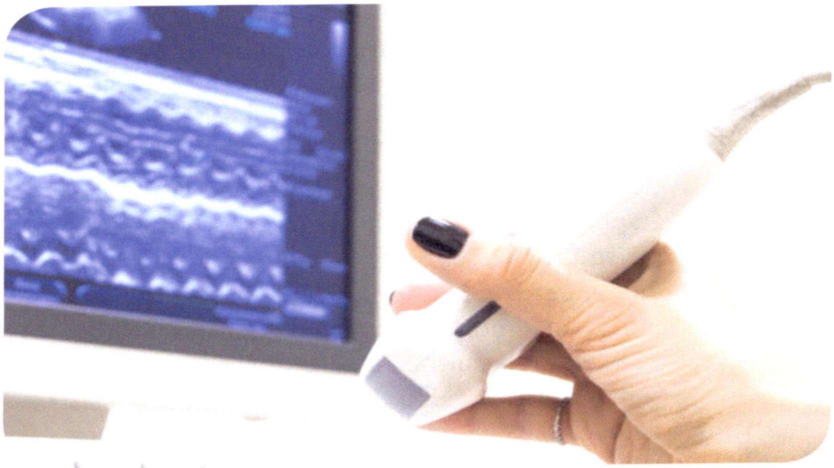

Introduction

Medical imaging has made it possible to see inside the body without surgery, which helps find and treat diseases sooner. Ultrasound is preferred among other modalities because it is safe, easy to use, and lets doctors see images as they happen. Utilizing high-frequency sound waves, ultrasound provides detailed images of soft tissues without exposing patients to ionizing radiation, making it an ideal initial imaging technique, especially in nephrology for assessing kidney health and transplantation outcomes (Singla *et al.*, 2022). Doppler imaging adds to ultrasound by showing the flow of blood and its direction, which is useful in finding vascular problems such as stenosis or thrombosis. They are all important in clinical work, and they keep improving as technology advances, helping doctors make better diagnoses and care for patients. As healthcare guidelines emphasize the integration of evidence-based imaging strategies, understanding the principles and applications of ultrasound and Doppler imaging is essential for

LEARNING OBJECTIVES

After studying this chapter, you will be able to:

1. Understand principles of ultrasound imaging;
2. Know applications of ultrasound imaging;
3. Focus on principles of doppler imaging;
4. Describe the clinical significance of Doppler imaging.

optimizing diagnostic and therapeutic decisions (Cosentino *et al.*, 2019).

Definition of Ultrasound Imaging

Medical imaging has advanced a lot to help with accurate diagnosis and better patient outcomes, and ultrasound imaging is now a commonly used non-invasive and flexible method in many clinics. Ultrasound imaging sends high-frequency sound waves into the body, and the echoes from tissues of different densities are used to create live pictures inside the body. It gives clinicians the ability to see organs, blood vessels, and tumors without using ionizing radiation on patients. Also, new ultrasound technologies, such as Doppler techniques, have allowed for assessing blood flow in blood vessels.

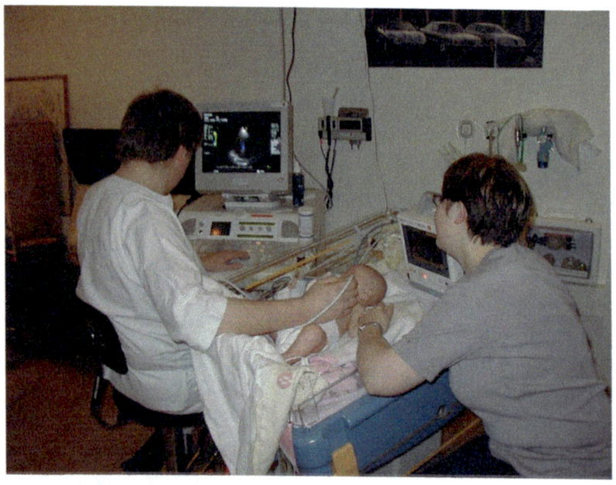

Figure 6.1. Ultrasound imaging utilizes high-frequency sound waves transmitted into the body to produce real-time images of internal structures by detecting the echoes reflected by tissues of varying densities.

Source: https://upload.wikimedia.org/wikipedia/commons/a/a7/Sonographer_doing_pediatric_echocardiography.JPG.

Enhancements in signal processing, including eigenvalue decomposition-based clutter filtering, have improved the sensitivity and resolution of blood flow detection without contrast agents, making ultrasound a powerful tool for detecting microvascular structures (Huang *et al.*, 2024). Additionally, innovative methods like superb microvascular imaging have demonstrated improved delineation of tumor boundaries during surgeries, illustrating ultrasound's critical role in both diagnostic and intraoperative environments (Cai *et al.*, 2024) (Figure 6.1).

Definition of Doppler Imaging

Medical imaging has improved a lot by using technology that helps doctors diagnose more accurately and learn about how the body functions. An example of this is Doppler imaging, which uses ultrasound to measure how the frequency of sound waves changes when they bounce off moving blood cells. The Doppler effect, which shifts the frequency of sound waves, helps clinicians observe and measure blood flow in vessels, giving important information about vascular health. Unlike regular ultrasound, Doppler ultrasound can show how blood flows in real time, which helps find conditions like arterial blockages and venous insufficiencies. It helps other imaging methods by giving information on how the body works, not just what it looks like, which improves patient care. While fusion imaging combines ultrasonography with other modalities to further diagnostic capabilities (Bellati *et al.*, 2018), Doppler imaging remains fundamental due to its noninvasive nature and immediate feedback. Because it is used in so many clinical settings, it is an important part of modern ultrasound.

Importance of Ultrasound in Medical Diagnostics

The development of new imaging methods has made it easier and more accurate to find different medical conditions early. Because it does not require surgery, shows images in real time, and is affordable, ultrasound is a key technology among these methods. As an example, using both clinical information and ultrasound results to assess postmenopausal bleeding helps doctors tell apart benign from malignant endometrial problems, which improves the accuracy of the diagnosis and decreases the need for invasive procedures. Doppler ultrasounds also play a big role in vascular medicine, since they provide a safe and inexpensive alternative to CT angiography, which is more invasive and uses radiation. In diagnosing peripheral arterial disease, Doppler ultrasound provides high sensitivity and specificity across different arterial segments, making it indispensable for initial assessment and ongoing monitoring (Malaichamy *et al.*, 2024). These examples underscore ultrasound's vital importance as a reliable diagnostic tool across various medical disciplines (Figure 6.2).

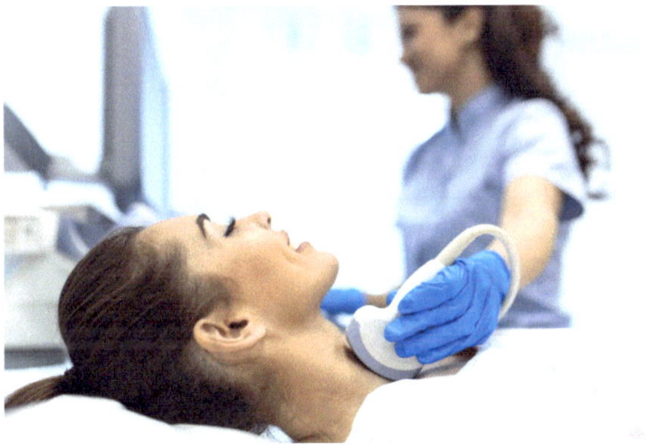

Figure 6.2. Advancements in imaging technologies have revolutionized diagnostic processes, allowing for earlier and more accurate detection of a variety of medical conditions.

Source: https://lotusdiagnostic.com/wp-content/uploads/2023/05/Non-Invasive-Imaging-scaled.webp.

Overview of Doppler Effect in Imaging

Medical imaging relies on the Doppler effect to show and measure how blood flows, which helps with the diagnosis of many health problems. Doppler imaging works by noticing changes in frequency in the ultrasound waves bounced off moving blood cells, which helps to see vascular hemodynamics in real time. Because of this detailed information, doctors can see how blood flows and is directed, which helps in diagnosing heart problems and checking if treatments are working. For example, the assessment of venous congestion using venous excess Doppler ultrasound can identify flow abnormalities predictive of kidney injury, illustrating how Doppler principles enhance organ-level evaluations beyond traditional methods (Koratala *et al.*, 2022). Additionally, Doppler imaging contributes to musculoskeletal assessments by detecting localized hypervascularity indicative of partial tendon ruptures, highlighting its versatility across medical specialties (Gatz *et al.*, 2020). They highlight how the Doppler effect greatly improves both the accuracy of diagnoses and patient management.

Applications of Ultrasound and Doppler Imaging

Better medical imaging technologies have made it possible to diagnose and monitor many conditions, especially in the areas of heart and pregnancy care. Noninvasive assessments are made possible by ultrasound and Doppler imaging, which allow doctors to see soft tissues and monitor blood flow.

They are very useful for finding problems in the blood vessels, such as stenosis, thrombosis, and aneurysms, and for keeping an eye on the development of the fetus and the placenta. Using Doppler techniques makes it easier to measure blood flow and its direction, which is important for detecting hypertension and peripheral artery disease. Besides, because they are in real time, they make it possible for doctors to decide quickly during procedures which is good for patients. Medical guidelines emphasize the importance of these tools in clinical workflows, highlighting their diagnostic accuracy and safety profiles when used by trained professionals in accordance with established standards (Cosentino *et al.*, 2019; Williams *et al.*, 2018) (Figure 6.3).

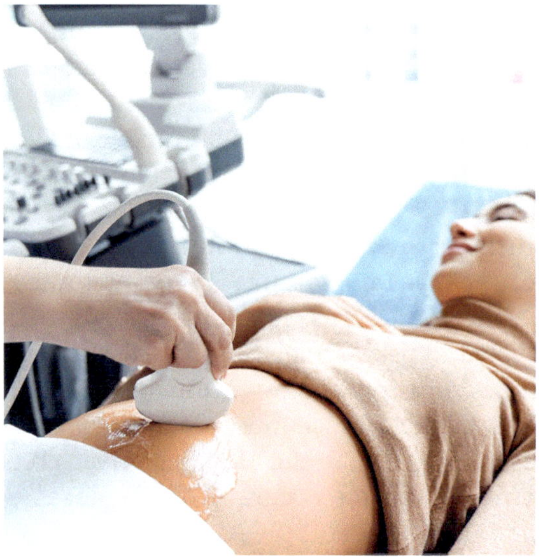

Figure 6.3. Ultrasound and Doppler imaging play a critical role in noninvasive assessments, allowing clinicians to visualize soft tissues and evaluate blood flow dynamics with precision.

Source: https://klinikaflebologii.pl/wp-content/uploads/2025/01/diagnostyka-ultrasonograficzna-klinika-flebologii-zaj.jpg.

Significance of Advancements in Imaging Technology

Because of the ongoing improvements in medical imaging, both diagnoses and patient care have improved, mainly in ultrasound and Doppler imaging. Innovations such as artificial intelligence integration have transformed image analysis by enhancing pattern recognition and automating quantitative assessments, thereby improving diagnostic precision and efficiency in liver imaging and other applications (Zhou *et al.*, 2019). They allow clinicians to do their job more easily and detect health problems earlier and more reliably. Furthermore, refined Doppler techniques contribute to a better understanding of physiological processes, exemplified by studies on endometrial receptivity where Doppler indices serve as biomarkers linked to pregnancy outcomes, although their predictive capabilities require further enhancement (Craciunas *et al.*, 2018). All of these improvements together help provide better, faster, and more personalized care, and they also give researchers new ways to study, highlighting the key role imaging plays in improving noninvasive diagnostics and healthcare.

6.1. Principles of Ultrasound Imaging

Learning Outcome

1. Understand basic physics of sound waves;
2. Explain the mechanism of ultrasound generation;
3. Focus on the interaction of ultrasound with tissues;
4. Learn the image formation process;
5. Identify types of ultrasound waves;
6. Know the equipment used in ultrasound imaging;
7. Focus on safety considerations in ultrasound;
8. List limitations of ultrasound technology;
9. Give a comparison with other imaging modalities.

Improvements in imaging technology have greatly increased what ultrasound can do, mainly because of ultrafast platforms. Although traditional ultrasound is widely used, it can only see things clearly in limited areas and at about 70 to 100 frames per second. On the other hand, ultrafast ultrasound captures many thousands of images every second, which makes it easier to see details and improves the accuracy of diagnosis. Because of these improvements, various advanced methods such as high-frequency ultrasound, contrast-enhanced ultrasound, shear wave elastography, and vector flow imaging can be used. Every modality helps in understanding vascular structures and the processes that cause diseases, providing clear insights into blood flow and vessel walls. Such innovations have practical implications in clinical scenarios, including the assessment and preparation of vascular access sites before surgical procedures (Ilaria *et al.*, 2021). Because of these principles, ultrasound imaging keeps growing, making it possible to diagnose more conditions than before.

6.1.1. Basic Physics of Sound Waves

It is important to learn about wave principles to see how ultrasound and Doppler imaging operate. Sound waves, unlike electromagnetic waves, need a medium such as air, liquid, or solid matter to travel in as vibrations of particles. Frequency, wavelength, and amplitude are important parameters in waves that decide how they interact with various materials.

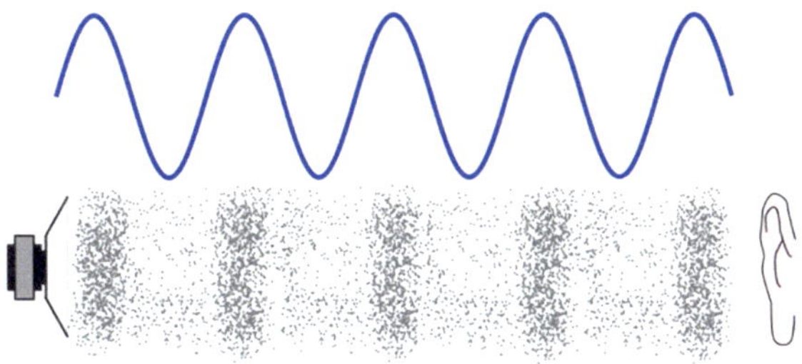

Figure 6.4. Sound waves, unlike electromagnetic waves, require a medium through which to propagate, traveling as mechanical vibrations of particles in air, liquid, or solid tissues.

Source: https://user-image.kinnu.xyz/d7d78a53-09a3-4379-8cd0-ab2a7838f386?s=0x0x100x100&w=1000.

Because ultrasound in medicine uses short-wavelength high-frequency waves, it provides detailed images. The propagation of these waves is affected by factors including acoustic impedance and attenuation, which determine the depth of penetration and clarity of the images produced (Ghafar *et al.*, 2024). Furthermore, when the source or reflector of these waves moves relative to the receiver, a Doppler shift in frequency occurs, providing valuable information about blood flow dynamics and tissue movement (Cowley *et al.*, 2017). Mastery of these basic physics concepts underpins the effective use and ongoing development of ultrasound technologies (Figure 6.4).

6.1.2. Mechanism of Ultrasound Generation

The basis of creating ultrasound waves is the piezoelectric effect, which allows certain crystals in the transducer to change electrical energy into vibrations. Alternating electrical current in these crystals makes them expand and contract very fast, sending out high-frequency sound waves that penetrate the body. They bounce off several interfaces and are detected by the same crystals in reverse, which turns them back into electrical signals for processing images. The mechanism's precision is very important because it helps detect small changes in wave frequency needed for both ultrasound and Doppler imaging to assess blood flow. New developments in transducers have made it possible for them to work over a wider range of frequencies, which leads to better and more detailed images. Recent developments even explore enhanced methods like contrast-enhanced ultrasound, expanding diagnostic capabilities while emphasizing safety and patient comfort (Cantisani *et al.*, 2016).

6.1.3. Interaction of Ultrasound with Tissues

The way ultrasound waves move through the body is influenced by many factors that affect the quality of the images and their usefulness for diagnosing. Ultrasound waves hitting different tissues cause reflection, refraction, scattering, and absorption, which may alter the intensity and quality of the image. Such interactions play a role in how we see anatomy and also in the way we interpret Doppler signals in blood flow. Moreover, advances in computational methods, such as machine learning, have been increasingly applied to optimize the interpretation of ultrasound data by better accounting for these tissue-specific interactions, enhancing both diagnostic precision and reliability in clinical settings (Iula *et al.*, 2022). Understanding the detailed interaction between ultrasound waves and tissues is important for better real-time imaging and more convenient ways to examine patients. The complexity of wave-tissue interaction underscores the importance of continued research aimed at refining ultrasound technology to maximize its clinical benefits (Aldžić *et al.*, 2013) (Figure 6.5).

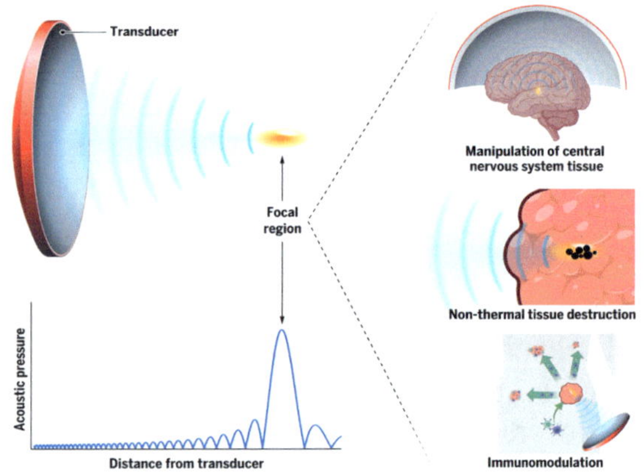

Figure 6.5. The passage of ultrasound waves through biological tissues is governed by complex interactions that influence image quality and diagnostic accuracy.

Source: https://www.science.org/cms/10.1126/science.adp7206/asset/20ddc8e9-76fd-4592-9f2d-7d43c588ab92/assets/images/large/science.adp7206-fa.jpg.

6.1.4. Image Formation Process

The ability of ultrasound imaging to show internal organs is based mainly on the process of image formation, which uses sound waves at very high frequencies. Sound waves from the ultrasound pulse meet tissues with different acoustic impedances, which leads to some of the sound waves being reflected and scattered back to the transducer. The returning echoes are changed into electrical signals, which are used to build a picture of the tissue inside the body. Advanced techniques like B-flow enhance this process by detecting specific artifacts, such as the twinkle artifact associated with microcalcifications, thereby improving diagnostic accuracy without reliance on Doppler shift information (Gazhonova *et al.*, 2024). Moreover, Doppler imaging complements this by analyzing frequency changes due to motion, such as blood flow, which is essential in assessing vascular and inflammatory processes, as seen in pancreatic pathology (O'reilly *et al.*, 2013). Because of these mechanisms, ultrasound and Doppler imaging are very precise in medical settings.

6.1.5. Types of Ultrasound Waves

The variety of ultrasound waves is very important for enhancing the effectiveness of ultrasound and Doppler imaging in diagnosis. Ultrasound waves are usually divided into continuous and pulsed waves, and each type is important for different reasons in medical imaging. Continuous waves have a steady frequency and amplitude, so they are best for measuring fast-moving blood using Doppler, and pulsed waves send short bursts that help locate problems more precisely at lower blood velocities. Also, the number of ultrasound waves per second determines how far they can go into the body and how clear the image is; higher frequencies produce ,more explicit pictures, but only go a short distance, while lower frequencies can see deeper, but the images are not as sharp. Advanced simulations integrating fluid-structure interactions have enabled the generation of synthetic ultrasound data reflective of physiological conditions, emphasizing the complex behavior of these waves in varied tissues and blood flow dynamics

(Degroote *et al.*, 2010). Understanding these wave types facilitates optimized imaging protocols, crucial for accurate vascular assessments (Figure 6.6).

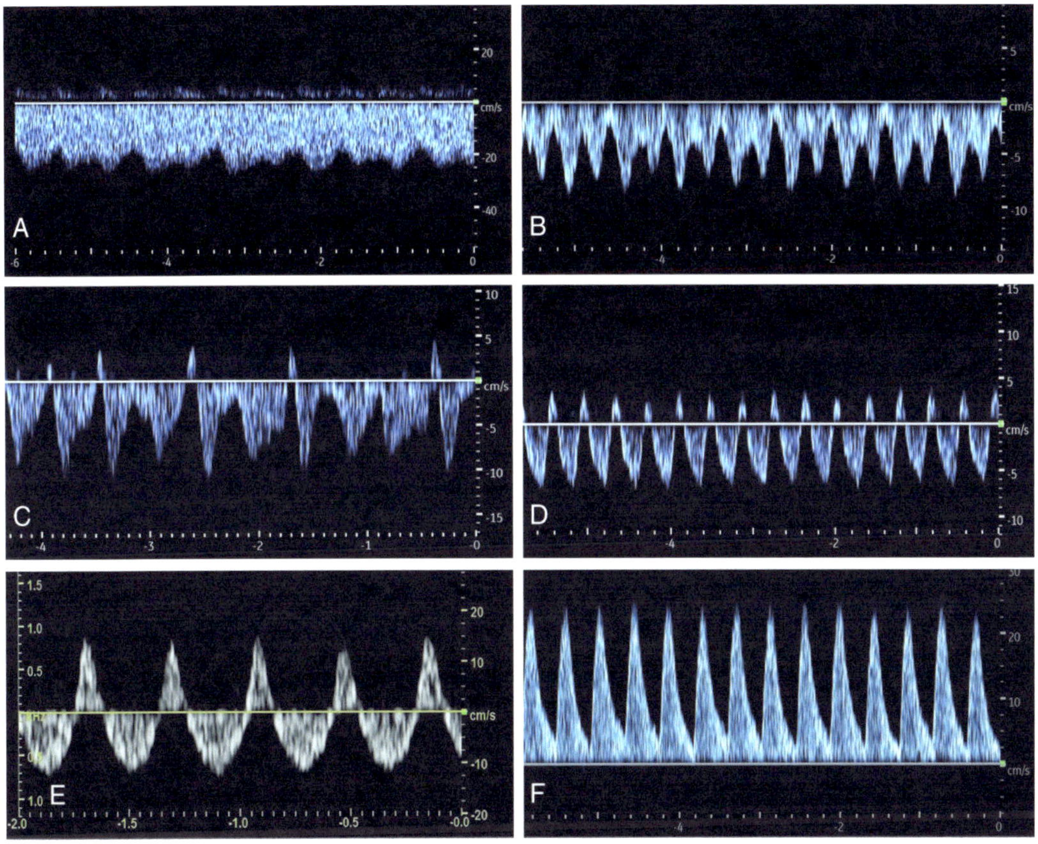

Figure 6.6. Ultrasound waves can be broadly classified into continuous and pulsed waves, with each type serving distinct purposes in medical imaging.

Source: https://www.ajnr.org/content/ajnr/44/6/707/F2.large.jpg.

6.1.6. Equipment Used in Ultrasound Imaging

Better ultrasound imaging has been made possible by continuous upgrades in both hardware and software, which have improved the accuracy and usefulness of doctors' diagnoses. These changes are mainly based on using advanced transducers that can send and receive high-frequency sound waves to build up images of what is inside the body. Modern ultrasound equipment now frequently incorporates innovative features such as Microvascular Ultrasound (MVUS), which enables the detection of slow-velocity blood flow within small vessels without contrast agents, thereby improving visualization of vascular patterns in organs like the liver and kidneys (Cannella *et al.*, 2023). Additionally, the evolution of Doppler technology, including both transthoracic and transesophageal methods, reflects decades of collaboration between engineers and clinicians, which has driven the optimization of sensitivity and resolution in flow imaging (Fraser *et al.*, 2022). Because of these advances, it is clear that a team approach helps improve ultrasound systems, allows them to be used in many medical fields and increases the accuracy of vascular imaging for better diagnosis.

6.1.7. Safety Considerations in Ultrasound

Even though ultrasound and Doppler imaging have advanced, making diagnosis much better, safety is still very important to avoid any negative results. The use of high-frequency transducers and prolonged exposure during procedures such as acoustic radiation force impulse (ARFI) elastography raises concerns about thermal tissue damage due to increased energy deposition. However, studies indicate that transient temperature rises observed during diagnostic pulses generally stay within the safety limits established by regulatory bodies like the FDA, with mechanical indices below harmful thresholds (Karaman, 2017). In neonatal care, transcranial Doppler ultrasound is applied cautiously to avoid cerebral ischemia, especially when evaluating collateral circulation before invasive procedures such as extracorporeal membrane oxygenation or cardiac surgery; this preoperative assessment has effectively minimized neurological complications (Reddan *et al.*, 2024). Continuous monitoring and adherence to established safety protocols are essential, and ongoing research is necessary to refine these guidelines, ensuring that the diagnostic benefits of ultrasound are balanced against any potential risks to patient safety (Figure 6.7).

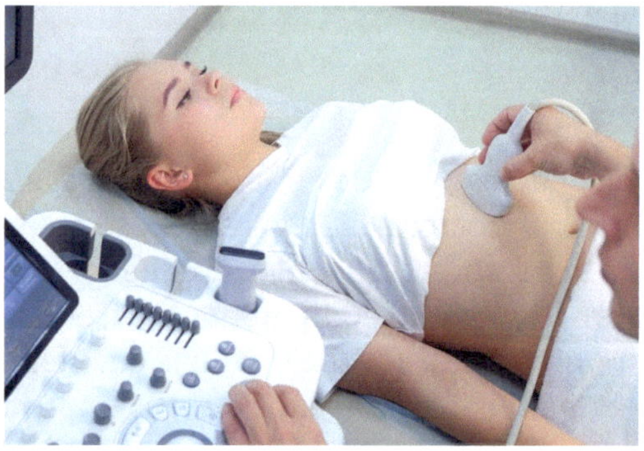

Figure 6.7. Acoustic radiation force impulse (ARFI) elastography.

Source: https://gulfcare-uae.com/assets/img/blog/arfi.jpg.

6.1.8. Limitations of Ultrasound Technology

Even though ultrasound is widely used and continues to improve, it has major limitations that affect its usefulness in medicine. One major challenge involves the accuracy of flow velocity estimations, which can suffer from artifacts, especially in regions with high spatial flow gradients or complex three-dimensional movements, leading to underestimations and angular deviations in measurements, as demonstrated in studies on neonatal cardiac flows using 2-D speckle tracking (Fadnes *et al.*, 2016). In addition, standard ultrasound has problems with sensitivity, a narrow viewing area, and reliance on the direction of blood flow, which can make it hard to assess the whole vascular system. Although new approaches combining high-frame-rate imaging with contrast agents show promise in addressing these issues, current technologies still struggle with depth penetration and flow visualization in small or tortuous vessels (Bazigou *et al.*, 2015). For this reason, ultrasound technology must keep improving to help in complicated medical cases.

6.1.9. Comparison with Other Imaging Modalities

Because of new technologies, clinicians have access to several medical imaging tools, each with its own set of pros and cons, which affect how they are used in different situations. Ultrasound and Doppler imaging stand out due to their noninvasive nature, use of nonionizing radiation, and ability to provide real-time visualization, which contrasts with modalities such as computed tomography (CT) and magnetic resonance imaging (MRI) that may involve ionizing radiation or higher costs. When examining kidneys, ultrasound can show their structure and function, especially blood supply and vessel health, and is usually the first test used for abnormal kidney function. Although

CT and MRI give detailed images and show more of the body, they are not as easy to use or safe for everyday or bedside use. Also, having a point-of-care ultrasound device means doctors can get instant information, which is not always possible with other imaging methods. Nonetheless, guidelines emphasize the importance of integrating multiple modalities as appropriate, considering patient-specific factors and updated clinical standards (Jean-Ricco *et al.*, 2017; Singla *et al.*, 2022) (Figure 6.8).

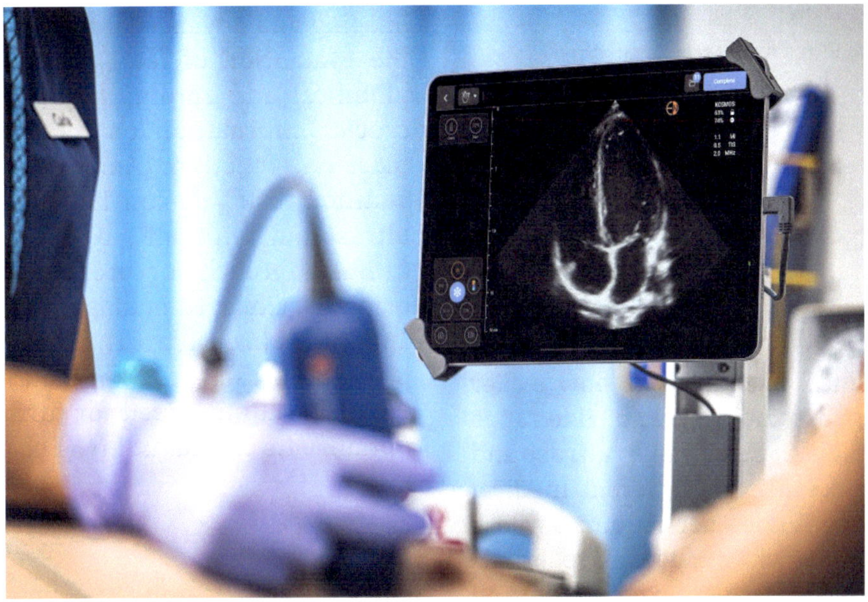

Figure 6.8. Point-of-care ultrasound devices.

Source: https://echonous.com/wp- content/ uploads/2024/10/2459298_Update ClinicalImage OnLifestyle Photo_090624-1.jpg.

Test Your Knowledge

1. What is the basic principle behind ultrasound imaging?
2. Where in the ultrasound system are the sound waves produced?
3. How do the number of images per second and the quality of the images relate in ultrasound imaging?

6.2. Applications of Ultrasound Imaging

Learning Outcome

1. Understand obstetric ultrasound;
2. Explain abdominal ultrasound;
3. Define cardiac ultrasound (echocardiography);
4. Focus on musculoskeletal ultrasound;
5. Describe vascular ultrasound;
6. Discuss pediatric ultrasound;
7. Know emergency ultrasound;
8. Explain therapeutic applications of ultrasound;
9. Understand the research applications of ultrasound.

With better medical imaging, it is now easier and safer to diagnose and oversee a wide range of health problems. Especially, ultrasound imaging is now essential in different medical situations because it does not require surgery and allows doctors to view images in real time. It is used in obstetrics to monitor the fetus and in cardiology to check the detailed structure and functioning of the heart. Also, recent advances such as elastography help doctors measure the stiffness of tissues, which is useful for finding and classifying diseases. Identifying causes of infertility in men, such as varicocele, is made possible by using scrotal ultrasound with Doppler, as these subtle vascular problems are usually not seen during a physical exam. Because the diagnosis is precise, it leads to fewer invasive procedures, which helps patients and improves their outcomes. Consequently, the versatility and evolving functionality of ultrasound imaging reaffirm its significance in modern medicine (Das, 2024; Oglat *et al.*, 2024).

6.2.1. Obstetric Ultrasound

Better imaging tools have greatly improved prenatal care by giving doctors a better view of the fetus and the mother. Among all the technologies, obstetric ultrasound is especially important because it lets doctors check on pregnancy in real time without being invasive. Because of ultrasound, doctors can now see the fetus, check its organs and spot any problems, which has led to better outcomes for mothers and babies. Notably, the integration of advanced Doppler technologies, such as microvascular imaging and advanced dynamic flow, enhances the evaluation of fetal circulation, including umbilical and cardiac blood flow, providing crucial information on fetal well-being and placental function (Amedu *et al.*, 2024). In addition, using fusion imaging, which unites ultrasound with MRI or CT, is becoming a useful approach for prenatal care. Although primarily explored in diagnostic gynecology, its application in obstetrics holds potential for more precise assessments of prenatal abnormalities, underscoring the need for further research to optimize its clinical utility (Bellati *et al.*, 2018).

6.2.2. Abdominal Ultrasound

Better ultrasound technology has made it possible to detect and evaluate internal problems in the abdomen more accurately. MVUS has become useful for spotting slow blood flow in small blood vessels, something that standard Doppler techniques may miss. MVUS helps clearly show the vessels in the liver and kidneys, which supports the accurate characterization and differentiation of tumors. Three-dimensional ultrasound imaging helps abdominal ultrasound by giving more detailed views of the organs, which is especially helpful for Asherman's syndrome and follicular vascularity. The integration of these imaging modalities within the abdomen highlights the ongoing evolution in ultrasound technology, underscoring its critical role not only in non-invasive diagnosis but also in guiding therapeutic interventions in complex vascular and organ-specific diseases (Bartolotta *et al.*, 2023) (Figure 6.9).

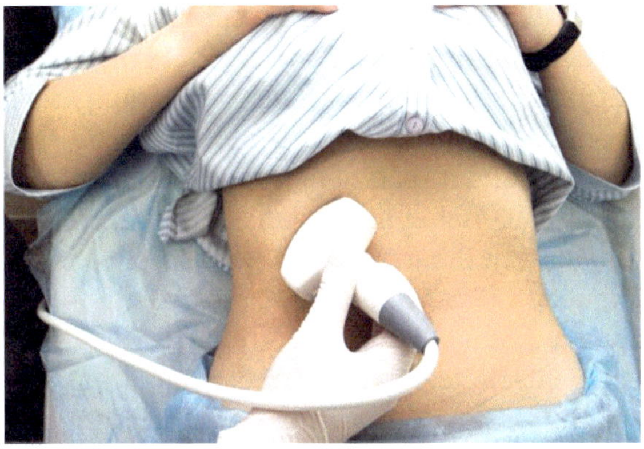

Figure 6.9. Abdominal ultrasound.

Source: https://cdn-apbgn.nitrocdn.com/TJhToCeBdthTVvVQvsfvpvDNSNjYOavZ/assets/images/optimized/rev-dc84968/ultrasound.ie/wp-content/uploads/2015/05/Abdominal-Ultrasound-Scans-Dublin-2.jpg.

6.2.3. Cardiac Ultrasound (Echocardiography)

New imaging techniques have greatly improved the way doctors check the heart's function, allowing them to find and treat complex heart problems without surgery. Among all these developments, echocardiography is especially important because it allows real-time viewing of the heart and its blood flow. For instance, contrast-enhanced transcranial color-coded Doppler (C-TCCD) has enhanced the detection of right-to-left shunts linked to patent foramen ovale (PFO), which are often implicated in cryptogenic stroke cases. This modality offers greater reliability compared to traditional transcranial Doppler by directly visualizing vascular anatomy and reducing interpretative errors (Ji *et al.*, 2023). Even so, the quality of images and Doppler measurements in echocardiography may be reduced by the way ultrasound waves are affected by different types of tissue. Such aberrations negatively affect resolution and signal-to-noise ratio, impacting both B-mode imaging and blood flow quantification modalities like pulsed wave Doppler and color flow imaging, thus underscoring the need for aberration correction techniques to optimize diagnostic accuracy (Fiorentini *et al.*, 2023).

6.2.4. Musculoskeletal Ultrasound

New imaging technology has greatly improved the ways doctors can diagnose problems with the skeletal and muscular systems. Musculoskeletal ultrasound is now considered useful because it can show soft tissue structures like muscles, tendons, ligaments, and nerves in real time. Unlike other tools, ultrasound gives clinicians the ability to watch anatomical movements as the body is in motion or under stress. Also, using Doppler imaging helps detect the blood flow changes that occur with inflammation or injury.

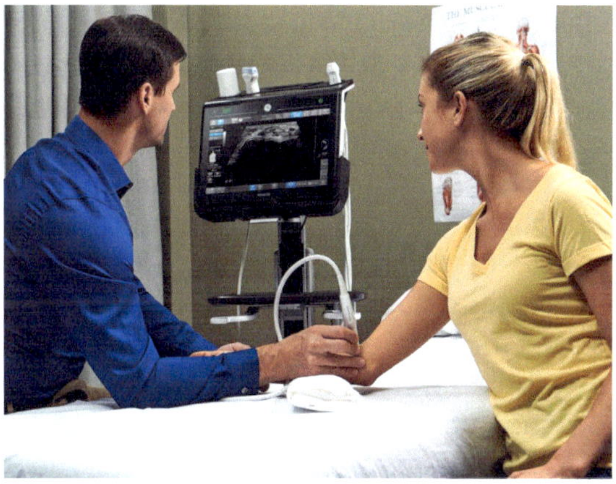

Figure 6.10. Musculoskeletal ultrasound.

Source: https://images-cdn.welcomesoftware.com/Zz04ZTc4YTBjOGNjNDcxMWVkODBmZDEy NmQxYmFmOWI1OQ==/venue- muskuloskeletal. webp.

Ultrasound elastography is a newer technique that helps by evaluating the tissue's stiffness, which gives important details about the condition of the tissue and any changes. This way of working helps doctors make correct diagnoses and choose the right interventions. Comprehensive atlases and detailed anatomical correlations aid practitioners in interpreting findings within a clinical context, ensuring that musculoskeletal ultrasound continues to advance as an indispensable modality in sports medicine and rheumatology (Snoj *et al.*, 2020; Taeymans, 2018) (Figure 6.10).

6.2.5. Vascular Ultrasound

New imaging techniques have made it much easier to diagnose and treat vascular diseases, and vascular ultrasound has become very important in this area. It combines traditional ultrasound with Doppler to show both the structure and the blood flow in blood vessels, helping doctors find stenosis, occlusions, and unusual blood flow. In peripheral vascular disease, vascular ultrasound helps doctors quickly and safely identify any issues, as the real-time information it provides is very important for treatment decisions. Although computed tomography angiography can offer more detailed anatomical visualization, especially in complex cases or elderly patients with advanced atherosclerosis, vascular ultrasound remains valuable due to its accessibility, cost-effectiveness, and safety profile, especially in pediatric populations (Sehar *et al.*, 2025). Additionally, innovations like ultrafast Doppler imaging extend the applicability of this technology to microvascular assessment in organs such as the kidney, highlighting its potential in monitoring renal vascular health without the need for contrast agents (Oh *et al.*, 2024).

6.2.6. Pediatric Ultrasound

New imaging technology has transformed how pediatric medicine makes diagnoses, providing safer and more convenient ways than before. In particular, ultrasound is widely used because it is non-invasive and does not use ionizing radiation, which is ideal for children. Its applications in pediatric orthopedics are extensive, ranging from detecting trauma-related injuries and developmental anomalies to guiding therapeutic procedures such as injections and biopsies, thereby minimizing complications and improving patient outcomes (Tzatzairis *et al.*, 2024). As well, pediatric neurosonography takes advantage of ultrasound's ability to be used anywhere and its safety to track brain conditions like hypoxic–ischemic encephalopathy and stroke immediately. Emerging techniques like contrast-enhanced ultrasound and elastography provide enhanced visualization of brain perfusion and tissue characteristics, broadening diagnostic capabilities in neurocritical care (Freeman *et al.*, 2022). Thus, pediatric ultrasound stands as a versatile and vital tool, blending diagnostic precision with patient safety in diverse clinical contexts (Figure 6.11).

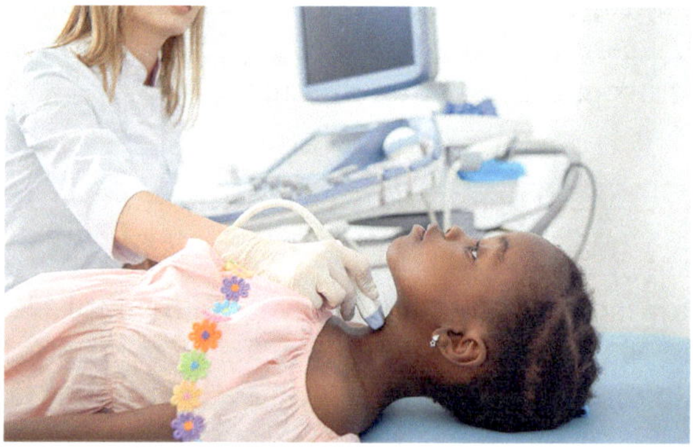

Figure 6.11. Pediatric ultrasound.

Source: https://www.acep.org/siteassets/sites/ultrasound/media/article-images/pediatricultrasound-800x495.jpg.

6.2.7. Emergency Ultrasound

In important clinical situations, having rapid and reliable diagnostic tools helps doctors decide on proper care and supports better patient outcomes. Emergency ultrasound has become very important at the bedside, as it quickly and safely images the heart, lungs, abdomen, and blood vessels. Because it is portable and can be used in real time, ultrasound is very useful when regular imaging is not possible. With emergency ultrasound, doctors can quickly find out about pneumothorax, pericardial tamponade, and intra-abdominal hemorrhage, which allows for prompt treatment. It is also important in managing the airway, checking the placement of the endotracheal tube, and checking blood flow to the brain after an injury. It does not take long to learn how to use competency, so its use can be adopted by many clinicians without much specialized training. Given its demonstrated efficacy, emergency ultrasound represents a transformative advancement in acute care diagnostics that integrates seamlessly with clinical assessments (Dinsmore *et al.*, 2022; Kalagara *et al.*, 2021).

6.2.8. Therapeutic Applications of Ultrasound

Ultrasound technology has changed a lot, so it is now used for both diagnosis and treatment, mainly for handling difficult medical conditions. Ultrasound-guided techniques in heart failure patients make it easy to find and monitor congestion, which allows doctors to adjust diuretic therapy and improve patient outcomes. This multiparametric approach combining lung ultrasound and venous Doppler analysis has demonstrated consistent prognostic value and therapeutic efficacy, thereby enhancing clinical decision-making and patient management across acute and chronic phases of heart failure (Gamarra *et al.*, 2025).

Ultrasound is now being used more often to examine respiratory muscles in critical care patients, which opens up new treatment options. Advanced ultrasound modalities provide real-time assessment of muscle dynamics and stiffness, informing ventilatory support strategies and rehabilitation efforts, which underscores the modality's expanding therapeutic potential (Dres *et al.*, 2025). These innovations exemplify the integrative role of ultrasound and Doppler imaging not only in diagnosis but also as indispensable tools in therapeutic regimes (Figure 6.12).

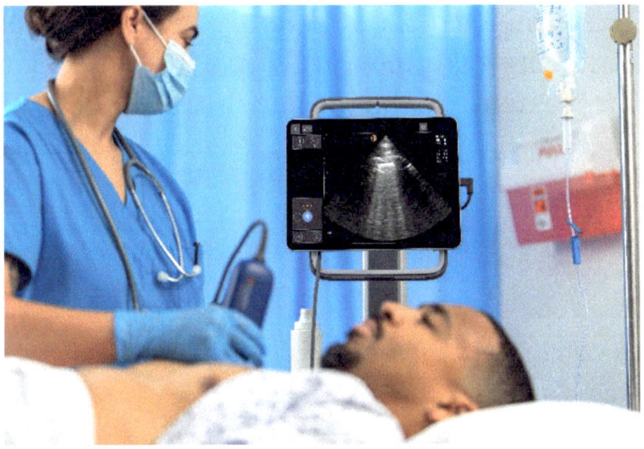

Figure 6.12. In heart failure patients, ultrasound-guided assessment enables accurate detection and monitoring of congestion, facilitating tailored diuretic therapy adjustments that improve patient outcomes and reduce hospital admissions.

Source: https://echonous.com/wp-content/uploads/2025/02/3.0_CC_EMed_Lung-859-Edit.jpg.

6.2.9. Research Applications of Ultrasound

Better imaging technology has made ultrasound more important in biomedical research by giving important information about both healthy and diseased processes in the body. In heart failure, using various ultrasound techniques, especially lung ultrasound and Doppler analysis, makes it easy to notice and control congestion, which is important for patient results. These methods offer a non-invasive, real-time assessment that supports prognostic evaluations and therapy adjustments, highlighting their growing clinical relevance (Gamarra *et al.*, 2025). Besides cardiovascular research, new technologies have been developed that use photoacoustic imaging with ultrasound microscopy to see the microenvironment of tumors. Thanks to this fusion, researchers can see the blood vessels and the oxygen levels in the tissue at the same time, which is important for understanding cancer growth and low oxygen levels. Furthermore, innovations such as deep learning-accelerated ultrasound localization microscopy have greatly enhanced acquisition speed, allowing longitudinal monitoring of tumor growth with sub-second frame rates (Zhao *et al.*, 2024). All in all, these improvements highlight how ultrasound is useful and continues to grow in many research areas.

Test Your Knowledge

1. What is the primary use of ultrasound in obstetrics?
2. What does ultrasound play in musculoskeletal imaging?

6.3. Principles of Doppler Imaging

Learning Outcome

1. Understand the Doppler effect;
2. Identify types of Doppler ultrasound;
3. Learn the mechanism of blood flow measurement;
4. Focus on signal processing in Doppler imaging;
5. Define factors affecting Doppler measurements;
6. Explain the equipment used in doppler imaging;
7. Describe safety considerations in doppler imaging;
8. List the limitations of Doppler technology;
9. Compare with other blood flow measurement techniques.

Better ultrasound technology has made it much easier to see blood flow, which is important for correct medical diagnosis. Doppler imaging works by detecting changes in frequency as the red blood cells move in vessels, so it can show how the blood vessels are working in real time. Still, traditional Doppler methods had trouble detecting slow or small blood vessels because they filtered out both low-velocity signals and motion artifacts. New methods, such as using unfocused plane waves and advanced 3D wall filtering, have improved the accuracy in telling apart tissue movement from blood flow. Because of these improvements, doctors can see microvascular structures directly, which makes their work more useful. Understanding these principles is crucial for optimizing Doppler imaging's application in healthcare, as illustrated in emerging ultrasound methods for both breast and ocular diagnostics (Mohindra *et al.*, 2024; Silverman, 2023).

6.3.1. Explanation of the Doppler Effect

Knowing how wave frequency changes when the source or observer moves is very important for medical imaging. This is called the Doppler effect, which explains how the frequency of a wave changes as the source and receiver move. Sound waves sent out by a transducer in ultrasound and Doppler imaging hit moving structures such as blood cells, which causes a shift in the frequency of the returning waves. After the frequency is altered, the machine converts it into velocity information, which allows doctors to check blood flow and identify potential issues. Doppler imaging helps doctors by measuring frequency shifts, which improves the accuracy of finding and monitoring heart problems. The integration of the Doppler effect in medical ultrasound exemplifies the intersection of physics with clinical application, highlighting the importance of precise guidelines to ensure reliable and reproducible imaging results (Baumgartner *et al.*, 2020; du Sert *et al.*, 2020) (Figure 6.13).

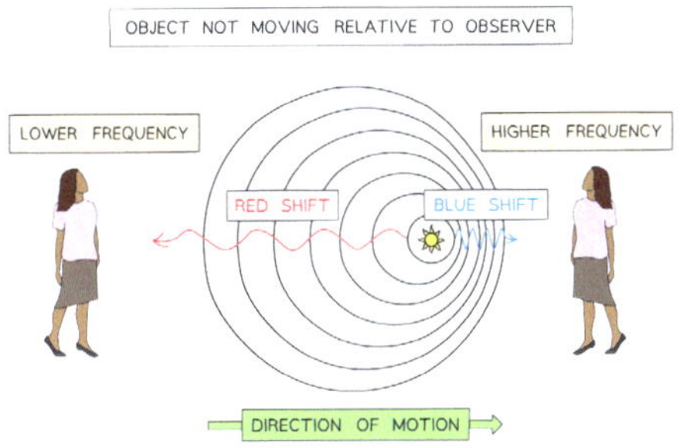

Figure 6.13. The Doppler effect describes this phenomenon, where the frequency of a wave changes relative to the motion between the source and the receiver.

Source: https://cdn.savemyexams.com/cdn-cgi/image/f=auto,width=3840/https://cdn.savemyexams.com/uploads/2024/07/6940_red-and-blue-shift-observer-answer.

6.3.2. Types of Doppler Ultrasound (Color, Spectral)

Improvements in medical imaging have made it much easier to study blood flow patterns without surgery, and Doppler ultrasound has been very important in this area. Color Doppler ultrasound uses color to show the direction and speed of blood flow on a grayscale image, which helps find problems in the blood vessels in real time. Spectral Doppler measures blood flow by showing how velocity changes over time, which allows for a detailed study of blood flow and related hemodynamic factors. Both color and spectral Doppler are used in clinical diagnostics: color Doppler helps map complicated blood vessels, while spectral Doppler gives accurate measurements of blood flow in the brain, which is important for diagnosis. Recent comparative studies highlight that imaging techniques such as transcranial color-coded Doppler yield more accurate cerebral artery velocity readings than non-imaging methods, underscoring the clinical relevance of color and spectral Doppler in vascular research and practice (Gunda *et al.*, 2024; Yao *et al.*, 2024).

6.3.3. Mechanism of Blood Flow Measurement

Because cardiac muscle contracts in a complicated way, it is difficult to accurately measure blood flow since the movement of the heart does not always match the way blood is released from it. Although imaging has made it easier to study heart activity indirectly, it is still hard to measure the mechanical excitation causing contraction.

Utilizing high-resolution, noninvasive modalities enables detection of minute velocity components, such as the mechanical wave-front propagation occurring milliseconds before electrical contraction onset, which correlates directly with myocardial activity and subsequent blood flow dynamics (Kanai *et al.*, 2010). Complementing this, ultrasonic techniques focused on analyzing backscattered signals through time-domain cross-correlation yield high spatial and temporal resolution velocity profiles within flowing biological fluids (Colin *et al.*, 2003). They make it possible to study the details of how blood flows and changes, which improves the accuracy of blood flow measurement. Together, these approaches underpin the mechanism by which ultrasound and Doppler imaging quantify dynamic intravascular flow, integrating mechanical and acoustic data to provide comprehensive vascular assessments (Figure 6.14).

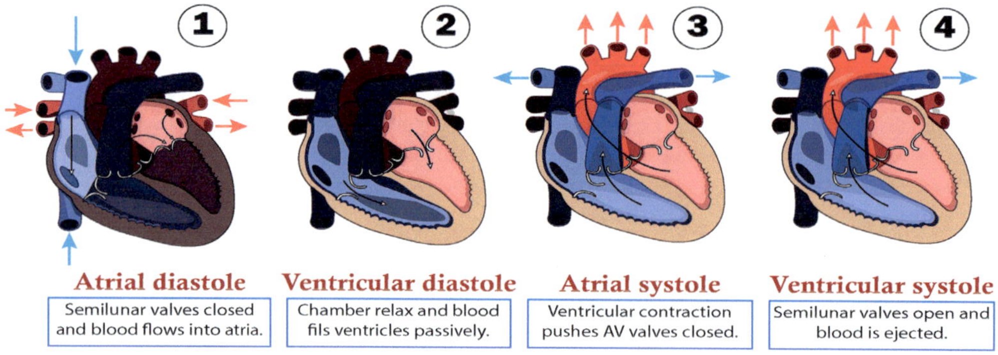

Figure 6.14. The intricacies of cardiac muscle contraction present significant challenges in accurately measuring blood flow, as the direction of myocardial contraction does not align straightforwardly with blood ejection dynamics.

Source: https://www.mdpi.com/mca/mca-29-00057/article_deploy/html/images/mca-29-00057-g001.png.

6.3.4. Signal Processing in Doppler Imaging

Because of new signal processing methods in Doppler imaging, ultrasound technology now provides much better images of blood flow. One critical challenge is the removal of clutter and noise that obscure microvascular flows, which has been addressed through innovative methods such as eigenvalue decomposition (EVD)-based clutter filtering. This approach enhances flow detection by applying spatial Gaussian windows to generate local data subsets, enabling high-definition imaging and reducing artifacts while maintaining computational efficiency, especially with GPU implementation (Huang *et al.*, 2024). Additionally, robust Principal Component Analysis (rPCA) methods, augmented with total variation regularization, have emerged to better separate low-rank tissue signals from sparse blood flow components. By incorporating spatial constraints, these advanced algorithms increase the sensitivity and contrast-to-noise ratio in ultrafast Doppler imaging, thereby effectively recovering microvascular details critical for clinical applications (Fang *et al.*, 2024). All these innovations show that using adaptive and localized signal processing is key to getting accurate Doppler images.

6.3.5. Factors Affecting Doppler Measurements

A number of technical and physiological elements can affect how accurate Doppler measurements are in ultrasound imaging. The angle of insonation is very important because Doppler frequency shifts are most accurate when the beam is parallel to the blood flow; any deviation may result in lower velocity measurements. If a patient moves or the transducer is not correctly positioned, artifacts may appear, and the signal might be weaker. Also, the tissues and vessels around the vessel can affect the extent of signal attenuation and scattering, which can change Doppler sensitivity. Settings for the instrument, such as filters, gain, and pulse repetition frequency, change the shape of the spectral waveform and how well the flow can be detected. The effects of ultrasound on tissue should be controlled based on the amount of power used and the duration of exposure, particularly in sensitive areas or early pregnancy, to follow ALARA rules. Because vascular flow can be complicated in diseases, it takes careful technique to detect changes in blood pressure. Implementation of standardized protocols and operator training significantly enhances measurement reliability and clinical relevance (Bilardo *et al.*, 2023). In hepatic vascular assessment, Doppler ultrasound facilitates comprehensive evaluation of flow dynamics and tissue stiffness, underscoring the modality's integrative diagnostic value (Gottardi *et al.*, 2018) (Figure 6.15).

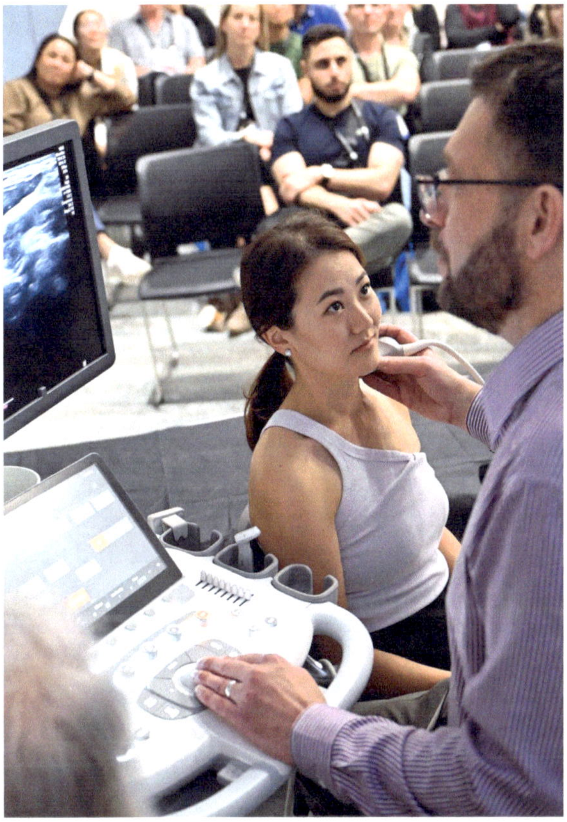

Figure 6.15. Accurate Doppler measurements in ultrasound imaging are influenced by a variety of technical and physiological factors that can impact diagnostic precision.

Source: https://assets.isu.pub/document-structure/240805064716-29da6fa7ca3277ee0560caca2f2e57a3/v1/38051ed231a02b18fd0c2273f08f08e1.jpeg.

6.3.6. Equipment Used in Doppler Imaging

The progress of Doppler imaging has greatly improved the accuracy with which doctors diagnose and treat patients in different fields of medicine. A key part of this progress is adding high-frequency transducers that can both send and receive ultrasound waves to look for blood flow changes in real time. Many modern Doppler instruments use B-mode ultrasound together with Doppler spectral analysis to give detailed vascular images and show the speed of blood flow. Because of portable and user-friendly equipment, point-of-care applications are now more common, especially for vascular access monitoring in hemodialysis patients, who require constant observation of their arteriovenous fistulas. Since the equipment is safe, non-invasive, and reduces the need for invasive procedures, different specialties in medicine now cooperate more in the clinic. Moreover, the development of endoscopic ultrasound-guided biopsy tools incorporates Doppler technology to minimize complications by avoiding vascular structures, thereby improving targeted liver lesion sampling (Shah *et al.*, 2019). The practical reliability and sensitivity of Doppler ultrasound underscore its essential role in vascular assessment and ongoing clinical surveillance (Mudoni *et al.*, 2016).

6.3.7. Safety Considerations in Doppler Imaging

During Doppler imaging, patient safety requires paying attention to several important points, mainly those involving ultrasound exposure. It is very important to train practitioners, since this helps them create and read images that are valid for diagnosis and reduce the risk. Whenever Doppler is used, especially for the eye, lung, or fetus, the exposure to ultrasound should be kept as low as possible to minimize potential harm. The need for accurate results should be balanced with the need for efficient imaging, which means adjusting the output and exposure time. Moreover, expanding the proficiency of healthcare providers through standardized curricula and certification can enhance the safe utilization of Doppler imaging, addressing increasing demand while maintaining quality of care (Moon *et al.*, 2017). Such safety protocols not only reduce potential tissue damage but also contribute to reducing reliance on more hazardous imaging modalities, underscoring the importance of safety in advancing patient-centered care (Abo *et al.*, 2019) (Figure 6.16).

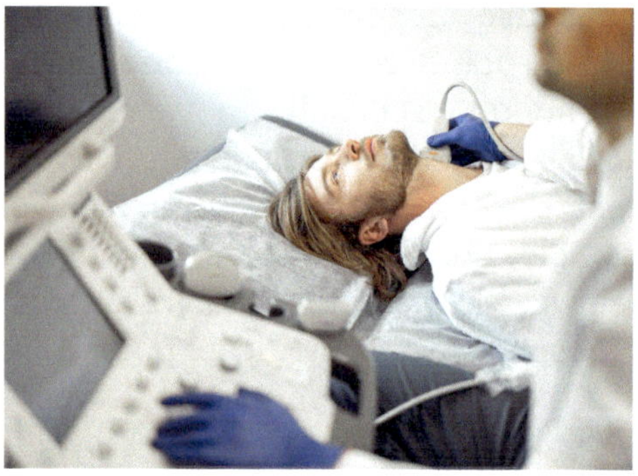

Figure 6.16. Ensuring patient safety during Doppler imaging necessitates careful consideration of several factors, particularly related to ultrasound exposure.

Source: https://sp-ao.shortpixel.ai/client/to_webp,q_glossy,ret_img/https://avicennacardiology.com/wp-content/uploads/2024/06/5623691b-ea54-474f-ae8e-c5cbffcf9cda.png.

6.3.8. Limitations of Doppler Technology

While Doppler technology has advanced a lot, some issues still affect how well it works in clinical settings. It is hard for traditional Doppler ultrasound to detect slow blood flow in small vessels because the filters used to remove motion artifacts also remove the signals from slow blood, which makes the technique less sensitive. Because of this, it is not always possible to accurately describe the blood vessels in the breast, which is important for diagnosis and judging the severity of a lesion. Besides, Doppler methods can be influenced by artifacts and the skills of the person operating the device, which may reduce the reliability and consistency of the results. Some of these issues are being solved by new tools such as microvascular imaging and Angio-PLUS, which can detect microvascular flow without contrast agents, though these are not widely used or understood by most practitioners. Thus, while Doppler imaging continues to evolve, its diagnostic potential is occasionally constrained by technical and interpretive challenges that require ongoing refinement and clinician education (Hafeez *et al.*, 2025; Mohindra *et al.*, 2024).

6.3.9. Comparison with Other Blood Flow Measurement Techniques

Improvements in vascular imaging are meant to make blood flow measurement more accurate and sensitive in medical diagnosis. The Angio-PLUS microvascular imaging technique is more effective than traditional color Doppler at showing slow-moving blood and thin vessels, which are important in telling apart malignant from benign breast masses. Angio-PLUS has demonstrated higher vascular scores and better diagnostic performance than conventional color Doppler, with increased sensitivity reaching 80% and specificity of 66.7%, thus facilitating more precise tumor characterization (Mohindra *et al.*, 2023). Also, using three-dimensional blood flow measurements with vector Doppler, transverse oscillation, and ultrasound speckle tracking, it is found that there are subtle differences in accuracy and bias among these methods. While ultrasound speckle tracking achieves minimal flow rate underestimation (-0.5%), other methods show larger errors, indicating ongoing challenges in replicating complex hemodynamics in clinical settings (Dumas *et al.*, 2021). All of this shows that ultrasound techniques are changing more than other methods used to measure blood flow.

Test Your Knowledge

1. What is the basic principle behind Doppler imaging?
2. What kind of movement causes the frequency to change in Doppler ultrasound?

6.4. Clinical Significance of Doppler Imaging

Learning Outcome

1. Understand role in cardiovascular diagnostics;
2. Assess vascular diseases;
3. Monitor fetal health;
4. Evaluate organ perfusion;
5. Detection of blood clots;
6. Know use in preoperative assessments;
7. Focus on postoperative monitoring applications;
8 Discuss research advancements in doppler imaging;
9. Describe future directions in Doppler technology.

New imaging technologies have greatly enhanced the accuracy of diagnosis and the treatment of patients for several medical problems. Doppler imaging is essential for assessing how well blood and tissues are flowing without the need for invasive testing. In breast oncology, Doppler ultrasound aids in differentiating malignant from benign lesions by evaluating parameters such as resistive index, systolic peak velocity, and vascularity patterns, with malignant lesions typically demonstrating higher vascularity and resistive indices (Rehman *et al.*, 2025).

Also, in peripheral vascular disease, Doppler ultrasound is important because it gives useful information about blood flow, making it a key first choice for diagnosing children, where reducing radiation is very important. However, when anatomical detail is paramount, such as in elderly patients with complex atherosclerotic changes, complementary imaging like computed tomography angiography is often necessary (Sehar *et al.*, 2025). For this reason, Doppler imaging is important in medicine because it supplies instant information about blood flow, which helps with early diagnosis, treatment, and better outcomes for patients.

6.4.1. Role in Cardiovascular Diagnostics

New non-invasive imaging methods have made it much easier to find and monitor cardiovascular diseases early. Doctors can use ultrasound and Doppler imaging to see the heart and blood vessels in action, which helps them understand the heart's function, any problems with valves, and vascular conditions. They are especially helpful in checking the speed of blood flow and the resistance of the vessels, which are key in the diagnosis of atherosclerosis, stenosis, and heart valve disorders. In addition, Doppler ultrasound checks how blood moves in the arteries, which supports the doctor in identifying and managing heart-related problems. As emphasized in clinical guidelines, combining ultrasound imaging with Doppler assessments offers a comprehensive approach to cardiovascular diagnostics by detecting both anatomical and functional impairments early, guiding timely therapeutic interventions, and improving patient outcomes (Cosentino *et al.*, 2019; Lees *et al.*, 2020) (Figure 6.17).

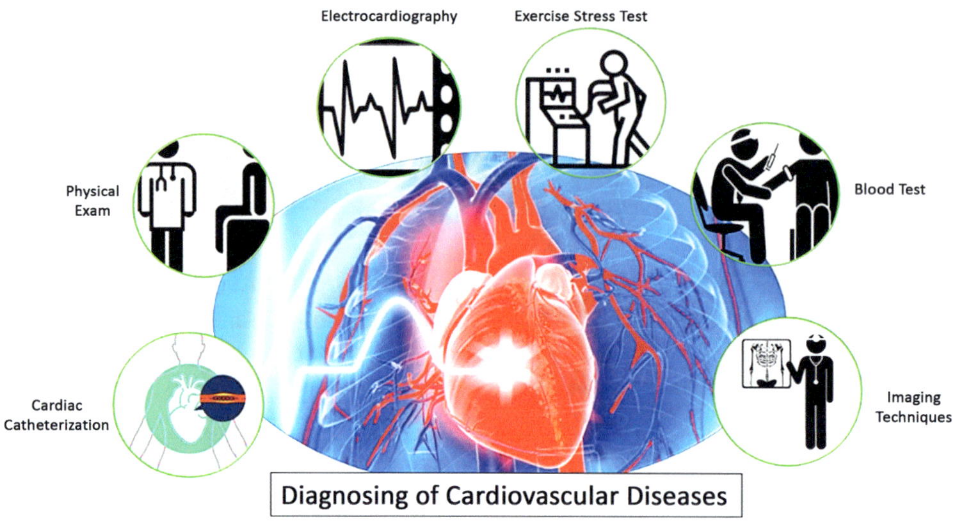

Figure 6.17. Advancements in non-invasive imaging techniques have significantly enhanced the capacity for early detection and monitoring of cardiovascular diseases.

Source: https://www.mdpi.com/chemosensors/chemosensors-09-00067/article_deploy/html/images/chemosensors-09-00067-g002.png.

6.4.2. Assessment of Vascular Diseases

New imaging tools have made it much easier to assess vascular diseases, mainly with the help of ultrasound and Doppler imaging. They give detailed information about the movement of blood and the condition of blood vessels, which makes it possible to detect and assess diseases early and accurately. Doppler ultrasound makes it possible to measure the speed and direction of blood flow, which helps doctors spot stenosis, occlusions, and unusual shunting in arteries and veins. Ultrasound imaging also makes it possible to see vascular structures without surgery, which helps diagnose aneurysms, clots, and problems with the vessel wall. When Doppler data is combined with anatomical images, it helps doctors make decisions, estimate risk, and plan treatment. Even though it is used broadly, it is still necessary to pay attention to patient-related details and technical issues to ensure accurate results. The integration of these imaging techniques continues to play a pivotal role in managing vascular diseases and optimizing patient outcomes (Lees *et al.*, 2020; Lorusso *et al.*, 2021).

6.4.3. Monitoring Fetal Health

Improvements in medical imaging have greatly helped clinicians monitor the health of unborn babies without having to do invasive procedures. Using ultrasound with Doppler techniques makes it possible to carefully examine fetal growth and blood flow, which helps find problems like intrauterine growth restriction. This condition, linked to smaller placental size and impaired umbilical artery flow, demands careful monitoring to mitigate adverse outcomes for both mother and fetus (Meyer *et al.*, 2018). Also, regularly examining the fetal heart rate with Doppler ultrasound makes it easier to find abnormalities early, but there are still some difficulties with the signal and interference. Despite limitations, Doppler ultrasound remains a preferred method in clinical settings due to its low cost and real-time feedback, facilitating timely interventions that reduce fetal morbidity and mortality risks (Gan *et al.*, 2011). Together, these imaging modalities constitute a cornerstone of modern fetal health monitoring (Figure 6.18).

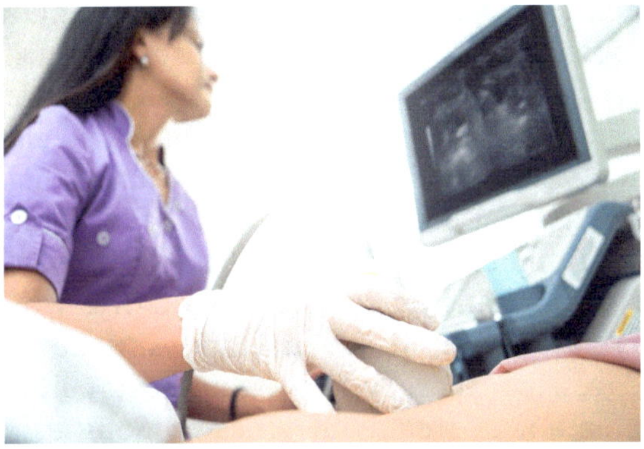

Figure 6.18. Ultrasound imaging, particularly when combined with Doppler techniques, allows for detailed evaluation of fetal development and blood flow dynamics, which are crucial in identifying complications such as intrauterine growth restriction.

Source: https://medanta.s3.ap-south-1.amazonaws.com/blogs/July2024/nOKBhHrRahHBSlnxzm0e6haaj3P84Y-metaRG9wcGxlciBVbHRyYXNvdW5kIGluIFByZWduYW5jeSBBc3Nlc3NpbmcgQmxvb2QgRmxvdyBmb3IgQmFieSdzIEhlYWx0aC5qcGc=-.jpg.

6.4.4. Evaluation of Organ Perfusion

New ultrasound technology makes it much easier to evaluate how well organs are receiving blood supply and functioning, without the need for surgery. Using traditional Doppler imaging, it is often hard to spot microvascular flow because of the movement of the patient and the way wall filters remove weak signals. Recent developments, such as ultrafast Angio PLanewave UltraSensitive (Angio-PL.U.S.) imaging, offer superior sensitivity in capturing subtle blood flow variations within small vessels, enabling detailed evaluation of intramuscular and organ microvascularity. This method has demonstrated comparability to conventional color Doppler flow imaging in quantifying blood perfusion while showing advantages in detecting regional asymmetries in tissue vascularity, suggesting promising clinical applications for monitoring disease progression and organ function (Miller *et al.*, 2024). Furthermore, noncontrast microvascular imaging techniques, exemplified by Angio-PLUS, refine the differentiation between tissue motion and blood flow without the need for contrast agents, broadening their utility in assessing pathological vascular changes, particularly in tumor evaluation (Mohindra *et al.*, 2024).

6.4.5. Detection of Blood Clots

The advancement of ultrasound technology has significantly enhanced the ability to detect and monitor blood clots, particularly in conditions such as deep vein thrombosis (DVT). If blood clots are not identified promptly, they can cause pulmonary embolism, which is why accurate imaging is very important. Using fibrinogen-mimicking fluoropeptide nanoemulsions in contrast-enhanced ultrasound imaging enables the visualization of thrombi by targeting activated platelets and showing live images of vessel blockages. This way of using drugs improves the clarity of Doppler ultrasound and can also prevent clots from growing further by binding to platelets, providing a combined treatment and diagnostic platform. Additionally, Doppler ultrasound delivers critical information on blood flow dynamics and vessel patency, facilitating the assessment of clot impact on circulation and guiding clinical intervention with greater precision (Bilardo *et al.*, 2023; Sloand *et al.*, 2021) (Figure 6.19).

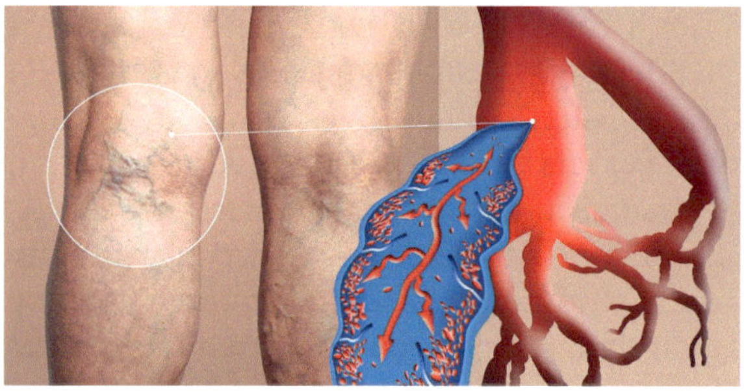

Figure 6.19. Deep vein thrombosis (DVT).

Source: https://s43932.pcdn.co/wp-content/uploads/sites/147/2024/01/Deep-Vein-Thrombosis-min-scaled.jpeg.optimal.jpeg.

6.4.6. Use in Preoperative Assessments

Proper assessments done before surgery make it safer and more likely that the patient will recover well, and an ultrasound with Doppler imaging is now a useful tool for this purpose. They allow surgeons to see blood vessels, soft tissues, and lesions clearly, so they can plan the surgery without cutting into the patient. Three-dimensional ultrasound imaging enhances the accuracy of volumetric and spatial assessments of pathological regions, facilitating more detailed mapping than traditional two-dimensional methods, which is essential for complex surgeries involving organs such as the thyroid or muscular systems (Shen *et al.*, 2024). Furthermore, contrast-enhanced echocardiography employing ultrasound-enhancing agents improves evaluation of cardiac function and blood flow dynamics, offering critical information about myocardial viability and intracardiac anatomy that guides cardiovascular surgeries (Albulushi *et al.*, 2024). In general, using ultrasound and Doppler imaging before surgery helps doctors make more confident diagnoses, avoid unexpected problems during the operation, and design better surgeries.

6.4.7. Postoperative Monitoring Applications

Thanks to better medical imaging, it is now simpler to track patients after surgery, mainly for cases where the patient's blood vessels are important. Free flaps in reconstructive surgery need ongoing and careful monitoring of blood flow to avoid ischemic problems. Recent innovations have focused on real-time ultrasound techniques utilizing compact, patch-type probes that enable continuous Doppler imaging of flap perfusion, ensuring early detection of blood flow disturbances and timely intervention to improve clinical outcomes (Kim *et al.*, 2025). Additionally, pulsed high-intensity focused ultrasound (pHIFU) combined with Doppler imaging offers a novel avenue for monitoring microbubble activity, which correlates with tissue damage and healing progression, thereby facilitating postoperative evaluation of treatment efficacy (Song *et al.*, 2024). Such integration of ultrasound and Doppler imaging provides clinicians with high-contrast, dynamic visualization of physiological changes, ultimately enhancing patient safety by allowing more accurate and immediate postoperative monitoring (Figure 6.20).

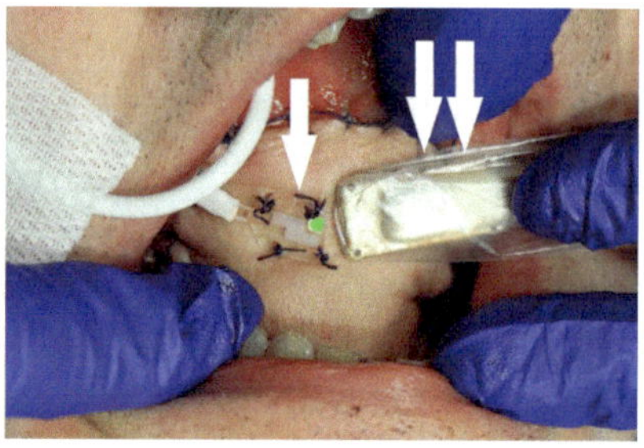

Figure 6.20. In reconstructive surgery, the viability of free flaps depends on continuous and precise assessment of blood flow to prevent ischemic complications.

Source: https://media.springernature.com/lw685/springer-static/image/art%3A10.1007%2Fs00784-023-05177-x/MediaObjects/784_2023_5177_Fig1_HTML.jpg.

6.4.8. Research Advancements in Doppler Imaging

Advancements in medical imaging have made Doppler imaging much better at showing and analyzing the movement of blood and tissues. Thanks to better hardware, data collection, and algorithms, these advances tackle the earlier issues with resolution and penetration depth. Significantly, using AI and deep learning has greatly improved how images are interpreted, helping doctors more accurately detect diseases and separate tissues in real time, which is crucial for making medical decisions. Furthermore, emerging approaches in image-guided microrobotics highlight the necessity for advanced Doppler imaging techniques capable of tracking minuscule therapeutic agents within complex biological environments, pushing the frontiers of minimally invasive interventions (Aziz *et al.*, 2020). The ongoing convergence of AI-driven analytics with 3D reconstruction and visualization promises to refine Doppler imaging's diagnostic precision, ultimately supporting tailored treatment planning and improved patient outcomes across various medical fields (Panayides *et al.*, 2020).

6.4.9. Future Directions in Doppler Technology

With new developments in biomedical engineering and material science, Doppler technology is expected to undergo significant changes, mainly because of the use of new signal processing and interface materials. Emerging methods in fetal health monitoring, such as non-invasive fetal electrocardiography, suggest potential synergies with Doppler ultrasound by enhancing the precision and reliability of cardiac signal extraction and anomaly classification, thereby extending Doppler's diagnostic capabilities in prenatal care (Li *et al.*, 2025). Concurrently, innovations in hydrogel-based human-machine interfaces offer promising avenues for improving the biocompatibility and mechanical flexibility of Doppler probes, potentially enabling more comfortable, long-term monitoring applications (Ullah *et al.*, 2025). Progress in conductive hydrogels and new fabrication methods could help Doppler devices operate better and be more flexible, which would make it easier for them to be used in biological tissues. With these multidisciplinary strategies, Doppler technology will gain from better signal quality and easier use, which will result in more accurate diagnostics and a wider range of medical uses.

Test Your Knowledge

1. What is the medical importance of using Doppler ultrasound to check blood flow in the arteries?
2. How is Doppler ultrasound used to watch for signs of atherosclerosis?

SUMMARY

Because of new imaging methods, it is now much easier to assess complicated physiological and anatomical issues with accuracy. Through the integration of innovative methods such as 4D-Flow MRI and vector flow Doppler ultrasound within controlled experimental settings, researchers have successfully characterized intricate hemodynamic phenomena, including flow patterns and pressure differentials in cardiac models, offering valuable insights into prosthetic valve performance (Stephan *et al.*, 2024). Similarly, the application of 3D ultrasound combined with Doppler angiography has proven instrumental in prenatal diagnosis by providing clear, spatially accurate depictions of fetal cardiac and vascular anatomy, facilitating early and reliable detection of anomalies without the need for mental reconstruction (Guindi *et al.*, 2020). They point out that ultrasound and Doppler imaging are helpful for diagnosis and also for gaining a better understanding of how the body works. Thus, using these advanced imaging techniques can lead to better clinical results by making diagnoses more accurate and enabling the selection of appropriate treatments.

Improvements in imaging have greatly improved how cardiovascular medicine diagnoses and monitors patients. Because they are non-invasive and can show cardiac structures and blood flow in real time, ultrasound and Doppler imaging are now important tools. They help assess the heart, its valves, and the blood vessels, which helps doctors make better treatment. Doppler imaging is important for checking blood flow and spotting abnormalities early, which can influence a patient's outcome. Still, it is important to keep improving imaging and interpretation guidelines to handle the challenges of congenital heart diseases. In addition, when different medical fields collaborate, imaging results and clinical care are better coordinated, which benefits patients. The evolving landscape of ultrasound and Doppler technology underscores the importance of ongoing education and guideline adherence, reinforcing professional responsibility in medical practice (Cosentino *et al.*, 2019; Rychik *et al.*, 2019).

KEY TERMS FROM THIS CHAPTER

- Ionizing radiation
- Kidney health
- Stenosis
- Diagnoses
- Superb microvascular imaging
- Noninvasive assessments
- Peripheral artery disease
- Electrical energy
- Nephrology
- Transplantation
- Thrombosis
- Microvascular structures
- Vascular hemodynamics
- Hypertension
- Artificial intelligence
- Transducers

CRITICAL THINKING QUESTIONS

1. **What idea is used by ultrasound imaging to create images?**
   a. Electromagnetic waves
   b. Ionizing radiation
   c. High-frequency sound waves
   d. Magnetic fields
2. **In Doppler ultrasound, what is primarily measured?**
   a. Tissue elasticity
   b. Blood flow velocity
   c. Bone density
   d. Tumor size
3. **Which Doppler ultrasound technique is most often used to look at blood flow in the arteries and veins?**
   a. Power Doppler
   b. Color Doppler
   c. Spectral Doppler
   d. Continuous-wave Doppler
4. **What is an advantage of ultrasound over CT or MRI?**
   a. It provides more detailed images of soft tissues
   b. It has no ionizing radiation
   c. It is better for detecting bone fractures
   d. It is ideal for imaging deep abdominal organs
5. **What frequency range is most often used for ultrasound imaging used in diagnosis?**
   a. 10–20 Hz
   b. 20–100 Hz
   c. 1–20 MHz
   d. 30–50 MHz

Short Answer Questions

1. What is the basic principle behind ultrasound imaging?
2. How does Doppler ultrasound differ from conventional ultrasound imaging?
3. What are the most common uses of Doppler ultrasound in examining the blood vessels?
4. Why is ultrasound better than CT and MRI in some situations?
5. What are the limitations of ultrasound imaging?
6. What part do contrast agents play in ultrasound imaging?
7. What is the process of a color Doppler ultrasound in depicting blood flow?
8. Which tissues on ultrasound are shown as hypoechoic, hyperechoic, or anechoic?
9. What risks and safety issues might occur during ultrasound imaging?

Answers to Critical Thinking Questions

1. (c); 2. (b); 3. (b); 4. (b); 5. (c)

REFERENCES

1. Abo, A., Abramowicz, J., Bigelow, T., Bigelow, A., *et al.* (2019). *Diagnostic Ultrasound Safety Review for Point-of-Care Ultrasound Practitioners.* https://core.ac.uk/download/286268919.pdf (accessed on 1st June 2025).
2. Albulushi, A., Xie, F., & Porter, T. R. (2024). Ultrasound enhancing agents in cardiovascular imaging: Expanding horizons beyond coronary arteries. *Cardiovascular Ultrasound, 22.* https://www.semanticscholar.org/paper/5e4d01fd43bc21460d60d4441ab351b150cc78cf (accessed on 1st June 2025).
3. Aldžić, A., Habeš, S., Obradović, Z., Ridžal, E., *et al.* (2013). *Air Pollution by Nitrogen Oxides in Sarajevo from 2005 to 2010.* https://core.ac.uk/download/73974384.pdf (accessed on 1st June 2025).
4. Amedu, C., Anyasor, E., Babington, E. A., Reeve, E., *et al.* (2024). *Non-Contrast Ultrasound Assessment of Blood Flow in Clinical Practice.* https://core.ac.uk/download/630478035.pdf (accessed on 1st June 2025).
5. Aziz, A., Pane, S., Iacovacci, V., Koukourakis, N., Czarske, J., Menciassi, A., Medina-Sánchez, M., *et al.* (2020). Medical imaging of microrobots: Toward *in vivo* applications. *ACS Nano, 14*, 10865–10893. https://doi.org/10.1021/acsnano.0c05530 (accessed on 1st June 2025).
6. Bartolotta, T. V., Cannella, R., Mazzola, M., Pilato, A., *et al.* (2023). *New Microvascular Ultrasound Techniques: Abdominal Applications.* https://core.ac.uk/download/587991931.pdf (accessed on 1st June 2025).
7. Baumgartner, H., De Backer, J., Babu-Narayan, S. V., Budts, W., Chessa, M., Diller, G. P., Lung, B., *et al.* (2020). 2020 ESC guidelines for the management of adult congenital heart disease. *European Heart Journal, 42*, 563–645. https://doi.org/10.1093/eurheartj/ehaa554 (accessed on 1st June 2025).
8. Bazigou, E., Eckersley, R. J., Leow, C., Tang, M., *et al.* (2015). Flow velocity mapping using contrast enhanced high-frame-rate plane wave ultrasound and image tracking: Methods and initial *in vitro* and *in vivo* evaluation. *Ultrasound in Medicine and Biology.* https://core.ac.uk/download/77002662.pdf (accessed on 1st June 2025).
9. Bellati, F., Caserta, D., Costanzi, F., De Marco, A., *et al.* (2018). Real-time virtual sonography in gynecology & obstetrics: Literature's analysis and case series. *Biomed J. Sci. & Tech. Res.* https://core.ac.uk/download/195777140.pdf (accessed on 1st June 2025).
10. Bilardo, C. M., Chaoui, R., Hyett, J., Kagan, K. O., Karim, J., Papageorghiou, A. T., Poon, L. C., *et al.* (2023). ISUOG practice guidelines (updated): Performance of 11–14-week ultrasound scan. *Ultrasound in Obstetrics and Gynecology, 61*, 127–143. https://doi.org/10.1002/uog.26106 (accessed on 1st June 2025).
11. Cai, S., Xing, H., Wang, Y., Wang, Y., Ma, W., Jiang, Y., Li, J., *et al.* (2024). Clinical application of intraoperative ultrasound superb microvascular imaging in brain tumors resections: Contributing to the achievement of total tumoral resection. *BMC Medical Imaging, 24.* https://www.semanticscholar.org/paper/dbe444514cb8d392220a07e6bbf22d3facd5c974 (accessed on 1st June 2025).
12. Cannella, R., Pilato, G., Mazzola, M., & Bartolotta, T. V. (2023). New microvascular ultrasound

techniques: Abdominal applications. *La Radiologia Medica, 128*, 1023–1034. https://doi.org/10.1007/s11547-023-01679-6 (accessed on 1st June 2025).

13. Cantisani, V., Deganello, A., Dietrich, C. F., Duran, C., *et al.* (2016). Role of contrast-enhanced ultrasound (CEUS) in pediatric practice: An EFSUMB position statement. https://core.ac.uk/download/74320188.pdf (accessed on 1st June 2025).
14. Colin, A., Ackerson, B., Bandyopadhyay, R., Barnes, K., Berson, A., Bohs, L., Bonnefous, O., *et al.* (2003). *High-Frequency Ultrasonic Speckle Velocimetry in Sheared Complex Fluids.* http://arxiv.org/abs/cond-mat/0311072 (accessed on 1st June 2025).
15. Cosentino, F., Grant, P. J., Aboyans, V., Bailey, C. J., Ceriello, A., Delgado, V., Federici, M., *et al.* (2019). 2019 ESC guidelines on diabetes, pre-diabetes, and cardiovascular diseases developed in collaboration with the EASD. *European Heart Journal, 41*, 255–323. https://doi.org/10.1093/eurheartj/ehz486 (accessed on 1st June 2025).
16. Cowley, M. J., & Hughes, S. W. (2017). *Teaching the Doppler Effect in Astrophysics.* http://arxiv.org/abs/1701.04478 (accessed on 1st June 2025).
17. Craciunas, L., Gallos, I., Chu, J., Bourne, T., Quenby, S., Brosens, J. J., & Coomarasamy, A. (2018). Conventional and modern markers of endometrial receptivity: A systematic review and meta-analysis. *Human Reproduction Update, 25*, 202–223. https://doi.org/10.1093/humupd/dmy044 (accessed on 1st June 2025).
18. Das, P. (2024). Application of scrotal ultrasound imaging in clinicopathologically suspected cases of male infertility – A prospective study in a peripheral medical college in West Bengal. *Asian Journal of Pharmaceutical and Clinical Research.* https://www.semanticscholar.org/paper/b6f63c59805c6d7c8a5f731aea5764a91c2bfecb (accessed on 1st June 2025).
19. De Gottardi, A., Berzigotti, A., Buscarini, E., & García-Criado, Á. (2018). Ultrasonography in liver vascular disease. *Ultraschall in der Medizin – European Journal of Ultrasound, 39*, 382–405. https://doi.org/10.1055/a-0647-1658 (accessed on 1st June 2025).
20. Degroote, J., Lovstakken, L., Segers, P., Swillens, A., *et al.* (2010). Synthetic vascular ultrasound imaging through coupled fluid-structure interaction and ultrasound simulations. https://core.ac.uk/download/55773067.pdf (accessed on 1st June 2025).
21. Dinsmore, M., & Venkatraghavan, L. (2022). Clinical applications of point-of-care ultrasound in brain injury: A narrative review. *Anesthesia, 77*, 69–77. https://doi.org/10.1111/anae.15604 (accessed on 1st June 2025).
22. Dres, M., Doorduin, J., Boussouar, S., & Bachasson, D. (2025). Advancements in imaging techniques for monitoring the respiratory muscles. *Critical Care, 29.* https://www.semanticscholar.org/paper/0859ca9cf5abec52dd7863107343442e1d20d682 (accessed on 1st June 2025).
23. Dumas, R., Riemer, K., Toulemonde, M., Lerendegui, M., Weinberg, P., Tang, M., & Varray, F. (2021). 4D ultrafast blood flow imaging comparison: Vector Doppler, transverse oscillation and speckle tracking. In *2021 IEEE International Ultrasonics Symposium (IUS).* https://www.semanticscholar.org/paper/e5ed100fddcee2549a1a069c708b2e79994a4674 (accessed on 1st June 2025).
24. Fadnes, S., Lovstakken, L., Rodriguez-Morales, A., Segers, P., *et al.* (2016). Assessing the performance of ultrafast vector flow imaging in the neonatal heart via multiphysics modeling

and *in vitro* experiments. *IEEE Transactions on Ultrasonics, Ferroelectrics, and Frequency Control.* https://core.ac.uk/download/74712692.pdf (accessed on 1st June 2025).

25. Fang, B., Li, H., & Chen, Y. (2024). Total variational robust PCA for ultrasound microvascular clutter filtering. In *2024 IEEE Ultrasonics, Ferroelectrics, and Frequency Control Joint Symposium (UFFC-JS).* https://www.semanticscholar.org/paper/b689fb1042b61c37e86bc46f383de39117a0e81b (accessed on 1st June 2025).

26. Fiorentini, S., Måsøy, S., & Avdal, J. (2023). Analysis of aberration effects on flow imaging and quantification in echocardiography. *IEEE Open Journal of Ultrasonics, Ferroelectrics, and Frequency Control, 3,* 194–202. https://www.semanticscholar.org/paper/dd49c075848014ffea40f0b9a7d6e1e3e6c0081a (accessed on 1st June 2025).

27. Fraser, A. G., Monaghan, M., Van Der Steen, A. F. W., & Sutherland, G. R. (2022). A concise history of echocardiography: Timeline, pioneers, and landmark publications. *European Heart Journal – Cardiovascular Imaging, 23,* 1130–1143. https://doi.org/10.1093/ehjci/jeac111 (accessed on 1st June 2025).

28. Freeman, C., & Hwang, M. (2022). Advanced ultrasound techniques for neuroimaging in pediatric critical care: A review. *Children, 9.* https://www.semanticscholar.org/paper/4b0149ab6c04163550113e4bfb29c7d790b57f66 (accessed on 1st June 2025).

29. Gamarra, A., Salamanca, J., Díez-Villanueva, P., Cuenca, S., Vázquez, J., Aguilar, R., Diego, G., *et al.* (2025). Ultrasound imaging of congestion in heart failure: A narrative review. *Cardiovascular Diagnosis and Therapy, 15,* 233–250. https://www.semanticscholar.org/paper/1a9c01d8df04709e9d76aed32a22483a72e9eba3 (accessed on 1st June 2025).

30. Gan, K. B., Zahedi, E., & Ali, M. (2011). Application of adaptive noise cancellation in transabdominal fetal heart rate detection using photoplethysmography. https://www.semanticscholar.org/paper/c03d7a58222c06d50d79905e5068d24542d59d7e (accessed on 1st June 2025).

31. Gatz, M., Spang, C., & Alfredson, H. (2020). Partial Achilles tendon rupture—A neglected entity: A narrative literature review on diagnostics and treatment options. *Journal of Clinical Medicine, 9,* 3380–3380. https://doi.org/10.3390/jcm9103380 (accessed on 1st June 2025).

32. Gazhonova, V. E., Popova, A. Y., & Mironova, E. V. (2024). Searching for a twinkling artefact in breast microcalcifications using B-flow ultrasonic non-doppler technology: A prospective study. *Diagnostic Radiology and Radiotherapy.* https://www.semanticscholar.org/paper/bf75821ad2af16da5ae2be1a29961717c9c64ea3 (accessed on 1st June 2025).

33. Ghafar, S. A., Haqiqullah, C., Jan, A. A., Nasratullah, M., *et al.* (2024). *Basics of Ultrasound and Its Use in Medicine: A Review Article.* https://core.ac.uk/download/620883361.pdf (accessed on 1st June 2025).

34. Guindi, W. E., Dreyfus, M., Carle, G., & Alassas, N. (2020). The additional diagnostic value of the three-dimensional 3D ultrasound and Doppler angiography imaging in the prenatal diagnosis of left isomerism. *Journal of Clinical Case Reports and Images.* https://www.semanticscholar.org/paper/78c80750eda0280c5797b5bb1d56e88348ebf3aa (accessed on 1st June 2025).

35. Gunda, S. T., Ng, T. K. V., Liu, T. Y., Chen, Z., Han, X., Chen, X., Pang, M., *et al.* (2024). A comparative study of transcranial color-coded Doppler (TCCD) and transcranial Doppler (TCD) ultrasonography techniques in assessing the intracranial cerebral arteries hemodynamics.

Diagnostics, 14. https://www.semanticscholar.org/paper/80f0faf5d3f26f862786275706495514a672b114 (accessed on 1st June 2025).

36. Hafeez, S. A., & M. R. (2025). Risk-adapted breast cancer screening: Combining DOT and ultrasound with AI to overcome mammography limitations. *2025 International Conference on Machine Learning and Autonomous Systems (ICMLAS)*. https://www.semanticscholar.org/paper/5fe88c29b6dc536986a8b266ca12ba1286f8450f (accessed on 1st June 2025).
37. Huang, C., Lok, U., Zhang, J., Liu, H., & Chen, S. (2024). Real-time adaptive and localized spatiotemporal clutter filtering for ultrasound small vessel imaging. https://www.semanticscholar.org/paper/8914f83a090ade6b29c268c4e8645a1a2a1ee89b (accessed on 1st June 2025).
38. Ilaria, F., Ilaria, P., & Meola, M. (2021). Advances in vascular anatomy and pathophysiology using high resolution and multiparametric sonography. *The Journal of Vascular Access*. https://core.ac.uk/download/566466881.pdf (accessed on 1st June 2025).
39. Iula, A., & Micucci, M. (2022). *Recent Advances in Machine Learning Applied to Ultrasound Imaging*. https://core.ac.uk/download/554193682.pdf (accessed on 1st June 2025).
40. Ji, M. H., & Seoung, Y. H. (2023). Right-to-left shunt evaluation in cardiac patent foramen ovale using bubble contrast transcranial color-coded Doppler: A cryptogenic stroke case. *Healthcare, 11*. https://www.semanticscholar.org/paper/c477655fdef8741df40065df6fa9b2ef176da4ca (accessed on 1st June 2025).
41. Kalagara, H., Coker, B. J., Gerstein, N. S., Kukreja, P., Deriy, L., Pierce, A., & Townsley, M. M. (2021). Point-of-care ultrasound (POCUS) for the cardiothoracic anesthesiologist. *Journal of Cardiothoracic and Vascular Anesthesia, 36*, 1132–1147. https://doi.org/10.1053/j.jvca.2021.01.018 (accessed on 1st June 2025).
42. Kanai, H., & Tanaka, M. (2010). *Visualization of Minute Mechanical-Excitation/Relaxation Wave-Front Propagation in Myocardial Tissue*. https://core.ac.uk/download/pdf/289399.pdf (accessed on 1st June 2025).
43. Karaman, E. (2017). Response to 'Safety of elastography applied to the placenta: Be careful with ultrasound radiation force.' *Journal of Obstetrics and Gynecology Research, 43*. https://www.semanticscholar.org/paper/cfef1eb8b22c33c9ab3feed5381ee9770da80994 (accessed on 1st June 2025).
44. Kim, Y., Kim, J. H., Ryu, Y. H., Ha, H., Lee, S. J., Lee, S. C., Lim, C., *et al.* (2025). Real-time ultrasound imaging system utilizing patch-type ultrasound probe for free-flap blood perfusion monitoring. *IEEE Sensors Journal, 25*, 8898–8906. https://www.semanticscholar.org/paper/81b8ef03687406c0f030160307863931f469d30a (accessed on 1st June 2025).
45. Koratala, A., & Reisinger, N. (2022). Venous excess Doppler ultrasound for the nephrologist: Pearls and pitfalls. *Kidney Medicine, 4*, 100482. https://doi.org/10.1016/j.xkme.2022.100482 (accessed on 1st June 2025).
46. Lees, C., Stampalija, T., Baschat, A., Da Silva, C. F., Ferrazzi, E., Figueras, F., Hecher, K., *et al.* (2020). ISUOG practice guidelines: Diagnosis and management of small-for-gestational-age fetus and fetal growth restriction. *Ultrasound in Obstetrics and Gynecology, 56*, 298–312. https://doi.org/10.1002/uog.22134 (accessed on 1st June 2025).

47. Li, X., Wan, J., & Peng, X. (2025). Review of non-invasive fetal electrocardiography monitoring techniques. *Sensors (Basel, Switzerland), 25.* https://www.semanticscholar.org/paper/e6a149a699291f9c5927aca8d610738302981b39 (accessed on 1st June 2025).

48. Lorusso, R., Shekar, K., MacLaren, G., Schmidt, M., Pellegrino, V., Meyns, B., Haft, J. W., *et al.* (2021). ELSO interim guidelines for venoarterial extracorporeal membrane oxygenation in adult cardiac patients. *ASAIO Journal, 67,* 827–844. https://doi.org/10.1097/mat.0000000000001510 (accessed on 1st June 2025).

49. Malaichamy, A., Pandian, V., Arumugam, T., & Ravipati, C. (2024). Advances in vascular imaging: A comparative analysis of Doppler ultrasound and multidetector CT for lower limb peripheral arterial disease diagnosis. *Cureus, 16.* https://www.semanticscholar.org/paper/37fb1b5999f23106732e74bf74b48b13669a65d2 (accessed on 1st June 2025).

50. Meyer, N., Schüler, T., & Zenclussen, A. (2018). High frequency ultrasound for the analysis of fetal and placental development *in vivo. Journal of Visualized Experiments: JoVE, 141.* https://www.semanticscholar.org/paper/4816bf40e479f79447fb7eed3666d4d4565b3173 (accessed on 1st June 2025).

51. Miller, T., Chambara, N., Ying, M. T. C., & Pang, M. (2024). Using ultrafast Angio planewave ultrasensitive and conventional Doppler imaging techniques to assess intramuscular blood perfusion in older adults. *BMC Medical Imaging, 24.* https://www.semanticscholar.org/paper/7243cde142fedf9311e2ad347dc5c9a5320c5664 (accessed on 1st June 2025).

52. Mohindra, N., & Soni, N. (2024). Ultrasound-based noncontrast microvascular imaging for evaluation of breast lesions: Imaging techniques and review of diagnostic criteria. *The Indian Journal of Radiology & Imaging, 34,* 702–713. https://www.semanticscholar.org/paper/fe11165c5d10a433a72a28bbc41ede3e5d0620fe (accessed on 1st June 2025).

53. Mohindra, N., Jain, N., Yadav, S., Agrawal, V., Mishra, P., Mishra, A., & Agarwal, G. (2023). Utility of ultrasound Angio-PLUS imaging for detecting blood flow in breast masses and comparison with color Doppler for differentiating benign from malignant masses. *Acta Radiologica, 64,* 2087–2095. https://www.semanticscholar.org/paper/b0f7011fcf2bbf4e8aa7b1b6b05fc834e1940a05 (accessed on 1st June 2025).

54. Moon, S. (2017). *Echocardiography Curriculum Development for Physician Assistants Using Entrustable Professional Activities.* https://core.ac.uk/download/215924737.pdf (accessed on 1st June 2025).

55. Mudoni, A., Caccetta, F., Caroppo, M., Musio, F., Accogli, A., Zacheo, M. D., Burzo, M., *et al.* (2016). Echo color Doppler ultrasound: A valuable diagnostic tool in the assessment of arteriovenous fistula in hemodialysis patients. *The Journal of Vascular Access, 17,* 446–452. https://www.semanticscholar.org/paper/99f55fa7dc3e30928310131f6812a218fa75fd50 (accessed on 1st June 2025).

56. O'Reilly, D., Rakonczay, Z., & Kylänpää, M. (2013). Acute and chronic pancreatic inflammation. *International Journal of Inflammation, 2012.* https://www.semanticscholar.org/paper/2d8541b04b7ee1b8b61c83673090e49eda905882 (accessed on 1st June 2025).

57. Oglat, A. A., & Abukhalil, T. (2024). Ultrasound elastography: Methods, clinical applications, and limitations: A review article. *Applied Sciences.* https://www.semanticscholar.org/paper/0bc80b40eaf5c4e7484d0c0537133c7ebebe57e9 (accessed on 1st June 2025).

58. Oh, D., Lee, D., Heo, J., Kweon, J., Yong, U., Jang, J., Ahn, Y. J., *et al.* (2024). Longitudinal vascular monitoring of acute and diabetic kidney diseases with 3D renal ultrafast ultrasound Doppler imaging. In *2024 IEEE Ultrasonics, Ferroelectrics, and Frequency Control Joint Symposium (UFFC-JS).* https://www.semanticscholar.org/paper/098a480c2222de50319ac15741082e7689bedf71 (accessed on 1st June 2025).

59. Panayides, A. S., Amini, A. A., Filipović, N., Sharma, A., Tsaftaris, S. A., Young, A. A., Foran, D. J., *et al.* (2020). AI in medical imaging informatics: Current challenges and future directions. *IEEE Journal of Biomedical and Health Informatics, 24*, 1837–1857. https://doi.org/10.1109/jbhi.2020.2991043 (accessed on 1st June 2025).

60. Percie Du, S. N., Ahluwalia, A., Alam, S., Avey, M. T., Baker, M., Browne, W. J., Clark, A., *et al.* (2020). Reporting animal research: Explanation and elaboration for the ARRIVE guidelines 2.0. *PLoS Biology, 18*, e3000411–e3000411. https://doi.org/10.1371/journal.pbio.3000411 (accessed on 1st June 2025).

61. Reddan, T., Malouf, M., Venugopal, P. S., & Powell, J. (2024). Pre-operative transcranial Doppler ultrasound assessment of cerebral collateral circulation in children undergoing Veno-arterial extracorporeal membrane oxygenation or cardiac surgery. *Journal of Medical Radiation Sciences.* https://www.semanticscholar.org/paper/dd583c3b2d39c5777c27f9961db93862334420bf (accessed on 1st June 2025).

62. Rehman, S., Alavi, S., Raheel, N., Yasin, A., Ameer, S., & Alavi, S. R. (2025). Usefulness of resistive index to differentiate benign from malignant breast lesions using color Doppler ultrasound. *Pakistan Postgraduate Medical Journal.* https://www.semanticscholar.org/paper/1b8551dd15d5605ce9b1b56ad7c5067a62338499 (accessed on 1st June 2025).

63. Ricco, J. B., Bartelink, M. L., Björck, M., Brodmann, M., Cohnert, T., Czerny, M., De Carlo, M., *et al.* (2017). 2017 ESC guidelines on the diagnosis and treatment of peripheral arterial diseases, in collaboration with the European Society for Vascular Surgery (ESVS). *European Heart Journal, 39*, 763–816. https://doi.org/10.1093/eurheartj/ehx095 (accessed on 1st June 2025).

64. Rychik, J., Atz, A. M., Celermajer, D. S., Deal, B. J., Gatzoulis, M. A., Gewillig, M., Hsia, T. Y., *et al.* (2019). Evaluation and management of the child and adult with Fontan circulation: A scientific statement from the American Heart Association. *Circulation, 140.* https://doi.org/10.1161/cir.0000000000000696 (accessed on 1st June 2025).

65. Sehar, A., Ashraf, R., Fatima, M., Akhtar, U., Saeed, F., & Sibtain, M. (2025). Comparison between Doppler ultrasound and computed tomography angiography in the diagnosis of peripheral vascular disease in different age groups. *Insights–Journal of Health and Rehabilitation.* https://www.semanticscholar.org/paper/7c503052297088435260ed124547da245aab3ca6 (accessed on 1st June 2025).

66. Shah, A., Al-Hanayneh, M., Chowdhry, M., Bilal, M., & Singh, S. (2019). Endoscopic ultrasound guided liver biopsy for parenchymal liver disease. *World Journal of Hepatology, 11*, 335–343. https://www.semanticscholar.org/paper/82c0eed4cd5a9ad387139cbd4278feb1c4abc1b8 (accessed on 1st June 2025).

67. Shen, E., Fan, K., Lu, Y., Chen, X., Li, C., Ma, X., Wu, T., *et al.* (2024). 3D multi-modality free-hand ultrasound imaging for medical research. *2024 IEEE International Symposium on Biomedical Imaging (ISBI).* https://www.semanticscholar.org/paper/c7cb411fca2eac22c3bd4390192e5713512f0554 (accessed on 1st June 2025).

68. Silverman, R. H. (2023). Principles of ophthalmic ultrasound. *Expert Review of Ophthalmology, 18*, 379–389. https://www.semanticscholar.org/paper/8121a8aceee821223ef8d8c9f03bf0b912e84640 (accessed on 1st June 2025).

69. Singla, R., Kadatz, M., Rohling, R., & Nguan, C. (2022). Kidney ultrasound for nephrologists: A review. *Kidney Medicine, 4*, 100464. https://doi.org/10.1016/j.xkme.2022.100464 (accessed on 1st June 2025).

70. Sloand, J. N., Rokni, E., Watson, C. T., Miller, M. A., Manning, K. B., Simon, J. C., & Medina, S. H. (2021). Ultrasound-responsive nanopeptisomes enable synchronous spatial imaging and inhibition of clot growth in deep vein thrombosis. *Advanced Healthcare Materials, 10*. https://doi.org/10.1002/adhm.202100520 (accessed on 1st June 2025).

71. Snoj, Ž., Wu, C. H., Taljanovic, M., Dumić-Čule, I., Drakonaki, E., & Klauser, A. (2020). Ultrasound elastography in musculoskeletal radiology: Past, present, and future. *Seminars in Musculoskeletal Radiology, 24*, 156–166. https://www.semanticscholar.org/paper/6369d66cce2681a8328807590ef15d770b7fb9f6 (accessed on 1st June 2025).

72. Song, M., Sapozhnikov, O., Khokhlova, V. A., Son, H., Totten, S., Wang, Y. N., & Khokhlova, T. D. (2024). Dynamic mode decomposition based Doppler monitoring of *de novo* cavitation induced by pulsed HIFU: An *in vivo* feasibility study. *Scientific Reports, 14*. https://www.semanticscholar.org/paper/4b1005dccee290993e8bad277de89b3856e573bf (accessed on 1st June 2025).

73. Stephan, H., Grefen, L., Clevert, D., Onkes, M., Ning, J., Thierfelder, N., Mela, P., *et al.* (2024). 4D-flow MRI and vector ultrasound in the *in vitro* evaluation of surgical aortic heart valves – A pilot study. *Journal of Cardiovascular Translational Research, 18*, 158–168. https://www.semanticscholar.org/paper/dd59a2f2bd37fe93923324fe6c75596213fba55c (accessed on 1st June 2025).

74. Taeymans, O. (2018). *Musculoskeletal Ultrasound: When Does it Make a Difference?* https://www.semanticscholar.org/paper/ade23b4d373003bde13b1e2b48e105389cd0655a (accessed on 1st June 2025).

75. Tzatzairis, T., Skarentzos, K., Grammatikos, C., Karamalis, C., Korakianitis, K., Kourempeles, R., & Drosos, G. (2024). Ultrasound applications in pediatric orthopedics. *Archives of Bone and Joint Surgery, 12*, 457–468. https://www.semanticscholar.org/paper/59925c2de86c06c9431d2c10ff413b9a2621bbc3 (accessed on 1st June 2025).

76. Ullah, A., Kim, D. Y., Lim, S. I., & Lim, H. R. (2025). Hydrogel-based biointerfaces: Recent advances, challenges, and future directions in human–machine integration. *Gels, 11*. https://www.semanticscholar.org/paper/e13f6aa43866f58a534a2f45d8dbea024b565217 (accessed on 1st June 2025).

77. Williams, B., Mancia, G., Spiering, W., Agabiti, R. E., Azizi, M., Burnier, M., Clement, D. L., *et al.* (2018). 2018 ESC/ESH guidelines for the management of arterial hypertension. *European Heart Journal, 39*, 3021–3104. https://doi.org/10.1093/eurheartj/ehy339 (accessed on 1st June 2025).

78. Yao, B., Yang, L., Evans, K. D., & Roll, S. C. (2024). Doppler sonography evaluation of median nerve intraneural blood flow: A systematic review. *Journal of Diagnostic Medical Sonography*. https://www.semanticscholar.org/paper/cbfe4bca5ca67bd75b5c2c91254ee765009a6770 (accessed on 1st June 2025).

COMPUTED TOMOGRAPHY (CT)

7

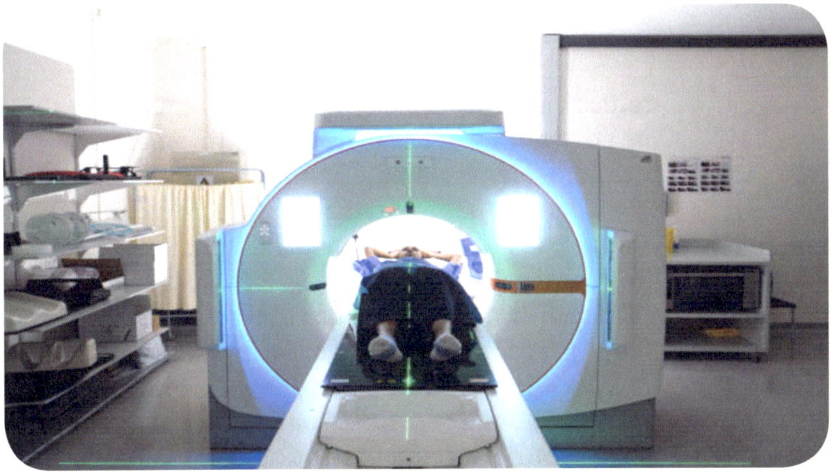

LEARNING OBJECTIVES

After studying this chapter, you will be able to:

1. Understand principles of computed tomography;
2. Know applications of CT in medical diagnostics;
3. Discuss the advantages and disadvantages of CT imaging;
4. Explain the future of computed tomography in diagnostics.

Introduction

With the help of medical imaging, doctors can now see detailed pictures of the inside of a person's body without having to do surgery. Among these imaging modalities, computed tomography (CT) has emerged as an indispensable tool in modern clinical practice due to its ability to produce cross-sectional images with high spatial resolution. Over recent years, innovations such as dual-energy CT (DECT) and photon-counting computed tomography (PCCT) have further expanded the diagnostic potential of CT by enhancing material differentiation and image quality while reducing radiation exposure. Improvements in technology allow doctors to view blood vessels and related problems more clearly and to measure the extent of disease in the tissue. As a result, CT imaging now plays a crucial role in diagnosing and managing a wide range of conditions, particularly in vascular and coronary artery diseases, where accurate and early detection significantly influences patient outcomes (Meloni *et al.*, 2024; Stański *et al.*, 2024).

Definition of Computed Tomography (CT)

New imaging techniques make it much easier to see inside the body, which helps doctors identify diseases more quickly and accurately. CT shows how technology is advancing by making use of X-rays and computers to produce images of the body from different directions. They supply much more information about bone, soft tissue, and blood vessels than X-rays can. The use of CT scans is important because they let doctors find tumors, infections, and structural problems, which helps with early diagnosis and better treatment plans. Moreover, CT imaging integrates structural data with physiological insights, broadening its diagnostic utility in diseases like chronic obstructive pulmonary disease (COPD), where spirometry alone may be insufficient (Lowe *et al.*, 2019). Despite concerns over cost and potential artifacts, the refinement of CT technology continues to enhance its role as an indispensable diagnostic tool across numerous medical disciplines (Pulumati *et al.*, 2023) (Figure 7.1).

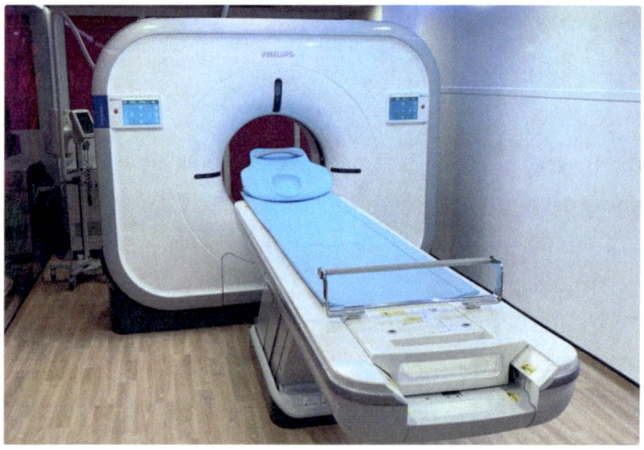

Figure 7.1. Modern diagnostic imaging has revolutionized the ability to visualize internal structures with remarkable clarity, enabling more accurate and timely identification of diseases.

Source: https://tichealth.co.uk/wp-content/uploads/2025/01/CT.webp.

Historical Development of Computed Tomography (CT) Technology

The progress of CT technology is a major development in diagnostic imaging, showing constant improvements since its invention. At first, CT was created in the early 1970s as a new way to see inside the body without using surgery. In the past, CT mainly did basic cross-sectional imaging, but with time, better technology made it possible to scan more quickly, see images more clearly, and build three-dimensional models, making it more useful for diagnosis. These advancements not only enhanced the detection of complex pathologies but also paved the way for integration with emerging technologies, including artificial intelligence, which further improved diagnostic accuracy and reduced false positives in conditions such as lung cancer (Kasaudhan *et al.*, 2024). Moreover, CT's role in mediastinal disease diagnosis has been profoundly augmented by minimally invasive procedures guided by CT imaging, demonstrating its pivotal contribution to both clinical workflow and patient outcomes (Dollin *et al.*, 2024). As a result, CT technology has greatly changed the way medical diagnostics are done.

Importance of Computed Tomography (CT) in Modern Diagnostics

Improvements in imaging have made it possible for doctors to quickly and safely get detailed pictures of the body. CT is very important in this change because it provides clear images that help doctors find and define diseases. Unlike ordinary radiography, CT gives a three-dimensional view, which is important for correct diagnosis and treatment planning, especially for congenital heart diseases. For instance, ECG-gated multidetector CT has proven invaluable in diagnosing rare adult presentations of congenital anomalies like total anomalous pulmonary vein drainage, offering precise anatomical detail that is essential for appropriate clinical management (Adamczyk *et al.*, 2018). Because of technology, CT images are now better, and patients get less radiation, which has made CT useful for a broader range of people. Being able to quickly obtain detailed diagnostic information is why CT is so important in medicine today.

Overview of Computed Tomography (CT) Imaging Process

CT imaging is precise because it changes raw data into detailed cross-sectional images, which helps doctors make accurate decisions. At first, X-rays rotate around the patient to take pictures from several angles. After that, these projections are reconstructed using advanced algorithms, for example, filtered back projection or iterative reconstruction, to produce two-dimensional slices of the inside of the body.

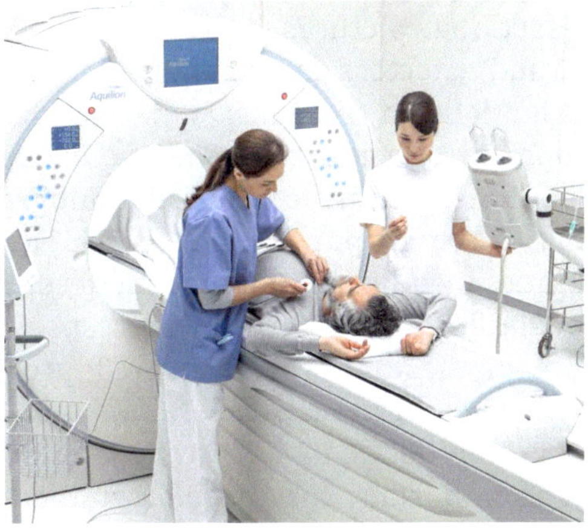

Figure 7.2. The precision of computed tomography (CT) imaging relies on a complex process that transforms raw data into detailed cross-sectional images, enabling accurate diagnosis and treatment planning.

Source: https://catalinaimaging.com/wp-content/uploads/2023/04/aquilion-prime-sp-enable-confident-diagnosis-1024x899.jpeg.

These slices can be further processed through advanced segmentation techniques like U-Net or nnU-Net, which enhance the delineation of structures such as tumors or lesions, thereby improving diagnostic accuracy and clinical decision-making (Palazzo *et al.*, 2024). The integration of these methods optimizes visualization, especially in challenging cases such as bone infections like osteomyelitis, where CT imaging provides critical information on infection extent and bone involvement (Gulyamov, 2024). This imaging process underscores CT's indispensable role in modern diagnostics by combining detailed anatomical visualization with advanced data processing (Figure 7.2).

Comparison with Other Imaging Modalities

There are now many types of medical imaging, and each one is useful for different situations due to its unique strengths and limitations. Compared to magnetic resonance imaging (MRI), CT offers faster acquisition times, making it preferable in emergency settings where rapid assessment is crucial. Because ultrasound relies on the skill of the operator and does not penetrate well, CT is better at looking at deep structures. Because of its high spatial resolution, CT can clearly show small details in bones and bleeding, which other methods may not be able to do as well. Positron emission tomography combined with CT (PET/CT), particularly with novel tracers like 18F-fluciclovine, offers functional imaging capabilities that inform treatment planning, as demonstrated in prostate cancer recurrence management, highlighting PET/CT's role in complementing anatomical detail provided by CT alone (Andriole *et al.*, 2018). However, echocardiography remains advantageous for cardiac imaging due to its portability and absence of radiation; yet, the risk of infection transmission in certain scenarios underscores the situational preference for CT or alternative modalities (Kirkpatrick *et al.*, 2020). All things considered, CT is different because it can provide fast results, clear images, and a wide range of diagnostic uses.

Current Trends in Computed Tomography (CT) Diagnostics

Recent advancements in computed tomography have significantly expanded its diagnostic capabilities, particularly through the development of photon-counting detector CT (PCD-CT), which offers enhanced image resolution and improved tissue differentiation. This cutting-edge technology has shown substantial promise in cardiac imaging, particularly for assessing coronary artery disease and atherosclerotic plaques, reflecting a rapidly increasing research focus from leading centers worldwide (Arachchige *et al.*, 2025). Concurrently, the integration of CT into infectious disease diagnostics marks another crucial trend; notably, the 2023 European Society of Cardiology guidelines endorse cardiac CT as a primary tool alongside echocardiography for identifying valvular and paravalvular lesions in infective endocarditis, underscoring its growing clinical importance (Petkovic *et al.*, 2024). These trends underscore a broader move toward multi-modal imaging strategies and precision diagnostics, where CT's role is continually refined and expanded through technological innovation and evidence-based validation, promising enhanced diagnostic accuracy and patient outcomes across diverse medical disciplines (Figure 7.3).

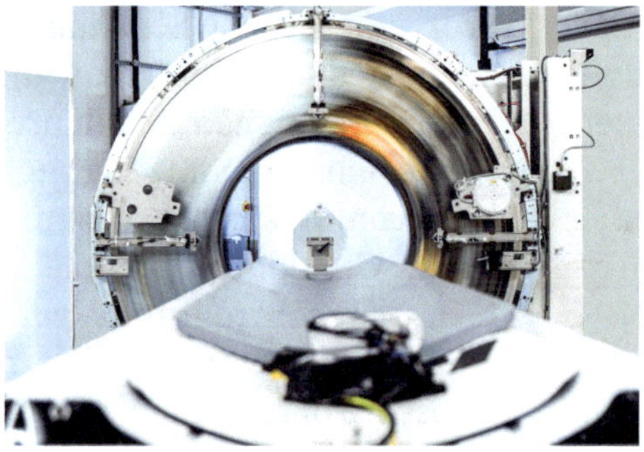

Figure 7.3. Photon-counting detector CT (PCD-CT).

Source: https://www.itnonline.com/sites/default/files/field/image/Siemens_Naeotom_Alpha_photon_counting_CT_2021.jpeg.

7.1. Principles of Computed Tomography (CT)

Learning Outcome

1. Understand basic physics of CT imaging;
2. Discuss the role of X-rays in CT scans;
3. Identify image reconstruction techniques;
4. Explain types of CT scanners;
5. Focus on contrast agents used in CT;
6. Know radiation dose considerations;
7. Focus on image quality factors;
8. Describe safety protocols in CT imaging;
9. Explain future developments in CT technology.

Advancements in imaging technologies have significantly enhanced diagnostic precision, particularly through innovations in computed tomography (CT). The basic idea of CT is to take cross-sectional pictures by rotating an X-ray source and detectors around the patient, which allows for detailed views inside the body. Recent developments such as dual-energy CT (DECT) and photon-counting computed tomography (PCCT) have expanded CT's diagnostic capabilities by utilizing different energy spectra and quantifying photon energies, respectively. Because of these improvements, CT provides clear tissue separation, uses less radiation, and offers better detail in both time and space, which is important for vascular studies and other medical uses. For example, using DECT to tell apart calcium and iodine makes it easier to diagnose mechanical jaundice, which depends on finding biliary obstructions. Combining these technological advances with comprehensive diagnostic procedures has improved outcomes and treatment planning in complex cases (Magomedov *et al.*, 2025; Stański *et al.*, 2024).

7.1.1. Basic Physics of Computed Tomography (CT) Imaging

Appreciating how CT imaging works is important

to see its value in diagnosis. CT imaging uses the fact that X-ray beams are absorbed differently by different tissues, which results in images that show the body's cross-sections. An X-ray source moves around the patient, and detectors measure the rays that pass through the body, which are then processed by algorithms to create clear images. As a result, it is possible to clearly see bones, soft tissues, and blood vessels, which is not possible with traditional two-dimensional X-rays. Moreover, advancements such as cone beam computed tomography (CBCT) have expanded applications, particularly in maxillofacial diagnostics, by providing three-dimensional detail crucial for accurate assessment and treatment planning (Alshomrani, 2024). Similarly, CT angiography utilizes these physical principles to identify coronary artery disease and vulnerable plaques, demonstrating how basic physics directly informs sophisticated clinical applications (Dimitriadis *et al.*, 2024) (Figure 7.4).

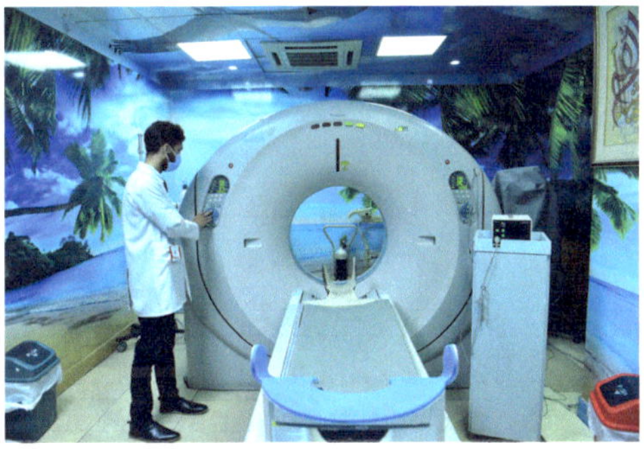

Figure 7.4. Understanding the fundamental physics behind computed tomography (CT) imaging is essential to appreciate its diagnostic capabilities.

Source: https://alnoordiagnostic.com/wp-content/uploads/2021/03/Service_Cityscan.jpg.

7.1.2. Role of X-rays in Computed Tomography (CT) Scans

X-rays, which are the main source of ionizing radiation in CT, have played a big role in its evolution. In CT scans, a narrow beam of X-rays passes through the patient while rotating and taking several images, which are then reassembled to show the inside of the body in 3D. It makes it possible to see tissues, organs, and pathological changes in great detail, which is not possible with standard X-ray imaging. Even though X-rays are helpful for diagnosis, the risk of exposure to radiation is still a worry, mainly for those who need many X-rays. Recent advancements integrating artificial intelligence have shown promise in minimizing radiation doses while maintaining image quality by optimizing X-ray beam parameters and post-processing techniques (David-Olawade *et al.*, 2025). Furthermore, the generation of synthetic X-ray data assists in improving imaging protocols without additional patient exposure, especially in specialized areas like dental imaging, enhancing diagnostic capabilities while maintaining safety (Sunilkumar *et al.*, 2024).

7.1.3. Image Reconstruction Techniques

New image reconstruction methods have made CT much more effective for diagnosis. They help to turn raw information from projections into detailed cross-sectional pictures needed for correct medical interpretation. Classical algorithms such as filtered backprojection (FBP) offer computational efficiency but can be limited by noise and artifacts. More sophisticated iterative methods, including maximum likelihood expectation maximization (MLEM), provide improved image quality by reducing noise and allowing corrections for physical factors, as demonstrated in specialized applications like polychromatic X-ray fluorescence CT imaging (Chen *et al.*, 2017). They are needed when you need to see the details of complicated anatomy or minor signs of disease. Furthermore, modern CT scanners often integrate ECG-gated techniques to optimize image reconstruction for dynamic regions, such as the heart, enabling precise visualization of congenital anomalies and vascular anatomy (Adamczyk *et al.*, 2018). These evolving reconstruction strategies continue to expand the clinical utility of CT by improving image accuracy while accommodating the unique challenges posed by diverse diagnostic requirements (Figure 7.5).

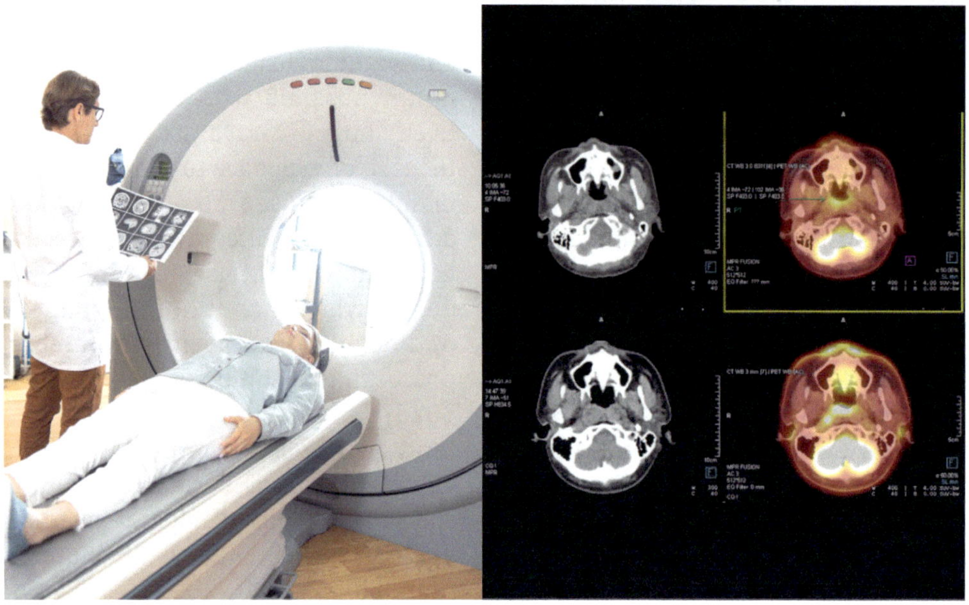

Figure 7.5. Advancements in image reconstruction techniques have significantly enhanced the diagnostic capabilities of computed tomography (CT).

Source: https://kiranpetct.com/wp-content/uploads/2024/04/How-CT-Scans-Work.png.

7.1.4. Types of Computed Tomography (CT) Scanners (e.g., Spiral, Multi-slice)

New imaging technology has made computed tomography much more useful in medicine, which has resulted in the creation of different types of CT scanners for different clinical uses. Among these, spiral (or helical) CT scanners represent a major innovation by acquiring continuous volumetric data during a single breath-hold, thus reducing motion artifacts and improving image quality. Multi-slice CT scanners make it possible to take multiple slices at once, making scans faster and images clearer, which helps doctors make better decisions about treatment. These scanners also enable more complex image reconstruction methods, which, when combined with emerging machine learning techniques, have the potential to further enhance diagnostic performance through intelligent data processing and analysis (Wang, 2016). Since its inception in the 1970s, CT technology has continually evolved, with improvements in scanner types playing a crucial role in expanding its diagnostic utility (Power *et al.*, 2016).

7.1.5. Contrast Agents used in Computed Tomography (CT)

Progress in computed tomography has been greatly helped by the creation of contrast agents that make images easier to read and diagnose. Iodine-based compounds have been the main choice for contrast materials because they are very effective at blocking X-rays. Still, new technologies make use of nanoparticles from gold, platinum, and lanthanides, which are denser and absorb more X-rays than the usual agents. They boost contrast resolution and are also colloidally stable and biocompatible, which is important for both patient safety and their removal from the body. Besides, photon-counting detectors allow the precise identification of various contrast agents at the same time by using their unique K-edge absorption. This innovation allows for accurate quantification and differentiation of contrast materials in complex diagnostic scenarios, thereby expanding the diagnostic potential of CT imaging in both clinical and preclinical settings (Ahmad *et al.*, 2023; Sotenskii *et al.*, 2024) (Figure 7.6).

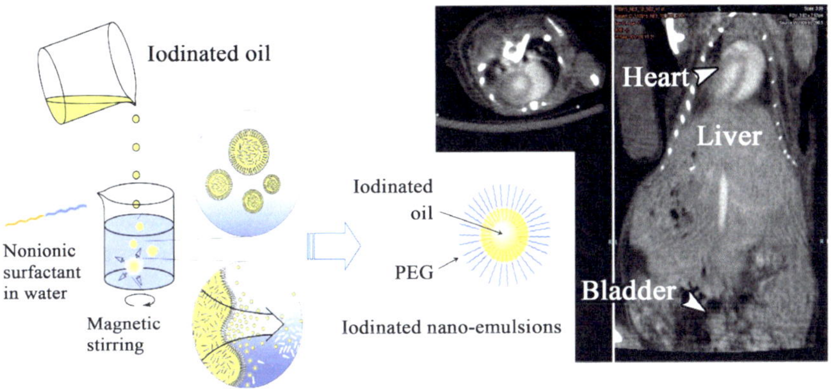

Figure 7.6. Traditionally, iodine-based compounds have dominated as contrast materials due to their effective X-ray attenuation.

Source: https://pub.mdpi-res.com/molecules/molecules-26-07063/article_deploy/html/images/molecules-26-07063-g008.png?1652257676.

7.1.6. Radiation Dose Considerations

It is very important in CT to protect patients and still get accurate results, because exposure to ionizing radiation in CT can be dangerous. Technological and imaging improvements are aimed at providing clear images and, at the same time, reducing the radiation patients receive. Recent developments in artificial intelligence (AI) have significantly contributed to this effort by enabling low-dose imaging techniques that reduce radiation without compromising image clarity, through sophisticated noise reduction and artifact elimination methods (Adeleke *et al.*, 2025). Moreover, standardized guidelines for patient preparation and imaging protocols further optimize radiation use by tailoring examinations to clinical needs and patient characteristics, thereby preventing unnecessary exposure (Avni *et al.*, 2016). Since CT is used more often in people who must have several scans, it is important to use these strategies to keep their long-term risks low, so radiation dose is a key factor in responsible radiology.

7.1.7. Image Quality Factors

Getting the best image quality in CT is necessary to improve how accurately diseases can be seen and assessed. The quality and usefulness of CT scans depend a lot on spatial resolution, contrast resolution, noise levels, and the way the scan is performed. For example, in the evaluation of bone strength and mineral density for osteoporosis diagnosis, high-resolution images enable precise biomechanical analysis through finite element methods, supporting accurate fracture risk assessment without additional testing (Bouxsein *et al.*, 2020). Also, if the images are not clear, it may be difficult to notice minor changes in the bones, as seen in studies about mild vertebral deformities that could show early osteoporotic fractures. Enhanced bone geometry and structural visualization through quantitative CT techniques further illustrate the critical role of image quality in distinguishing between varying degrees of skeletal deterioration (Boutroy *et al.*, 2010). Therefore, controlling image acquisition and processing variables directly affects CT's effectiveness in diagnostics, particularly in complex assessments requiring detailed anatomical and functional information (Figure 7.7).

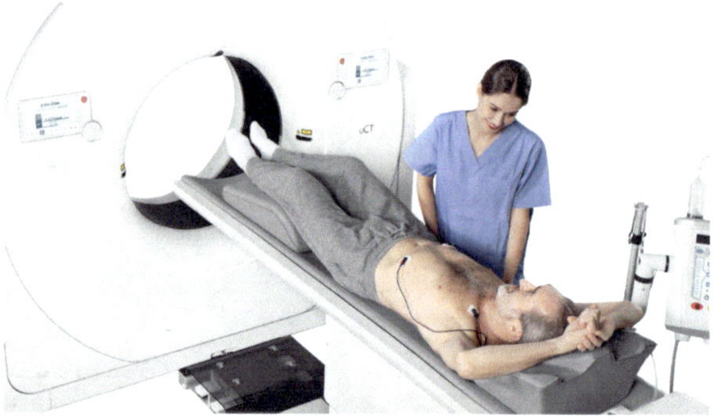

Figure 7.7. Achieving optimal image quality in computed tomography (CT) is essential to enhance diagnostic accuracy and ensure reliable clinical assessments.

Source: https://amrichealth.com/wp-content/uploads/2024/01/Untitled-design-18.png.

7.1.8. Safety Protocols in Computed Tomography (CT) Imaging

Better medical imaging has improved the accuracy of disease detection, but it also means that safety is very important for patients. The major safety issue in CT is keeping patients away from too much ionizing radiation, which can cause radiation-related health issues. To overcome this, safety protocols advise using the best scanning settings, using dose modulation, and only scanning the essential parts of the body. Recent developments have demonstrated the role of artificial intelligence in enhancing these protocols by enabling low-dose imaging with maintained or improved image quality, thus balancing diagnostic efficacy with patient safety (Adeleke *et al.*, 2025). Additionally, complementary techniques like microwave tomography offer alternative approaches for specific scenarios, such as monitoring thermal ablation treatments, potentially reducing reliance on repeated CT scans and further mitigating radiation exposure (Cavagnaro *et al.*, 2018). It is very important to use these safety strategies to make sure CT is used safely in diagnostics.

7.1.9. Future Developments in Computed Tomography (CT) Technology

The field of medical imaging is being shaped by progress in computed tomography, which offers more accurate and tailored ways to diagnose patients. Key innovations such as PCCT enhance image quality by increasing spatial and temporal resolution, enabling detailed assessments of cardiovascular structures and facilitating early disease detection through advanced texture and radiomics analysis (Ayx *et al.*, 2025). They are important for improving patient outcomes, as they enable effective risk management and tracking of treatment progress. In musculoskeletal imaging, DECT has expanded its utility beyond gout diagnosis, incorporating low-dose protocols combined with sophisticated reconstruction algorithms to maintain image quality while reducing radiation exposure (Ulas *et al.*, 2024). Also, advanced four-dimensional CT methods let doctors examine joint instabilities and ligament injuries in motion, giving them more detailed information about different conditions. Together, these technological advancements herald a more refined diagnostic era, integrating functional and structural data to enhance clinical decision-making and personalized treatment planning (Ayx *et al.*, 2025; Ulas *et al.*, 2024) (Figure 7.8).

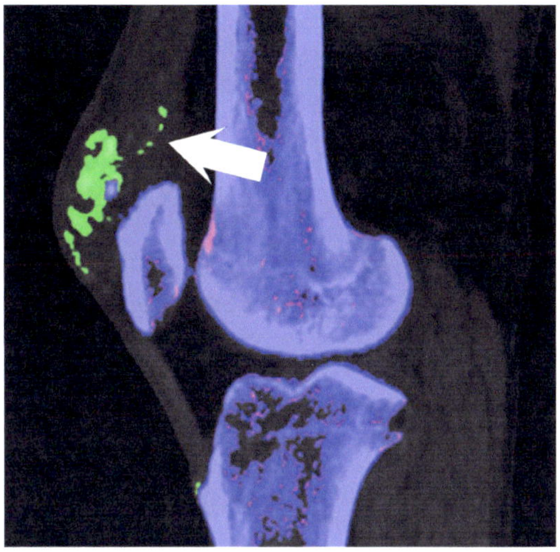

Figure 7.8. In musculoskeletal imaging, dual-energy CT (DECT) has expanded its utility beyond gout diagnosis, incorporating low-dose protocols combined with sophisticated reconstruction algorithms to maintain image quality while reducing radiation exposure.

Source: https://media.springernature.com/lw685/springer-static/image/art%3A10.1007%2Fs00256-024-04856-4/MediaObjects/256_2024_4856_Fig4_HTML.jpg.

Test Your Knowledge

1. What is the reason for using contrast agents in CT imaging?
2. Which contrast agents are most often used in CT scans?

7.2. Applications of Computed Tomography (CT) in Medical Diagnostics

Learning Outcome

1. Understand CT in oncology for tumor detection;
2. Know the use of CT in trauma assessment;
3. Explain the role of CT in cardiovascular imaging;
4. Discuss the role of CT in pulmonary diagnostics;
5. Perform CT in gastrointestinal evaluations;
6. Describe neurological applications of CT;
7. Know CT-guided biopsies and interventions;
8. Discuss pediatric considerations in CT diagnostics;
9. List the limitations of CT in certain conditions.

New imaging methods have greatly improved the accuracy and efficiency of medical diagnostics, and CT has been very important in this process. CT scans give detailed images of cross-sections, helping doctors diagnose injuries, cancer, vascular problems, and infections. The integration of digital radiography has further improved image quality while reducing exposure to radiation compared to traditional film-based methods, thereby increasing patient safety and diagnostic reliability (Rayyani *et al.*, 2024). Moreover, the development of automatic preprocessing and segmentation pipelines, such as those employed in AutoCT, has facilitated more precise localization and quantitative analysis of pathological features within the images (Bai *et al.*, 2023). They make it easier for doctors to work and also help artificial intelligence improve the accuracy of diagnoses. Therefore, CT imaging is still necessary because it brings together clinical knowledge and the latest technology to help patients.

7.2.1. Computed Tomography (CT) in Oncology for Tumor Detection

New developments in medical imaging have helped doctors find cancer sooner and with greater accuracy, which results in better outcomes for patients. CT is very important in oncology because it allows doctors to see the size, position, and relationship of tumors to other tissues.

Because CT scans produce very clear cross-sectional images, clinicians are able to see tumors that are not easy to detect with other techniques, which helps with accurate staging and monitoring of cancer. When combined with functional imaging techniques, such as PET and CT, it further refines tumor characterization, improving diagnostic confidence and treatment planning (Mishra, 2024). Nevertheless, radiation is a problem, so new technologies are needed to help protect patients and make the most of medical scans. Overall, CT remains indispensable in oncological diagnostics, underpinning the effective detection and management of various cancers (Figure 7.9).

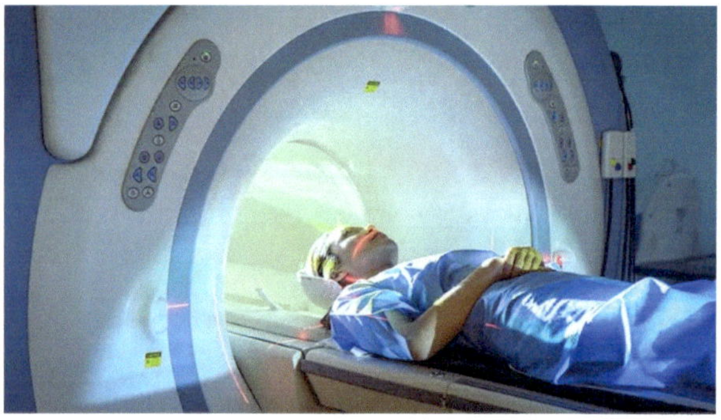

Figure 7.9. Computer tomography (CT) remains indispensable in oncological diagnostics, underpinning the effective detection and management of various cancers.

Source: https://images.everydayhealth.com/images/cancer/cancer-diagnosis-and-tests-722x406.jpg?sfvrsn=b53cc840_3.

7.2.2. Use of Computed Tomography (CT) in Trauma Assessment

Properly assessing trauma helps save lives and prevent serious health problems, and new imaging technologies have greatly changed the way things are done in the clinic. Because of its ability to produce clear images fast, CT is now widely used to check for injuries at different sites at the same time. Using multi-slice CT scanners enables doctors to quickly scan the whole body in the initial trauma survey, which helps detect serious conditions that could be missed with regular X-rays and limited imaging. The REACT-2 trial underscores the clinical importance of immediate total-body CT, highlighting its potential to improve diagnostic accuracy and patient outcomes by streamlining trauma work-up without compromising resuscitation efforts (Prokop *et al.*, 2012). Additionally, CT plays a pivotal role in monitoring complex musculoskeletal sequelae post-injury, such as post-traumatic myositis ossificans, where its ability to identify lesion maturity guides treatment decisions (Cesarec *et al.*, 2020). This means that adding CT to trauma care protocols is a major change towards faster and more accurate diagnosis.

7.2.3. Computed Tomography (CT) for Cardiovascular Imaging

The use of new technology in cardiology has made it easier to diagnose properly and keep patients safe. One important advancement is PCCT, which swaps traditional energy-integrating detectors for photon-counting detectors that transform X-ray photons into electrical signals. This shift allows for superior image quality through enhanced spatial resolution, improved contrast differentiation, and reduced artifacts, while concurrently lowering radiation exposure—a critical consideration in vulnerable populations such as pediatric patients (Arachchige *et al.*, 2025). Moreover, cardiovascular computed tomography angiography (CTA) has evolved beyond simple visualization of vascular lumen changes. Applications today use 3D printing for personalized anatomy, advanced 3D images with virtual and augmented reality, and CT scans to assess heart function. These innovations, supported by the integration of artificial intelligence, expand the clinical utility of CTA from early diagnosis to prognostication and individualized treatment planning, thereby improving overall patient management in cardiovascular disease (Sun, 2024) (Figure 7.10).

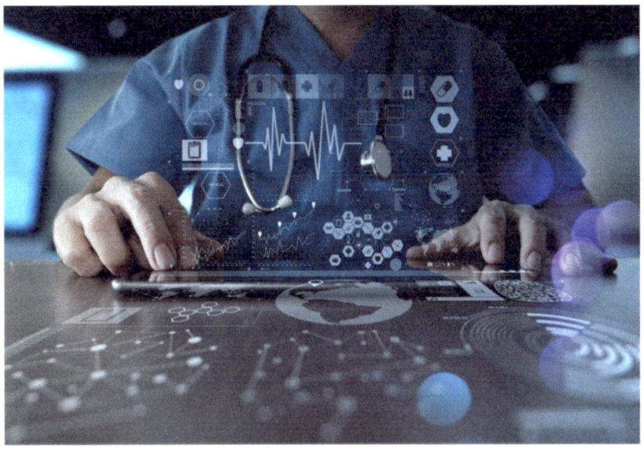

Figure 7.10. Emerging technological advancements have significantly transformed cardiovascular imaging, enhancing both diagnostic accuracy and patient safety.

Source: https://d2jx2rerrg6sh3.cloudfront.net/images/Article_Images/ImageForArticle_22572_16533781526443229.jpg.

7.2.4. Role of Computed Tomography (CT) in Pulmonary Diagnostics

New imaging methods have made it possible to detect lung problems more accurately and in greater detail, and CT scans are now a key tool for this purpose. CT is better than traditional radiography at finding interstitial lung diseases, pulmonary embolisms, and malignancies because it produces clear cross-sectional images. The integration of automated segmentation techniques, such as deep learning models applied in cardiovascular and pulmonary structures, further optimizes the diagnostic process by enabling precise delineation of anatomical features, which is essential for assessing complex thoracic pathologies (Al'Aref *et al.*, 2020). Besides, as CT technology keeps improving, scans are completed more quickly, with less radiation, and the images are still of high quality, which benefits both patients and their health. Pictures and illustrations of these new technologies prove how important CT is in modern lung medicine, especially for quick and correct diagnoses.

7.2.5. Computed Tomography (CT) in Gastrointestinal Evaluations

Advanced imaging techniques are often needed to correctly diagnose problems of the digestive system. CT is critical here since it produces detailed pictures that make it possible to find any structural issues, blockages, or problems with blood vessels. For example, in cases of dysphagia where external esophageal compression is suspected, CT angiography can reveal vascular variations such as an aberrant right subclavian artery, enabling precise diagnosis and appropriate surgical intervention (Cella *et al.*, 2020).

Furthermore, CT combined with other imaging modalities, like positron emission tomography in oncology, helps characterize tumor microenvironments and evaluate therapeutic responses, although clinical tumor targeting may vary from preclinical observations (Dehdashti *et al.*, 2017). These capabilities underscore CT's importance in gastrointestinal evaluations, allowing clinicians to not only detect but also monitor disease progression, thereby improving patient management and outcomes within diagnostic protocols (Figure 7.11).

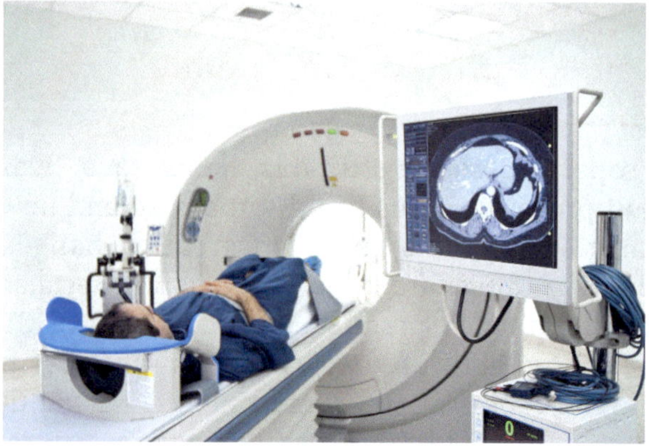

Figure 7.11. Computed tomography (CT) plays a pivotal role in this context, offering high-resolution cross-sectional images that assist in identifying structural abnormalities, obstructions, and vascular anomalies.

Source: https://www.touchstoneimaging.com/wp-content/uploads/2024/01/AdobeStock_53156310-scaled.jpeg.

7.2.6. Neurological Applications of Computed Tomography (CT)

Better imaging tools have greatly improved how CT is used for neurological diagnostics. CT helps doctors quickly and clearly see inside the head, so it is important for the first evaluation of emergencies like stroke, head injury, and bleeding in the brain. Recent developments like DECT and PCCT have further refined the modality's capabilities by improving tissue differentiation and reducing radiation exposure, which are particularly beneficial in vascular and soft tissue evaluation within the brain (Stański *et al.*, 2024). Besides, using CT guidance for interventions has expanded the role of CT in therapy, enabling precise biopsies and targeted procedures in difficult areas of the brain, thus reducing the risk of invasive actions. While certain high-risk procedures, like splenic biopsies demonstrating CT-guided tract sealing techniques, illustrate the potential for broader neurological applications, the focus remains on maximizing safety and diagnostic yield (Segger *et al.*, 2024). These innovations underscore CT's indispensability in modern neurological practice.

7.2.7. Computed Tomography (CT)-Guided Biopsies and Interventions

New imaging methods have greatly improved the precision and safety of diagnosing with tissue sampling and less invasive treatments. Using CT guidance for biopsies helps doctors see the target clearly and accurately, so they do not have to insert the needle more than once, which also helps reduce pain for the patient. The integration of robotic assistance systems, such as MAXIO, has further refined these procedures by facilitating improved planning and needle navigation, leading to fewer punctures, lower radiation exposure, and enhanced diagnostic yield compared to conventional manual techniques (Kumar *et al.*, 2025). Moreover, CT imaging plays a critical role in identifying subtle pathological features, as seen in complex infections like abdominal actinomycosis, where CT detection of abscesses, fistulae, or foreign bodies informs both biopsy guidance and treatment decisions (Krailertmongkol *et al.*, 2025). These developments underscore CT's pivotal role in improving interventional outcomes and patient management through detailed visualization and precise intervention (Figure 7.12).

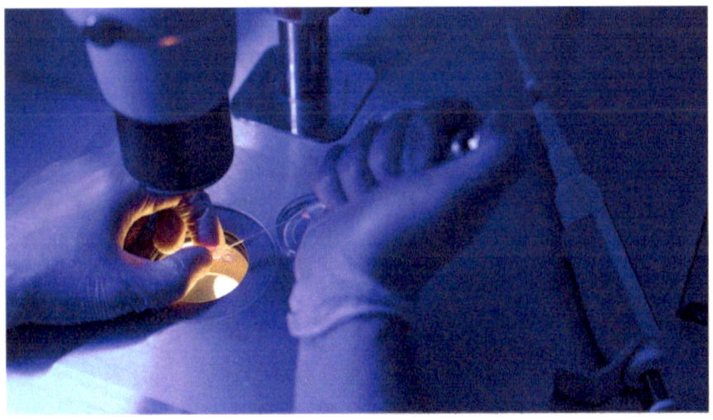

Figure 7.12. Computer tomography (CT)-guided biopsies.

Source: https://neumarksurgery.com/wp-content/uploads/lung-biopsy.jpeg.

7.2.8. Pediatric Considerations in Computed Tomography (CT) Diagnostics

It is important in medical imaging for pediatrics to consider the special needs of children to ensure the correct diagnosis and safety of the patients. Since children are more sensitive to radiation, it is essential to try to use the lowest amount possible during CT scans. Because children are so sensitive, their scanning parameters, such as tube current and voltage, need to be adjusted according to their size and age. Advances in artificial intelligence have played a pivotal role in developing low-dose imaging techniques without compromising image quality, thereby significantly reducing potential radiation risks for young patients (Adeleke *et al.*, 2025). Also, using specialized shielding and sedation methods improves both the patient's comfort and the quality of the images taken during procedures. It is very important to consider these points for children to avoid long-term risks from radiation and still get good test results. Using these strategies highlights how CT diagnostics are changing, by balancing new technology with patient care.

7.2.9. Limitations of Computed Tomography (CT) in Certain Conditions

Although CT is very useful in medicine, it has some clear limitations for certain health problems. For example, CT's sensitivity in detecting subtle brain abnormalities such as cerebral microbleeds (CMB) is inferior compared to magnetic resonance imaging (MRI), particularly susceptibility-weighted imaging, which can better identify early or small vascular lesions. This reduced sensitivity poses challenges in comprehensive cerebrovascular assessments, especially when intracranial calcifications and CMB coexist, complicating diagnostic accuracy and prognostication (Chang *et al.*, 2019). Furthermore, while CT scans opportunistically evaluate bone strength and mineral density, their application in osteoporosis diagnosis requires additional specialized analyses, like biomechanical computed tomography (BCT), to supplement traditional bone density scans. These advanced techniques highlight CT's indirect role rather than being a standalone solution for skeletal integrity assessments (Bouxsein *et al.*, 2020). So, although CT is very useful, it is sometimes necessary to use other imaging methods in certain conditions to ensure proper patient management.

Test Your Knowledge

1. What conditions are commonly diagnosed using CT imaging in the abdomen?
2. How is CT used in the evaluation of trauma patients?

7.3. Advantages and Disadvantages of Computed Tomography (CT) Imaging

Learning Outcome

1. Know high-resolution imaging capabilities;
2. Talk about how CT scans are faster than many other imaging methods;
3. Define the non-invasive nature of CT diagnostics;
4. Explain comprehensive imaging of complex structures;
5. Identify risks associated with radiation exposure;
6. Focus on the cost considerations of CT scans;
7. Describe the accessibility of CT technology;
8 Know potential for misdiagnosis or over-reliance;
9. Understand ethical considerations in CT usage.

Improvements in imaging have led to better diagnosis, and CT is now important because it creates clear cross-sectional images and three-dimensional views. Because CT imaging has very high spatial resolution, it makes it easy to see the details of bone structures and the mouth, which helps in making important decisions in dental implantology and oral surgery. Additionally, CT scans reduce magnification errors common in traditional radiographs and facilitate multiplanar analysis, providing comprehensive diagnostic information (Jurić *et al.*, 2023).

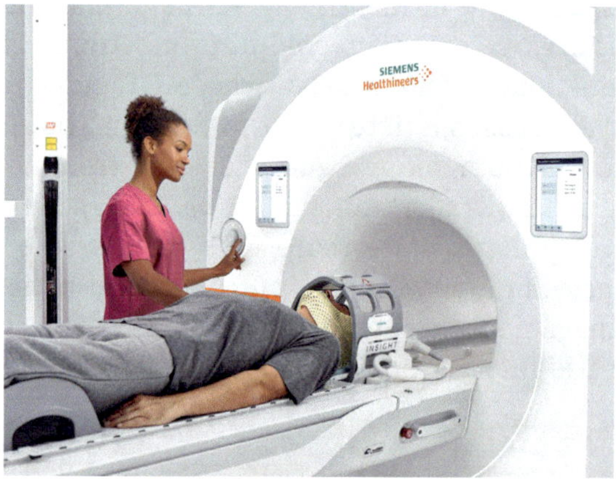

Figure 7.13. CT scans may exhibit limited soft tissue contrast and susceptibility to motion artifacts, potentially compromising image quality.

Source: https://marketing.webassets.siemens-healthineers.com/1800000004245995/fd2bb67c6eb2/v/17365b3e078f/siemens_mri-in-therapy_magnetom-rt-pro-edition-for-magnetom-vida_container-1_1800000004245995.jpg.

7.3.1. High-resolution Imaging Capabilities

The development of computed tomography has greatly improved how precisely doctors can make diagnoses. With PCD-CT, there is now the ability to see anatomical structures in great detail, surpassing the capabilities of traditional CT. This is particularly evident in applications like bone microarchitecture analysis, where PCD-CT offers simultaneous qualitative and quantitative assessment of mineral composition, enabling more sensitive and accurate diagnoses of conditions such as osteoporosis (Bhattarai *et al.*, 2023). Besides imaging bones, higher spatial resolution now helps with cardiac and pulmonary exams, which rely on seeing fine details to catch early signs of disease. The integration of hardware advancements, including optimized tube current modulation and sophisticated image reconstruction algorithms, further refines image clarity while mitigating radiation exposure (Lell *et al.*, 2023). With these new technologies, CT can take very detailed images that help doctors make accurate decisions.

7.3.2. Speed of Computed Tomography (CT) Scans Compared to Other Modalities

Imaging technology has been improved to cut down on scan times, which helps both doctors and patients. CT scans are quicker than MRI and conventional radiography, which makes it possible to get detailed cross-sectional images in less time. Having this speed is very useful in emergency situations, since a quick diagnosis can save lives. While modalities like SPECT/CT offer valuable functional and anatomical information, their combined imaging sequences generally require longer scan times; however, adjustments in CT protocols within SPECT/CT have facilitated reduced radiation doses and more efficient imaging without compromising diagnostic quality (Eseonu *et al.*, 2024). CT is much faster than MRI, since it can scan the whole body in seconds to minutes, while MRI takes a much longer time. These advantages highlight CT's pivotal role in diagnostics, balancing speed and image resolution while maintaining patient safety, a factor emphasized in developing diagnostic reference levels for radiological practice (Sina *et al.*, 2024) (Figure 7.14).

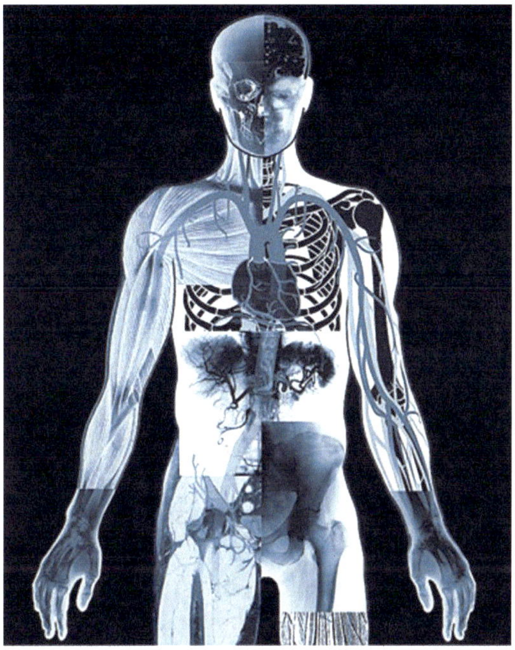

Figure 7.14. While modalities like SPECT/CT offer valuable functional and anatomical information, their combined imaging sequences generally require longer scan times.

Source: https://spectrum.ieee.org/media-library/image.jpg?id=25572177&width=980.

7.3.3. Non-invasive Nature of Computed Tomography (CT) Diagnostics

As medical imaging has improved, more importance is given to making patients comfortable while still ensuring accurate results, which makes non-invasive methods very important. This is demonstrated by CT, which supplies clear cross-sectional images without requiring surgery. Unlike invasive approaches that may cause infection or take a long time to recover from, CT allows doctors to quickly and easily view internal structures, which helps with finding and staging diseases early. For instance, in bladder cancer management, CT plays a crucial role in diagnosis and staging, complementing cystoscopy by identifying malignant lesions without physical intrusion into the body (Halpern *et al.*, 2018). Similarly, in diagnosing bone lesions such as aneurysmal bone cysts, CT enhances reliability by revealing internal characteristics like fluid levels and septa, which might be missed through traditional imaging techniques (Bekiesińska-Figatowska *et al.*, 2009). Having these features makes CT a valuable non-invasive way to diagnose, since it provides good detail about the body and keeps patients comfortable and safe.

7.3.4. Comprehensive Imaging of Complex Structures

Because of new imaging technology, doctors can now view and analyze small anatomical structures with great detail and accuracy. CT is different in this way because it gives clear images of all layers in the body, making it possible to assess complex areas such as blood vessels and bones. Modern methods such as multidetector CT and advanced post-processing, which use multiplanar reconstruction, maximum intensity projection, and volume rendering, make it easier to view delicate illnesses and their positions among dense or overlapping tissues. For example, in the evaluation of pulmonary thromboembolism, these imaging modalities facilitate the accurate identification of intraluminal filling defects and vascular occlusions, thereby improving diagnostic confidence and treatment planning (Ravula *et al.*, 2024). Similarly, CT-guided interventions targeting musculoskeletal pain capitalize on precise anatomical delineation to deliver minimally invasive treatments, underscoring the modality's role in both diagnosis and management (Batra *et al.*, 2025). Such comprehensive imaging capabilities contribute significantly to improved patient outcomes by supporting accurate diagnosis and tailored therapeutic approaches (Figure 7.15).

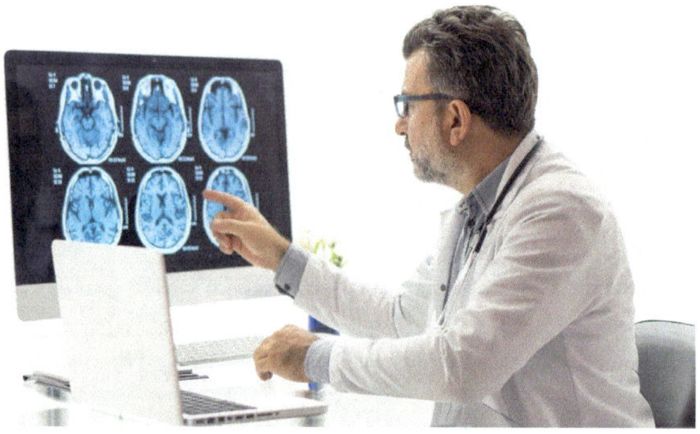

Figure 7.15. Techniques like multidetector CT and sophisticated post-processing methods—including multiplanar reconstruction, maximum intensity projection, and volume rendering.

Source: https://www.postdicom.com/images/blog-posts/Advanced%20Image%20Processing%20-%20Presented%20by%20PostDICOM.jpg.

7.3.5. Risks Associated with Radiation Exposure

Improvements in medical imaging have greatly improved the ability to diagnose, but the risk of ionizing radiation is still a big issue. Being exposed to radiation, mainly from CT scans, can increase the risk of cancer over a lifetime, mainly for people who have to undergo imaging often. Modern research shows that third-generation dual-source CT systems can reduce radiation exposure by up to 50%, keeping image quality high and bringing down effective dose to about 2.0 mSv, which helps lower the risk of cancer. This is different from the higher doses given by earlier CT machines, which added to people's radiation exposure. In addition, using artificial intelligence in imaging has the potential to reduce radiation exposure by reducing noise and optimizing imaging settings, so patients are protected and the diagnosis is still correct. Nevertheless, despite technological improvements, careful consideration of radiation risks remains essential in clinical decision-making to balance diagnostic benefits against potential long-term harm (Adeleke *et al.*, 2025; Brix *et al.*, 2020).

7.3.6. Cost Considerations of Computed Tomography (CT) Scans

The use of advanced imaging technologies in clinical diagnostics tends to have major financial effects that should be carefully considered. Because CT scans require expensive equipment, upkeep, and trained staff, they are not always affordable. CT scans are accurate for diagnosing diseases, which helps doctors make decisions and reduces costs from wrong or delayed treatment, but they are still very expensive to set up and use.

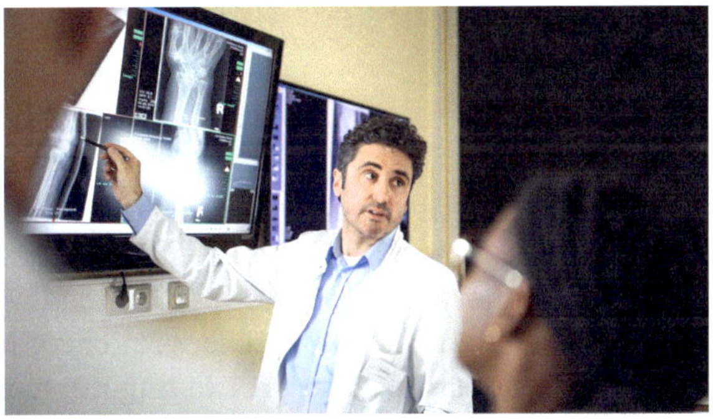

Figure 7.16. Computed tomography (CT) scans, widely valued for their detailed cross-sectional imaging capabilities, pose particular cost considerations due to the need for specialized equipment, maintenance, and skilled personnel.

Source: https://www.postdicom.com/images/blog-posts/Advanced%20Image%20Processing(2)%20-%20Presented%20by%20PostDICOM.jpg.

Also, using CT imaging too much or for the wrong reasons can cause healthcare costs to rise unnecessarily. To achieve both cost-efficiency and good clinical results, one must follow guidelines that guide use, limit unnecessary tests, and use alternative imaging when possible. When making this balance, patient outcomes, exposure to radiation, and the use of healthcare resources are all very important. Consequently, cost assessments of CT scans must align with broader healthcare policies and ethical frameworks to ensure sustainable and equitable diagnostic practices (Authors Task Force Members *et al.*, 2014; Mathijssen, 2020) (Figure 7.16).

7.3.7. Accessibility of Computed Tomography (CT) Technology

New imaging technologies have improved how modern diagnoses are made, but not all healthcare facilities can use them. Although CT is known for its clear images and key part in finding cardiac masses, it is not always available equally to everyone. The lack of good infrastructure, high costs, and not enough technical skills can keep many areas from using AI. However, ongoing developments, including novel reconstruction methods exemplified by Anisotropic X-ray Dark-Field Tomography (AXDT), promise enhanced imaging capabilities with improved efficiency and noise performance, potentially lowering barriers to access through more practical and stable implementations (Frank *et al.*, 2025). The integration of CT as a routine clinical tool is vital, as its detailed diagnostic output directly impacts patient management and outcomes (Joudar *et al.*, 2025). Ensuring everyone has equal access to CT is important for its benefits to be accessible everywhere in the world.

7.3.8. Potential for Misdiagnosis or Over-reliance

Even though CT imaging is very advanced, it is still possible for doctors to make the wrong diagnosis. Often, diagnostic errors happen because it is difficult to interpret results and because CT findings are trusted too much without checking other clinical signs. For instance, an overdependence on CT scans can lead to misclassifications, as seen in complex conditions like clavicle fractures, where radiological inaccuracies contributed to significant diagnostic discrepancies between fracture types (Bakir *et al.*, 2025). Such mistakes harm patient care and also hinder large-scale data analyses and AI from working effectively. Additionally, in regions with limited healthcare infrastructure, such as Sub-Saharan Africa, resource constraints and insufficient training exacerbate these risks, highlighting systemic vulnerabilities when CT diagnoses are taken at face value without comprehensive assessment (Banson *et al.*, 2024). Consequently, while CT is invaluable, cautious integration with clinical judgment remains essential to mitigate misdiagnosis and avoid detrimental over-reliance (Figure 7.17).

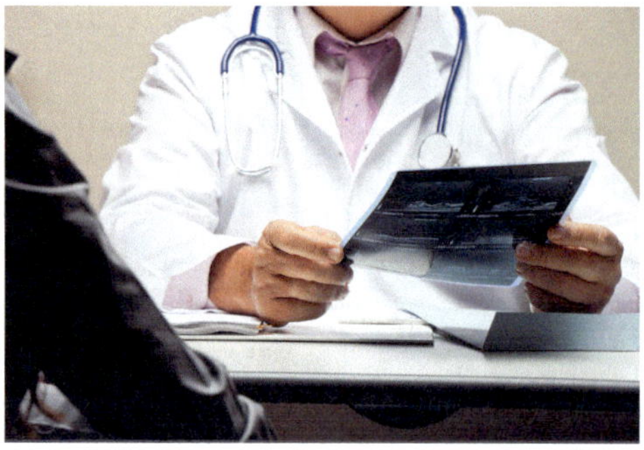

Figure 7.17. Diagnostic errors in Computer Tomography (CT) findings.

Source: https://www.fronzutolaw.com/wp-content/uploads/2019/06/diagnostic-imaging-errors.jpg.

7.3.9. Ethical Considerations in Computed Tomography (CT) Usage

The fast growth of CT technology has made diagnosis easier, but it also calls for careful ethical consideration. It is very important to weigh the benefits of treatment against the possible risks, such as radiation, for patient safety and informed consent. Healthcare professionals should make sure patients understand the reason for performing a CT scan, especially if other ways of imaging are possible. This is crucial for vulnerable populations, including the elderly or those with chronic conditions, who may face cumulative radiation risks or complications linked to preexisting devices like cardiac implantable electronic devices (Lyon *et al.*, 2022). Also, some groups may not be able to use CT diagnostics because the healthcare system is not always accessible to everyone. Ethical practice requires regularly checking if a treatment is needed, to prevent overuse that can cause extra healthcare expenses and harm. Medical professionals must navigate these issues carefully, adhering to best practices that prioritize patient welfare and autonomy (Zeppenfeld *et al.*, 2022).

Test Your Knowledge

1. What dangers come from the ionizing radiation used in CT scans?
2. How can the amount of radiation used in CT scans be lowered?
3. What are the main differences in what CT and MRI can show?

7.4. Future of Computed Tomography in Diagnostics

Learning Outcome

1. Learn innovations in CT technology;
2. Explain the integration of artificial intelligence in CT analysis;
3. Focus on advances in radiation dose reduction;
4. Discuss the development of portable CT devices;
5. Know the role of CT in personalized medicine;
6. Explain expansion of CT applications in preventive care;
7. Describe global disparities in CT access;
8 Understand research trends in CT imaging;
9. Identify future challenges and opportunities.

New imaging and data processing systems are going to make CT much more accurate and effective in diagnosing diseases. Emerging techniques, such as automated specimen handling and enhanced image capture modalities, promise to reduce the time and complexity involved in producing high-resolution, multidimensional scans, which will improve diagnostic accuracy and facilitate broader clinical applications (Adcock *et al.*, 2017). Additionally, the integration of probabilistic models and Bayesian frameworks into CT data analysis can provide deeper insights by incorporating uncertainties and prior knowledge to more accurately interpret complex biological structures, advancing personalized medicine and targeted therapeutic strategies (Appel *et al.*, 2010). All of these updates allow for better image capture, better blending of data, and more reliable interpretation, which will make CT diagnostics more comprehensive and flexible for various medical needs in the future. As a result, CT will probably move forward through the use of robotics, computational intelligence, and advanced imaging physics in combination.

7.4.1. Innovations in Computed Tomography (CT) Technology

New medical imaging technologies have greatly improved how doctors diagnose patients, and CT is being pushed further by these innovations. The integration of CT data with augmented reality (AR) and virtual reality (VR) has introduced immersive three-dimensional visualization, facilitating more precise surgical planning and patient-specific treatment strategies. This interdisciplinary approach enhances the interpretability of imaging by merging theoretical research with practical applications, thus elevating the potential for improved healthcare outcomes (Ziyad *et al.*, 2024). At the same time, medical image processing advances use neural networks and fuzzy logic, which help improve the segmentation, classification, and enhancement of CT images. These computational techniques refine diagnostic accuracy and allow for seamless integration of imaging with other patient data, supporting a more holistic understanding of pathology (Yadav *et al.*, 2024). Together, these innovations underscore the evolving nature of CT technology, highlighting its pivotal role in advancing medical diagnostics and personalized care (Figure 7.18).

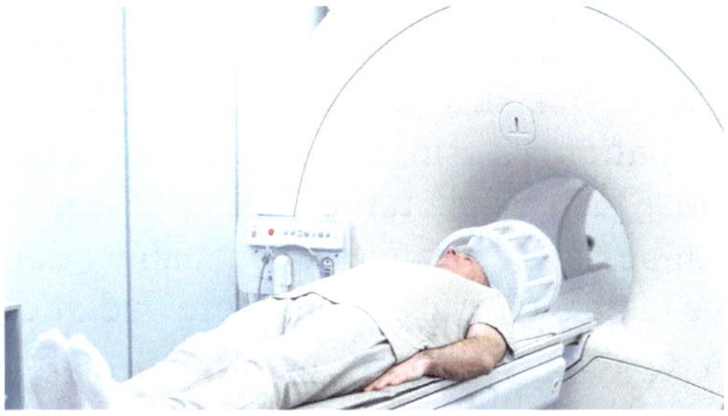

Figure 7.18. Advancements in medical imaging have significantly transformed diagnostic capabilities, with emerging technologies pushing the boundaries of Computed Tomography (CT).

Source: https://medicalbuyer.co.in/wp-content/uploads/2024/03/Rethinking-MRI-to-provide-the-reach-that-it-deserves.jpg.

7.4.2. Integration of Artificial Intelligence (AI) in Computed Tomography (CT) Analysis

Medical imaging has improved a lot due to advances in technology, mainly in making diagnoses more accurate. An important change is using AI with CT scans, which has helped doctors detect and describe abnormalities in the lungs. AI-assisted systems seem to help detect more cases and lower the number of false negatives, which is important for quick and accurate diagnosis. Still, the first use of AIs has shown that there is a temporary drop in accuracy and an increase in false positives, which means radiologists need to be well-trained and use AIs consistently to maximize their benefits. Also, by automating image analysis, AI helps reduce the effects of operator variation, much like machine learning models in echocardiography have shown expert performance and better consistency. This integration signifies a pivotal step toward augmenting radiological diagnostics and elevating patient care standards (Liu *et al.*, 2025; Maturi *et al.*, 2025).

7.4.3. Advances in Radiation Dose Reduction

Innovations in technology have greatly changed diagnostic imaging, especially in dealing with the radiation risk in CT scans. New imaging systems, such as photon-counting CT scanners, are important because they allow doctors to see detailed images with less radiation. It helps doctors diagnose more accurately and protects people from the lasting health effects of ionizing radiation, which is still a main concern in hospitals. With AI, scanning protocols can be adjusted for each patient, and images can be monitored in real time, which reduces the amount of radiation used. They go along with wider efforts to use gentle and eco-friendly methods that do not affect the image quality. In dental and maxillofacial surgery, for instance, these improved imaging capabilities support more precise preoperative evaluations and minimally invasive interventions, ultimately enhancing patient safety and treatment outcomes (Adadzi *et al.*, 2024; Husain *et al.*, 2023) (Figure 7.19).

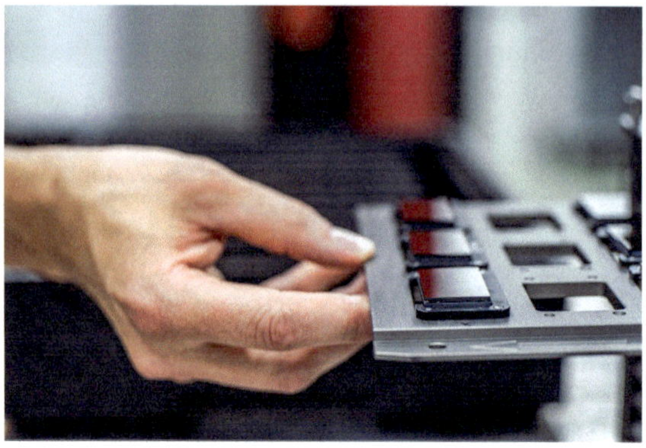

Figure 7.19. Enhanced imaging modalities, such as photon-counting computed tomography (CT) scanners, have emerged as pivotal tools that enable higher-resolution images while concurrently lowering the radiation dose patients receive.

Source: https://www.itnonline.com/sites/default/files/inline-images/Siemens_Naeotom_Alpha_photon-counting_boards_CT%20.jpeg.

7.4.4. Development of Portable Computed Tomography (CT) Devices

Because of new developments in medical imaging, it is now more important to have flexible and accessible diagnostic tools, leading to the creation of portable CT devices. Conventional CT scanners are not very portable, are expensive, and require special facilities, which makes them unavailable in many emergency or remote sites. The miniaturization of NDT technologies in other industries highlights the feasibility of compact, mobile imaging systems that maintain high performance despite size reduction (Addepalli *et al.*, 2018). In hospitals and clinics, using a portable CT device can allow doctors to take images at the bedside, which is very useful for quick diagnosis and treatment choices in urgent or non-surgical cases. Additionally, integrating real-time monitoring capabilities with portable CT scanners can enhance procedural outcomes, similar to how emerging imaging modalities monitor thermal ablation in clinical treatments (Cavagnaro *et al.*, 2018). So, portable CT is a major step forward in providing flexible and efficient diagnostics to meet the needs of modern healthcare.

7.4.5. Role of Computed Tomography (CT) in Personalized Medicine

Better imaging technology has allowed personalized medicine to be used in more ways for both diagnosis and treatment. CT, which can quickly give detailed information about the body, is very important in this new approach.

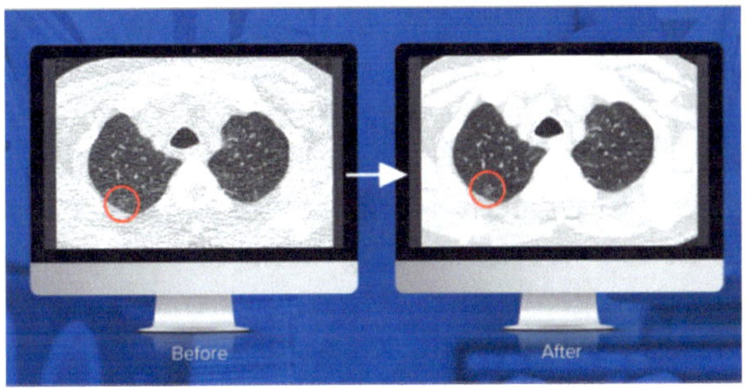

Figure 7.20. The incorporation of artificial intelligence (AI) in computed tomography (CT) imaging has further enhanced personalized medicine by enabling low-dose protocols that reduce radiation exposure without compromising image quality.

Source: https://www.itnonline.com/sites/default/files/field/image/CT_noise_PixelShine.jpg.

By integrating CT data with functional imaging modalities such as Positron Emission Tomography (PET), clinicians gain comprehensive insights into a patient's unique pathology, facilitating precise disease characterization and targeted treatment planning (Mishra, 2024). Moreover, the incorporation of AI in CT imaging has further enhanced personalized medicine by enabling low-dose protocols that reduce radiation exposure without compromising image quality, thus ensuring patient safety while maintaining diagnostic accuracy (Adeleke *et al.*, 2025). Because of these improvements, imaging protocols can now be tailored to each patient, which helps with diagnostics and minimizes risks. As a result, CT's evolving capabilities contribute substantially to the personalization of care, improving clinical outcomes through more accurate and patient-centered diagnostics (Figure 7.20).

7.4.6. Expansion of Computed Tomography (CT) Applications in Preventive Care

Better imaging technology has broadened the range of diagnostic tools in healthcare, especially in preventive measures that try to find disease before symptoms start. It used to be that CT was mainly used to find existing conditions, but now it is also used to help prevent them. Better imaging tools enable doctors to spot mild pathological changes sooner, which helps with early treatment and slows the progress of chronic diseases.

Notably, the integration of specialized CT methods, such as Cone-Beam CT in dentistry, exemplifies this shift by enabling detailed visualization of oral structures with minimized radiation exposure, thereby supporting early detection of dental and maxillofacial abnormalities (Chikorde *et al.*, 2024). Thanks to this expansion, CT is useful for confirming diseases, assessing risks, and monitoring patients, which all help improve patient outcomes by allowing for individual preventive care. As CT improves, it is predicted to be used more often for early detection and prevention, helping to provide complete healthcare.

7.4.7. Global Disparities in Computed Tomography (CT) Access

Even though CTs are recognized for their usefulness in diagnosis, they are not available to everyone, which points to big healthcare inequalities around the world. There is not enough CT equipment in many low- and middle-income countries, which leads to delays or inaccurate or incomplete imaging. Because CT is less accessible, managing patients is less effective, and health outcomes are poorer than in places where CT is used more often. Also, there are situations where the same treatment is used too much, but in places with fewer resources, it is not used enough, which highlights problems in the system and following guidelines.

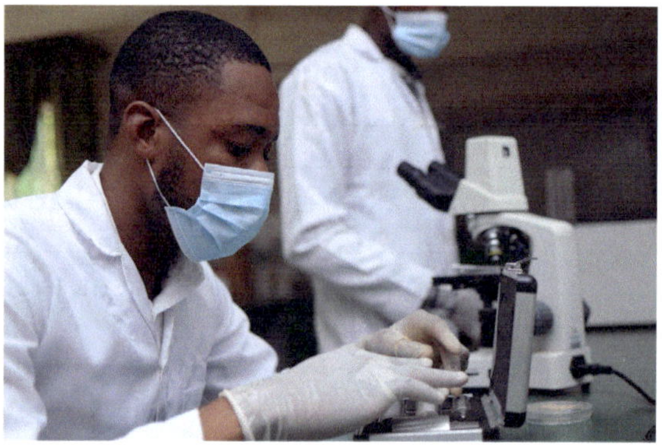

Figure 7.21. Many low- and middle-income countries lack sufficient computed tomography (CT) infrastructure, resulting in delays or a complete absence of timely and accurate diagnostic imaging.

Source: https://cancerworld.net/wp-content/uploads/2022/09/PathologyServicesAfrica.jpg.

For instance, excessive CT scans in cases of mild head injury have raised concerns about unnecessary radiation exposure and healthcare costs, emphasizing the need for judicious utilization worldwide (Saran *et al.*, 2024). Meanwhile, in oncology diagnostics, CT protocols such as computed tomography with water enema and intravenous contrast have been proven effective for tumor staging, yet such advanced applications remain out of reach for many populations (Suárez Oceguera *et al.*, 2024). Addressing these disparities necessitates coordinated efforts to improve infrastructure, training, and equitable resource distribution (Figure 7.21).

7.4.8. Research Trends in Computed Tomography (CT) Imaging

Improvements in medical imaging have helped doctors make more accurate diagnoses, and CT has become very important in medical care. CT imaging research aims to improve image quality while lowering radiation exposure, which benefits patients. Dual-energy CT and photon-counting detectors are being noticed for their ability to give more accurate details about the tissues and their functions. Furthermore, integration with other imaging modalities like PET and MRI offers complementary data that enhances diagnostic confidence, especially in cancer detection and staging (Halpern *et al.*, 2018). Work is being done to create new contrast agents and biomarkers that make it easier to identify and distinguish lesions. Also, upgrades in CT hardware, such as better focal spot technology, help to improve image quality and reduce the time needed for scanning. All of these trends in research reflect a complete effort to make CT scans more useful and to address their limitations.

7.4.9. Future Challenges and Opportunities

AI is helping to solve previous problems in CT diagnostics, for example, by reducing the amount of radiation and making image processing more efficient. The integration of AI-driven low-dose imaging techniques aims to maintain high diagnostic quality while significantly reducing patient radiation risks, presenting a critical opportunity for safer imaging practices (Adeleke *et al.*, 2025). Furthermore, AI-powered semantic segmentation methods enhance the precision of anatomical delineation in CT scans, facilitating faster and more accurate data annotation, which could revolutionize clinical workflows and research protocols (Bolocko *et al.*, 2024). Even so, such advancements can lead to extra challenges, including the need to manually verify results, ethical issues with AI, and the need for significant computing power and rules from regulators. Handling these matters is important for the wider use of AI in healthcare. AI and CT imaging coming together can greatly improve how diagnoses are made, protect patients, and simplify radiology practices, but it also requires handling both technical and ethical challenges.

Test Your Knowledge

1. What is special about 3D CT imaging, and how is it applied in medicine?
2. What are the recent changes in protecting people from radiation during CT scans?

SUMMARY

Thanks to new medical imaging, diagnoses are now more precise and efficient, and CT is at the head of these developments. CT scans give clear pictures of the body in sections, which makes it easier to spot many medical conditions and plan the proper treatment. Moreover, recent integration with artificial intelligence techniques has enriched the interpretative capabilities of CT scans, offering explainability and enhanced diagnostic confidence through sophisticated machine learning models (Yang *et al.*, 2021). This synergy is particularly evident in urgent health crises, such as the COVID-19 pandemic, where CT imaging combined with AI-driven analysis accelerated diagnostic workflows and improved patient outcomes (Jamshidi *et al.*, 2020). Because of this, CT is still a key diagnostic method, always improving with new technology to satisfy the increasing needs of healthcare and help doctors make better decisions for their patients.

New developments in medical imaging have improved diagnosis, and CT is very important in many areas of medicine. Throughout the discussion, the strengths of CT in detecting intricate anatomical details and evaluating pathological changes have been emphasized, particularly in oncological settings such as renal cell carcinoma, where its ability to identify extrarenal fat invasion is critical despite some limitations in sensitivity and specificity (Ma *et al.*, 2025). The chapter also highlighted the adaptation of CT protocols during the COVID-19 pandemic to minimize infection risks while maintaining diagnostic efficacy, underscoring the importance of standardized operating procedures and thorough radiographic interpretation (Sunawari *et al.*, 2024). In short, CT is still a key tool for diagnosis, since it provides clear images and ensures safety during the procedure. Even with some limits, such as how diagnostic results depend on the size of samples and infection control, continuous research and updates to protocols are expected to enhance CT's accuracy and usefulness in medical diagnostics, ensuring it remains important.

KEY TERMS FROM THIS CHAPTER

- Dual-energy CT (DECT)
- Chronic obstructive pulmonary disease (COPD)
- ECG-gated multidetector
- Iterative reconstruction
- 18F-fluciclovine
- Maximum likelihood expectation maximization
- Photon-counting computed tomography
- Congenital heart diseases
- Filtered back projection
- Osteomyelitis
- Cone beam computed tomography (CBCT)

CRITICAL THINKING QUESTIONS

1. **What is the primary principle behind Computed Tomography (CT)?**
   a. X-ray beams allow doctors to make detailed images that show inside the body.
   b. Images of the inside of the body are made by using sound waves
   c. Radioactive tracers are injected to visualize tissues.
   d. Electromagnetic fields are used to create body images.
2. **What is the main reason for the rotating gantry in a CT scanner?**
   a. It houses the detector array.
   b. It produces high-frequency sound waves.
   c. It spins to allow the machine to send and receive X-rays from many different angles.
   d. It monitors patient movement.
3. **In a CT scan, the resulting images are called:**
   a. Tomograms
   b. Echograms
   c. Radiographs
   d. SPECT images
4. **Which of the following is a key advantage of multidetector CT (MDCT) over traditional single-detector CT?**
   a. Faster image acquisition
   b. Lower radiation dose
   c. Higher image resolution
   d. It does not require intravenous contrast agents
5. **What is a usual purpose for using contrast agents in CT scans?**
   a. To visualize soft tissue structures with better clarity
   b. To reduce the amount of radiation required
   c. To enhance the imaging of bone structures
   d. To improve patient comfort during the scan

Short Answer Questions

1. What is the primary technology used in Computed Tomography (CT) to create images?
2. How does a CT scanner make images that show different parts of the body at once?
3. For what reason is the rotating gantry used in a CT scanner?
4. Why is CT imaging able to give more detailed results than conventional X-ray?
5. What is the principle behind image reconstruction in CT?

Answers to Critical Thinking Questions

1. (a); 2. (c); 3. (a); 4. (a); 5. (a)

REFERENCES

1. Adadzi, J., Anderson, II. J., Azi, C. I., Carsrud, *et al.* (2024). Transformative advancements in diagnostic imaging: Reducing risks, enhancing accuracy, and promoting sustainability. https://core.ac.uk/download/621451782.pdf (accessed on 1st June 2025).
2. Adamczyk, P., Czekajska-Chehab, E., Drop, A., Siek, *et al.* (2018). Total anomalous pulmonary vein drainage in a 60-year-old woman diagnosed in an ECG-gated multidetector computed tomography: A case report and review of literature. https://core.ac.uk/download/160736705.pdf (accessed on 1st June 2025).
3. Adcock, M., Anderson, S., Fisher, N., La Salle, *et al.* (2017). *Towards High-Throughput 3D Insect Capture for Species Discovery and Diagnostics.* http://arxiv.org/abs/1709.02033 (accessed on 1st June 2025).
4. Addepalli, B., Broberg, D., Ditchburn, R., Garnier, C., Jolly, M., Li, *et al.* (2018). A review of miniaturized non-destructive testing technologies for in-situ inspections. *Procedia Manufacturing.* https://core.ac.uk/download/323306202.pdf (accessed on 1st June 2025).
5. Adeleke, S., Adeleke, S., Akpan, A. O., Akpan, *et al.* (2025). *AI-Driven Advances in Low-Dose Imaging and Enhancement—A Review.* https://core.ac.uk/download/647986101.pdf (accessed on 1st June 2025).
6. Ahmad, M., Liu, S., Tegafaw, T., Al Saidi, A. K. A., Zhao, D., Liu, Y., Nam, S. W., *et al.* (2023). Heavy metal-based nanoparticles as high-performance X-ray computed tomography contrast agents. *Pharmaceuticals, 16.* https://www.semanticscholar.org/paper/3a8ec0fd7872aea3642a699bd04e702068c31711 (accessed on 1st June 2025).
7. Al'Aref, S. J., Andreini, D., Baskaran, L., Bax, *et al.* (2020). Automatic segmentation of multiple cardiovascular structures from cardiac computed tomography angiography images using deep learning. https://core.ac.uk/download/323311060.pdf (accessed on 1st June 2025).
8. Al-Haj, H. A., Bosshard, F. A., Schmidt, V., Stadlinger, *et al.* (2023). *Imaging in Third Molar Surgery: A Clinical Update.* https://core.ac.uk/download/611956219.pdf (accessed on 1st June 2025).
9. Al-Haj, H. A., Piccirelli, M., Stadlinger, B., Valdec, *et al.* (2022). Magnetic resonance imaging for preoperative diagnosis in third molar surgery: A systematic review. https://www.zora.uzh.ch/id/eprint/218367/1/ZORA_s11282_022_00611_4.pdf (accessed on 1st June 2025).
10. Alshomrani, F. (2024). Cone-beam computed tomography (CBCT)-based diagnosis of dental bone defects. *Diagnostics, 14.* https://www.semanticscholar.org/paper/af760686afe50319dd91b115bea0cf94ca55532e (accessed on 1st June 2025).
11. Andriole, G. L., Kostakoğlu, L., Chau, A., Duan, F., Mahmood, U., Mankoff, D. A., Schuster, D. M., *et al.* (2018). The impact of positron emission tomography with ^{18}F-fluciclovine on the treatment of biochemical recurrence of prostate cancer: Results from the LOCATE trial. *The Journal of Urology, 201*, 322–331. https://doi.org/10.1016/j.juro.2018.08.050 (accessed on 1st June 2025).
12. Appel, L., Betram, J., Blackwell, B., Dewar, *et al.* (2010). *Model Data Fusion: Developing Bayesian Inversion to Constrain Equilibrium and Mode Structure.* http://arxiv.org/abs/1002.3189 (accessed on 1st June 2025).

13. Authors Task Force Members, Erbel, R., Aboyans, V., Boileau, C., Bossone, E., Di Bartolomeo, R., Eggebrecht, H., *et al.* (2014). 2014 ESC guidelines on the diagnosis and treatment of aortic diseases. *European Heart Journal, 35*, 2873–2926. https://doi.org/10.1093/eurheartj/ehu281 (accessed on 1st June 2025).
14. Avni, F., Bhatnagar, G., Cronin, C. G., Hoeffel, C., *et al.* (2016). The first joint ESGAR/ESPR consensus statement on the technical performance of cross-sectional small bowel and colonic imaging. https://core.ac.uk/download/98339549.pdf (accessed on 1st June 2025).
15. Ayx, I., Bauer, R., Schönberg, S. O., & Hertel, A. (2025). Cardiac radiomics analyses in times of photon-counting computed tomography for personalized risk stratification in the present and in the future. *RoFo: Fortschritte auf dem Gebiete der Röntgenstrahlen und der Nuklearmedizin*. https://www.semanticscholar.org/paper/98974d0b6c0b64ed50c2dab1dff69ce597a7b20f (accessed on 1st June 2025).
16. Bai, Z., Bouchard, K. E., Essiari, A., Perciano, R., *et al.* (2023). *AutoCT: Automated CT Registration, Segmentation, and Quantification*. http://arxiv.org/abs/2310.17780 (accessed on 1st June 2025).
17. Bakir, M. S., Claudé, L. S., Ekkernkamp, A., Gümbel, D., *et al.* (2025). Erroneous classification and coding as a limitation for big data analyses: Causes and impacts illustrated by the diagnosis of clavicle injuries. https://core.ac.uk/download/642859832.pdf (accessed on 1st June 2025).
18. Banson, M., Buckman, V., Darko, K., Totimeh, T., *et al.* (2024). Neuro-oncology access in Sub-Saharan Africa: A literature review of challenges and opportunities. https://core.ac.uk/download/613721197.docx (accessed on 1st June 2025).
19. Batra, V., Spalkit, S., Bugata, S. K., Chari, R., & Batta, N. S. (2025). Ultrasound and computed tomography-guided interventions for the hip joint and pelvis: Comprehensive imaging review. *Indian Journal of Musculoskeletal Radiology*. https://www.semanticscholar.org/paper/f0ca66da320ff69040cacefd7c1dff538c7f53e0 (accessed on 1st June 2025).
20. Bekiesińska-Figatowska, M., Brągoszewska, H., Iwanowska, B., Klepacka, M., *et al.* (2009). *The Symptomatology of Aneurysmal Bone Cyst: The Value of Diagnostic Imaging*. https://core.ac.uk/download/161629234.pdf (accessed on 1st June 2025).
21. Bhattarai, A., Tanaka, R., Yeung, A. W. K., & Vardhanabhuti, V. (2023). Photon-counting CT material decomposition in bone imaging. *Journal of Imaging, 9*, 209–209. https://doi.org/10.3390/jimaging9100209 (accessed on 1st June 2025).
22. Bolocko, K., Edelmers, E., Kazoka, D., Pilmane, M., *et al.* (2024). *Automatization of CT Annotation: Combining AI Efficiency with Expert Precision*. https://core.ac.uk/download/618266624.pdf (accessed on 1st June 2025).
23. Boutroy, S., Bouxsein, M. L., Crawford, R. P., DeLong, M. E., Eckstein, F., *et al.* (2010). Relation of vertebral deformities to bone density, structure, and strength. https://core.ac.uk/download/323080767.pdf (accessed on 1st June 2025).
24. Bouxsein, M. L., Clarke, B. L., Cosman, F., Keaveny, T. M., *et al.* (2020). Biomechanical computed tomography analysis (BCT) for clinical assessment of osteoporosis. https://core.ac.uk/download/323308619.pdf (accessed on 1st June 2025).
25. Brix, G., Gawlitza, J., Haubenreisser, H., Henzler, T., *et al.* (2020). COPD imaging on a 3rd generation dual-source CT: Acquisition of paired inspiratory-expiratory chest scans at an

overall reduced radiation risk. https://core.ac.uk/download/382461302.pdf (accessed on 1st June 2025).

26. Cavagnaro, M., Crocco, L., Lopresto, V., Pinto, R., *et al.* (2018). Monitoring thermal ablation via microwave tomography: An *ex vivo* experimental assessment. *Diagnostics*. https://core.ac.uk/download/195776752.pdf (accessed on 1st June 2025).
27. Cella, S., Esposito, S., Fanelli, U., Gismondi, P., Iannarella, R., Meoli, A., Vincenzi, F. (2020). An unusual dysphagia for solids in a 17-year-old girl due to a lusoria artery: A case report and review of the literature. *Int. J. Environ. Res. Public Health*. https://core.ac.uk/download/521222237.pdf (accessed on 1st June 2025).
28. Cesarec, G., & Martinec, S. (2020). Power Doppler usage for early diagnostics and follow-up of post-traumatic myositis ossificans: A case report. *Med. Jad.* https://core.ac.uk/download/322933239.pdf (accessed on 1st June 2025).
29. Chang, P., Cho, A. H., Chow, D., Fisher, M., *et al.* (2019). *Cerebral Microbleeds in a Stroke Prevention Clinic.* https://core.ac.uk/download/323075566.pdf (accessed on 1st June 2025).
30. Chen, M., Deng, L., He, P., Jiang, H., *et al.* (2017). Monte Carlo simulation for polychromatic X-ray fluorescence computed tomography with sheet-beam geometry. *International Journal of Biomedical Imaging*. https://core.ac.uk/download/188807521.pdf (accessed on 1st June 2025).
31. Chikorde, K., Dalal, R., Rajan, M., Rodda, S., *et al.* (2024). *CBCT in Modern Dentistry: Transforming Diagnosis and Treatment Planning.* https://core.ac.uk/download/620886933.pdf (accessed on 1st June 2025).
32. David-Olawade, A. C., Olawade, D., Vanderbloemen, L., Rotifa, O. B., Fidelis, S. C., Egbon, E., Akpan, A. O., *et al.* (2025). AI-driven advances in low-dose imaging and enhancement—A review. *Diagnostics, 15*. https://www.semanticscholar.org/paper/44051b152f1c9fdf0599bfc6f3bf4a45b07ac104 (accessed on 1st June 2025).
33. Dehdashti, F., Freimark, B. D., Frye, J., Frye, S., *et al.* (2017). First-in-man evaluation of 124I-PGN650: A PET tracer for detecting phosphatidylserine as a biomarker of the solid tumor microenvironment. *Molecular Imaging*. https://core.ac.uk/download/129070165.pdf (accessed on 1st June 2025).
34. Dimitriadis, K. S., Pyrpyris, N., Theofilis, P., Mantzouranis, E., Beneki, E., Kostakis, P., Koutsopoulos, G., *et al.* (2024). Computed tomography angiography identified high-risk coronary plaques: From diagnosis to prognosis and future management. *Diagnostics, 14*. https://www.semanticscholar.org/paper/912f4b43619f358413952ba4be40b5d81da7e4e8 (accessed on 1st June 2025).
35. Dollin, Y., Munoz, P. J. A., Sung, L., Hasteh, F., Fortich, M., Lopez, A., Van, N. K., *et al.* (2024). Diagnostic modalities in the mediastinum and the role of bronchoscopy in mediastinal assessment: A narrative review. *Mediastinum, 8*. https://www.semanticscholar.org/paper/2c377dd4106d429590803a477f326a11c64975d8 (accessed on 1st June 2025).
36. Eseonu, K., Oduoza, U., Robinson, P., Easty, M. J., Nadarajah, R., & Biassoni, L. (2024). Bone scintigraphy with SPECT/CT in pediatric patients with neck and back pain in comparison with other imaging modalities: The experience of a tertiary pediatric referral center. *Nuclear Medicine Communications, 45*, 278–286. https://www.semanticscholar.org/paper/ad14cad4d3ed73edc25f57405920ec34195296d4 (accessed on 1st June 2025).

37. Frank, D., Höfs, C., & Lasser, T. (2025). *Statistical Reconstruction for Anisotropic X-Ray Dark-Field Tomography*. ArXiv, abs/2501.03160. https://www.semanticscholar.org/paper/8b6e2445afe1d15b29bf7ed11dfb9704a374860e (accessed on 1st June 2025).

38. Gulyamov, Y. (2024). Brief overview of modern methods of radiological diagnostics of osteomyelitis. *Traumatology and Orthopedics of Kazakhstan*. https://www.semanticscholar.org/paper/19092393f41047c6747a77667c01181a2e2481b1 (accessed on 1st June 2025).

39. Halpern, E. J., Kim, S., Salmanoglu, E., Thakur, M., *et al.* (2018). *A Glance at Imaging Bladder Cancer.* https://core.ac.uk/download/227055407.pdf (accessed on 1st June 2025).

40. Jamshidi, M., Lalbakhsh, A., Talla, J., Peroutka, Z., Hadjilooei, F., Lalbakhsh, P., Jamshidi, M., *et al.* (2020). Artificial intelligence and COVID-19: Deep learning approaches for diagnosis and treatment. *IEEE Access, 8*, 109581–109595. https://doi.org/10.1109/access.2020.3001973.

41. Joudar, I., Nasri, S., Kamaoui, I., & Skiker, I. (2025). Cardiac computed tomography for cardiac masses: A necessity or a luxury? *The Journal of International Medical Research, 53*. https://www.semanticscholar.org/paper/5335b2cc41b4d124019ee3b12798bb4272853403 (accessed on 1st June 2025).

42. Jurić, B., & Matijaš, T. (2023). *The Role of CBCT in the Field of Dental Implantology*. https://core.ac.uk/download/580133359.pdf (accessed on 1st June 2025).

43. Kasaudhan, H., Shukla, K. K., Kushwaha, R., Sharma, K., Gupta, U., & Sharma, A. (2024). Early detection and analysis of lung cancer using artificial intelligence. *2024 IEEE International Conference on Computing, Power and Communication Technologies (IC2PCT), 5*, 1470–1474. https://www.semanticscholar.org/paper/b1094dae257bacd86cfa58d298ac5857a4235365 (accessed on 1st June 2025).

44. Kirkpatrick, J. N., Mitchell, C., Taub, C., Kort, S., Hung, J., & Swaminathan, M. (2020). ASE statement on protection of patients and echocardiography service providers during the 2019 novel coronavirus outbreak: Endorsed by the American College of Cardiology. *Journal of the American Society of Echocardiography, 33*, 648–653. https://doi.org/10.1016/j.echo.2020.04.001 (accessed on 1st June 2025).

45. Krailertmongkol, T., Muangsomboon, K., Na Songkhla, N., Thiravit, S., & Muangsomboon, S. (2025). Clinical features and computed tomography (CT) findings in abdominal actinomycosis: A retrospective review. *The ASEAN Journal of Radiology*. https://www.semanticscholar.org/paper/ee6ecfd66d20a89afd97f3754c7423d35f3dcc6e (accessed on 1st June 2025).

46. Kumar, A. A., Kannappan, S., & Geetha, G. (2025). Clinical experiences with robotic computed tomography-guided interventions: A comparison with manual technique. *Asian Journal of Medical Sciences*. https://www.semanticscholar.org/paper/2539706c9ed2cd923d3090a310662ee44f44cfec (accessed on 1st June 2025).

47. Lell, M., & Kachelrieß, M. (2023). Computed tomography 2.0. *Investigative Radiology*. https://doi.org/10.1097/rli.0000000000000995.

48. Liu, W., Wu, Y., Zheng, Z., Bittle, M., Yu, W., & Kharrazi, H. (2025). Enhancing diagnostic accuracy of lung nodules in chest computed tomography using artificial intelligence: Retrospective analysis. *Journal of Medical Internet Research, 27*. https://www.semanticscholar.org/paper/5cbb9bcf96f68d232432991b75a75f323046c196 (accessed on 1st June 2025).

49. Lowe, K., Regan, E. A., Anzueto, A., Austin, E., Austin, J. H. M., Beaty, T. H., Benos, P. V., *et al.* (2019). COPDGene® 2019: Redefining the diagnosis of chronic obstructive pulmonary disease. *Chronic Obstructive Pulmonary Diseases: Journal of the COPD Foundation, 6*, 384–399. https://doi.org/10.15326/jcopdf.6.5.2019.0149 (accessed on 1st June 2025).

50. Lyon, A. R., López-Fernández, T., Couch, L. S., Asteggiano, R., Aznar, M. C., Bergler-Klein, J., Boriani, G., *et al.* (2022). 2022 ESC guidelines on cardio-oncology developed in collaboration with the European Hematology Association (EHA), the European Society for Therapeutic Radiology and Oncology (ESTRO) and the International Cardio-Oncology Society (IC-OS). *European Heart Journal, 43*, 4229–4361. https://doi.org/10.1093/eurheartj/ehac244 (accessed on 1st June 2025).

51. Ma, J., Yuan, E., Feng, S., Yao, J., He, C., Chen, Y., & Song, B. (2025). Diagnostic performance of CT for extrarenal fat invasion in renal cell carcinoma: A meta-analysis and systematic review. *Insights into Imaging, 16*. https://www.semanticscholar.org/paper/ca4e3bee5ce9296c0c298beeff0f9fcc10c219d5 (accessed on 1st June 2025).

52. Magomedov, M., Magomedov, H. M., & Magomedov, A. A. (2025). Mechanical jaundice and principles of modern diagnostics. *Medicus*. https://www.semanticscholar.org/paper/8a679cbb0817927d8912863095909d56963f1a99 (accessed on 1st June 2025).

53. Mathijssen, I. M. J. (2020). Updated guideline on treatment and management of craniosynostosis. *Journal of Craniofacial Surgery, 32*, 371–450. https://doi.org/10.1097/scs.0000000000007035 (accessed on 1st June 2025).

54. Maturi, B., Dulal, S., Sayana, S., Ibrahim, A., Ramakrishna, M., Chinta, V., Sharma, A., *et al.* (2025). Revolutionizing cardiology: The role of artificial intelligence in echocardiography. *Journal of Clinical Medicine, 14*. https://www.semanticscholar.org/paper/f3527c4918000ddee71202d360a9b2bd13156a6c (accessed on 1st June 2025).

55. Meloni, A., Maffei, E., Positano, V., Clemente, A., De Gori, C., Berti, S., La Grutta, L., *et al.* (2024). Technical principles, benefits, challenges, and applications of photon counting computed tomography in coronary imaging: A narrative review. *Cardiovascular Diagnosis and Therapy, 14*, 698–724. https://www.semanticscholar.org/paper/cedacb89c36ed454b05f51079c585fd85ca8836a (accessed on 1st June 2025).

56. Mishra, A. (2024). *PET/CT Scan: Bridging Metabolic and Anatomical Imaging*. https://core.ac.uk/download/622189017.pdf (accessed on 1st June 2025).

57. Palazzo, S., Zambetta, G., & Calbi, R. (2024). An overview of segmentation techniques for CT and MRI images: Clinical implications and future directions in medical diagnostics. *Medical Imaging Process & Technology*. https://www.semanticscholar.org/paper/9d1721bfd41fd24c8b0cf688a7d9dc78d9447b3f (accessed on 1st June 2025).

58. Perera, M. A. A. S., & Verma, Y. (2025). Role of photon-counting computed tomography in pediatric cardiovascular imaging. *World Journal of Clinical Pediatrics, 14*. https://www.semanticscholar.org/paper/97695ab1fffe5f87d20b94f2c4b68926e4241a90 (accessed on 1st June 2025).

59. Perera, M. A. A. S., Catapano, F., Lisi, C., El Choueiri, J., Pellicanò, F., Figliozzi, S., Politi, L., *et al.* (2025). Trends in clinical cardiac photon-counting detector CT research: A comprehensive bibliometric analysis. *Diagnostics, 15*. https://www.semanticscholar.org/paper/66c221c3c1c08c4aed5875261a7c0effc27aa376 (accessed on 1st June 2025).

60. Petkovic, A., Menković, N., Petrović, O., Bilbija, I., Nisevic, M., Radovanovic, N., Stanisavljević, D., *et al.* (2024). Imaging in infective endocarditis—Current opinions and trends in cardiac computed tomography. *Diagnostics, 14*. https://www.semanticscholar.org/paper/e7016adbf7dd6a0a5bc592797aa842a6a272797e (accessed on 1st June 2025).

61. Power, S., Moloney, F., Twomey, M., James, K., O'Connor, O. J., & Maher, M. M. (2016). Computed tomography and patient risk: Facts, perceptions and uncertainties. *World Journal of Radiology, 8*, 902. https://doi.org/10.4329/wjr.v8.i12.902.

62. Prokop, A., Salim, A., Leidner, B., Leidner, B., Beuker, J. A., Smith, C. M., *et al.* (2012). A multicenter, randomized controlled trial of immediate total-body CT scanning in trauma patients (REACT-2). https://core.ac.uk/download/pdf/8732652.pdf (accessed on 1st June 2025).

63. Pulumati, A., Pulumati, A., Dwarakanath, B. S., Verma, A., & Papineni, R. V. (2023). Technological advancements in cancer diagnostics: Improvements and limitations. *Cancer Reports, 6*. https://doi.org/10.1002/cnr2.1764 (accessed on 1st June 2025).

64. Ravula, P., Mohanakrishnan, A., Muralidharan, Y., Kanadasan, K., & Natarajan, P. (2024). The role of advanced post-processing techniques in computed tomography pulmonary angiography for the accurate diagnosis of pulmonary thromboembolism: A retrospective study. *Cureus, 16*. https://www.semanticscholar.org/paper/cb1821ebf1fcbddae18a500100c3fab8d21ca9b0 (accessed on 1st June 2025).

65. Rayyani, A. A., Shalalni, A. A., Radwan, A. H., Shibli, K. A., Jabin, J. Y., Mokli, M. A. Y., Mabuj, J. M., *et al.* (2024). Digital X-ray imaging: Emphasis can be placed on developments in digital X-ray technologies and their applications in diagnosis and treatment. *Journal of Positive Psychology & Wellbeing*. https://core.ac.uk/download/616775625.pdf (accessed on 1st June 2025).

66. Saran, M., Arab-Zozani, M., Behzadifar, M., Gholami, M., Azari, S., Bragazzi, N., & Behzadifar, M. (2024). Overuse of computed tomography for mild head injury: A systematic review and meta-analysis. *PLOS ONE, 19*. https://www.semanticscholar.org/paper/c20714c7d6c281a89e3972784309e0d259334abb (accessed on 1st June 2025).

67. Segger, L., Lerchbaumer, M., Collettini, F., Hamm, B., Fleckenstein, F., Fehrenbach, U., Gebauer, B., *et al.* (2024). Percutaneous computed tomography (CT) fluoroscopy-guided biopsy of the spleen using fibrin glue as a sealant. *Diagnostics, 14*. https://www.semanticscholar.org/paper/79413a92ceb2fa4599d34c5a0ec312b7427ee9d5 (accessed on 1st June 2025).

68. Sina, S., Kardan, M. R., Karimi, A. H., Bahreinipour, M., Rakeb, Z., Sadeghi, M. H., Nazari, J. M. A., *et al.* (2024). National diagnostic reference levels (DRLs) for general and interventional radiography, mammography, and CT scan based on the latest surveys in Iran. *Radioprotection*. https://www.semanticscholar.org/paper/b100adb4c5bce55608e61c7636479cb9f973980b (accessed on 1st June 2025).

69. Sotenskii, R., Rozhkov, V. A., Shashurin, D. A., Suslova, E., & Chelkov, G. (2024). Novel algorithm for qualitative and quantitative material analysis by the K-edges for photon-counting computed tomography. *Journal of Instrumentation, 19*. https://www.semanticscholar.org/paper/b216f80a3f9711a770bdbc87ff5f5de7006d3111 (accessed on 1st June 2025).

70. Stański, M., Michałowska, I., Lemanowicz, A., Karmelita-Katulska, K., Ratajczak, P., Sławińska, A., Serafin, Z. (2024). Dual-energy and photon-counting computed tomography in vascular

applications—Technical background and post-processing techniques. *Diagnostics, 14*. https://www.semanticscholar.org/paper/d1d253a652a1b4c8e4afac189fe91873fd7c5688 (accessed on 1st June 2025).

71. Suárez, O. J., De La Cruz De, O. A., Ortega, D. Y., & Salas De La, C. Y. (2024). Computed tomography hydroenema as a diagnostic alternative for colon tumors. *Health Leadership and Quality of Life*. https://www.semanticscholar.org/paper/a352453e4ec0e6c93b7fab6b2291543b65a1a2dc (accessed on 1st June 2025).

72. Sun, Z. (2024). Cardiovascular computed tomography in cardiovascular disease: An overview of its applications from diagnosis to prediction. *Journal of Geriatric Cardiology, 21*(5), 550–576. https://www.semanticscholar.org/paper/045ab8f2d03472d15d6bde146fedaaf57e808072 (accessed on 1st June 2025).

73. Sunawari, A. L., Rahimi, A., Saadiah, A., *et al.* (2024). A policy examination of COVID-19 impact on the radiology department standard operating procedures (SOPs): The Malaysian experience. *Malaysian Journal of Science Health & Technology*. https://www.semanticscholar.org/paper/6903516f15353f954c77580592fa9c8e644e38bd (accessed on 1st June 2025).

74. Sunilkumar, A. P., Parida, B. K., & You, W. (2024). Recent advances in dental panoramic X-ray synthesis and its clinical applications. *IEEE Access, 12*, 141032–141051. https://www.semanticscholar.org/paper/bcb43567eb995e8d721b9407dfc762ad8aee8a4d (accessed on 1st June 2025).

75. Ulas, S., & Diekhoff, T. (2024). Computed tomography—Current status and future directions for arthritis imaging. *Therapeutic Advances in Musculoskeletal Disease, 16*. https://www.semanticscholar.org/paper/400ac30dba4cbdfe4eaeb9c6c56bdece66818d81 (accessed on 1st June 2025).

76. Wang, G. (2016). A perspective on deep imaging. *IEEE Access, 4*, 8914–8924. https://doi.org/10.1109/access.2016.2624938 (accessed on 1st June 2025).

77. Yadav, P., Lokhande, A., Prasanna, B. L., & Thorat, G. (2024). Conceptual importance of imaging and signal processing in the medical science. In *2024 International Conference on Healthcare Innovations, Software and Engineering Technologies (HISET)*. https://www.semanticscholar.org/paper/58d2c820d6e4c4ac0ade0de4d21e05d6f78e13cf (accessed on 1st June 2025).

78. Yang, G., Ye, Q., & Xia, J. (2021). Unbox the black-box for the medical explainable AI via multi-modal and multi-center data fusion: A mini-review, two showcases and beyond. *Information Fusion, 77*, 29–52. https://doi.org/10.1016/j.inffus.2021.07.016 (accessed on 1st June 2025).

79. Zeppenfeld, K., Tfelt-Hansen, J., Riva, M., Winkel, B. G., Behr, E. R., Blom, N. A., Charron, P., *et al.* (2022). 2022 ESC guidelines for the management of patients with ventricular arrhythmias and the prevention of sudden cardiac death. *European Heart Journal, 43*, 3997–4126. https://doi.org/10.1093/eurheartj/ehac262 (accessed on 1st June 2025).

80. Ziyad, N., Yoosaf, S., Prabha, N., & Nair, N. V. (2024). Visualizing MRI & CT scans using mixed reality. In *2024 IEEE 12th Region 10 Humanitarian Technology Conference (R10-HTC)*. https://www.semanticscholar.org/paper/445c09cd73c589c81b1272ca530c8591accb4964(accessed on 1st June 2025).

MAGNETIC RESONANCE IMAGING (MRI)

8

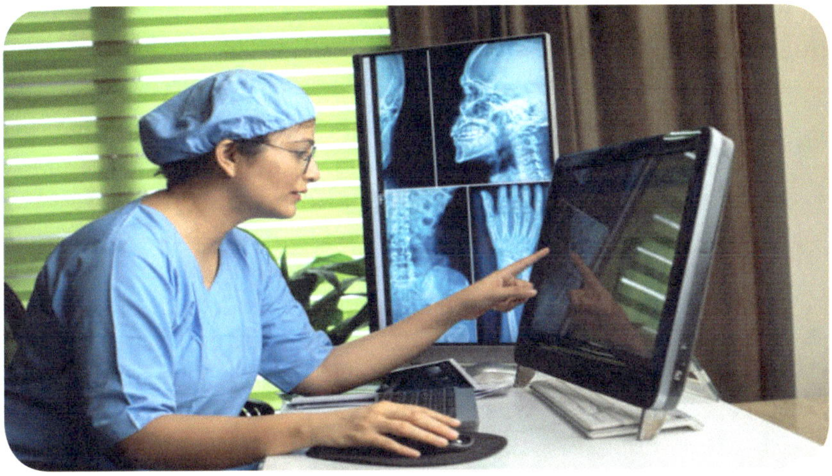

LEARNING OBJECTIVES

After studying this chapter, you will be able to:

1. Understand principles of MRI technology;
2. Explain clinical applications of MRI;
3. Focus on safety and risks associated with MRI;
4. Describe innovations and future directions in MRI.

Introduction

With modern medical imaging, doctors can see inside the body in detail that was not possible before. Among these technologies, Magnetic Resonance Imaging (MRI) stands out for its exceptional ability to produce detailed images of soft tissues without ionizing radiation. From the beginning, MRI has been important for diagnosing many conditions, such as problems in the brain and muscles, because it provides clear and distinct images. But the usual way of analyzing MRI images is subjective, which can cause differences in interpretation and sometimes result in incorrect diagnoses. To address these challenges, recent developments incorporate artificial intelligence techniques, including machine learning and deep learning, to enhance image processing, lesion detection, and tumor classification, thereby improving diagnostic accuracy and efficiency (Dong, 2024). Furthermore, innovations in image reconstruction have introduced unsupervised deep learning models that accelerate processing speed while maintaining quality, overcoming limitations related to data availability and computational demand (Wu *et al.*, 2024).

Definition of Magnetic Resonance Imaging (MRI)

New medical technology has improved how doctors look inside the body and see its structures in great detail. Magnetic Resonance Imaging is one of the most important innovations because it provides detailed images of soft tissues, organs, and other parts of the body without surgery or other invasive methods.

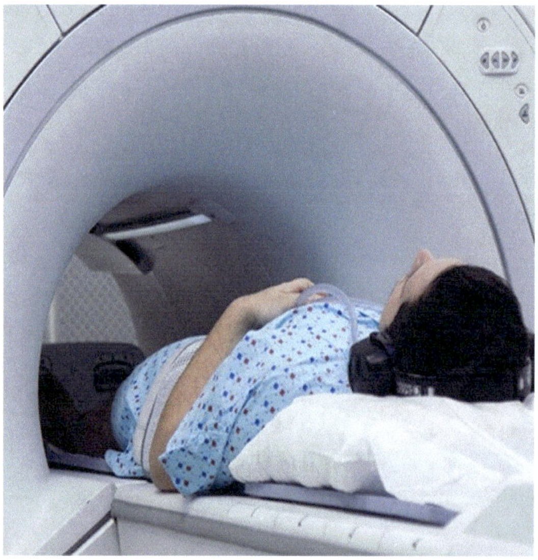

Figure 8.1. MRI captures anatomical and physiological information by detecting the alignment and relaxation of hydrogen protons in the body's water molecules.

Source: https://burtominternational.com/wp-content/uploads/2024/02/1.5-Tesla-MRI-2.jpg.

MRI is different from ionizing radiation-based techniques because it uses signals from the position and movement of hydrogen protons in water. This way, doctors can see the fine details needed for correct diagnosis and planning treatments. Additionally, with the integration of cutting-edge techniques such as feature tracking and tissue mapping, MRI has expanded its utility beyond mere visualization, offering quantitative assessments of tissue deformation and characterization of pathological changes (Sclafani *et al.*, 2024). The synergy between MRI and emerging technologies, including artificial intelligence, further enhances the precision and efficiency of image analysis, demonstrating the modality's evolving role in modern medical practice (Fıçıcı *et al.*, 2023) (Figure 8.1).

Historical development of Magnetic Resonance Imaging (MRI) Technology

Bringing physics into medical technology greatly changed how diagnostic imaging was done. At the beginning, things like blood pressure devices and X-rays were developed, which made it possible for MRI to be invented. This combination of scientific fields led to the MRI, which started as basic equipment and grew to produce highly detailed images of the inside of the body without using ionizing radiation. By doing this, the accuracy of diagnosis went up, and the risk of health problems from earlier images was lowered. Recent innovations, including ultra-high-field MRI scanners, further enhance resolution while minimizing patient exposure to potentially harmful effects, representing a crucial advancement over conventional techniques (Adadzi *et al.*, 2024; Myers *et al.*, 2021). Moreover, the incorporation of artificial intelligence in MRI facilitates real-time image analysis, personalized protocols, and improved workflow efficiency, underscoring the dynamic and ongoing evolution of MRI technology in the medical field (Adadzi *et al.*, 2024).

Importance of Magnetic Resonance Imaging (MRI) in Modern Medicine

Diagnostic tools have changed clinical medicine a lot, and MRI is now considered one of the most important. Alongside other modalities such as endoscopy and computed tomography, MRI offers a non-invasive method that provides detailed, high-contrast images of soft tissues, aiding in the accurate diagnosis of complex conditions, particularly in fields like gastroenterology (Belousova *et al.*, 2024). MRI can show both normal and abnormal structures in the body without using ionizing radiation, which makes it safer for patients and provides the necessary details for planning treatment. Despite its apparent benefits, patient awareness regarding MRI procedures and their health implications remains limited, with many experiencing discomfort or anxiety during scans (Sumon *et al.*, 2024). Improving how patients are educated and communicated with is very important for better MRI use. Overall, MRI's ability to integrate multiple imaging contrasts and its role in comprehensive diagnostic approaches solidifies its importance within modern medicine (Belousova *et al.*, 2024) (Figure 8.2).

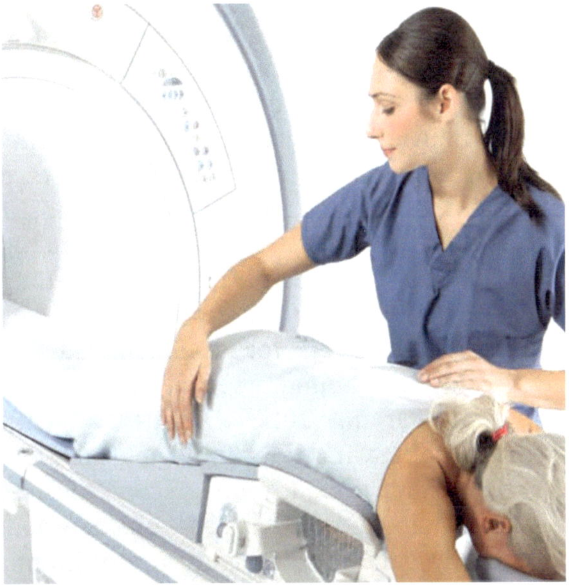

Figure 8.2. Advancements in diagnostic technologies have profoundly transformed clinical medicine, with magnetic resonance imaging (MRI) emerging as a crucial tool among them.

Source: https://burtominternational.com/wp-content/uploads/2024/02/1.5-Tesla-MRI-5.jpg.

Overview of How Magnetic Resonance Imaging (MRI) Works

MRI produces detailed pictures inside the body by using nuclear magnetic resonance, in which hydrogen nuclei are made to respond to a strong magnetic field and radiofrequency pulses. When pulses are given, the protons are excited and then release energy as they go back to their normal position, which sensors pick up and process into images. How these images appear and what they show depends on the tissues and the magnetic environment, and this can be improved by the use of contrast agents. Traditional metal-based agents like gadolinium and manganese have advanced imaging clarity but raise concerns related to toxicity and accumulation, prompting research into safer, non-metallic alternatives with promising biocompatibility and biodegradability despite challenges in sensitivity and stability (Wang *et al.*, 2025). This dynamic interplay of physics, chemistry, and technology underscores MRI's unparalleled capacity to reveal anatomical and functional details critical to medical diagnosis (Gallucci *et al.*, 2024).

Comparison with Other Imaging Techniques

Because of new imaging technologies, diagnostic tools can be used in more ways than just magnetic resonance imaging. For instance, dual-energy computed tomography (DECT) has demonstrated remarkable efficacy in detecting bone marrow edema, achieving sensitivity and specificity comparable to MRI when assessing vertebral compression fractures, with water-HAP decomposition techniques closely mirroring MRI's depiction of edema areas (Yao *et al.*, 2025). Meanwhile, AI-assisted iterative algorithm protocols in accelerated fast spin-echo MRI have significantly reduced scan times without compromising image quality or diagnostic accuracy, particularly in musculoskeletal evaluations such as knee imaging, indicating potential benefits over standard MRI sequences (Liu *et al.*, 2024). Such developments show that MRI is flexible and ahead in the market, but they also point out that DECT can be a good alternative in specific clinical cases. For this reason, deciding between MRI and other imaging methods depends on considering diagnostic accuracy, the speed of results, and the ability to see certain tissues, which makes personalized imaging strategies crucial in healthcare.

Common Applications of Magnetic Resonance Imaging (MRI)

Thanks to new imaging technology, especially magnetic resonance imaging, diagnosis has improved a lot in medicine. MRI is used in many medical areas because it creates detailed images without using ionizing radiation.

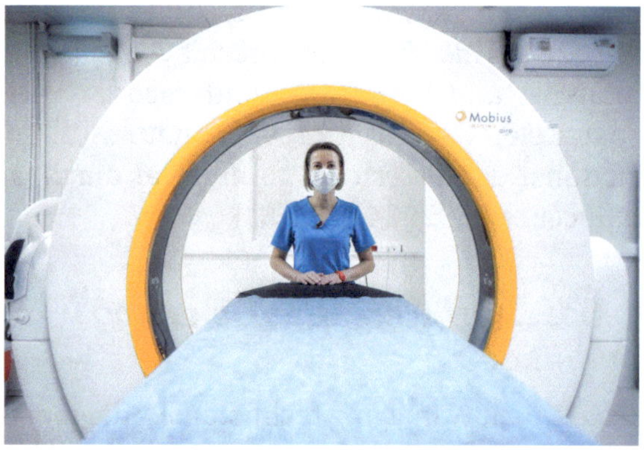

Figure 8.3. Magnetic resonance imaging (MRI) is widely employed across various medical specialties due to its ability to generate high-resolution images without ionizing radiation.

Source: https://www.laiic.com/cdn/shop/articles/mri_machines_explained_2041x.png?v=1677552565.

Some common uses are in neurological tests, which help detect brain tumors, stroke, and multiple sclerosis, and in imaging the muscles and joints to locate abnormalities and injuries. MRI is also very important for cardiovascular imaging since it gives clear images of the heart and its blood vessels. The integration of deep learning models has further enhanced the diagnostic accuracy and efficiency of MRI by improving image analysis, reducing human error, and enabling faster interpretation of complex cases (Slimane *et al.*, 2025). Moreover, MRI is instrumental in biomedical engineering fields, supporting both therapeutic planning and monitoring by offering precise localization, classification, and segmentation of anatomical features, which aligns with broader trends in medical image processing and analysis (Yadav *et al.*, 2024) (Figure 8.3).

Safety Considerations in Magnetic Resonance Imaging (MRI)

Both patients and staff must be protected by having protocols that cover all the hazards and risks in magnetic resonance imaging. Because MRI uses strong magnets and radiofrequency waves, there is a risk of projectile accidents, thermal injuries, and problems with implants, which is especially important for pediatric patients who might need sedation and might have unique implant issues. Establishing a robust safety culture through structured screening, zoning regulations, staff training, and emergency preparedness is crucial for minimizing adverse events and maintaining a secure environment (Alkhulaifat *et al.*, 2025). Additionally, the integration of advanced technologies, including AI-based predictive models, underscores the need to balance innovation with safety considerations by carefully validating imaging protocols and adjusting for patient variability to prevent diagnostic errors or unintended consequences (Zhang, 2025). It is very important to value safety, be honest, and take responsibility to get the most out of MRI while keeping everyone safe.

Limitations of Magnetic Resonance Imaging (MRI)

Even though MRI is highly advanced, there are some problems that affect its usefulness in medicine. For instance, functional MRI techniques, such as perfusion and diffusion imaging, enhance tumor characterization but often face challenges due to tissue heterogeneity and overlapping features between benign and malignant lesions, limiting their standalone diagnostic reliability (Drapé *et al.*, 2013). Moreover, while multiparametric MRI (mpMRI) of the prostate demonstrates high sensitivity in detecting clinically significant cancers, the interpretation of negative mpMRI results remains problematic.

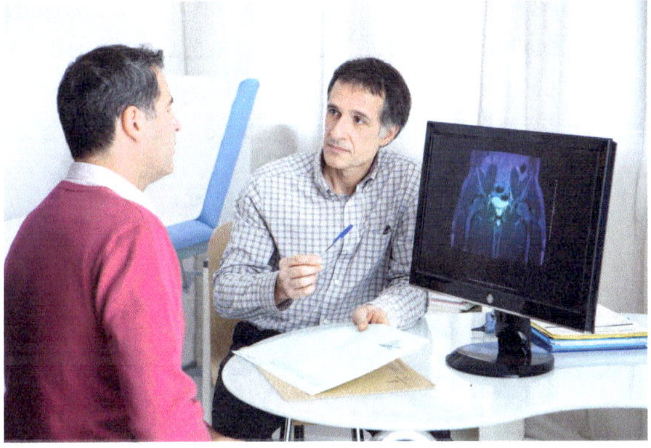

Figure 8.4. While multiparametric MRI (mpMRI) of the prostate demonstrates high sensitivity in detecting clinically significant cancers, the interpretation of negative mpMRI results remains problematic.

Source: https://cdn.prod.website-files.com/63bf3f41c3bc69578d823f01/64aed675097bb4d04ed4e792_prostate%20mri.jpg.

Negative findings do not conclusively exclude disease, necessitating supplementary procedures like systematic biopsies, particularly in younger patients with suspicious clinical markers such as elevated prostate-specific antigen levels (Barchetti *et al.*, 2018). Because MRI requires special equipment and skills, not everyone can use it and its results may not be the same every time which makes it more of an additional tool than a main one for diagnosis. These factors collectively underscore the need for cautious evaluation of MRI findings within broader clinical contexts (Figure 8.4).

Future Trends in Magnetic Resonance Imaging (MRI) Technology

Improvements in technology are always affecting medical imaging, and in MRI, they are expected to lead to better diagnosis and a better experience for patients. Advances in MRI technology such as ultra-high-field machines, make it possible to find changes in the body that could not be seen before. Additionally, the integration of artificial intelligence (AI) and machine learning algorithms is anticipated to streamline image acquisition and interpretation, reducing scan times while increasing diagnostic accuracy. New, mobile and affordable MRI systems are becoming available to help people in remote or poorly equipped areas. Moreover, hybrid imaging technologies that combine MRI with other modalities, such as positron emission tomography (PET), will provide more comprehensive anatomical and functional information. They fit with the general trend toward minimally invasive and patient-focused healthcare. These promising directions underscore ongoing research focused on improving both technological capabilities and clinical outcomes in MRI applications (Hendi *et al.*, 2023; Welch *et al.*, 2012).

8.1. Principles of Magnetic Resonance Imaging (MRI) Technology

Learning Outcome

1. Understand basic physics of magnetic fields;
2. Explain role of radiofrequency pulses;
3. Know image formation process;
4. Identify types of MRI sequences;
5. Focus on contrast agents used in MRI;
6. Discuss signal-to-noise ratio in MRI;
7. Describe importance of magnetic field strength;
8. Define artifacts in MRI imaging;
9. Know advances in MRI technology.

Better MRI technology has led to sharper images and easier processing which has made it more useful for diagnosis. MRI relies on controlling hydrogen protons in the body with strong magnets and radio waves and these signals are then turned into detailed pictures. They are so precise because of advanced algorithms and methods that separate various body parts and disease changes. With the help of deep learning, recent computational methods have made MRI segmentation more accurate so that doctors can rely on fewer annotated images for diagnosis. They handle difficulties with limited data by applying self-supervised and semi-supervised methods which improves how MRI is used in medical imaging of the heart and brain. As MRI technology continues to evolve, these principles underpin efforts to improve image clarity and diagnostic reliability, strengthening its role as a non-invasive, radiation-free imaging modality in medicine (Liu *et al.*, 2024; Rabah *et al.*, 2024).

8.1.1. Basic Physics of Magnetic Fields

Magnetic fields are important in MRI because they interact with atomic nuclei to give clear images. Magnetic fields influence charged particles and moving electric currents, according to electromagnetism which helps the nuclear spins line up in the strong static magnetic field produced by the MRI scanner. Because of this alignment, a net magnetization vector is formed, and applying radiofrequency pulses disturbs it, which leads to detectable signals as nuclei return to their original state. The complexities of these interactions not only facilitate image formation but also introduce various physical risks, such as induced electric currents and heating effects, which must be carefully managed in clinical settings to ensure patient safety (Panych *et al.*, 2018). Moreover, precise control and measurement of magnetic fields enable advanced techniques like beamforming for improved signal localization, contributing to the high temporal and spatial resolution characteristic of neuroimaging modalities related to MRI (Kim *et al.*, 2021) (Figure 8.5).

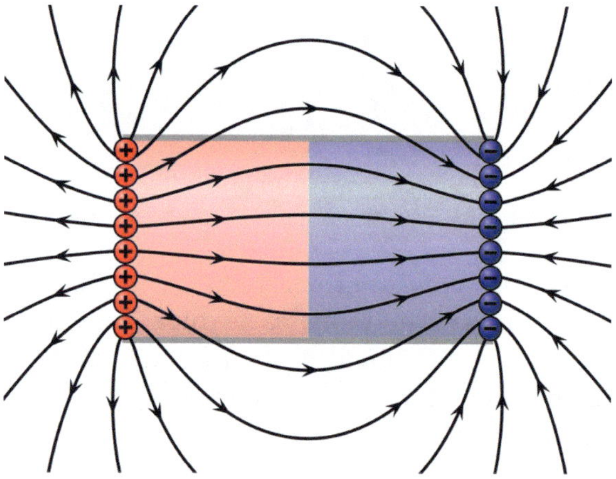

Figure 8.5. Understanding the behavior of magnetic fields is fundamental to the operation of Magnetic Resonance Imaging (MRI), as these fields interact intricately with atomic nuclei to produce detailed images.

Source: https://7cad390533514c32acc8-75d23ce06fcfaf780446d85d50c33f7b.ssl.cf6.rackcdn.com/sc/1708308253-normal-magnetic-field.jpg.

8.1.2. Role of Radiofrequency Pulses

The intricacies of Magnetic Resonance Imaging hinge on the precise manipulation of hydrogen protons within the body, a process fundamentally facilitated by radiofrequency (RF) pulses. Pulses of energy are applied to the protons, which disturbs the alignment of the protons and makes them move away from their equilibrium when a strong magnetic field is present. This excitation and subsequent relaxation of protons generate the signals that form detailed images, thus underscoring the essential influence of RF pulses on image quality and diagnostic clarity (Hiremath, 2023). Advances in RF pulse design, notably through artificial intelligence-driven methodologies like DeepRF, have introduced innovative waveform configurations that optimize energy use and enhance magnetization control, promising improved imaging outcomes and reduced operational costs (Shin *et al.*, 2021). Because MRI technology is advancing, improving RF pulses is still essential, since it helps make the method more adaptable and efficient for medical use.

8.1.3. Image Formation Process

In MRI, images are made by the interaction of nuclear magnetic moments with external magnetic fields, which shows detailed pictures of the inside of the body. At first, the patient is put in a strong, even magnetic field that helps the protons in the body line up. Radiofrequency pulses disturb the protons' alignment, which makes them give off signals as they go back to their normal state. The signals sent out are picked up and processed to make contrast images. The ability of MRI to noninvasively visualize water content and tissue characteristics at a micrometer scale allows for precise monitoring of physiological and pathological processes, as demonstrated in studies of embolism formation and recovery in plant stems (Ahrens *et al.*, 2013). Additionally, advancements such as Fusion Imaging combine MRI data with ultrasonography, enhancing diagnostic accuracy in complex fields like gynecology (Bellati *et al.*, 2018). Thus, the formation of MRI images is a sophisticated process integrating physics and computational techniques to provide critical clinical insights (Figure 8.6).

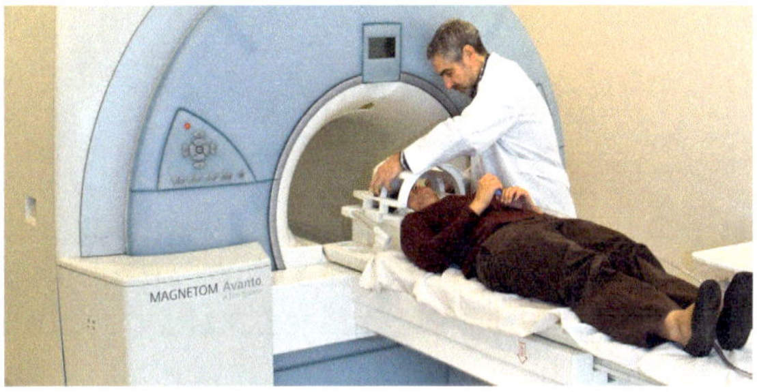

Figure 8.6. Radiofrequency pulses then perturb alignment, causing the protons to emit signals as they return to their equilibrium state.

Source: https://images.theconversation.com/files/29647/original/gxp3tcjs-1377055247.jpg?ixlib=rb-4.1.0&rect=292%2C399%2C2459%2C1194&q=45&auto=format&w=1356&h=668&fit=crop.

8.1.4. Types of Magnetic Resonance Imaging (MRI) Sequences

Knowing the details of different MRI sequences helps improve the accuracy of diagnosis and choose the right imaging plan for different cases. MRI sequences manipulate parameters such as repetition time (TR) and echo time (TE) to highlight different tissue contrasts, enabling the differentiation of anatomical structures and pathological changes. Usually, T1-weighted images are taken to highlight anatomy and fat, T2-weighted images to highlight fluids and swelling and proton density images to show both clearly. Advanced sequences such as diffusion-weighted imaging (DWI) and functional MRI (fMRI) offer insights into cellular density and brain activity, respectively. Moreover, the integration of contrast agents, notably in core-shell nanoparticle forms, has enhanced the capability of MRI to detect molecular and cellular phenomena (Jenjob *et al.*, 2020). In addition, MRI protocols must consider specific patient factors, especially during pandemics, where imaging prioritization and protective measures are paramount to minimize risk, underscoring the role of tailored and judicious use of MRI sequences (Kirkpatrick *et al.*, 2020).

8.1.5. Contrast Agents used in Magnetic Resonance Imaging (MRI)

The progress of MRI technology depends a lot on developing contrast agents that help improve the quality and focus of images. Mainly, contrast agents used in MRI are gadolinium-based and they help identify tissues by changing the way they relax. Recent research shows that carbon nanotubes linked to organic molecules may be used as new MRI contrast agents. They have better binding properties and can be customized which helps produce more detailed images and accurate diagnostics.

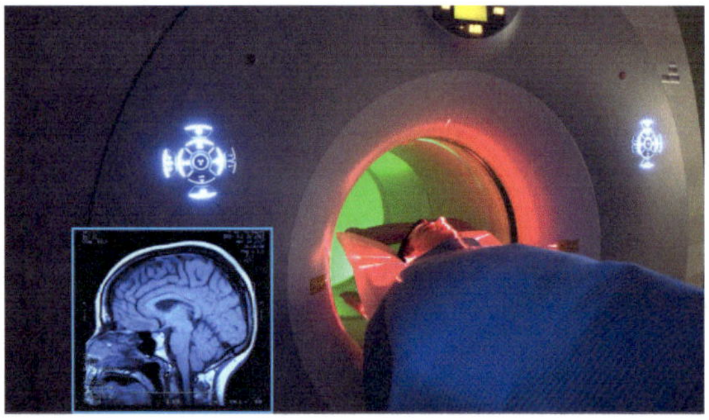

Figure 8.7. MRI contrast agents.

Source: https://cdn.labmanager.com/assets/articleNo/5088/iImg/32764/c655703a-980c-40e7-8773-0cd2c3696bdc-feb15-2018-nibib-1-istock-mri.jpg.

Computational studies using dispersion-corrected Density Functional Theory have shown that interactions between carbon nanotubes and aromatic molecules significantly influence adhesion strength and, consequently, imaging efficacy (Lado-Touri Iño, 2023). Additionally, multifunctional nanomaterials engineered with fluorescent tags and metal cores offer integrated diagnostic and therapeutic capabilities, especially in challenging applications like brain imaging, while emphasizing biocompatibility and minimal toxicity (Thangam *et al.*, 2021). Such innovations promise to revolutionize MRI by enhancing both visualization and personalized disease management (Figure 8.7).

8.1.6. Signal-to-noise Ratio in Magnetic Resonance Imaging (MRI)

Achieving high-quality magnetic resonance imaging hinges significantly on optimizing the signal-to-noise ratio (SNR), which directly influences image clarity and diagnostic reliability. Issues like electromagnetic interference and flaws in equipment can reduce SNR, which causes images to be distorted or not informative. Addressing these issues involves strategies such as narrowing receiver bandwidth, careful planning of scanning parameters, and editing corrupted k-space data to mitigate interference effects, as shown in studies involving adapted clinical scanners for specialized imaging tasks like sodium MRI (Tarasova *et al.*, 2024). Moreover, advancements in MRI technology, including the employment of ultra-high-field 7 Tesla systems, have shown promise in enhancing SNR and spatial resolution. Yet, their adoption remains limited by practical constraints such as high costs and operational complexities (Radojewski *et al.*, 2024). In addition, even though higher field strengths improve imaging, more studies are needed to address these problems and prove that they are useful for clinical use.

8.1.7. Importance of Magnetic Field Strength

The accuracy and clarity of MRI images are very much affected by the strength of the magnetic field used during the scan. Improved signal-to-noise ratios due to stronger magnetic fields improve the visibility of fine details in images. This is particularly critical when analyzing complex structures or subtle physiological changes, such as quantifying liver fat content in patients with hepatic steatosis, where precise measurement can influence diagnostic outcomes and treatment strategies (Kavanaugh *et al.*, 2017). Additionally, higher magnetic field strengths enable faster image acquisition, making dynamic monitoring of internal processes more feasible, as seen in 3D analysis of porous media and fluid flow within biological systems (Haynes *et al.*, 2012). Yet, there are some practical problems, for example, the cost can rise, and it becomes more difficult to handle higher field strengths. Yet, the key role magnetic field strength has in improving MRI's usefulness for diagnosis and research makes it very important in both clinical and experimental settings.

8.1.8. Artifacts in Magnetic Resonance Imaging (MRI) Imaging

The quality and usefulness of magnetic resonance images are often reduced by artifacts that show up in the images. They are caused by patient motion, the limits of the equipment, and the physical limitations of imaging. Advanced reconstruction techniques have been developed to mitigate such errors; for instance, novel calibration-less parallel imaging methods simultaneously estimate coil profiles and image content, thereby reducing artifacts caused by data inconsistencies and undersampling while maintaining rapid acquisition speeds (Holme *et al.*, 2018). However, emerging contrast mechanisms such as RASER imaging introduce new complexities; despite offering enhanced contrast through cooperative nonlinear interactions, these methods generate artifacts like amplitude distortions and side lobes that extend beyond the imaging domain (Adams *et al.*, 2022). Understanding and addressing these artifact sources is crucial for refining MRI techniques, ensuring that enhanced image contrast does not come at the expense of compromised image reliability, ultimately facilitating more accurate clinical assessments (Figure 8.8).

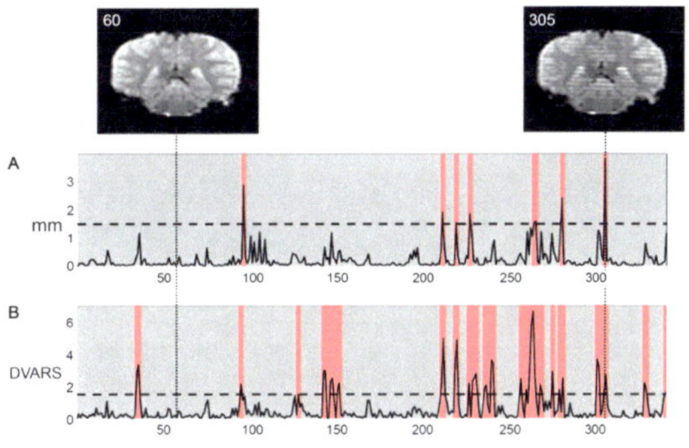

Figure 8.8. The fidelity of magnetic resonance imaging is frequently challenged by artifacts that compromise image quality and diagnostic accuracy.

Source: https://www.frontiersin.org/files/Articles/221501/fneur-08-00232-HTML/image_m/fneur-08-00232-g001.jpg.

8.1.9. Advances in Magnetic Resonance Imaging (MRI) Technology

Innovations in quantum technology and advanced computing have made magnetic resonance imaging much better at diagnosing conditions. Using quantum principles has made it possible to enhance both the resolution and sensitivity of imaging which aids in seeing soft tissues and small changes in the body more accurately. The advanced hardware and software taking advantage of quantum coherence and spin dynamics allow these improvements to go beyond the limits of traditional MRI. Quantum sensors and advanced radiofrequency coils help images be taken more quickly and with less noise which benefits both patients and the speed of the process. Ongoing research programs are exploring how quantum electromechanical systems and coherent quantum electronics can be harnessed to push MRI technology further, potentially transforming it into a tool with unparalleled precision and versatility in clinical settings (MacFarlane *et al.*, 2002). While challenges remain, these advances underscore a promising future, affirming MRI's continued evolution as a cornerstone of medical imaging (Berry *et al.*, 2016).

Test Your Knowledge

1. For what reason are gradient coils used in MRI scanners?
2. In what situations are MRI contrast agents indicated?

8.2. Clinical Applications of Magnetic Resonance Imaging (MRI)

Learning Outcome

1. Understand neurological imaging;
2. Explain musculoskeletal imaging;
3. Focus on cardiovascular imaging;
4. Learn oncological imaging;
5. Discuss abdominal and pelvic imaging;
6. Understand pediatric applications of MRI;
7. Define functional MRI (fMRI);
8. Describe diffusion-weighted imaging;
9. Discuss MRI in preoperative planning.

Advancements in imaging technologies have significantly enhanced the diagnostic capabilities within clinical medicine, especially in the context of neurological and cardiovascular disorders. fMRI, particularly resting-state fMRI, has become instrumental in identifying functional biomarkers that aid in diagnosing and prognosticating neurological diseases, leveraging large multisite datasets despite challenges related to data heterogeneity (Yang *et al.*, 2022). Additionally, four-dimensional (4D) flow MRI represents a major leap forward in cardiovascular imaging by offering comprehensive visualization and quantification of hemodynamic parameters beyond traditional two-dimensional methods. This enables detailed assessment of blood flow dynamics, wall shear stress, and pressure gradients, which are crucial for understanding cardiac and vascular pathologies (Zhuang *et al.*, 2021). This shows that MRI is flexible and central to improving patient care through detailed and non-invasive images, which help doctors create personalized treatment plans for many medical conditions.

8.2.1. Neurological Imaging

Thanks to new imaging tools, neurology now offers much better ways to see the brain and its workings. MRI at 7 Tesla has improved the ability to distinguish between tissues, which has made the diagnosis more accurate. Because of this, it is possible to detect small changes in the brain that are not seen with traditional methods, which helps improve both diagnosis and treatment in neurological diseases. For example, in pediatric neuroimaging, 7 T MRI demonstrates feasibility despite concerns about safety and patient comfort, indicating its potential to revolutionize clinical practice and research in younger populations (Arachchige *et al.*, 2024). In addition, the use of advanced MRI methods, such as resting-state functional MRI and magnetic resonance spectroscopy, gives useful information about the changes in the brain that happen in epilepsy. These innovations, sometimes combined with machine learning approaches, improve presurgical planning and treatment monitoring, underscoring MRI's pivotal role in personalized neurological care (Desale *et al.*, 2024) (Figure 8.9).

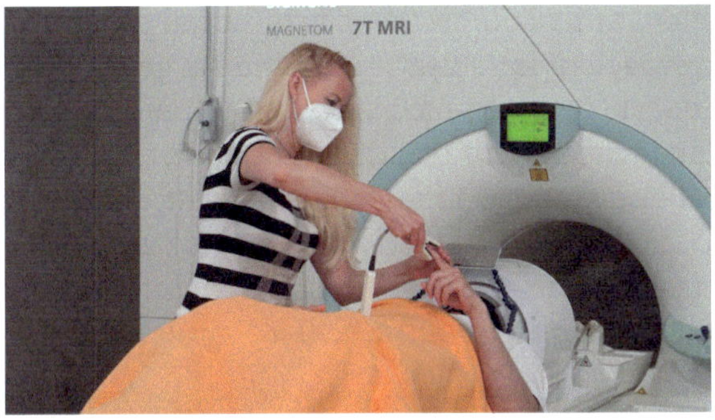

Figure 8.9. Magnetic resonance imaging (MRI), particularly at high magnetic field strengths such as 7 Tesla, has pushed the boundaries of diagnostic accuracy by offering superior resolution and tissue contrast.

Source: https://cloudfront.jove.com/CDNSource/teasers/62142.jpg.

8.2.2. Musculoskeletal Imaging

Better imaging technologies have greatly improved how doctors diagnose different medical conditions, especially those related to complex tissue structures. Because the musculoskeletal system is made up of bones, muscles, and connective tissues, it is very challenging to image using medical technology. MRI is now the top choice for imaging musculoskeletal problems because it gives clear images without using ionizing radiation. Emerging diffusion MRI techniques have shown promise in detecting subtle microstructural changes in bone, such as those associated with osteoporosis, expanding the diagnostic scope beyond conventional imaging (Capuani *et al.*, 2015). Additionally, the integration of MRI with therapeutic technologies like MRI-guided focused ultrasound surgery offers a cutting-edge combination of precise imaging and minimally invasive treatment for musculoskeletal disorders, facilitating real-time monitoring and targeted intervention (Albisinni *et al.*, 2015). All of these improvements stress the key part MRI plays in diagnosis and new approaches to musculoskeletal care.

8.2.3. Cardiovascular Imaging

Better imaging methods have greatly improved how cardiovascular diseases are diagnosed and managed, and cardiovascular MRI is very important in this process. It is possible to see the structure and function of the heart in great detail, allowing clinicians to tell which areas are still healthy and which are not. Beyond viability assessment, cardiovascular MRI provides crucial insights into the underlying etiology of various cardiac disorders, guiding treatment decisions and prognostic evaluations (Yilmaz *et al.*, 2011). For ST-segment elevation myocardial infarction, cardiovascular MRI is now essential for assessing new therapies that aim to reduce the infarct size and prevent harmful changes in the heart. Multiparametric mapping techniques further enhance understanding of myocardial edema, microvascular obstruction, and hemorrhage, showcasing the complex pathophysiological changes post-infarction (Arai *et al.*, 2018). Consequently, cardiovascular MRI stands as an essential, non-invasive tool that improves clinical outcomes and expands the scope of cardiac imaging beyond traditional limitations (Figure 8.10).

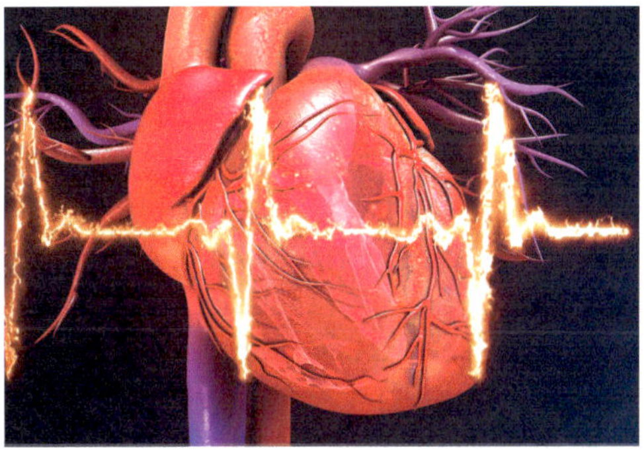

Figure 8.10. Cardiovascular MRI provides crucial insights into the underlying etiology of various cardiac disorders.

Source: https://www.acc.org//-/media/Non-Clinical/Images/2023/06/CARDIOLOGY/28/Heart-Failure-1200x800.jpg.

8.2.4. Oncological Imaging

Better imaging tools have greatly improved both diagnosis and treatment in oncology, mainly because of MRI. Unlike standard imaging, multiparametric MRI uses different techniques to better understand how a tumor looks and works, a capability not available with traditional scans. Diffusion-weighted MRI (DW-MRI) exemplifies this by capturing microstructural variations within cancerous tissues, enabling differentiation based on cellular density and vascularization—key features in tumor characterization and treatment monitoring. Thanks to new techniques in DW-MRI, such as intravoxel incoherent motion and diffusion kurtosis imaging, it is now possible to map microstructures and correlate them well to histological findings, which improves the accuracy of diagnosis. Also, because MRI does not use ionizing radiation, it is safer for repeated use in patients with cancer than CT scans. Despite these advancements, challenges in standardization and accessibility persist, underscoring the need for continued research and training to fully realize MRI's potential in oncological imaging (Fokkinga *et al.*, 2023; Masino *et al.*, 2024).

8.2.5. Abdominal and Pelvic Imaging

Improved imaging methods have greatly improved the way abdominal and pelvic conditions are diagnosed by revealing detailed information about their structures and problems. Because MRI can clearly show soft tissues and does not use ionizing radiation, it is very useful in these areas. With this method, doctors can detect various problems, for example, tumors, inflammation, and abnormalities in blood vessels, which support their decisions. Moreover, the integration of hybrid imaging technologies like PET/MRI further enriches the diagnostic process by combining metabolic and anatomical information, thus improving the characterization of pelvic and upper abdominal tumors and inflammation (Sollini *et al.*, 2018). Such innovations complement traditional diagnostic approaches found in Ayurvedic surgery, where modern imaging modalities now augment the visualization and treatment planning rooted in ancient medical knowledge (Das *et al.*, 2024). Collectively, these advances reinforce MRI's critical role in comprehensive abdominal and pelvic imaging (Figure 8.11).

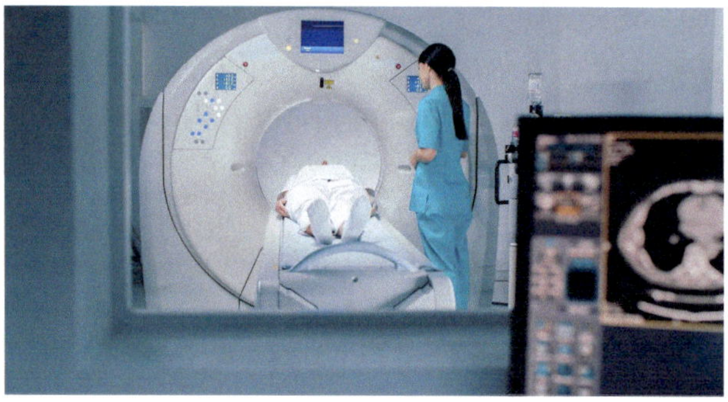

Figure 8.11. Advancements in imaging techniques have profoundly transformed the diagnostic landscape for abdominal and pelvic conditions, offering unparalleled insights into complex anatomical and pathological states.

Source: https://www.diagnopein.com/img/Radiology/CT%20SCAN%20machine%20wit%20patients.jpg.

8.2.6. Pediatric Applications of Magnetic Resonance Imaging (MRI)

Improvements in imaging have greatly changed how pediatric care is provided, particularly through the use of MRI. Hybrid PET/MRI in children with malignant musculoskeletal tumors has made it easier to stage the disease and monitor treatment since it combines metabolic information from PET with MRI's excellent soft-tissue images. This fusion not only improves diagnostic accuracy but also reduces ionizing radiation exposure, a critical consideration for pediatric patients requiring repeated imaging over time (de Heras *et al.*, 2024). Apart from oncology, multi-parametric and multi-nuclear MRI can now be used to non-invasively assess the whole kidney function in children. These innovative methods evaluate tissue characteristics such as perfusion, oxygenation, and fibrosis and reveal metabolic processes at the cellular level, supporting early disease detection and personalized management without relying on invasive biopsies or radiation (de Mul *et al.*, 2024). All of these uses of MRI in children point to a major change in how medical imaging is done for childhood illnesses.

8.2.7. Functional MRI (fMRI)

Because of improvements in magnetic resonance imaging, doctors can now see the body's structures and their function. fMRI is notable among these tools because it can detect blood oxygen changes in the brain, which helps connect specific brain regions to their functions. Unlike anatomical MRI, fMRI helps researchers and clinicians study the brain's blood flow, which makes it possible to study mental functions, brain diseases, and healing after injury. This technique leverages the blood-oxygen-level-dependent (BOLD) contrast, which reflects alterations in deoxyhemoglobin concentration during neural activation. Because fMRI has both high spatial and temporal resolution, it allows doctors to study brain function without surgery, which greatly helps in making diagnoses and choosing treatments. Moreover, developments in simultaneous multimodal imaging, such as combining PET with MRI, are poised to further enrich functional assessment by merging metabolic and anatomical data, highlighting the evolving versatility of MRI technologies (Sabbaghan *et al.*, 2025). Although primarily focused on neurological applications, functional imaging principles are increasingly influencing other MRI domains, demonstrating MRI's dynamic role in comprehensive biomedical investigation (Press *et al.*, 2025) (Figure 8.12).

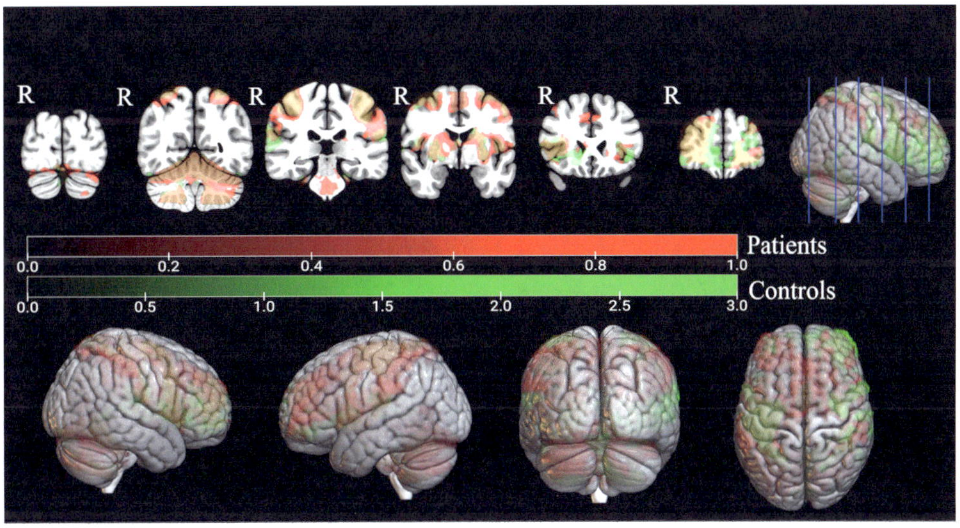

Figure 8.12. The integration of high spatial and temporal resolution in functional MRI (fMRI) facilitates noninvasive exploration of brain function, significantly enhancing diagnostic and therapeutic strategies.

Source: https://www.researchgate.net/publication/344754492/figure/fig2/AS:948471934767105@1603144739106/fMRI-activation-maps-during-the-right-hand-finger-tapping-clusters-are-marked-in-red-for.png.

8.2.8. Diffusion-weighted Imaging (DWI)

The development of DWI has made it possible to see the structure of tissues at an excellent level. It distinguishes itself by being sensitive to changes in cellular structure and number, which is why it is very useful for early diagnosis and distinguishing between diseases. For instance, in neurological disorders, DWI facilitates the identification of microstructural degeneration and connectivity disruptions that traditional MRI methods might miss, enhancing diagnostic accuracy and enabling improved monitoring of disease progression (Ortega-Robles *et al.*, 2025). Similarly, in oncological applications, DWI combined with apparent diffusion coefficient (ADC) mapping enhances the detection and characterization of malignancies, such as carcinoma of the gallbladder, by distinguishing between benign and malignant tissues based on water diffusion patterns (Dudhe *et al.*, 2024). So, DWI is a major advancement for MRI because it provides valuable numbers that help guide diagnosis and treatment decisions.

8.2.9. Magnetic Resonance Imaging (MRI) in Preoperative Planning

Planning before surgery is essential, and precise images are needed to help choose the best treatment options. Because of its ability to clearly show soft tissues and use many imaging techniques, MRI has become an important tool for this purpose. For example, in endometrial cancer, MRI combining T2-weighted imaging with DWI or dynamic contrast-enhanced MRI (DCE-MRI) significantly enhances the assessment of myometrial invasion depth, which is crucial for determining the extent of surgery needed. Studies demonstrate that T2WI combined with either DWI or DCE-MRI achieves much higher diagnostic accuracy compared to T2WI alone, guiding surgical decisions more effectively without additional contrast administration when using DWI (Raja *et al.*, 2024). Similarly, in breast cancer, while preoperative MRI provides detailed tumor visualization, its routine use may increase mastectomy rates without improving survival or reducing reoperation rates, highlighting the importance of balancing imaging benefits against clinical outcomes during surgical planning (Mota *et al.*, 2023) (Figure 8.13).

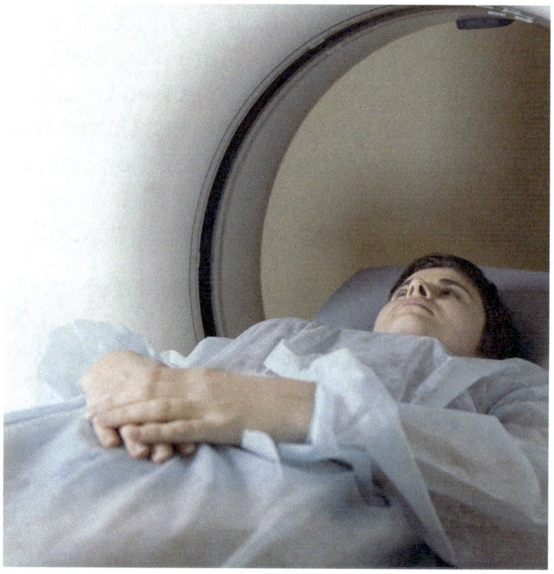

Figure 8.13. Magnetic resonance imaging (MRI) in preoperative planning.

Source: https://www.medica.de/medicacache/picf/8/0/4/9/273015535117 59/MRT_Bildgebung_panthermedia-net-craig-robinson-sharepic_facebook_1200x1200-.jpg.

Test Your Knowledge

1. What are the usual reasons doctors order a brain MRI?
2. How is MRI used in spinal cord evaluation?
3. What is the role of MRI in musculoskeletal imaging?

8.3. Safety and Risks Associated with Magnetic Resonance Imaging (MRI)

Learning Outcome

1. Learn contraindications for MRI;
2. Identify risks of claustrophobia;
3. Know the safety of contrast agents;
4. Discuss potential effects of magnetic fields;
5. Focus on patient screening protocols;
6. Describe the role of MRI technologists in safety;
7. Define guidelines for MRI in special populations;
8. Perform emergency procedures during MRI;
9. Identify long-term effects of MRI exposure.

The progress in MRI technology has helped medical diagnostics, but it has also made people with implanted devices and electrodes more at risk. It has been demonstrated that intracranial electrodes may cause risks by applying mechanical pressure, heating tissue, and delivering electrical stimulation during MRI scans because of their interaction with magnetic and radiofrequency fields. Experimental evaluations have revealed that excessive tissue heating can occur, but these effects can be mitigated through specific precautions like limiting specific absorption rates and careful positioning of electrodes and cables, ensuring temperature increases remain within safe margins (Allen *et al.*, 2010). Additionally, while historically MR imaging was contraindicated for patients with pacemakers and implantable cardioverter-defibrillators (ICDs), recent improvements in device design and protective measures have allowed select patients to safely undergo MRI scans under controlled conditions (Ariel *et al.*, 2005). Because of this, it is necessary to keep researching and use strict safety measures to ensure MRI is used safely and effectively in medicine.

8.3.1. Contraindications for Magnetic Resonance Imaging (MRI)

Although MRI is very useful for diagnosis, its risks must be considered by paying attention to the list of contraindications to keep patients safe. A main worry is about metal implants or foreign objects, which could be moved or heated by the strong magnetic fields. For instance, specific breast biopsy clips have been rigorously assessed for safety in ultra-high-field 7 Tesla MRI scanners, demonstrating minimal magnetic susceptibility and negligible heating effects, thereby confirming their compatibility when appropriate imaging protocols are followed (Dong *et al.*, 2024). Additionally, particular patient populations require vigilance; although MRI appears generally safe even for vulnerable groups such as preterm infants, standard protocols remain essential to monitor vital signs and mitigate any risks during scanning (Falsaperla *et al.*, 2024). Ultimately, contraindications for MRI encompass a spectrum of considerations, including device safety, patient condition, and scanner specifications, all critical to optimizing imaging efficacy while minimizing harm (Figure 8.14).

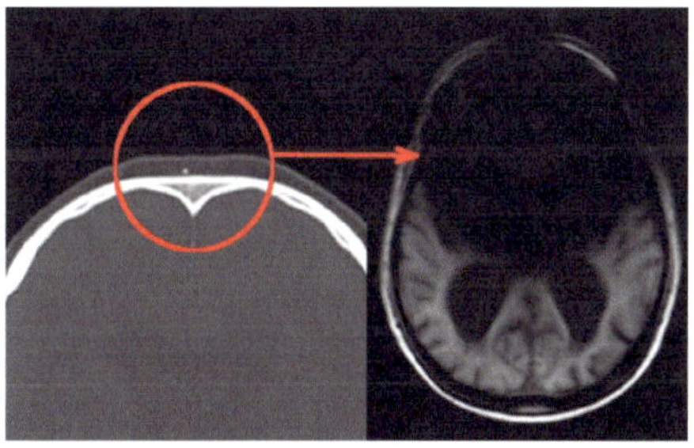

Figure 8.14. Metallic implants or foreign bodies, which may interact adversely with the strong magnetic fields, potentially causing displacement or heating.

Source: https://www.researchgate.net/publication/334168340/figure/fig2/AS:1086083811029007@1635953967255/Interactions-of-an-MRI-scanner-and-a-small-metal-foreign-body-The-size-of-the-foreign.jpg.

8.3.2. Risks of Claustrophobia

Having to lie inside the tight space of an MRI scanner can make patients feel very anxious, especially those who are claustrophobic, which can reduce the effectiveness of the test. Patients who feel claustrophobic might move a lot, which can create motion artifacts that reduce the accuracy of the imaging and the test results. Having to remain still and confined in a narrow tube for a long time causes many patients' distress, which is a significant problem with MRI technology. Although alternatives such as oral contrast agent-assisted ultrasound are being explored to lessen the reliance on MRI for certain diagnoses, especially in resource-limited settings, these approaches are not universally applicable (Ji *et al.*, 2024). Having claustrophobia can be uncomfortable for patients, and it sometimes causes the scan to be incomplete, which requires the procedure to be repeated, raising costs and delaying the diagnosis. Balancing the superior diagnostic capabilities of MRI with patient tolerance remains a critical consideration, especially compared to faster and less confining modalities such as CT, which may be preferred in acute settings despite lower soft tissue resolution (Shah *et al.*, 2024).

8.3.3. Safety of Contrast Agents

Contrast agents have played a big role in improving the image quality and accuracy of MRI results. Because of their effectiveness and low toxicity, gadolinium-based compounds have been the preferred choice for a long time and are well known for their safety. As a result, more attention is being given to gadolinium staying in body tissues and the chance of nephrogenic systemic fibrosis in at-risk individuals, which has led to the search for other agents. One promising substitute is manganese (II)-based contrast agents, which exhibit favorable physicochemical properties and a more benign toxicity profile. Recent studies demonstrate that Mn (II)-disubstituted symmetrical complexes with dithiocarbamate ligands offer comparable relaxivity and contrast enhancement to gadolinium agents when tested at clinical magnetic field strengths. This suggests manganese complexes could provide a safer option, reducing adverse effects associated with gadolinium without compromising imaging quality (Boschi *et al.*, 2023). Continued evaluation of such alternatives is critical for optimizing patient safety in MRI diagnostics (Figure 8.15).

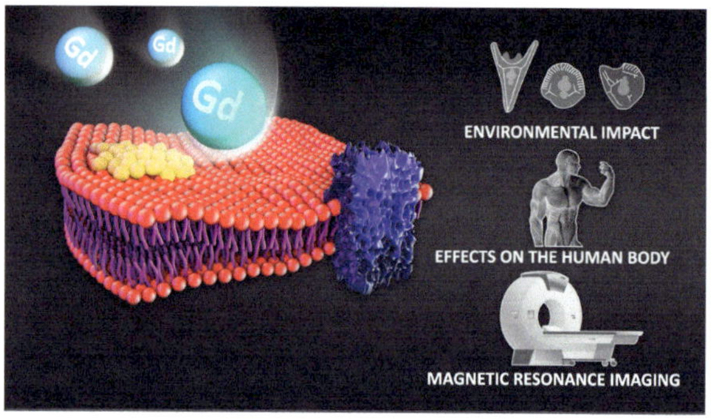

Figure 8.15. Gadolinium-based compounds have long been favored due to their effectiveness and relatively low toxicity, establishing a well-documented safety profile.

Source: https://pub.mdpi-res.com/molecules/molecules-25-05762/article_deploy/html/images/molecules-25-05762-ag.png?1607485031.

8.3.4. Potential Effects of Magnetic Fields

MRI technology involving magnetic fields brings up issues about safety at work and the quality of the images produced. Because of the strong static magnetic fields in MRI, the movement of people nearby can lead to the creation of electric fields in the body, which may be dangerous for workers who are often close to the scanners. Studies employing motion analysis in simulated MRI workspaces have demonstrated that induced electric fields remain below thresholds set by European safety directives, suggesting current operational protocols effectively mitigate these risks for radiographers and cleaners (Abbate *et al.*, 2021). Furthermore, advancements in ultrahigh field MRI, such as 7 Tesla systems, enhance signal-to-noise ratios and imaging resolution, yet also present challenges, including inhomogeneous magnetic fields and increased energy absorption in tissues (Lawrence *et al.*, 2013). Because of these difficulties, it is important to regularly review the effects of magnetic fields in MRI to ensure both safety and good diagnostic results.

8.3.5. Patient Screening Protocols

Using the right patient screening approach helps make the most of MRI and prevents unneeded procedures and risks.

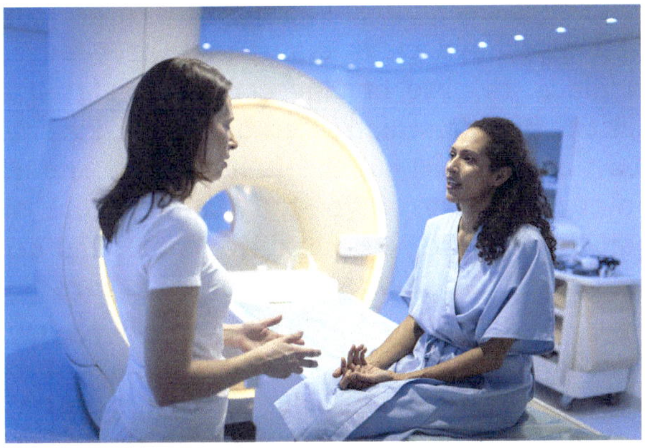

Figure 8.16. Prior to undergoing magnetic resonance imaging (MRI), patients must be evaluated for contraindications such as implanted metallic devices, claustrophobia, or renal impairment related to contrast agents.

Source: https://www.health.com/thmb/MAawMgTvQYXyPZ9EpnRmKXyjaNM=/1500x0/filters:no_upscale():max_bytes(150000):strip_icc()/Health-GettyImages-1318505557-7cff218737e84f778729d7ae6fb359ea.jpg.

People having an MRI should be tested for conditions that may prevent the procedure, such as metal implants, fear of being in small spaces, or kidney problems with contrast agents. In the context of prostate cancer, multiparametric MRI (mpMRI) has become a critical tool for initial assessment, facilitating better detection and localization compared to traditional biopsy methods. Screening protocols that incorporate mpMRI can enhance accuracy by identifying significant lesions and guiding targeted biopsies, thus reducing overdiagnosis and overtreatment associated with less specific tests (Cabarrus *et al.*, 2017). Furthermore, mpMRI's reliability in correlating with histopathologic findings at radical prostatectomy highlights its importance in patient selection and treatment planning (Duncan *et al.*, 2018). Incorporating these advanced imaging techniques into screening guidelines improves clinical outcomes and personalized management strategies (Figure 8.16).

8.3.6. Role of Magnetic Resonance Imaging (MRI) Technologists in Safety

Patient safety during magnetic resonance imaging is achieved through careful preparation and constant monitoring, which are mainly the duties of MRI technologists. They have to assess patients for conditions such as claustrophobia, implanted devices, and other safety concerns, because these can impact whether the imaging procedure can be done safely and successfully. For instance, patients with cardiac implantable electronic devices require special protocols to prevent adverse events, necessitating technologists' familiarity with device-specific guidelines to safely conduct scans without compromising device function (Lanz *et al.*, 2024). Additionally, technologists play a critical role in managing patient comfort and communication, which can reduce scan cancellations and improve completion rates, especially when addressing common concerns like claustrophobia and physical discomfort (Manuweera *et al.*, 2024). Being skilled in technology and patient care helps them handle risks, ensure safety, and carry out accurate imaging in many different clinical settings.

8.3.7. Guidelines for Magnetic Resonance Imaging (MRI) in Special Populations

It is important to use modified guidelines when doing magnetic resonance imaging on pediatric and anxious adult patients. In pediatric cases, preoperative MRI plays a crucial role in assessing anatomical parameters, like tendon cross-sectional area and thickness, to predict autograft suitability before anterior cruciate ligament reconstruction, highlighting the need for precise imaging protocols that accommodate developmental differences and minimize scanning time (Vivekanantha *et al.*, 2024).

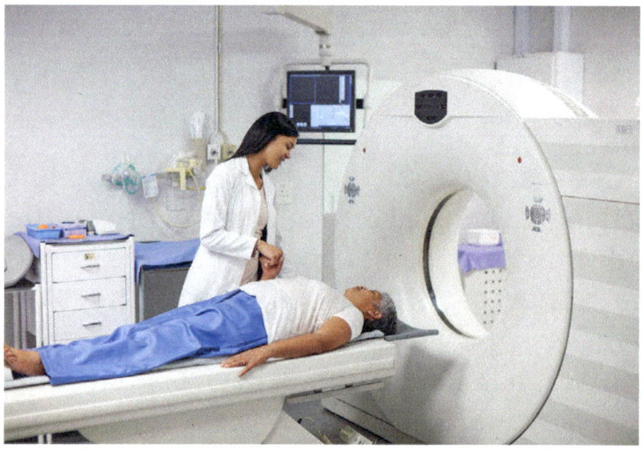

Figure 8.17. For adults who may experience anxiety or require immobility during the procedure, sedation strategies involving agents such as fentanyl, butorphanol, and midazolam must be carefully selected based on their pharmacological profiles, balancing effective sedation with patient safety.

Source: https://www.verywellhealth.com/thmb/6IlSVz9YaHxZ5KUTWcFID0XmVHg=/1500x0/filters:no_upscale():max_bytes(150000):strip_icc()/it-ll-be-over-before-you-know-it-512702076-599cf073aad52b001104b457.jpg.

For adults who may experience anxiety or require immobility during the procedure, sedation strategies involving agents such as fentanyl, butorphanol, and midazolam must be carefully selected based on their pharmacological profiles, balancing effective sedation with patient safety (Verma *et al.*, 2024). Overall, these guidelines emphasize individualized planning, including sedation administration and imaging parameter adjustments, to optimize MRI outcomes across diverse patient groups, ultimately improving both comfort and diagnostic accuracy in special populations (Figure 8.17).

8.3.8. Emergency Procedures During Magnetic Resonance Imaging (MRI)

Because of the special risks during magnetic resonance imaging, it is important to prepare well and have clear emergency procedures in place. In case of emergency, such as if a patient becomes distressed or has an adverse reaction to contrast, the first priority should be to get them out of the scanner bore as quickly and safely as possible. People who can spot signs of patient discomfort and have the right knowledge are important for dealing with these situations. Following the standard ways of screening and monitoring also helps prevent emergencies. Emergency response plans must also account for potential complications in vulnerable populations, including infants and young children, whose physical risks during MRI procedures may be less predictable and require tailored interventions (Downie *et al.*, 2009). Institutions are encouraged to implement standardized guidelines and continuous training to uphold safety standards and improve emergency readiness during MRI scans (Seibert *et al.*, 2018).

8.3.9. Long-term Effects of Magnetic Resonance Imaging (MRI) Exposure

Since MRI is widely used in medical diagnostics, especially on adolescents, there have been studies into how it may affect the body over the long term. Experiments with animal models have found that being exposed to MRI during adolescence, along with using substances, can cause sex-related changes in how the brain is connected. For instance, male rats exposed to cannabis vapors during adolescence exhibited significant changes in both functional and structural brain networks detectable through MRI in adulthood, suggesting that MRI can reveal lasting neurodevelopmental impacts that are potentially sex-specific, while females showed minimal changes (Marinho *et al.*, 2024). Besides, the progress in MRI has helped create drug delivery systems such as thermosensitive liposomes filled with chemotherapeutics, which can be released on demand by MRI conditions. These innovations highlight MRI's dual diagnostic and therapeutic roles, yet they emphasize the need to continually assess safety profiles to mitigate any adverse long-term biological effects (Alawak *et al.*, 2019) (Figure 8.18).

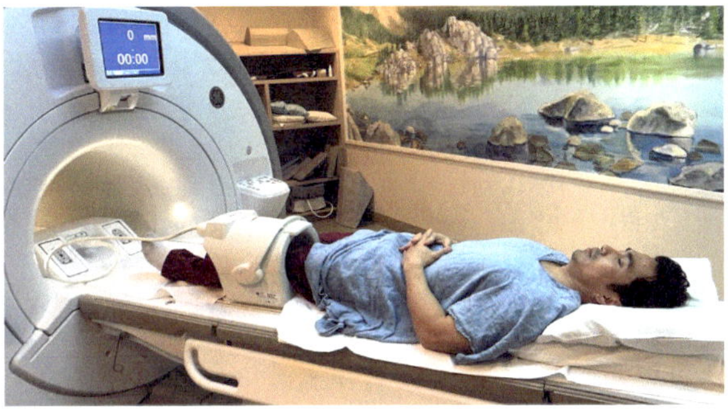

Figure 8.18. The utilization of MRI technology in medical diagnostics has prompted investigations into its long-term effects on biological systems, particularly due to its widespread use in vulnerable populations such as adolescents.

Source: https://health.ucdavis.edu/radiology/images/MYMRI%20ICONS/MR%20Neuro/Joe%20Photos/kneepatient840.jpg.

Test Your Knowledge

1. What are the absolute contraindications for MRI?
2. Why are metal implants a concern in MRI environments?

8.4. Innovations and Future Directions in Magnetic Resonance Imaging (MRI)

Learning Outcome

1. Understand the development of portable MRI machines;
2. Explain advances in imaging speed and resolution;
3. Learn integration of AI in MRI analysis;
4. Discuss new contrast agents and techniques;
5. Focus on MRI-guided interventions;
6. Describe hybrid imaging technologies;
7. Understand research in functional and molecular imaging;
8. Know the expansion of MRI applications in telemedicine;
9. Identify future challenges in MRI technology.

Medical imaging technology is always advancing, which improves the way healthcare is diagnosed and treated. This trend is shown by using MRI with other imaging methods and new technologies, which help doctors see and diagnose problems more clearly. For instance, the combination of MRI with computed tomography (CT) alongside augmented reality (AR) and virtual reality (VR) facilitates the creation of interactive, three-dimensional models that can revolutionize surgical planning and medical education, thereby improving patient outcomes and clinical efficiency (Ziyad *et al.*, 2024). Also, since it is important to spot complex diseases such as pancreatic ductal adenocarcinoma early, new developments in MRI screening are needed. By developing non-invasive, cost-effective biosensors and refining MRI protocols, researchers aim to overcome current limitations related to accessibility, specificity, and time constraints, ultimately contributing to earlier diagnoses and improved prognoses (Sharma *et al.*, 2025). They prove that MRI will continue to be a key and developing tool in medicine.

8.4.1. Development of Portable Magnetic Resonance Imaging (MRI) Machines

The progress made in imaging technology has had a significant impact on Magnetic Resonance Imaging, especially by making portable MRI machines possible. Traditional MRI systems are very effective, but their big size, high price, and complicated infrastructure make them less available in remote or poor areas. New ideas in magnets, processing signals, and machine learning have helped shrink parts of the machine while maintaining its accuracy and picture quality. Because they are portable, these devices can be used more easily at the bedside, in emergencies, and in the field. Moreover, integrating advanced computational methods, including Convolutional Neural Networks, has improved image reconstruction and interpretation, enabling real-time diagnostic support outside conventional clinical environments (Dhami *et al.*, 2008; Firdaus *et al.*, 2024). The ongoing refinement of portable MRI technology marks a pivotal shift toward democratizing advanced medical imaging, potentially transforming healthcare delivery by extending its reach beyond specialized hospital settings to broader populations (Figure 8.19).

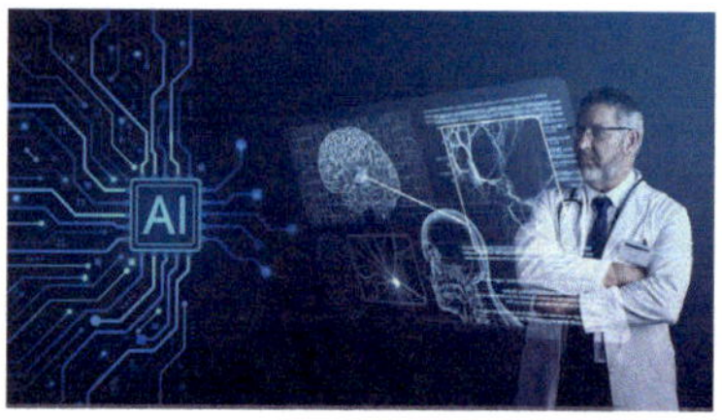

Figure 8.19. Moreover, integrating advanced computational methods, including Convolutional Neural Networks, has improved image reconstruction and interpretation, enabling real-time diagnostic support outside conventional clinical environments.

Source: https://trendsresearch.org/wp-content/uploads/2025/03/AI-in-Mapping-Neural-Pathways-for-Neuroscience.jpg.

8.4.2. Advances in Imaging Speed and Resolution

MRI is always being improved because there is a strong demand for faster scanning without sacrificing the quality of the images. With compressed sensing and parallel imaging, data collection is now much faster, so scans can be done quickly for clinical use with high resolution. Also, ultrahigh-field MRI machines produce better signal-to-noise ratios, making it easier to spot fine anatomical differences and contrast, which are important for early detection of diseases. Even with the improvements, it is still difficult to balance the speed of imaging and its resolution, especially because of artifacts and contrast agent issues at higher field strengths. Newer advanced nanoprobes are proving useful in improving sensitivity and specificity, which helps produce clearer images at ultrahigh fields. Also, using machine learning algorithms makes it possible to automate quality control, which guarantees that the images are of high quality and reliable. Collectively, these advancements underscore a transformative era in MRI, characterized by enhanced diagnostic accuracy and efficiency (Du *et al.*, 2022; Patel *et al.*, 2024).

8.4.3. Integration of Artificial Intelligence (AI) in Magnetic Resonance Imaging (MRI) Analysis

Advances in computing have greatly changed medical imaging, especially by adding artificial intelligence to magnetic resonance imaging analysis. With advanced machine learning and deep learning, AI can detect and describe anomalies in MRI scans faster and more accurately than usual. Because of this merger, it is now easier to find and classify important features that help doctors make more precise medical decisions. But using AI in healthcare is not always easy; since many AI models are not transparent, this can be concerning for their level of understanding and trustworthiness by clinicians. To address this, explainable AI (XAI) frameworks such as Local Interpretable Model-agnostic Explanations (LIME) are being developed and validated to ensure the reliability and transparency of AI-driven insights, thereby increasing clinician confidence and adoption. Overall, the integration of AI in MRI analysis promises significant advancements in patient care, offering more accurate diagnosis and personalized treatment strategies (Khosravi *et al.*, 2024; Md. Hassan *et al.*, 2024) (Figure 8.20).

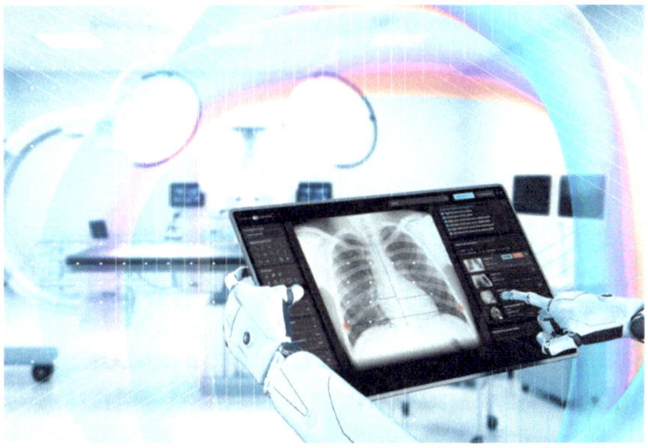

Figure 8.20. Artificial Intelligence (AI) enhances the detection and characterization of anomalies within magnetic resonance imaging (MRI) scans with greater speed and accuracy than traditional methods.

Source: https://www.bgosoftware.com/blog/wp-content/uploads/2024/02/bgo-software-blog-post-size-Role-of-AI-no-title.png.

8.4.4. New Contrast Agents and Techniques

More and more, new ideas in magnetic resonance imaging focus on improving both the quality of the images and the ability to diagnose accurately. Using magnetic nanoparticles as contrast agents helps the vascular half-life, which results in much better images. Their magnetic properties, which are unique to nanoparticles, make them visible under a magnetic field so that doctors can spot fine details of the body more clearly. Also, the size of particles is very important for their function, and smaller particles, about 10 nm across, tend to remain in the body for longer than larger ones. Moreover, applying coatings or dopants to these particles improves their biocompatibility and performance, reduces problems with the materials, and increases safety for clinical use. Alongside these chemical improvements, novel imaging techniques such as parallel imaging and high-capacity gradients facilitate faster acquisition times and higher spatial resolution, collectively advancing MRI's diagnostic power (Eskandari & Kosar, 2020; Nameghi *et al.*, 2016).

8.4.5. Magnetic Resonance Imaging (MRI)-guided Interventions

Because of recent improvements in imaging, minimally invasive procedures can now be used in more cases, and MRI is playing a key role in guiding them. When compared to computed tomography and ultrasonography, MRI gives better contrast for soft tissues and the ability to view images from many directions, which is very useful for discovering lesions in bones and soft tissues. By seeing things more clearly, the doctor can accurately track devices and identify lesions, which helps make musculoskeletal interventions more successful. Although MRI traditionally faced challenges such as motion sensitivity and prolonged acquisition times, the advent of fast imaging sequences has addressed these limitations, thereby increasing its suitability for real-time procedural guidance (Ahrar *et al.*, 2018). Their ability to image anatomy without using ionizing radiation is leading to more MRI-guided interventions, which can be just as good or better than ultrasound guidance in some cases. As the demand for safer, more complex interventional techniques grows, MRI's role in therapeutic procedures is expected to expand, alongside considerations for patient sedation and safety protocols (Bhagavatula *et al.*, 2018) (Figure 8.21).

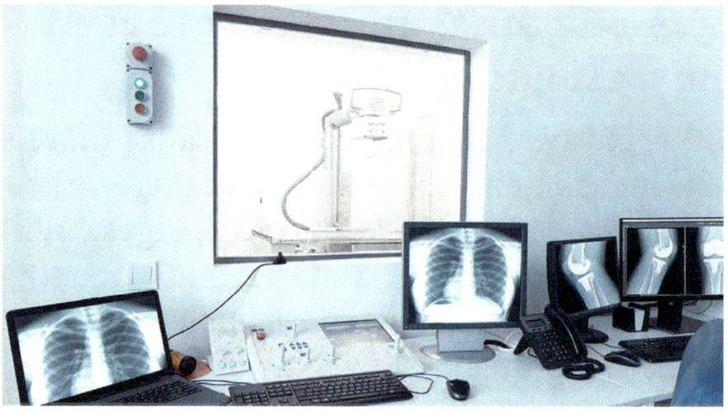

Figure 8.21. MRI-guided interventions are gaining prevalence due to their ability to provide detailed anatomical insights without ionizing radiation.

Source: https://medicalbuyer.co.in/wp-content/uploads/2024/07/Leveraging-cutting-edge-innovations-to-revolutionize-diagnostics.jpg.

8.4.6. Hybrid Imaging Technologies

Because of new developments in medical imaging, several imaging methods are now combined, making it possible to use hybrid imaging to improve the accuracy of disease diagnosis. This is especially true for the combination of PET and MRI, which allows both anatomical and functional details to be gathered in one session. The combination uses MRI's ability to clearly show soft tissues and PET's view of metabolic and molecular changes, giving a full picture of what is happening in the body. In oncology, neurology, and cardiology, such systems have proven useful by helping to identify and describe pathological changes at an earlier stage. Even so, the high costs and technical difficulties involved are keeping many from using these drugs. Continued innovation and clinical validation are critical to overcoming these limitations and maximizing the benefits of hybrid imaging technologies within personalized medicine frameworks (Alsaedi *et al.*, 2024; Rabah *et al.*, 2024).

8.4.7. Research in Functional and Molecular Imaging

Better imaging tools have made it possible to study biological activities and functions in detail, which is very helpful for understanding diseases and their treatments. Especially, using MRI with PET and optoacoustic imaging has allowed for the gathering of different data sets that show both anatomical and physiological changes at the same time. This way of combining MRI, PET, and optoacoustic methods provides a full understanding of diseases inside the body. Research efforts have focused on developing novel contrast agents, including chemical dyes and nanoparticles, which improve the sensitivity and specificity of these combined imaging platforms, especially in small animal brain studies (Ji *et al.*, 2021). Moreover, the emergence of integrated PET/MRI systems facilitates simultaneous data acquisition, though challenges like artifact-free imaging remain under active investigation (Cherry *et al.*, 2008). Such advances are set to change how research and clinical diagnostics are done by improving imaging at the functional and molecular levels.

8.4.8. Expansion of Magnetic Resonance Imaging (MRI) Applications in Telemedicine

Because of technology, healthcare systems now offer more remote diagnostic services, mainly through telemedicine. Because of telemedicine, MRI, which was typically done in hospitals, is now available to people living in areas far from hospitals. This expansion is propelled by innovations in artificial intelligence, which enhance image processing, interpretation accuracy, and workflow efficiency, thus enabling real-time remote consultations and diagnoses (Najjar, 2023). Furthermore, the synergy between AI and the Internet of Medical Things (IoMT) facilitates seamless data transmission and remote operation of MRI systems, making high-quality imaging accessible beyond conventional clinical environments (Manickam *et al.*, 2022). They make it possible for more people to use important diagnostic tools and help patients by reducing wait times, and eliminating the need to go to a clinic. Consequently, the expansion of MRI applications in telemedicine represents a transformative step in contemporary healthcare, amalgamating imaging technology with intelligent systems to deliver more personalized and timely care (Figure 8.22).

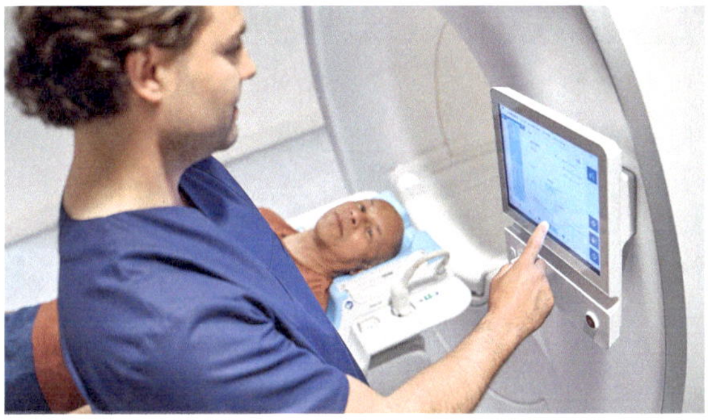

Figure 8.22. Magnetic Resonance Imaging (MRI), traditionally confined to hospital settings, is increasingly leveraged in telemedicine to extend specialized diagnostic services to geographically underserved populations.

Source: https://www.philips.com/c-dam/corporate/innovation-and-you/global/sep-2022/2-operational-efficiency.jpg.

8.4.9. Future Challenges in Magnetic Resonance Imaging (MRI) Technology

Even with great progress in imaging, MRI encounters several challenges that need to be addressed to improve its usefulness and availability in healthcare. A main issue is to cut down scan times without sacrificing image quality, which usually needs new hardware and advanced image reconstruction methods. It is still very important to make sure patients feel comfortable and have less movement during scans, especially children and the elderly. The integration of artificial intelligence offers promising solutions for optimizing imaging protocols and reducing errors, yet issues of algorithm generalizability and regulatory approval persist, complicating widespread clinical adoption (David-Olawade *et al.*, 2025). Besides, if MRI devices could be made both cheaper and portable, they would be much more accessible in places with few resources, but at present, there are technical and engineering barriers to doing so. Ultimately, overcoming these challenges is essential for MRI to continue evolving as a noninvasive, precise diagnostic tool within an increasingly competitive and technologically complex medical imaging landscape (Mahfuz *et al.*, 2024).

Test Your Knowledge

1. How is artificial intelligence being integrated into MRI interpretation?
2. How are MRI scan times being reduced at present?

SUMMARY

It is clear from considering the progress and uses of magnetic resonance imaging that MRI is a key tool in both medical care and research. Its non-invasive nature and capacity for detailed imaging have revolutionized diagnostic capabilities, particularly in areas such as liver fat quantification, which holds significant implications for understanding and treating hepatic steatosis on a global scale (Kavanaugh *et al.*, 2017). The evolution of MRI, including thoughtful adaptations such as the renaming to dissociate from misleading associations, highlights the ongoing balance between scientific progress and public perception (Goldberg *et al.*, 2007). Also, even though MRIs are very helpful, making sure incidental findings are handled properly avoids causing unneeded stress or unnecessary actions. As MRI is improved and used more, it will help both patients and scientists, highlighting its key role in both medical practice and research.

New developments in magnetic resonance imaging have made it much more useful in clinical practice, especially for diagnosing and treating rectal cancer. Traditional MRI methods have made it easier to identify and monitor cancer stages, though it is still difficult to find tumors early, assess the risk, and predict how well treatment will work. The use of advanced functional MRI techniques such as diffusion kurtosis imaging and amide proton transfers-weighted MRI, with radiomics and artificial intelligence, is expected to help better identify and predict outcomes in tumors. AI-based algorithms have shown they can lessen artifacts, reconstruct images, and lower the amount of contrast agent needed, which results in better image quality and safety for patients. Even with these progresses, there are still issues with understanding how these models work and their ability to be used in different situations, which means more research is needed to make them common in daily use. Overall, these developments collectively point toward a future where MRI's diagnostic and predictive power is greatly enhanced, facilitating tailored and more effective treatment strategies (Gong *et al.*, 2025; Melazzini *et al.*, 2025).

KEY TERMS FROM THIS CHAPTER

- Image processing
- Artificial intelligence
- Magnetic field
- Hydrogen nuclei
- Gadolinium
- Sensitivity
- Market
- Perfusion
- Hydrogen protons
- Nuclear magnetic resonance
- Radiofrequency pulses
- Protons
- Manganese
- Knee imaging
- Human error
- Diffusion imaging

CRITICAL THINKING QUESTIONS

1. **What is the primary physical principle behind MRI?**
   a. Ionizing radiation
   b. Ultrasound reflection
   c. Nuclear magnetic resonance
   d. Photoelectric effect
2. **Why are certain nuclei preferred in clinical MRI because they are found in high amounts in the body?**
   a. Carbon-12
   b. Hydrogen (protons)
   c. Oxygen
   d. Phosphorus
3. **Which electromagnetic field is necessary for MRI to work?**
   a. Infrared
   b. Microwave
   c. Strong magnetic field
   d. Gamma rays
4. **What does T1-weighted MRI primarily highlight?**
   a. Fluid content
   b. Fatty tissue
   c. Bone
   d. Air
5. **In what way do contrast agents improve MRI scans?**
   a. Reduce scan time
   b. Enhance tissue contrast
   c. Increase magnetic field strength
   d. Eliminate motion artifacts

Short Answer Questions

1. How does nuclear magnetic resonance contribute to MRI imaging?
2. What types of tissues are best visualized using MRI?
3. Why do clinicians most often focus on hydrogen when using MRI?
4. What is the role of the radiofrequency (RF) pulse in MRI?
5. In what ways do T1- and T2-weighted sequences change the contrast of images?

Answers to Critical Thinking Questions

1. (c); 2. (b); 3. (c); 4. (b); 5. (b)

REFERENCES

1. Abbate, B. F., Acri, G., Caputo, V., Durante, S., Gallias, K. K., Gurrera, D., Iacoviello, G., *et al.* (2021). *Experimental and Modeling Analyses of Human Motion Across the Static Magnetic Field of an MRI Scanner.* https://core.ac.uk/download/638994878.pdf (accessed on 1st June 2025).
2. Adadzi, J., Anderson, II. J., Azi, C. I., Carsrud, *et al.* (2024). Transformative advancements in diagnostic imaging: Reducing risks, enhancing accuracy, and promoting sustainability. *Eur. J. Med. Health Res.* https://core.ac.uk/download/621451782.pdf (accessed on 1st June 2025).
3. Adams, A., Appelt, S., Chekmenev, E. Y., Fleischer, *et al.* (2022). RASER MRI: Magnetic resonance images formed spontaneously exploiting cooperative nonlinear interaction. *Science Advances.* https://core.ac.uk/download/534983585.pdf (accessed on 1st June 2025).
4. Ahrar, K., Sabir, S., Yevich, S., Sheth, R., Ahrar, J., Tam, A., & Stafford, J. (2018). MRI-guided interventions in musculoskeletal system. *Topics in Magnetic Resonance Imaging, 27*, 129–139. https://www.semanticscholar.org/paper/38d348015ab66d463e48ece52dd3dcbc00d3193b (accessed on 1st June 2025).
5. Ahrens, E. T., Melcher, P. J., & Zwieniecki, M. A. (2013). Analysis of spatial and temporal dynamics of xylem refilling in *Acer rubrum* L. using magnetic resonance imaging. *Front Plant Sci.* https://core.ac.uk/download/323069059.pdf (accessed on 1st June 2025).
6. Rabah Al , A. A. A., Binmhusien, M. A., Alotaibi, M. H., & Almalki, B. A. (2024). Magnetic resonance imaging (MRI): Principles, applications, and clinical utility. *Journal of Advances and Scholarly Researches in Allied Education.* https://www.semanticscholar.org/paper/0dc3a9ffe2517f26fe2594acd535b16220255bd6 (accessed on 1st June 2025).
7. Alawak, M. (2019). *Immuno Magnetic Thermosensitive Liposomes for Cancer Therapy.* https://core.ac.uk/download/288436500.pdf (accessed on 1st June 2025).
8. Albisinni, U., Battista, G., Bazzocchi, A., Catalano, *et al.* (2015). *MRI-Guided Focused Ultrasound Surgery in Musculoskeletal Diseases: The Hot Topics.* https://core.ac.uk/download/98341478.pdf (accessed on 1st June 2025).
9. Alkhulaifat, D., Vidal, L., Larsen, E., Serai, S. D., Sinti-Ycochea, M., Mecca, P., Orfe, L., *et al.* (2025). MRI safety—developing the right culture. *Pediatric Radiology.* https://www.semanticscholar.org/paper/71cc274e3255feeba7a1dcbe8beae9440ca36b19 (accessed on 1st June 2025).
10. Allen, P. J., Carmichael, D. W., Lemieux, L., McEvoy, *et al.* (2010). *Feasibility of Simultaneous Intracranial EEG-fMRI in Humans: A Safety Study.* https://core.ac.uk/download/1688787.pdf (accessed on 1st June 2025).
11. Alsaedi, M. H., Joman, F. M. H., Alraddadi, A. F. M., Alharbi, H. N. B. S., Al Amry, M. A. R., Alazhri, H. K., Almaghamsi, M. S., *et al.* (2024). Advancements in magnetic resonance imaging: A systematic review of emerging technologies and clinical applications. *Journal of Ecohumanism.* https://www.semanticscholar.org/paper/566b3fea0146abdc39d670d3498b72fe4ffc6394 (accessed on 1st June 2025).
12. Arai, A. E., Berry, C., Bulluck, H., Dharmakumar, R., *et al.* (2018). Cardiovascular magnetic resonance in acute ST-segment-elevation myocardial infarction: Recent advances, controversies, and future directions. Circulation. https://core.ac.uk/download/158367890.pdf (accessed on 1st June 2025).

13. Barchetti, F., Barchetti, G., Campa, R., Catalano, *et al.* (2018). Negative multiparametric magnetic resonance imaging for prostate cancer: What's next? *European Urology*. https://core.ac.uk/download/154948010.pdf (accessed on 1st June 2025).

14. Bellati, F., Caserta, D., Costanzi, F., De Marco, *et al.* (2018). Real-time virtual sonography in gynecology & obstetrics: Literature's analysis and case series. *Biomed J. Sci. & Tech. Res.* https://core.ac.uk/download/195777140.pdf (accessed on 1st June 2025).

15. Belousova, A. A., Milchakova, E. M., Ogarkova, K. I., Kalakutok, Z. A., Agaloyan, S. V., Makaeva, A. A., Mustafaeva, S. E., *et al.* (2024). Modern high-tech approaches to the diagnosis of gastrointestinal diseases. *Cardiometry*. https://www.semanticscholar.org/paper/214c4f4669bcaae613d48f785791279d54d69371 (accessed on 1st June 2025).

16. Slimane Ben, J., Maqbool, A., Alshammari, A., Choukaier, D., Elsayed, M. S., & Ahmed, R. (2025). Deep learning applications in medical image analysis: Enhancing radiology with automated diagnostic tools. *Communications on Applied Nonlinear Analysis*. https://www.semanticscholar.org/paper/87d6cb5190208ffb5e6fb152763136c6cafffd70 (accessed on 1st June 2025).

17. Berry, C., & Mangion, K. (2016). *Advances in Magnetic Resonance Imaging of the Myocardial Area at Risk and Salvage.* https://core.ac.uk/download/46559873.pdf (accessed on 1st June 2025).

18. Bhagavatula, S., Patel, B., Tuncali, K., Silverman, S., & Shyn, P. (2018). Magnetic resonance imaging and ultrasound-guided percutaneous interventional radiology procedures. *Oxford Medicine Online*. https://www.semanticscholar.org/paper/9088aee7cab18fe60b240fd534f20a15d491f740 (accessed on 1st June 2025).

19. Boschi, A., Calderoni, F., Capozza, M., Carnevale, A., Cazzola, E., Del Bianco, L., Esposito, J., *et al.* (2023). Development and evaluation of the magnetic properties of a new manganese (II) complex: A potential MRI contrast agent. *International Journal of Molecular Sciences*. https://core.ac.uk/download/597836997.pdf (accessed on 1st June 2025).

20. Cabarrus, M. C., & Westphalen, A. C. (2017). Multiparametric magnetic resonance imaging of the prostate—a basic tutorial. *Transl. Androl. Urol.* https://core.ac.uk/download/323063417.pdf (accessed on 1st June 2025).

21. Capuani, S., Iundusi, R., Manenti, G., Tarantino, *et al.* (2015). Focus on diffusion MR investigations of musculoskeletal tissue to improve osteoporosis diagnosis: A brief practical review. *BioMed Research International*. https://core.ac.uk/download/pdf/53866903.pdf (accessed on 1st June 2025).

22. Cherry, S. R., Jacobs, R. E., & Louie, A. Y. (2008). *The Integration of Positron Emission Tomography with Magnetic Resonance Imaging.* https://core.ac.uk/download/4877286.pdf (accessed on 1st June 2025).

23. Das, N. K., & Panday, S. D. (2024). Integrating radiological diagnostic tools in Shalya Tantra: Advancements and clinical applications. *International Journal for Multidisciplinary Research*. https://www.semanticscholar.org/paper/1d88e90cfb6fb61dc23f6171453f317bfab502a2 (accessed on 1st June 2025).

24. David-Olawade, A. C., Olawade, D., Vanderbloemen, L., Rotifa, O. B., Fidelis, S. C., Egbon, E., Akpan, A. O., *et al.* (2025). AI-driven advances in low-dose imaging and enhancement—A review. *Diagnostics, 15*. https://www.semanticscholar.org/paper/44051b152f1c9fdf0599bfc6f3bf4a45b07ac104 (accessed on 1st June 2025).

25. De Mul, A., Schleef, M., Filler, G., McIntyre, C. W., & Lemoine, S. (2024). *In vivo* assessment of pediatric kidney function using multi-parametric and multi-nuclear functional magnetic resonance imaging: Challenges, perspectives, and clinical applications. *Pediatric Nephrology, 40*, 1539–1548. https://www.semanticscholar.org/paper/02495526d1ea03c8b9331f30f957d9cc43bfc6fe (accessed on 1st June 2025).

26. Desale, P., Dhande, R., Parihar, P., Nimodia, D., Bhangale, P. N., & Shinde, D. (2024). Navigating neural landscapes: A comprehensive review of magnetic resonance imaging (MRI) and magnetic resonance spectroscopy (MRS) applications in epilepsy. *Cureus, 16*. https://www.semanticscholar.org/paper/af7e40d432fb8f49784f39b492f7a27b0cdf5a65 (accessed on 1st June 2025).

27. Dhami, S. (2008). *Strategic Analysis of the Commercialization Potential of a Novel Algorithm.* https://core.ac.uk/download/638896345.pdf (accessed on 1st June 2025).

28. Dong, L. (2024). Research on artificial intelligence-assisted magnetic resonance imaging: A review. *Science and Technology of Engineering, Chemistry and Environmental Protection.* https://www.semanticscholar.org/paper/09c72e6c97b3a5bd83cbb1b7b6ad4393ec86a3a3 (accessed on 1st June 2025).

29. Dong, W., Ramchandran, K., Galloy, A., Nino, M. A., Kleingartner, M., Piaszynski, J., Raghavan, M. L., *et al.* (2024). Safety clearance and artifact testing of a nitinol breast biopsy clip in an ultra-high resolution (7 Tesla) magnetic resonance imaging environment. *Indian Journal of Radiology and Imaging.* https://www.semanticscholar.org/paper/4c5fe3f2f00ca100be0ad2f51df4d2aa21efc340 (accessed on 1st June 2025).

30. Downie, J., & Schmidt, M. (2009). Safety first: Recognizing and managing the risks to child participants in magnetic resonance imaging research. https://core.ac.uk/download/568216330.pdf (accessed on 1st June 2025).

31. Drapé, J.-L. (2013). *Advances in Magnetic Resonance Imaging of Musculoskeletal Tumors.* https://core.ac.uk/download/pdf/82501950.pdf (accessed on 1st June 2025).

32. Du, H., Wang, Q., Liang, Z., Li, Q., Li, F., & Ling, D. (2022). Fabrication of magnetic nanoprobes for ultrahigh-field magnetic resonance imaging. *Nanoscale.* https://www.semanticscholar.org/paper/d30ee96fee97f8d7d5312b54fd4f22bb758ca6c1 (accessed on 1st June 2025).

33. Dudhe, S., Mishra, G., Parihar, P., Shinde, D., & Kumari, A. (2024). MRI-based evaluation of carcinoma gallbladder using apparent diffusion coefficient (ADC) and diffusion weighted imaging (DWI). *F1000Research.* https://www.semanticscholar.org/paper/87ed54a32f9f4f8e197f614ce43a235801984c54 (accessed on 1st June 2025).

34. Duncan, I., Goldman, H., Harding, C., McGirr, *et al.* (2018). Accuracy of multiparametric magnetic resonance imaging to detect significant prostate cancer and index lesion location. https://core.ac.uk/download/213607798.pdf (accessed on 1st June 2025).

35. Eskandari, K. (2020). *Magnetic Nanoparticles to Improve the Contrast of Magnetic Resonance Imaging.* https://core.ac.uk/download/483639534.pdf (accessed on 1st June 2025).

36. Falsaperla, R., Marino, S., Ganci, N., Leone, G., Romano, C., Tropea, A., Romeo, P., *et al.* (2024). Magnetic resonance imaging in preterm infant: A systematic review on clinical procedure safety. *Topics in Magnetic Resonance Imaging: TMRI, 33*(1), e0310. https://www.semanticscholar.org/paper/439ad50cc32f4d8b31d22bfe562aadfd5c17c38f (accessed on 1st June 2025).

37. Fıçıcı, C., Koçak, O., & Telatar, Z. (2023). Definition and classification of heart diseases from data obtained with echocardiography Doppler. In *2023 Medical Technologies Congress (TIPTEKNO)*. https://www.semanticscholar.org/paper/e656d554f393408c60c6771f9ab360f65f7c8fac (accessed on 1st June 2025).

38. Fokkinga, E. P., Hernandez-Tamames, J., Ianuş, A., Nilsson, M., Tax, C., Pérez-López, R., & Grussu, F. (2023). Advanced diffusion-weighted MRI for cancer microstructure assessment in body imaging, and its relationship with histology. *Journal of Magnetic Resonance Imaging: JMRI*. https://www.semanticscholar.org/paper/bb6534c835839facd3ce090ea56749b13f62153c (accessed on 1st June 2025).

39. Gallucci, J., Secara, M., Chen, O., Oliver, L. D., Jones, B. D. M., Marawi, T., Foussias, G., *et al.* (2024). A systematic review of structural and functional magnetic resonance imaging studies on the neurobiology of depressive symptoms in schizophrenia spectrum disorders. *Schizophrenia, 10*. https://www.semanticscholar.org/paper/5491a4a40426dfc1900b5ebdea74bf3a531f4c94 (accessed on 1st June 2025).

40. Goldberg, S. (2007). *MRIs and the Perception of Risk*. https://core.ac.uk/download/70373833.pdf (accessed on 1st June 2025).

41. Gong, X., Ye, Z., Shen, Y., & Song, B. (2025). Enhancing the role of MRI in rectal cancer: Advances from staging to prognosis prediction. *European Radiology*. https://www.semanticscholar.org/paper/7bff8daa0c3eac8398a92ce6b580c843f6d2c426 (accessed on 1st June 2025).

42. Hassan, M. R., Hassan, M. M., & Rahman, M. A. (2024). Comparative analysis of LIME and shape analysis techniques in prostate cancer MRI interpretation. In *2024 International Conference on Engineering and Emerging Technologies (ICEET)*. https://www.semanticscholar.org/paper/3241713646d769faffde2e2392b3d6fb6e411828 (accessed on 1st June 2025).

43. Haynes, H., & Holmes, W. M. (2012). Imaging sediment structure: The emerging use of magnetic resonance imaging (MRI) for 3D analysis of sediment structures and internal flow processes. https://core.ac.uk/download/16458489.pdf (accessed on 1st June 2025).

44. Hendi, A. A. H., Bakri, E. G., Dohali, A. A., Thubab, A. A., Ogdi, K. M., Rajhi, H. A., Alharbi, O. A., *et al.* (2023). Development of medical imaging techniques: A review of technological advances in the field of medical imaging, such as magnetic resonance imaging (MRI), computed tomography (CT), and ultrasound imaging (ultrasound). *Journal of Positive Psychology & Wellbeing*. https://core.ac.uk/download/616775441.pdf (accessed on 1st June 2025).

45. Hiremath, S. (2023). Magnetic resonance imaging (MRI): Principles, system, engineering considerations for image optimization, and medical applications. *Progress in Medical Sciences*. https://www.semanticscholar.org/paper/80c7e64367a7599ea51ee3361722f6bc9d18bfde (accessed on 1st June 2025).

46. Holme, H. C. M., Lustig, M., Ong, F., Rosenzweig, *et al.* (2018). *ENLIVE: An Efficient Nonlinear Method for Calibration Less and Robust Parallel Imaging*. http://arxiv.org/abs/1706.09780.

47. Jenjob, R., Phakkeeree, T., & Crespy, D. (2020). Core–shell particles for drug-delivery, bioimaging, sensing, and tissue engineering. *Biomaterials Science, 8*, 2756–2770. https://doi.org/10.1039/c9bm01872g (accessed on 1st June 2025).

48. Ji, B., Ni, R., Ni, R., Shi, X., Kong, Y., & Guan, Y. (2021). Multimodal contrast agents for optoacoustic brain imaging in small animals. *Front. Bioeng. Biotechnol.* https://core.ac.uk/download/482641269.pdf (accessed on 1st June 2025).

49. Ji, J., Shi, X., Xia, Y., Gao, L. Y., Luo, N., Ma, L., Pan, A., *et al.* (2024). Can cereal-based oral contrast agents-assisted ultrasound become an alternative to non-contrast magnetic resonance imaging (MRI) in radiological follow-up for pancreatic cystic lesions? *Quantitative Imaging in Medicine and Surgery, 14*, 5602–5609. https://www.semanticscholar.org/paper/8a52747d0e975efdb9e1ffe7444168c2270f63d2 (accessed on 1st June 2025).

50. Kavanaugh, R. (2017). MRI overview for fat quantification in non-alcoholic fatty liver disease in the clinical and research settings. https://open.bu.edu/bitstream/2144/24022/5/Kavanaugh_bu_0017N_12875.pdf (accessed on 1st June 2025).

51. Khosravi, P., Mohammadi, S., Zahiri, F., Khodarahmi, M., & Zahiri, J. (2024). AI-enhanced detection of clinically relevant structural and functional anomalies in MRI: Traversing the landscape of conventional to explainable approaches. *Journal of Magnetic Resonance Imaging: JMRI*. https://www.semanticscholar.org/paper/6eb628bf6a0cee980846a1e2c3bd7640d18022f5 (accessed on 1st June 2025).

52. Kim, J. A., & Davis, K. (2021). Magnetoencephalography: Physics, techniques and applications in the basic and clinical neurosciences. *Journal of Neurophysiology*. https://www.semanticscholar.org/paper/cf9ce5275ac945dbb515aca35c134dd1d1632621 (accessed on 1st June 2025).

53. Kirkpatrick, J. N., Mitchell, C., Taub, C., Kort, S., Hung, J., & Swaminathan, M. (2020). ASE statement on protection of patients and echocardiography service providers during the 2019 novel coronavirus outbreak: Endorsed by the American College of Cardiology. *Journal of the American Society of Echocardiography, 33*, 648–653. https://doi.org/10.1016/j.echo.2020.04.001 (accessed on 1st June 2025).

54. Lado-Touriño, I. (2023). Molecular modelling of aromatic interactions between pyrene derivatives and carbon nanotubes: Materials for biomedical applications. *Polycyclic Aromatic Compounds, 44*, 2966–2979. https://www.semanticscholar.org/paper/ac8266807f1b211187cb842a58e1203c027fc3b4 (accessed on 1st June 2025).

55. Lanz, H., Strauß, K., Höpler, J., Kraft, M., Hoffmann, S., Binzenhöfer, L., Gade, N., *et al.* (2024). Safety of magnetic resonance imaging in patients with cardiac implantable electronic devices. *Journal of Cardiovascular Development and Disease, 11*. https://www.semanticscholar.org/paper/3494be777fbcdb796aa9d3a537cd6e525afd6fd2 (accessed on 1st June 2025).

56. Liu, H., Chen, Y., Zhang, M., Bu, H., Lin, F., Chen, J., Xiao, M., *et al.* (2024). Feasibility of knee magnetic resonance imaging protocol using artificial intelligence-assisted iterative algorithm protocols: Comparison with standard MRI protocols. *Frontiers in Medicine, 11*. https://www.semanticscholar.org/paper/77d9bd698c1d998361385f05d475899aca6472c4 (accessed on 1st June 2025).

57. Liu, Z., Kainth, K., Zhou, A., Deyer, T., Fayad, Z., Greenspan, H., & Mei, X. (2024). A review of self-supervised, generative, and few-shot deep learning methods for data-limited magnetic resonance imaging segmentation. *NMR in Biomedicine*. https://www.semanticscholar.org/paper/a69c737b3d2a902a9aaa06effe01f991215520b8 (accessed on 1st June 2025).

58. MacFarlane, A. G. J., Milburn, G. J., Dowling, J. P., Kwiet, P., & Liang, W. (2002). *Quantum Technology: The Second Quantum Revolution*. http://arxiv.org/abs/quant-ph/0206091 (accessed on 1st June 2025).

59. Mahfuz, M. M. H., Baladi, E., & Ahmed A. K. (2024). Microstrip patch antennas for breast tumor/cancer cell detection–Challenges, designs, and future opportunities: A review. *IEEE*

Access, 12, 172297–172324. https://www.semanticscholar.org/paper/9282a42dfed23c4ba5a8c0c5fef0f956063b1105 (accessed on 1st June 2025).

60. Manickam, P., Mariappan, S. A., Murugesan, S. M., Hansda, S., Kaushik, A., Shinde, R. B., & Thipperudraswamy, S. P. (2022). Artificial intelligence (AI) and internet of medical things (IoMT) assisted biomedical systems for intelligent healthcare. *Biosensors, 12*, 562. https://doi.org/10.3390/bios12080562 (accessed on 1st June 2025).

61. Manuweera, T., Karunakaran, K., Baechler, C., Rosales, J., Kleckner, A. S., Rosenblatt, P. Y., Ciner, A., *et al.* (2024). Barriers and facilitators for participation in brain magnetic resonance imaging (MRI) scans in cancer research: A feasibility and acceptability analysis. *Research Square*. https://www.semanticscholar.org/paper/ee2e61f2c3e6ef3500bbbaeab172e059b6036f21 (accessed on 1st June 2025).

62. Marinho, P. (2024). Differential effects of cannabis vapor constituents on brain connectivity: Exploring the long-term effects of adolescent exposure. https://core.ac.uk/download/621600712.pdf (accessed on 1st June 2025).

63. Masino, F., Eusebi, L., Montatore, M., Muscatella, G., Gifuni, R., Ferrara, V., Marcellini, M., *et al.* (2024). Fundamentals of dual energy CT and its emerging applications in bladder cancer. *Digital Diagnostics*. https://www.semanticscholar.org/paper/916a7aecddf44ea6eca3e3fe1648160204708a5e (accessed on 1st June 2025).

64. Melazzini, L., Bortolotto, C., Brizzi, L., Achilli, M., Basla, N., D'Onorio De Meo, A., Gerbasi, A., *et al.* (2025). AI for image quality and patient safety in CT and MRI. *European Radiology Experimental, 9*. https://www.semanticscholar.org/paper/0befd0874fb932c0fcc9cd374837421c26afc442 (accessed on 1st June 2025).

65. Mota, B., Reis, Y. N., De Barros, N., Cardoso, N. P., Mota, R., Shimizu, C., Tucunduva, T. C. De. M., *et al.* (2023). Effects of preoperative magnetic resonance image on survival rates and surgical planning in breast cancer conservative surgery: Randomized controlled trial (BREAST-MRI trial). *Breast Cancer Research and Treatment, 198*, 447–461. https://www.semanticscholar.org/paper/d64b6c507fd4f3ba27c59e1c319672f1e7d0af7f (accessed on 1st June 2025).

66. Myers, N. (2021). *Historical Interface of Physics and Medicine*. https://core.ac.uk/download/427316571.pdf (accessed on 1st June 2025).

67. Najjar, R. (2023). Redefining radiology: A review of artificial intelligence integration in medical imaging. *Diagnostics, 13*, 2760. https://doi.org/10.3390/diagnostics13172760 (accessed on 1st June 2025).

68. Nameghi, A. G., & Zoriasatain, S. (2016). *Techniques Used to Increase the Resolving Power of Magnetic Resonance Images*. https://core.ac.uk/download/478458963.pdf (accessed on 1st June 2025).

69. Ortega-Robles, E., De Celis, A. B., Cantillo-Negrete, J., Carino-Escobar, R., & Arias-Carrión, O. (2025). Advanced magnetic resonance imaging for early diagnosis and monitoring of movement disorders. *Brain Sciences, 15*. https://www.semanticscholar.org/paper/fbaaaa774a259321d7e7f5f1afb233921ff0cba3 (accessed on 1st June 2025).

70. Panych, L., & Madore, B. (2018). The physics of MRI safety. *Journal of Magnetic Resonance Imaging, 47*. https://www.semanticscholar.org/paper/80600de8a7edff5a3e2225a3da406062c557323a (accessed on 1st June 2025).

71. Patel, K., & Gupta, S. (2024). Evaluating machine learning-based automatic quality assurance of magnetic resonance images in healthcare system. In *2024 2nd International Conference on Advances in Computation, Communication and Information Technology (ICAICCIT), 1*, 443–449. https://www.semanticscholar.org/paper/b5e60495092a2dea156ddb8ec922d2e5dadaedc8 (accessed on 1st June 2025).

72. Perera, M. A. A. S., & Politi, L. (2024). Potential applications of 7 Tesla magnetic resonance imaging in pediatric neuroimaging: Feasibility and challenges. *World Journal of Clinical Pediatrics, 13.* https://www.semanticscholar.org/paper/2a2d3fc6a8cd4d5f414f9c8c3e1894b2d38159c9 (accessed on 1st June 2025).

73. Plaza De, L. H. I., García, C. L., Quílez, C. E., Camacho-Arias, M., Cárdenas, S. M. Del. P., & Martel, V. J. (2024). Positron emission tomography-magnetic resonance imaging applications in pediatric musculoskeletal tumors. *Quantitative Imaging in Medicine and Surgery, 14*, 7825–7838. https://www.semanticscholar.org/paper/d06e80758b9d186811bf041afc9c05bdd421b528 (accessed on 1st June 2025).

74. Press, B., Cho, J., & Kirsch, A. (2025). Magnetic resonance urogram in pediatric urology: A comprehensive review of applications and advances. *International Braz. J. Urol., 51*(3). https://www.semanticscholar.org/paper/db496a66873e096a4a7a9a965d1f5644531fa9d1 (accessed on 1st June 2025).

75. Radojewski, P., Piredda, G., Bonanno, G., Lövblad, K., Vargas, M. I., Sutter, R., Nanz, D., *et al.* (2024). Assessment of the available evidence for the use of 7-Tesla (T) magnetic resonance imaging (MRI) in neurological and musculoskeletal disorders, with comparison to 3-T and 1.5-T MRI: A systematic scoping review. *European Journal of Neurology, 32*. https://www.semanticscholar.org/paper/aa9d5f913df6f6532407b00b9bd87ba100ac9642 (accessed on 1st June 2025).

76. Raja, S., Sharma, P. K., Subramonian, S. G., Ravipati, C., & Natarajan, P. (2024). Enhancing preoperative assessment of endometrial cancer: The role of diffusion-weighted magnetic resonance imaging in evaluating myometrial invasion. *Cureus, 16*. https://www.semanticscholar.org/paper/bcfc0938b47113d53c3a2287d0c1cf5987cf4839 (accessed on 1st June 2025).

77. Roguin, A., & Nair, P. (2005). *Magnetic Resonance Imaging in Patients with ICDs and Pacemakers*. https://core.ac.uk/download/pdf/86359.pdf (accessed on 1st June 2025).

78. Sabbaghan, M., Nigam, S., Kasabasic, I., Manepalli, M., Wang, P., & Fan, J. (2025). The development and challenges of PET/MRI dual-modality imaging probes—An update. *Journal of Magnetic Resonance Imaging: JMRI*. https://www.semanticscholar.org/paper/80c5fea03a3a4d935edc3ea6189224706aa8956c (accessed on 1st June 2025).

79. Sclafani, M., Tini, G., Musumeci, B., Cianca, A., Maestrini, V., Cacciotti, L., & Arcari, L. (2024). Advanced cardiovascular magnetic resonance imaging in Takotsubo syndrome: Update on feature tracking and tissue mapping. *Current Cardiovascular Imaging Reports*. https://www.semanticscholar.org/paper/e8210d118c6c0de2cd6d3765dcac0926e633198b (accessed on 1st June 2025).

80. Seibert, A. J., Baird, C. T., Clements, J. B., De Boer, *et al.* (2018). AAPM medical physics practice guideline 10.a.: Scope of practice for clinical medical physics. *Journal of Applied Clinical Medical Physics.* https://core.ac.uk/download/286729023.pdf (accessed on 1st June 2025).

81. Shah, L., Khan, A. A., Fazal, R., Gul, H., Azam, G., & Afridi, P. (2024). Evaluation of acute

intracerebral hemorrhage using computed-tomography and magnetic resonance imaging from tertiary care hospital Peshawar. *Journal of Health and Rehabilitation Research*. https://www.semanticscholar.org/paper/6162e2cd1d1116d09b66e8c101080b382de12017 (accessed on 1st June 2025).

82. Sharma, N., Srivastava, S., Kurian, N. K., Crescent, B. A. R., Deekshi, D., Angira, A., & Ali, S. (2025). Transforming pancreatic cancer diagnosis: Conventional methods, challenges, and future innovations. *Exon*. https://www.semanticscholar.org/paper/c9ff991b0f90e4a9bf11d892724f9796d8911cd5 (accessed on 1st June 2025).

83. Shin, D., Kim, Y., Oh, C. H., An, H., Park, J., Kim, J. G., & Lee, J. (2021). Deep reinforcement learning-designed radiofrequency waveform in MRI. *Nature Machine Intelligence, 3*, 985–994. https://www.semanticscholar.org/paper/34bb6cb4b6478a31a6ef470ca6dd89aa5896fc14 (accessed on 1st June 2025).

84. Sollini, M., Berchiolli, R., Kirienko, M., Rossi, A., Glaudemans, A., Slart, R., Slart, R., *et al.* (2018). PET/MRI in infection and inflammation. *Seminars in Nuclear Medicine, 48*(3), 225–241. https://www.semanticscholar.org/paper/e3d962808a3d9f5c807e0931bb94e2bfced0c144 (accessed on 1st June 2025).

85. Lawrence St. , K. S., Wang, D. J. J., Wang, R., Xue, *et al.* (2013). *Turbo-FLASH Based Arterial Spin Labeled Perfusion MRI at 7 T*. https://core.ac.uk/download/323077044.pdf (accessed on 1st June 2025).

86. Sumon, S., Rahman, M., Ahamed, M., Sikder, M., Abedin, M., & Akanda, A. (2024). Knowledge, attitude and practice (KAP) and health impacts of MRI among the patients attending MRI in Dhaka City. *International Journal of Medical Imaging*. https://www.semanticscholar.org/paper/f18067ca88944652ef8f542c71bd73e4860f46f0 (accessed on 1st June 2025).

87. Tarasova, A. A., Anisimov, N., Pavlova, O. S., Gulyaev, M., & Pirogov, Y. (2024). Magnetic resonance imaging at low signal-to-noise ratio, electromagnetic interferences and hardware imperfections. *Electromagnetic Waves and Electronic Systems*. https://www.semanticscholar.org/paper/af4008a79bbafb9f1b98b0e0bab82ddab4702db8 (accessed on 1st June 2025).

88. Thangam, R., Paulmurugan, R., & Kang, H. (2021). Functionalized nanomaterials as tailored theranostic agents in brain imaging. *Nanomaterials, 12*. https://www.semanticscholar.org/paper/97e20221331ac0d6f8487a2247fb28e2022d8d10 (accessed on 1st June 2025).

89. Verma, N., & Dahake, J. S. (2024). Evaluating sedation strategies for magnetic resonance imaging: A comprehensive review of intravenous fentanyl, butorphanol, and midazolam in adult and pediatric populations. *Cureus, 16*. https://www.semanticscholar.org/paper/05e94632eb4b2e262cdf773a8b3a425f879ab040 (accessed on 1st June 2025).

90. Vivekanantha, P., Sun, B., Parasu, N., & de Sa, D. (2024). Magnetic resonance imaging can predict hamstring or quadriceps tendon autograft diameter in pediatric or adolescent anterior cruciate ligament reconstruction: A systematic review. *Journal of Pediatric Orthopedics*. https://www.semanticscholar.org/paper/dd807cb561b011678f304a540e10ca1dff2bb00e (accessed on 1st June 2025).

91. Wang, Y., Ma, X., Zhang, Y., Yang, Y., Wang, P., Chen, T., Gao, C., *et al.* (2025). Insights into non-metallic magnetic resonance imaging contrast agents: Advances and perspectives. *Small*. https://www.semanticscholar.org/paper/b07da02a983da472c7232dd7c26b9bf7ef3032bd (accessed on 1st June 2025).

92. Welch, A., Platt, B., Billings, S., Borchelt, D., Brankack, J., Drzezga, A., Dubois, B., *et al.* (2012). FDG-PET imaging, EEG and sleep phenotypes as translational biomarkers for research in Alzheimer's disease. *Biochemical Society Transaction*. https://core.ac.uk/download/370450.pdf (accessed on 1st June 2025).

93. Wu, Z., & Li, X. (2024). Adaptive knowledge distillation for high-quality unsupervised MRI reconstruction with model-driven priors. *IEEE Journal of Biomedical and Health Informatics, 28*, 3571–3582. https://www.semanticscholar.org/paper/a9bb872ef1a63d4d3ff2a331da86ddac6a91bac0 (accessed on 1st June 2025).

94. Yadav, P., Lokhande, A., Prasanna, B. L., & Thorat, G. (2024). Conceptual importance of imaging and signal processing in the medical science. In *2024 International Conference on Healthcare Innovations, Software and Engineering Technologies (HISET)*. https://www.semanticscholar.org/paper/58d2c820d6e4c4ac0ade0de4d21e05d6f78e13cf (accessed on 1st June 2025).

95. Yang, J., Wang, Q., Tao, T., Niu, S., & Liu, M. (2022). Deep hash with optimal transport-based domain adaptation for multisite MRI retrieval. *Wireless Communications and Mobile Computing*. https://www.semanticscholar.org/paper/b0f1b213956ef20dd12f0b262b54f9efea3a5d3e (accessed on 1st June 2025).

96. Yao, R., Zhu, X., Zhou, D., Yang, L., Yu, H., Zhang, R., Yu, T., *et al.* (2025). Fast kilovoltage peak-switching dual-energy computed tomography water-hydroxyapatite decomposition for detecting vertebral compression fracture-related bone marrow edema: A comparison with magnetic resonance imaging. *Quantitative Imaging in Medicine and Surgery, 15*, 2270–2279. https://www.semanticscholar.org/paper/471b886b834eab020b1b02f2cc5fbfd4aac7e117 (accessed on 1st June 2025).

97. Yilmaz, A., Zagrosek, A., Aletras, A. H., Caforio, A. L., Maceira, A. M., Sievers, B., Gange, C. A., *et al.* (2011). *Contrast-Enhancement Cardiac Magnetic Resonance Imaging Beyond the Scope of Viability*. https://core.ac.uk/download/pdf/8559501.pdf (accessed on 1st June 2025).

98. Zhang, Y. (2025). Enhancing rectal cancer liver metastasis prediction: Magnetic resonance imaging-based radiomics, bias mitigation, and regulatory considerations. *World Journal of Gastrointestinal Oncology, 17*. https://www.semanticscholar.org/paper/7fd4f92e462f214b01666d0e725a946ca9bd1dd2 (accessed on 1st June 2025).

99. Zhuang, B., Sirajuddin, A., Zhao, S., & Lu, M. (2021). The role of 4D flow MRI for clinical applications in cardiovascular disease: Current status and future perspectives. *Quantitative Imaging in Medicine and Surgery, 11*(9), 4193–4210. https://www.semanticscholar.org/paper/ae425bfe7b2ecb510b71d3dcf7ffeeccb6746809 (accessed on 1st June 2025).

100. Ziyad, N., Yoosaf, S., Prabha, N., & Nair, N. V. (2024). Visualizing MRI & CT scans using mixed reality. In *2024 IEEE 12th Region 10 Humanitarian Technology Conference (R10-HTC)*. https://www.semanticscholar.org/paper/445c09cd73c589c81b1272ca530c8591accb4964 (accessed on 1st June 2025).

NUCLEAR MEDICINE AND PET-CT

9

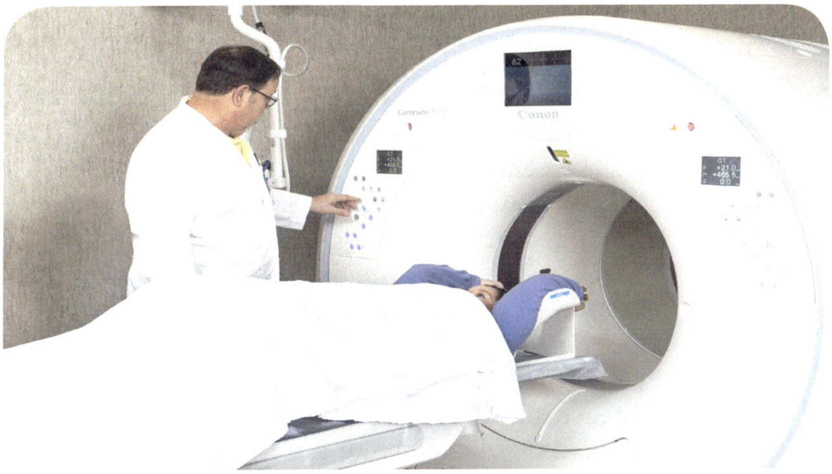

LEARNING OBJECTIVES

After studying this chapter, you will be able to:

1. Identify principles of nuclear medicine;
2. Explain PET-CT technology;
3. Concentrate on using nuclear medicine and PET-CT in medical settings;
4. Learn safety and ethical considerations.

Introduction

The use of modern medical imaging has greatly improved how diseases, especially cancer, are handled. Among these innovations, nuclear medicine, coupled with positron emission tomography-computed tomography (PET-CT), has emerged as a vital tool for detecting, staging, and monitoring malignancies with high precision. Because this technique combines functional and anatomical information, doctors can study metabolic processes as well as the structure of the body. For instance, in prostate cancer, PET-CT utilizing prostate-specific membrane antigen (PSMA) targeting tracers has enhanced diagnostic accuracy and treatment planning, with artificial intelligence further improving image interpretation and predictive capabilities (Tapper *et al.*, 2024). Similarly, in pediatric oncology, nuclear medicine advances, including novel PET tracers, have improved the detection of neuroblastoma metastases where traditional methods fall short, offering superior resolution and whole-body assessment (Samim *et al.*, 2021). It outlines how the use of nuclear medicine and PET-CT has changed clinical practice by bringing in new technologies to improve disease diagnosis and patient treatment.

Definition of Nuclear Medicine

The use of new medical imaging methods has greatly improved how doctors diagnose and check treatments, especially by showing what happens in the body without removing tissue. One of these is nuclear medicine, which makes use of radioactive materials to both find and treat diseases by focusing on specific organs or cells. Radiopharmaceuticals are given, and the gamma rays or positrons they produce are detected by PET-CT scanners, giving information about how the body functions in addition to its structure.

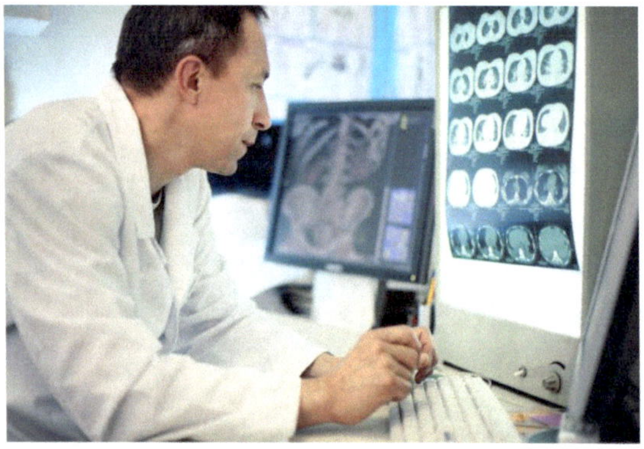

Figure 9.1. Nuclear medicine stands out as a specialized branch that utilizes radioactive substances to diagnose and treat various diseases by targeting specific organs or cellular functions.

Source: https://cdn-prod.medicalnewstoday.com/content/images/articles/248/248735/radiologist.jpg.

Nuclear medicine's capacity to image metabolic activity, receptor status, or blood flow offers clinicians critical information for managing conditions such as cancer, cardiovascular diseases, and neurological disorders (Lyon *et al.*, 2022). In neurooncological contexts, for instance, nuclear medicine complements MRI by delineating tumor metabolism and response to therapy, as detailed in guidelines established by leading professional societies (Law *et al.*, 2018). Therefore, nuclear medicine represents a vital intersection of molecular biology and clinical imaging, facilitating personalized and precise patient care (Figure 9.1).

Overview of Positron Emission Tomography combined with Computer Tomography (PET-CT) Technology

Improvements in imaging technology have greatly changed how medical diagnosis and treatment are done today. Among these innovations, PET-CT technology stands out by combining the metabolic imaging capabilities of positron emission tomography (PET) with the anatomical detail provided by computed tomography (CT). Because of this combination, clinicians can find abnormal metabolic activity in the body more accurately, which improves the detection, staging, and treatment of diseases. Especially in cancer care, PET-CT helps identify tumors by noticing their glucose uptake or by checking for Prostate-Specific Membrane Antigen in prostate cancer. Integration of artificial intelligence and machine learning further refines image analysis, improving diagnostic accuracy and outcome prediction through advanced algorithms like convolutional neural networks and radiomics (Boussios *et al.*, 2024). Using PET-CT together allows for accurate targeting of treatments and checking their effects, which is why it is so important in nuclear medicine today.

Importance of Nuclear Medicine in Healthcare

With better imaging technology, doctors can now find illnesses earlier and design treatments that are more suited to each case. Nuclear medicine is different from other innovations because it can show how organs and tissues work, which other imaging methods do not always reveal. Using radiopharmaceuticals, PET-CT in nuclear medicine helps to see how metabolic processes change, which reveals important details about a patient's disease and how it responds to treatment. In oncology, cardiology, and neurology, the ability to judge physiological function is very important since early diagnosis and proper staging play a major role in patient outcomes. Besides, because nuclear medicine is minimally invasive and exposes patients to less radiation, it is safer and more comfortable for them. The integration of PET-CT in clinical practice exemplifies how nuclear medicine bridges diagnostic precision with personalized care, underscoring its indispensable role in contemporary healthcare systems (Figure 9.2).

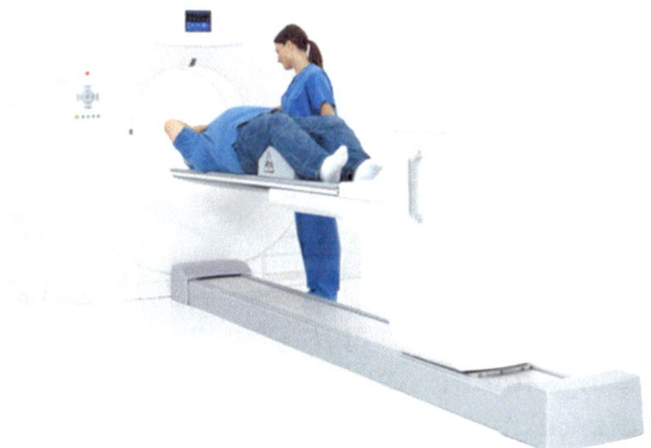

Figure 9.2. The integration of PET-CT in clinical practice exemplifies how nuclear medicine bridges diagnostic precision with personalized care, underscoring its indispensable role in contemporary healthcare systems.

Source: https://ddnmrc.com/image/nuclear.png.

Historical Development of Nuclear Medicine

Nuclear medicine developed mainly because of the discoveries of radioactivity and diagnostic imaging at the start of the 20th century. Wilhelm Röntgen and Marie Curie were the first to show that radioactive substances could be used to study the body without surgery. At the same time, important medical advances such as organ transplantation were made possible by new imaging methods, which improved results for patients and reduced risks after surgery. With time, radioactive tracers and imaging techniques worked together to create advanced systems like PET-CT. Mixing functional and anatomical imaging is a major step forward, making it possible to accurately identify and treat tumors in oncology. Ongoing developments seek to surmount limitations such as spatial resolution and radiation exposure, emphasizing a future where personalized diagnostics and therapies increasingly rely on this integrated approach (Benjamens *et al.*, 2020; Carsrud *et al.*, 2024).

Role of Imaging in Diagnosis and Treatment

Improvements in medical technology have greatly changed the methods for finding and treating diseases, and imaging has been key in this change. Especially, PET imaging used together with CT scans has improved early detection and monitoring of conditions like cancer and Alzheimer's disease. Doctors use these images to see the body's structure and function, which helps them diagnose and plan treatment for each patient. Even though PET and CT are very useful, they are not without problems, such as exposing patients to radiation and being expensive. New imaging tools, for example, Near Infrared Chemical Imaging Microspectroscopy and Fluorescence spectroscopic techniques, may help find disease at the single-cell or molecular level, which may improve sensitivity and reduce costs. However, these novel methods remain underfunded despite their potential to dramatically improve early diagnosis and patient outcomes (Baianu, 2011) (Figure 9.3).

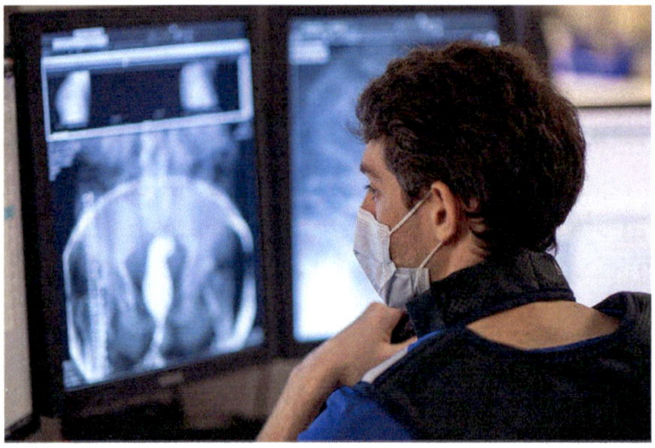

Figure 9.3. In particular, nuclear medicine techniques such as Positron Emission Tomography (PET) combined with Computed Tomography (CT) have enhanced the early detection and monitoring of conditions like cancer and Alzheimer's disease.

Source: https://my.clevelandclinic.org/-/scassets/images/org/care-pages/endo-path-img/imaging-care-feature.jpg.

Significance of Positron Emission Tomography combined with Computer Tomography (PET-CT) in Modern Medicine

New technologies in diagnostic imaging have greatly improved how complex medical problems are handled, especially by providing both anatomical and functional information. PET-CT demonstrates this combination by supplying both metabolic and structural details, which improves the accuracy of diagnosis and treatment planning. In neurological disorders such as acute ischemic stroke, PET-CT has demonstrated its ability to identify hypometabolic regions corresponding to infarctions and surrounding penumbra, critical for tailoring interventions and predicting outcomes (Bochev *et al.*, 2014). Similarly, in oncology, PET-CT's sensitivity in detecting hypermetabolic lesions aids in identifying both primary tumors and metastatic disease, as seen in cases of solitary fibrous tumor/hemangiopericytomas, where the modality assists in monitoring recurrence and spreads (Aparici *et al.*, 2018). PET-CT is important in modern medicine because it improves diagnosis, aids in treatment decision-making, and provides better prognostic information in many clinical fields.

9.1. Principles of Nuclear Medicine

Learning Outcome

1. Understand basic concepts of radioactivity;
2. Identify types of radiopharmaceuticals;
3. Explain the mechanism of action in nuclear imaging;
4. Know safety protocols in nuclear medicine;
5. Explain the comparison with other imaging modalities;
6. Focus on the role of gamma cameras;
7. Learn the importance of dosimetry;
8. Discuss advances in radiopharmaceutical development;
9. Know ethical considerations in nuclear medicine.

The use of both physiological and anatomical information is a major progress in diagnostic imaging, mainly in nuclear medicine. Nuclear medicine methods give different information compared to CT or MRI, revealing what is happening inside the body at the cellular and metabolic levels, which helps detect early signs of disease before any structural changes are seen. This feature is important for PET-CT, which uses positron emission tomography to see metabolic changes and CT to show the bodyis structure. Nuclear medicine depends on giving radiopharmaceuticals, which produce gamma rays that are detected by special cameras to see the body's processes. Because some diagnostic and treatment procedures use high levels of radiation, it is very important to strictly follow safety procedures to protect patients and operators. Optimizing these safety measures improves clinical outcomes while minimizing risks, supporting cost-effective and responsible use of nuclear medicine technology (Singh *et al.*, 2022; Soliman *et al.*, 2018).

9.1.1. Basic Concepts of Radioactivity

Knowing the basic rules of radioactivity is necessary to understand its applications in nuclear medicine and PET-CT imaging. Radioactivity means that unstable atomic nuclei will decay on their own and emit radiation as alpha, beta, or gamma particles. Because of this process, radioactive tracers can be followed inside the body without surgery. In particular, PET depends on positron-emitting radionuclides to produce detailed images of cellular and metabolic activities. The choice of radionuclide and its chemical properties significantly impact imaging efficacy and therapeutic potential, with radiometals such as gallium-68 and zirconium-89 offering versatile coordination chemistry for designing targeted probes (Jussing *et al.*, 2022). Furthermore, the optimization of radiotracer behavior in small-animal models has advanced preclinical imaging research, facilitating the development of novel diagnostic agents and therapeutic monitoring tools (Bankstahl *et al.*, 2015). This foundational knowledge underpins the continual evolution of PET-CT technology in personalized medicine (Figure 9.4).

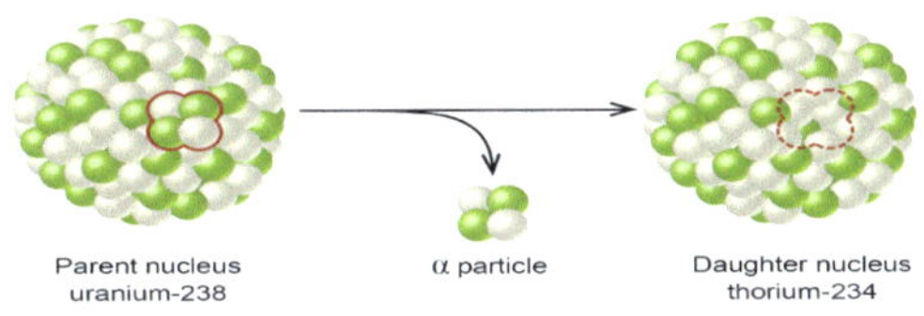

Figure 9.4. Radioactivity involves the spontaneous decay of unstable atomic nuclei, emitting radiation in the form of alpha, beta, or gamma particles.

Source: https://opentextbc.ca/chemistry/wp-content/uploads/sites/150/2016/05/CNX_Chem_21_03_Reaction1.jpg.

9.1.2. Types of Radiopharmaceuticals

Improvements in nuclear medicine have led to more types of radiopharmaceuticals, which help in the accurate diagnosis and treatment of many diseases. Radiopharmaceuticals are mainly grouped according to their radionuclide and carrier properties, which decide if they are used for diagnosis or treatment. To see physiological and molecular processes, diagnostic agents often use gamma-emitting isotopes for SPECT and positron-emitting isotopes for PET. Unlike diagnostic radiopharmaceuticals, therapeutic ones usually contain beta or alpha emitters to send radiation only to diseased areas. Monoclonal antibodies labeled with radionuclides exemplify this approach, offering targeted imaging and therapy tailored to specific cancer antigens or immune modulation pathways, which enhances personalized treatment strategies (Auletta *et al.*, 2016). Furthermore, the emerging field of theranostics combines diagnostic and therapeutic functions within a single radiopharmaceutical, facilitating precise treatment planning and real-time monitoring of response, particularly in oncology and inflammatory diseases (Kashyap *et al.*, 2020). This shows that a variety of radiopharmaceuticals is essential for the progress of nuclear medicine and PET-CT.

9.1.3. Mechanism of Action in Nuclear Imaging

Nuclear imaging provides detailed information about physiology and molecules because it uses radioactive tracers. After introducing the tracers, which give off positrons or gamma rays, they gather in specific tissues because of the body's metabolic or receptor activities. The radiation is detected by advanced scanners, like PET-CT machines, which make images that show how the body is working instead of just its structure. Using this approach, diseases, mainly cancer, can be found and staged earlier, since it detects metabolic changes before any noticeable structural changes take place. Advances in technology and standardized practice guidelines, developed through collaborative efforts of organizations represented in initiatives like those discussed by the European Association of Nuclear Medicine Technologist Committee and its American counterparts, have further refined image acquisition and interpretation protocols, enhancing diagnostic precision and patient care standards in nuclear medicine (Hogg *et al.*, 2011). The integration of imaging physics, tracer biochemistry, and computational reconstruction techniques exemplifies the complexity and sophistication underpinning this mechanism (Figure 9.5).

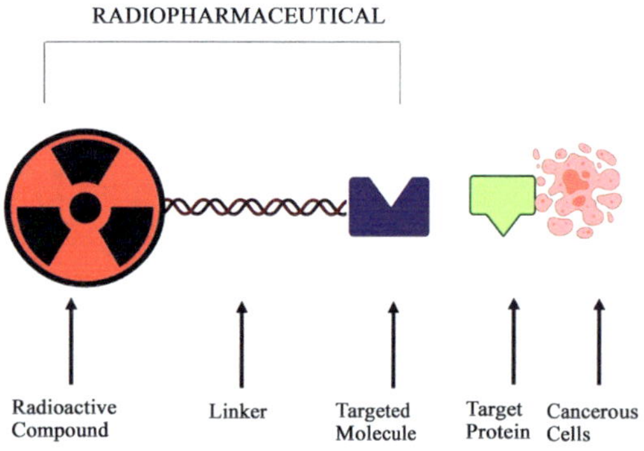

Figure 9.5. The capability of nuclear imaging to provide detailed physiological and molecular information stems from its unique mechanism of action involving radioactive tracers.

Source: https://media.springernature.com/lw685/springer-static/image/art%3A10.1186%2Fs40001-023-01627-0/MediaObjects/40001_2023_1627_Figa_HTML.png.

9.1.4. Safety Protocols in Nuclear Medicine

It is very important in nuclear medicine to have strict safety measures to prevent both patients and staff from getting too much radiation. Given the reliance on radiotracers such as those used in positron emission tomography-computed tomography (PET-CT), strict adherence to handling, storage, and disposal guidelines is essential. All facilities should make sure their staff are trained on how to avoid contamination, the use of shielding, and what to do in emergencies. Patient safety improves when the right dose is given and when medical staff keep an eye on the patient to weigh the positives of diagnosis against the risks of radiation. Additionally, current guidelines emphasize multidisciplinary collaboration to optimize safety measures across imaging and therapeutic applications, reflecting advancements highlighted in prostate cancer management and targeted systemic therapies (Ajani *et al.*, 2022; Lowrance *et al.*, 2023). New radiopharmaceuticals must be integrated carefully, since safety considerations are constantly evolving and require us to keep updating our protocols to achieve the best results without compromising safety.

9.1.5. Comparison with Other Imaging Modalities

New technologies in medical imaging have greatly improved how diseases are found, but every type of imaging has its own benefits and drawbacks for decision-making. Compared to conventional imaging techniques such as computed tomography (CT) and magnetic resonance imaging (MRI), PET-CT uniquely combines metabolic and anatomical information, providing superior sensitivity in detecting biochemical changes before structural abnormalities become apparent. Although CT provides clear images of bones and MRI shows soft tissue well, both fail to give the needed information for early detection and following treatment responses. In oncology, cardiology, and neurology, PET-CT is beneficial because metabolic activity is an important sign to look for. Additionally, emerging imaging technologies enhance visualization at cellular and molecular levels, facilitating novel therapies like stem cell treatment, where imaging guides cell implantation and monitors outcomes (Jokerst *et al.*, 2016). Even so, problems such as radiation exposure and cost are still issues that ionizing techniques have to deal with.

9.1.6. Role of Gamma Cameras

Nuclear medicine depends on accurate imaging methods that let doctors view what is happening inside the body without surgery. These cameras are fundamental in this area by detecting gamma rays from radiopharmaceuticals in patients, which allows for detailed images of how body organs function and interact. Besides diagnostics, they help with drug development and monitoring therapy by monitoring the distribution of radiotracers in animal models in real time. For instance, gamma scintigraphy has been instrumental in evaluating drug delivery systems and tumor targeting in animal studies, allowing for refined pharmacokinetic analyses and ethical reduction in animal use (Pawar *et al.*, 2024).

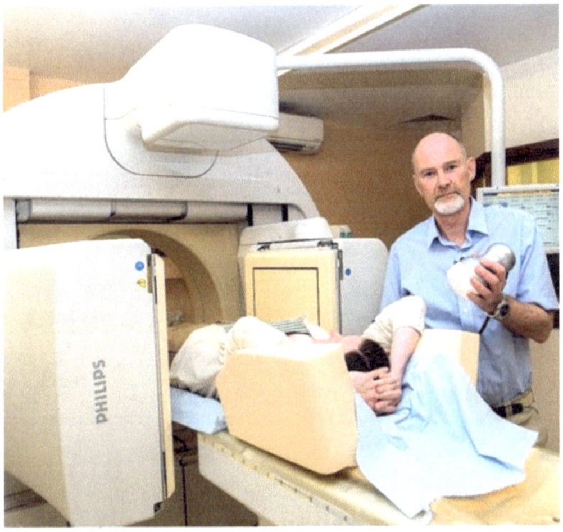

Figure 9.6. Gamma cameras serve as a cornerstone in this domain by detecting gamma radiation emitted from radiopharmaceuticals administered to patients, creating detailed images of organ function and molecular activity.

Source: https://www.bnms.org.uk/resource/resmgr/news_&_press_office/news/alan_perkins_gamma_camera_ra.jpg.

Additionally, observations from nationwide clinical surveys emphasize how modern gamma camera technologies, including those integrated into single photon emission computed tomography (SPECT) and combined SPECT/CT systems, contribute critically to optimizing patient doses and improving diagnostic accuracy across a range of nuclear medicine procedures (Skovorodko *et al.*, 2022). Thus, gamma cameras are indispensable for bridging clinical application and research innovation in nuclear medicine imaging (Figure 9.6).

9.1.7. Importance of Dosimetry

It is important to measure radiation dose accurately to help patients in nuclear medicine, mainly during PET-CT scans, which use radioactive drugs. Dosimetry helps doctors make sure that the benefits of the test are not outweighed by the risks by adjusting the amount of radiation given and avoiding unnecessary exposure. It is necessary for the safety and success of PET-CT scans, since patient characteristics such as metabolism and organ sensitivity can affect how much radiation they receive. Also, the use of dosimetry makes it easier to create standard protocols, which increases the consistency of nuclear medicine results across different institutions. It is also important for personalized medicine by allowing doctors to adjust the dose for patients who may be vulnerable such as children or those with health problems. Mapping the location of radiation in the body is important for improving how radiotherapy is planned and helps protect patients, which highlights the essential part dosimetry plays in nuclear medicine.

9.1.8. Advances in Radiopharmaceutical Development

New radiopharmaceuticals have played a major role in driving changes in how nuclear medicine is practiced. Using monoclonal antibodies labeled with radioactive isotopes is now possible, which helps target specific antigens that control angiogenesis and the immune system. Because of this, PET-CT imaging can now detect and diagnose diseases more precisely without the need for surgery. In addition, using radiolabeled antibodies makes it possible to assess the antigen status of each cancer lesion which helps decide on personalized therapy and monitor how the treatment is working. This progress supports the integration of biological therapies with nuclear imaging, offering new avenues for patient management and improving outcomes in oncology and beyond (Auletta *et al.*, 2016). These advances underscore the growing synergy between molecular biology and nuclear medicine in refining diagnostic accuracy and therapeutic efficacy (Figure 9.7).

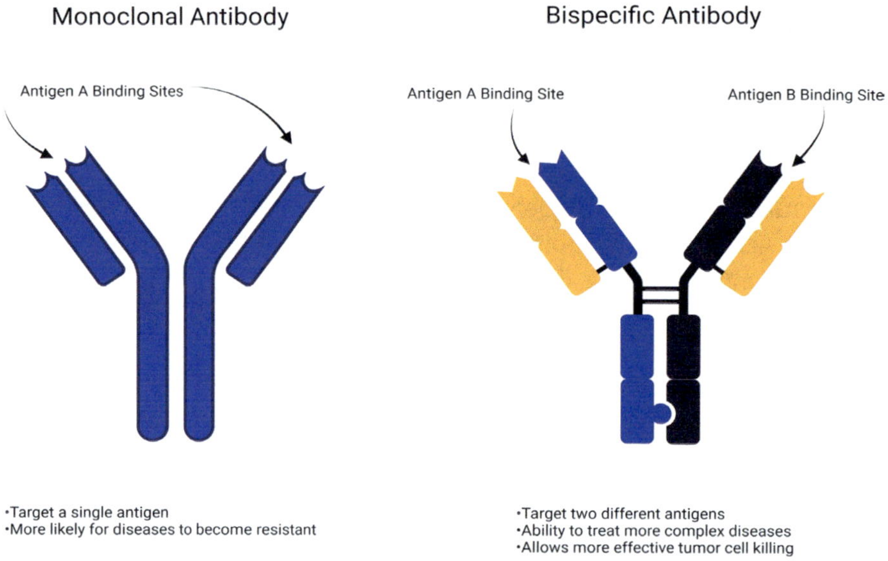

Figure 9.7. Radiolabeled antibodies provide valuable tools for evaluating the antigenic status of individual cancer lesions, facilitating personalized therapy decisions and effective monitoring of treatment responses.

Source: https://www.cell.com/cms/10.1016/j.isci.2022.105326/asset/5e1e112e-f353-4013-93de-dc7ead9ea53e/main.assets/gr6_lrg.jpg.

9.1.9. Ethical Considerations in Nuclear Medicine

Improvements in nuclear medicine, mainly PET-CT imaging, have changed how diseases are diagnosed and treated, but they also raise many ethical issues that require attention. Patient safety is very important, as using radioactive tracers means people may be exposed to ionizing radiation, so strict rules are needed to reduce the risks. Patient autonomy is protected by making sure that the benefits, risks, and alternatives are clearly explained to the patient. In addition, not all people can use these advanced technologies because they are expensive and not always available, which creates health inequalities. Additionally, the integration of novel techniques, such as stem cell tracking discussed in regenerative medicine, underscores the need for ethical guidelines in experimental settings to balance innovation with patient welfare (Jokerst *et al.*, 2016). It is also necessary to handle and dispose of radioactive materials properly to keep both the healthcare workers and the environment safe.

Test Your Knowledge

1. What is the primary principle behind nuclear medicine imaging?
2. What allows a PET scan to spot metabolic activity in the body?

9.2. Positron Emission Tomography combined with Computer Tomography (PET-CT) Technology

Learning Outcome

1. Give an overview of PET imaging and CT imaging;
2. Know integration of PET and CT technologies;
3. List the advantages of PET-CT over separate modalities;
4. Explain clinical applications of PET-CT;
5. Focus on the limitations and challenges of PET-CT;
6. Identify future trends in PET-CT technology;
7. Explain the role of artificial intelligence in PET-CT;
8. Describe patient preparation and procedure.

With new developments in biomedical imaging, it is now much easier to find and watch the progress of complex diseases at the molecular level. Among these innovations, PET-CT technology stands out by combining the metabolic and functional data obtained from positron emission tomography (PET) with the detailed anatomical information provided by CT. Combining these techniques makes it possible to precisely locate any physiological problems, which is important for managing ischemic heart disease. When CT is used with PET, the images become clearer, and it becomes easier to distinguish between different types of tissue, which improves how accurately a diagnosis can be made. In preclinical research, small animal models, particularly mice, benefit from dedicated PET/CT scanners that facilitate noninvasive assessment of myocardial perfusion and metabolism, as well as other pathophysiological processes, including inflammation and apoptosis (Brunetti *et al.*, 2012). Because PET-CT is expensive and not widely available compared to other nuclear imaging, its ability to reduce early deaths from heart disease makes it increasingly important in healthcare globally.

9.2.1. Overview of Positron Emission Tomography (PET) Imaging

Improvements in medical imaging have made it much easier to identify and deal with different diseases, mainly cancer. PET imaging, together with CT, has made a major difference in nuclear medicine by giving detailed information about both function and anatomy. PET imaging operates through the detection of radioactive tracers, such as those targeting prostate-specific membrane antigen (PSMA), allowing clinicians to visualize molecular processes in vivo with high sensitivity. Because of this integration, staging, choosing treatments, and monitoring diseases such as prostate cancer are done more accurately. Also, the use of artificial intelligence and machine learning in PET/CT imaging has improved its ability to interpret images and predict outcomes. These technological strides underscore PET imaging's critical role in personalized medicine by enhancing the understanding of disease biology and optimizing patient care (Boussios *et al.*, 2024) (Figure 9.8).

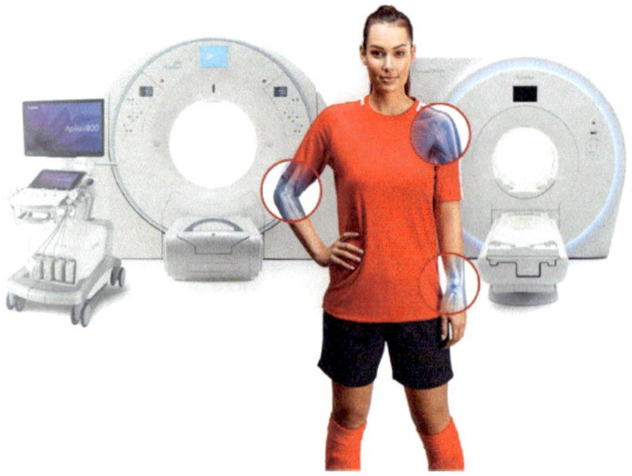

Figure 9.8. Positron Emission Tomography (PET) imaging, combined with computed tomography (CT), represents a pivotal development in nuclear medicine by providing detailed functional and anatomical information simultaneously.

Source:.

Thanks to better medical imaging, both diagnoses and patient care have significantly improved, mainly because functional and anatomical images are now combined. This progress is shown by combining PET with CT, which lets doctors see both the activity and the structure of tumors. Combining these methods improves the way staging, treatment planning, and response evaluation are performed in oncology, since ambiguity can occur when only one method is used. Using PET-CT technology together makes it easier for staff, reduces the number of times patients move between scanners, and shortens the overall scan time, which makes patients more comfortable and compliant. Moreover, adherence to standardized practice guidelines ensures that the integration maintains high-quality imaging and safety standards essential in nuclear medicine (Seibert *et al.*, 2018). The use of PET-CT, which combines energy use with images of the body, reflects how different fields are now combined in medicine.

9.2.2. Advantages of Positron Emission Tomography combined with Computer Tomography (PET-CT) Over Separate Modalities

By combining PET and CT, nuclear medicine has made a major advance by allowing metabolic and anatomical images to be taken together. PET and CT working together make it possible to find the exact location of any abnormalities seen on a PET scan, which improves the accuracy of diagnosis. For instance, current-generation PET-CT scanners equipped with multiple detector CT can acquire high-resolution volumetric datasets that surpass traditional imaging methods in evaluating pulmonary metastases, improving lesion characterization without additional contrast agents (Basu *et al.*, 2017).

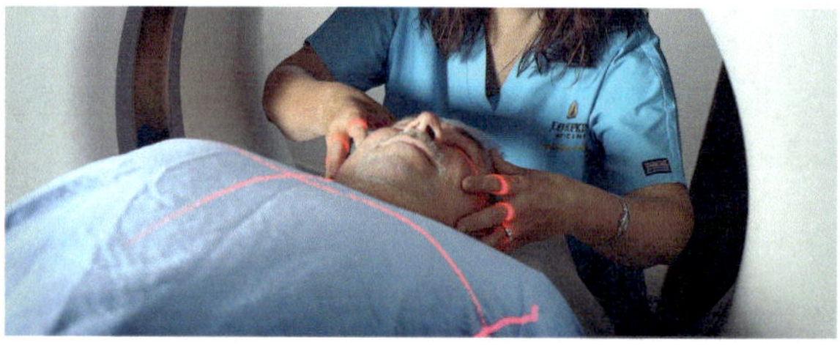

Figure 9.9. The integration of positron emission tomography (PET) with computed tomography (CT) represents a significant advancement in nuclear medicine by combining metabolic and anatomical imaging into a single modality.

Source: https://www.hopkinsmedicine.org/-/media/images/health/2_-treatment/radiology/pet_hero.jpg?h=500&iar=0&mh=500&mw=1300&w=1297&hash=17DEAF64746EF998C711DF9AC7A249CE.

Moreover, PET-CT offers the advantage of reduced radiation exposure and enhanced workflow efficiency compared to separate imaging procedures, as adjustments in CT parameters and PET radiopharmaceutical doses have successfully minimized overall patient dose, particularly in vulnerable populations such as pediatric patients (Kerrie *et al.*, 2025). These combined benefits underscore PET-CT's superiority in disease detection, staging, and therapeutic monitoring, consolidating its role as an indispensable tool in modern clinical practice (Figure 9.9).

9.2.3. Clinical Applications of Positron Emission Tomography combined with Computer Tomography (PET-CT)

Better medical imaging has greatly helped with the diagnosis and treatment of diseases, mainly cancer and disorders affecting the brain. PET-CT has become very important in clinical settings because it can show both the structure and function of the body simultaneously. With this technique, it is easier to find cancer, stage it, and assess treatment results, which supports better care for each patient. Also, PET-CT helps with early detection of Alzheimer's by discovering specific changes in brain metabolism, which enables early treatment. Although PET-CT is used widely, it has some disadvantages, like exposing patients to radiation and high expenses, which is why scientists are working on finding new methods that improve its benefits. Nonetheless, its clinical significance remains indisputable, contributing to improved patient outcomes and exemplifying the importance of nuclear medicine in modern diagnostics (Baianu, 2011).

9.2.4. Limitations and Challenges of Positron Emission Tomography combined with Computer Tomography (PET-CT)

Better imaging technology has made it easier to diagnose, but there are still some limits that stop PET-CT scans from being perfect.

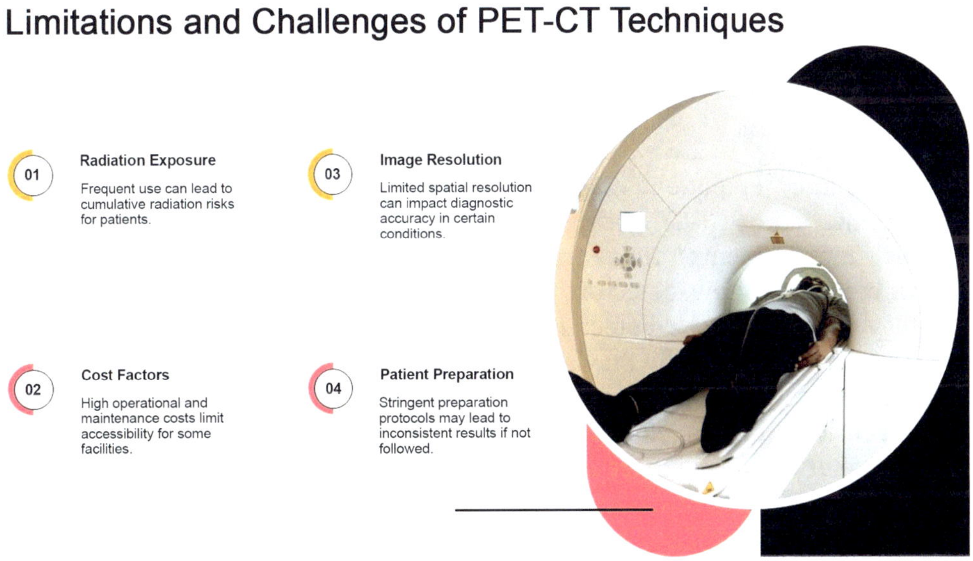

Figure 9.10. Advancements in imaging technologies have vastly improved diagnostic capabilities, yet inherent limitations impede the full potential of PET-CT scans.

Source: https://www.slideteam.net/media/catalog/product/cache/1280x720/c/o/comprehensive_insights_from_pet_ct_imaging_techniques_ppt_sample_st_ai_slide11.jpg.

There is a major problem due to the fact that nuclear medicine physicians and radiologists may interpret images differently, which can change the reliability of the diagnosis. Because specialized PET tracers, including PSMA for prostate cancer, are used more often, there is a greater need for experts to interpret them, but the number of qualified people is not enough. Also, AI tools for image analysis look promising, but they still have to overcome issues like lack of validation by other groups, limited future studies, and requiring more data from different centers to be reliable. Because of these challenges, AI is not widely used in PET-CT practices, which means more thorough research and validation are needed. Additionally, technical factors such as spatial resolution constraints and the potential for artifacts affect image quality and diagnostic confidence (Belal *et al.*, 2023) (Figure 9.10).

9.2.5. Future Trends in Positron Emission Tomography combined with Computer Tomography (PET-CT) Technology

Nuclear medicine imaging is always working to improve the accuracy of patient diagnoses and patient outcomes, and PET-CT is expected to make major improvements. New trends are focusing on combining new detectors and digital technology to improve the detection of diseases early and where in the body they occur. Innovations such as silicon photomultipliers and cadmium–zinc–telluride (CZT) detectors promise superior energy resolution and compact designs, facilitating more patient-friendly devices with shorter acquisition times and reduced radiation doses. Also, using iterative reconstruction algorithms with resolution recovery is expected to improve the quality and quantification abilities of images. These developments mirror advancements observed in related modalities like SPECT/CT, which have demonstrated enhanced clinical impact through improved detector efficiency and camera design (AlSaadi *et al.*, 2024). Such technological evolution, supported by interdisciplinary research and engineering, anticipates a future where PET-CT systems will be faster, more accurate, and widely accessible, reinforcing their role in personalized medicine and targeted therapies (Dhami *et al.*, 2008).

9.2.6. Role of Artificial Intelligence (AI) in Positron Emission Tomography combined with Computer Tomography (PET-CT)

Medical imaging has always tried to improve how accurately and efficiently complex procedures like PET-CT can be done. The use of AI in PET-CT technology greatly improves the accuracy of image analysis and registration in nuclear medicine.

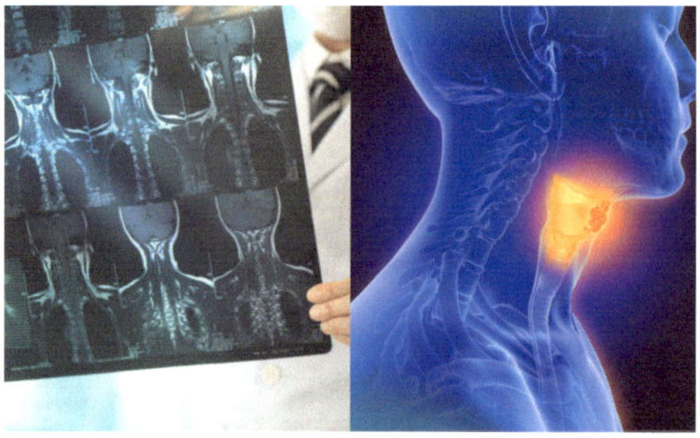

Figure 9.11. Advancements in medical imaging have consistently aimed to enhance diagnostic accuracy and efficiency, particularly in complex modalities like PET-CT.

Source: https://kiranpetct.com/wp-content/uploads/2025/01/FAPI-PETCT-in-Head-and-Neck-Cancers.png.

AI algorithms enable the alignment of multi-sensor PET and CT images captured at different times or positions, thereby improving the clarity and interpretability of anatomical and functional data crucial for diagnosis and treatment planning (Nag *et al.*, 2017). Also, AI can detect small changes in the body, such as mild inflammation or hidden infections, that are hard to see with the naked eye. By mining the abundant quantitative data from molecular imaging, AI tools not only boost sensitivity but also promise to predict patient outcomes and long-term risks, expanding the clinical utility of PET-CT beyond current capabilities (Aarntzen *et al.*, 2022). These innovations underscore AI's pivotal role in optimizing nuclear medicine diagnostics and personalized patient care (Figure 9.11).

9.2.7. Patient Preparation and Procedure

It is very important to make sure patients are prepared well and that all steps in the procedure are smooth for successful PET-CT imaging in nuclear medicine. Patients usually fast before receiving 18F-FDG to prevent other sugars from competing for uptake, which improves the accuracy of the tracer. The procedure involves precise dosing, with technologists required to handle and administer radioactive substances efficiently to limit radiation exposure, as demonstrated by studies tracking extremity doses during preparation and administration phases (Ramanathan *et al.*, 2024).

The time between the injection and the imaging is also set to ensure the tracer is well distributed and the images are clear. Advanced PET-CT systems, like the Biograph Vision Quadra, have been validated for clinical use due to their ability to produce high-quality diagnostic images with shorter scan times, thus reducing patient discomfort and motion artifacts during the procedure (Roya *et al.*, 2024). All these steps and measures together help improve the accuracy of diagnosis and protect patients in nuclear medicine.

Test Your Knowledge

1. Which radiopharmaceutical is most often used in PET scans?
2. What effects do combining PET and CT scans have on improving diagnosis?

9.3. Clinical Applications of Nuclear Medicine and Positron Emission Tomography combined with Computer Tomography (PET-CT)

Learning Outcome

1. Understand oncology applications;
2. Explain cardiology applications;
3. Focus on neurology applications;
4. Define infectious disease diagnosis;
5. Focusing on assessment of treatment response;
6. Describe the role in personalized medicine;
7. Know pediatric applications;
8. Describe research applications in nuclear medicine;
9. Learn case studies demonstrating efficacy.

Thanks to improved diagnostic imaging, important diseases like cancer and Alzheimer's can now be diagnosed earlier and managed better, which makes nuclear medicine and PET-CT essential in today's healthcare. Such technologies apply nuclear science to observe how molecules and cells work, and they are more sensitive than traditional imaging. PET-CT helps find the location of a tumor and also checks its activity and functions, which is important for proper diagnosis, staging, and assessing treatment effectiveness. Even though they have well-defined roles, problems with cost, image resolution, and patient radiation remain, which is why scientists are looking into other methods like Near Infrared Chemical Imaging and fluorescence spectroscopy for earlier detection. However, restricted funding for such innovative diagnostic approaches hampers the advancement of early cancer and Alzheimer's identification, underscoring the need for increased clinical and research support to fully realize nuclear medicine's potential impact on patient outcomes (Baianu, 2011).

9.3.1. Oncology Applications

Thanks to the progress in nuclear medicine, detecting and treating cancer has become much easier, and imaging techniques provide important information about tumors and their response to treatment. PET/CT is commonly seen as the best imaging method in oncology, but SPECT is still important in many clinical situations around the world. Recent advances in SPECT technology, such as improved collimator designs and novel radiotracers targeting specific cancer mechanisms, have expanded its applications beyond traditional bone scanning to include imaging angiogenesis and apoptosis, crucial processes in tumor progression and treatment evaluation (Adak *et al.*, 2012). When functional imaging is added to CT data, it helps make diagnosis and treatment monitoring more accurate, which improves personalized cancer care. These developments underscore the complementary roles of nuclear imaging modalities in oncology, particularly where resource limitations influence technology deployment (Figure 9.12).

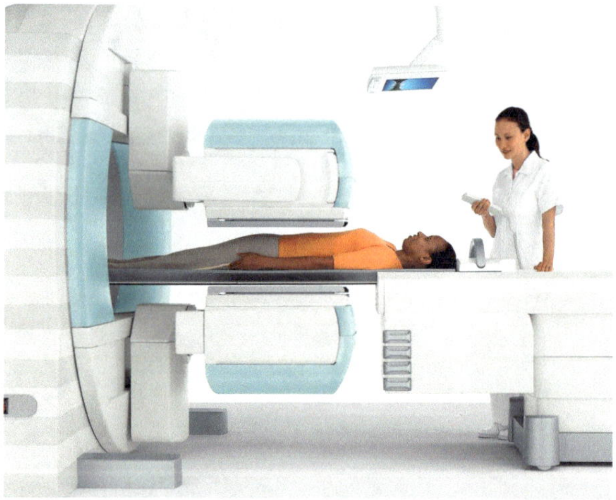

Figure 9.12. Single-photon emission computed tomography (SPECT) technology.

Source: https://kiranpetct.com/wp-content/uploads/2022/07/spect-ct-scan.jpg.

9.3.2. Cardiology Applications

Globally, cardiovascular diseases are a major cause of death, and this is a big problem for healthcare systems, mainly in low- and middle-income countries where 75% of such deaths occur. To deal with this, we need advanced tools for early detection and sorting patients by risk level. PET/CT in nuclear medicine is now widely used in cardiology since it supplies clear images of how the heart is functioning and using energy. Even though myocardial SPECT is commonly used, PET/CT offers much better image quality and the ability to measure accurately, which supports the diagnosis of ischemic heart disease and many other heart diseases. Even though PET/CT is very useful in medicine, it is not used more widely because it is expensive and scanners are not always easy to find, mainly for oncology. Even so, using PET/CT more in cardiology could greatly help manage patients and support the United Nations' target of lowering premature cardiovascular deaths by 30% by 2030.

9.3.3. Neurology Applications

Improvements in diagnostic imaging have greatly changed how neurological evaluations are done, giving us a better understanding of brain function and diseases. Nuclear medicine with PET-CT is especially useful for noticing metabolic changes that can be seen before structural changes show up on other types of scans. PET-CT plays a key role in diagnosing Alzheimer's disease by mapping amyloid plaques and measuring glucose use in the brain, which helps start treatment early.

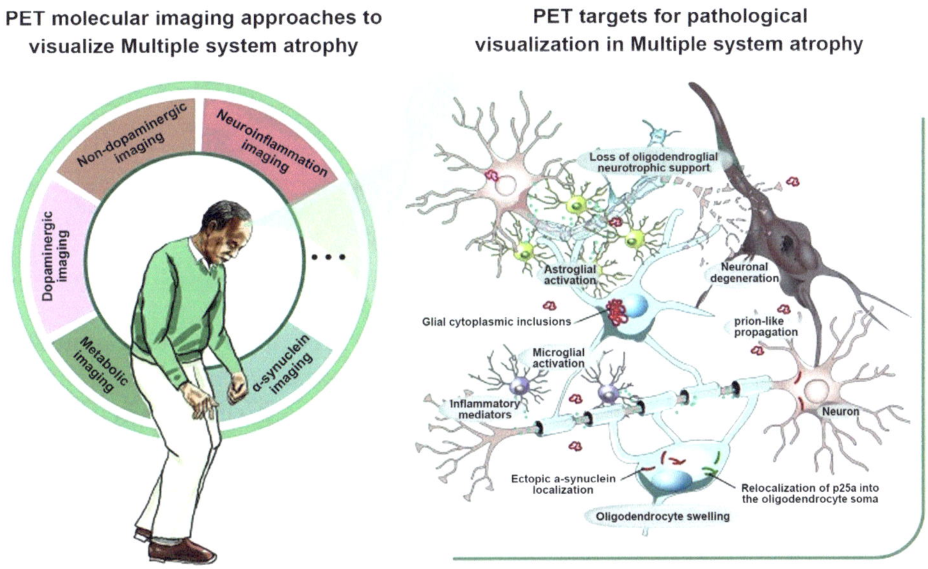

Figure 9.13. PET-CT aids in mapping amyloid plaques and assessing cerebral glucose metabolism, thereby facilitating early intervention.

Source: https://ars.els-cdn.com/content/image/1-s2.0-S0969996125000440-gr1.jpg.

PET-CT also helps a lot in epilepsy evaluation by finding the exact location of the seizure focus, which helps guide surgery when medications do not work. Using these modalities together provides more accurate diagnoses and better management of patients, according to recent studies that showed better identification and description of lesions. Consequently, nuclear medicine and PET-CT continue to play a critical role in advancing neurology practice (Figure 9.13).

9.3.4. Infectious Disease Diagnosis

New imaging methods have greatly changed how complex medical conditions, especially infectious diseases, are diagnosed when conventional methods do not clearly show the problem. Nuclear medicine, especially through 18F-fluorodeoxyglucose positron emission tomography combined with computed tomography (F-18 FDG PET/CT), offers a valuable tool in this regard. Clinicians can use this technique to spot metabolic changes linked to both sterile inflammation and septic infections, which helps them understand the presence, scope, and severity of infectious processes. It can be used in many conditions, for example, osteomyelitis, prosthetic joint infections, endocarditis, and systemic sarcoidosis, making it easier to diagnose these problems sooner. Also, combining PET/CT with MRI technologies may help improve the accuracy of diagnoses and patient management. Collaborative efforts to establish standardized protocols aim to harmonize these techniques across centers, underscoring their increasing clinical relevance in infectious disease diagnostics (Albano *et al.*, 2021; Glaudemans *et al.*, 2015).

9.3.5. Assessment of Treatment Response

Imaging technology progress has helped a lot in assessing the success of cancer treatments, mainly thanks to nuclear medicine and PET-CT. Even though bone scans have been a mainstay for staging and monitoring bone metastases, their lack of sensitivity and specificity makes it hard to quickly assess the response to treatment in prostate cancer. Innovative imaging techniques such as single-photon emission computed tomography combined with computed tomography and PET tracers targeting bone and tumor-specific markers offer enhanced detection capabilities; however, conclusive evidence supporting their superiority in therapy response monitoring remains limited (Azad *et al.*, 2016). In the field of neuro-oncology, PET scans using somatostatin receptor ligands are highly sensitive and specific for detecting meningiomas and help distinguish tumor recurrence from post-therapy changes, which improves the way treatment responses are evaluated. Furthermore, standardized protocols for PET imaging and theragnostic approaches in meningioma treatment underscore the evolving role of nuclear medicine in accurately determining treatment outcomes and guiding subsequent clinical decisions (Albert *et al.*, 2024) (Figure 9.14).

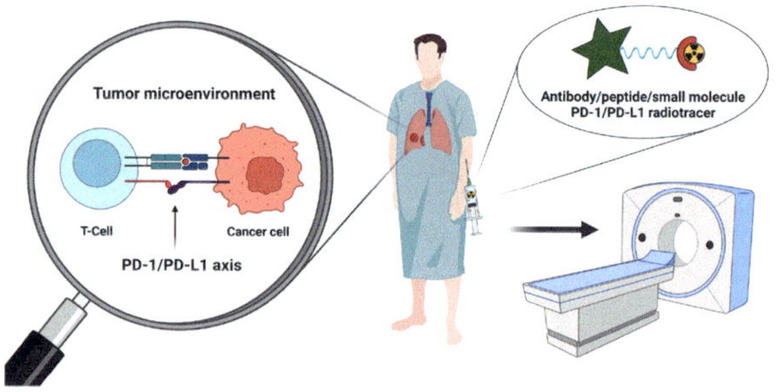

Figure 9.14. Innovative imaging techniques such as single-photon emission computed tomography combined with computed tomography and PET tracers targeting bone and tumor-specific markers offer enhanced detection capabilities.

Source: https://pub.mdpi-res.com/pharmaceuticals/pharmaceuticals-15-00747/article_deploy/html/images/pharmaceuticals-15-00747-ag.png?1655704960.

9.3.6. Role in Personalized Medicine

With new imaging technology, clinicians can now handle disease diagnosis and treatment more effectively, mainly in oncology, where tumors are not all the same. PET-CT in nuclear medicine helps to see both the structure and the activity of tumors, which supports a better understanding of the tumor and its environment.

Various radiopharmaceuticals make it possible to assess tumor heterogeneity without surgery, which is very important for designing individual treatment plans. PET-CT allows doctors to tell apart different tumor types and check the effectiveness of treatment, which leads to better patient outcomes. Also, the addition of new tracers and AI-based image analysis methods is expected to improve the sensitivity and specificity of PET-CT in personalized medicine. These developments underscore the modality's indispensable role in precision healthcare, ultimately improving prognosis through targeted interventions and dynamic treatment adjustments (Islam *et al.*, 2025; Jain *et al.*, 2025).

9.3.7. Pediatric Applications

The use of advanced medical imaging has made it much easier to diagnose complex diseases in children, since their symptoms can be vague and hard to understand. Using PET-CT in nuclear medicine provides a special benefit by joining metabolic and anatomical details, which is very important for pediatric patients because of their size and developing systems. The use of [F-18]FDG PET/CT has been increasingly adopted to identify and monitor inflammatory and infectious diseases in children, providing a noninvasive and comprehensive approach to detect sites of pathology that might otherwise remain elusive through conventional imaging. PET/MRI also shows promise because it can reduce the amount of radiation given to children, which is very important in their care. The importance of standardized protocols and interpretation criteria for pediatric applications ensures consistent and reliable results across institutions, facilitating effective treatment planning and follow-up in this vulnerable population (Albano *et al.*, 2021) (Figure 9.15).

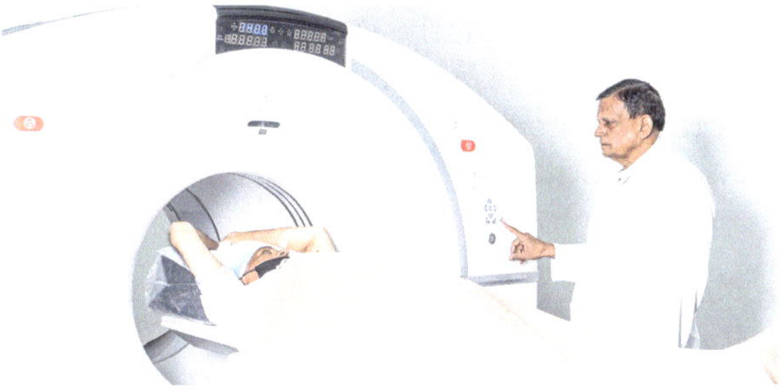

Figure 9.15. Nuclear medicine techniques, particularly positron emission tomography combined with computer tomography (PET-CT), offer a unique advantage by combining metabolic and anatomical information, which is crucial in pediatric patients due to their smaller size and developing physiology.

Source: https://bmchrc.org/speciality/6673ef6e2df71Nuclear%20Medicine.webp.

9.3.8. Research Applications in Nuclear Medicine

New developments in medical imaging have greatly changed the way diseases are diagnosed by providing important information about what happens at the molecular and cellular levels. Nuclear medicine is very important because it uses radioactive tracers and advanced imaging techniques such as PET and CT to detect and monitor pathological changes. Besides traditional imaging, research in nuclear medicine now includes Near Infrared Chemical Imaging Microspectroscopy and fluorescence spectroscopy, which make it possible to detect at the level of individual cells or molecules. These emerging modalities promise enhanced resolution and lower costs, addressing limitations associated with traditional nuclear imaging methods, including patient radiation exposure and imaging resolution challenges (Baianu, 2011). Early detection of critical diseases such as Alzheimer's disease and cancer is a priority for clinical research, underscoring the potential of nuclear medicine to improve therapeutic outcomes significantly (Baianu, 2011). More investment and research are necessary to make sure these innovative diagnostic tools are fully used in healthcare.

9.3.9. Case Studies Demonstrating Efficacy

Case studies showing the practical uses of PET-CT imaging have greatly boosted progress in nuclear medicine. One compelling example involves the use of positron emission tomography to monitor tumor activity and treatment response in patient-derived xenograft models, particularly in gastrointestinal stromal tumors (GIST). These studies demonstrate PET-CT's capacity to detect metabolic changes in tumors, providing critical insights that correlate strongly with histological findings, thus validating imaging as a reliable surrogate for disease progression and therapeutic efficacy in vivo (Babicky *et al.*, 2014). Additionally, in regenerative medicine, imaging techniques have enhanced the understanding of stem cell therapy by enabling real-time tracking and assessment of cell implantation and function, offering a non-invasive method to evaluate regenerative outcomes and improve treatment protocols (Jokerst *et al.*, 2016). All these case studies strengthen the idea that nuclear medicine and PET-CT are key to both targeted cancer therapies and many biomedical uses.

Test Your Knowledge

1. In what situations is PET-CT most often used in oncology?
2. What role does PET-CT play in finding out about heart disease?
3. How is PET-CT employed to find and follow up on cancer that comes back?

9.4. Safety and Ethical Considerations

Learning Outcome

1. Understand radiation exposure and risk management;
2. Focus on informed consent in nuclear medicine;
3. Know regulatory guidelines and standards;
4. Discuss patient privacy and data security;
5. Explain the environmental impact of nuclear medicine;
6. Describe ethical dilemmas in radiopharmaceutical use;
7. Focus on training and certification for practitioners;
8. Explain the public perception of nuclear medicine;
9. Understand future directions in ethical practices.

Improvements in nuclear medicine, such as those seen in PET-CT imaging, have boosted accuracy in diagnosis and monitoring of treatments, but they also require careful consideration of safety and ethics. Because radiopharmaceuticals are used, there must be strict rules to keep radiation exposure low for patients and staff and to ensure they are effective. Ethics in health care also addresses informed consent, privacy, and ensuring that these advanced technologies are given out in an equitable manner. Clinical research management plays a pivotal role in addressing these concerns by implementing standardized protocols and monitoring outcomes, thus fostering responsible innovation within nuclear medicine (Petisca *et al.*, 2024). Moreover, non-invasive imaging techniques are crucial in tracking cellular therapies, ensuring both therapeutic efficacy and patient safety throughout treatment processes (Jokerst *et al.*,

2016). For this reason, making sure PET-CT brings benefits without compromising patient welfare and ethics is still a top priority in advancing nuclear medicine.

9.4.1. Radiation Exposure and Risk Management

Good communication and patient awareness are essential for managing the risks of radiation exposure in nuclear medicine, especially in PET-CT imaging. Although these procedures help find problems, the radiation they use is not always well understood by patients, which can affect their decision-making and risk management. Studies reveal that a significant portion of nuclear medicine patients lack awareness of the radiation doses involved and receive insufficient information from existing educational materials (Drey *et al.*, 2019).

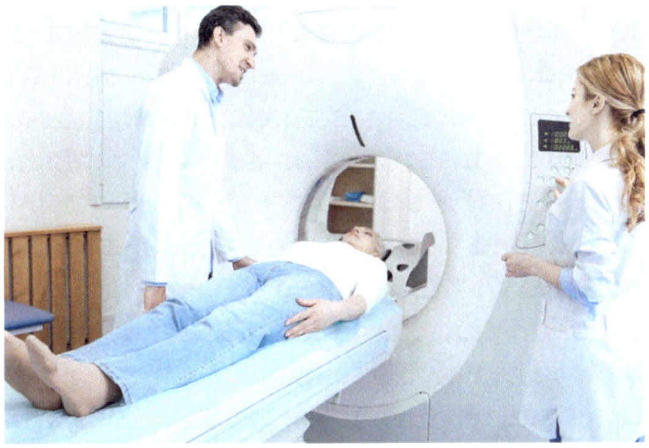

Figure 9.16. Proper communication and patient understanding are critical components in managing the risks associated with radiation exposure in nuclear medicine, particularly in positron emission tomography combined with computer tomography (PET-CT) imaging.

Source: https://sjra.com/wp-content/uploads/2022/12/CT-Technologists-Disucssing-Medical-Imaging-Process-With-Female-Patient-1.webp.

Additionally, research indicates that only a minority of patients can accurately compare their exposure to standard radiation dose benchmarks, and many express a desire for clearer, more detailed explanations within informational leaflets (Drey *et al.*, 2020). The study points out that better communication with patients, designed together, is necessary for clear and legal practices. Improving patient education not only supports ethical practice but also mitigates anxiety and encourages informed decision-making in clinical nuclear imaging (Figure 9.16).

9.4.2. Informed Consent in Nuclear Medicine

It is very important to get informed consent in nuclear medicine because the procedures in PET-CT can be complex and hard for patients to grasp. Patients must be clearly informed about the diagnostic procedures, including the use of radiopharmaceuticals and associated radiation exposure, which may vary depending on the modality, such as 68Ga-PSMA-11 PET/CT for prostate cancer recurrence or 82Rubidium PET-MPS for coronary artery disease detection (Ceci *et al.*, 2019; Lambelle, 2017). Telling patients about the benefits and risks allows them to make informed decisions about their care. Trust and compliance are encouraged, which are necessary for correctly diagnosing and planning treatment. Because these imaging procedures are advanced, the patient should be told about their risks, the amount of radiation involved, and what the results might show. So, informed consent is essential for good patient care in nuclear medicine.

9.4.3. Regulatory Guidelines and Standards

For nuclear medicine to be safe and effective, especially in PET-CT imaging, following the proper regulations and standards is very important. They are created to make sure patients get high-quality care, are safe from radiation, and the diagnosis is accurate. Professional organizations such as the American Association of Physicists in Medicine (AAPM) play a critical role in developing medical physics practice guidelines that undergo rigorous consensus and public review to reflect current scientific knowledge and clinical needs. They divide practices into those that are required and those that are suggested, to show what medical physicists must do and what they can do in different situations. This structured approach enables regulatory bodies and accrediting institutions to enforce safety and quality assurance measures effectively, thereby advancing patient care and professional accountability within nuclear medicine disciplines (Seibert *et al.*, 2018) (Figure 9.17).

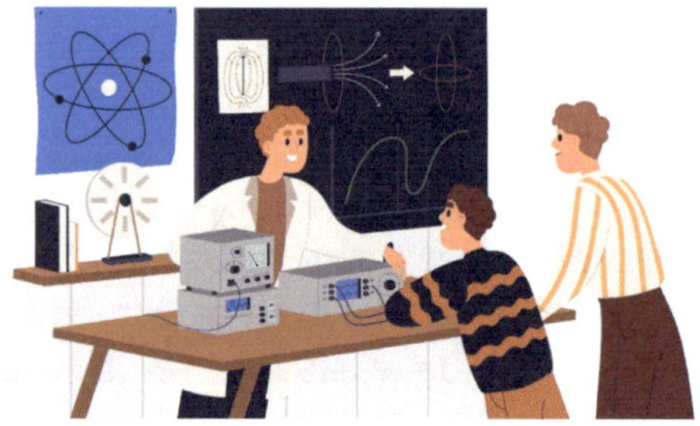

Figure 9.17. Ensuring the safety and efficacy of nuclear medicine practices, particularly in PET-CT imaging, depends heavily on adherence to established regulatory guidelines and standards.

Source: https://www.versantphysics.com/wp-content/uploads/2024/09/T.-Morgan.jpg.

9.4.4. Patient Privacy and Data Security

The addition of PET-CT imaging to nuclear medicine has greatly improved the accuracy of diagnoses and the care given to patients. Still, these improvements create new issues about patient privacy and the safety of health data, since many sensitive medical details are now kept digitally. Keeping this data confidential and accurate is very important, both to follow the rules and to keep patients trusting the system. Strong cybersecurity, which involves encryption, secure access controls, and frequent audits, should be used to prevent any breaches that might expose personal health information. Furthermore, adherence to professional guidelines and practice standards set forth by organizations like the American Association of Physicists in Medicine supports the protection of patient data throughout imaging processes (Seibert *et al.*, 2018). Because imaging archives and digital records are growing, institutions should make sure their data security frameworks keep up with advancements in technology to address risks effectively.

9.4.5. Environmental Impact of Nuclear Medicine

Using PET-CT imaging more widely has greatly improved the ability to diagnose and treat patients in nuclear medicine. Nevertheless, the progress made creates new environmental problems that we should pay more attention to. Water and soil can be contaminated if the radioactive waste produced by using radioactive isotopes in nuclear medicine is not handled properly. The energy-demanding ways of making isotopes add to greenhouse gas emissions, which affect the environment. It is important to have strong waste management procedures, such as proper storage, to mitigate these risks. Also, scientists are working on new radiotracers that have shorter life spans, hoping to lessen environmental risks without affecting their diagnostic effectiveness. Addressing these concerns is critical for balancing the medical benefits of PET-CT with ecological responsibility, ensuring that advancements in nuclear medicine do not come at an undue cost to the environment (Figure 9.18).

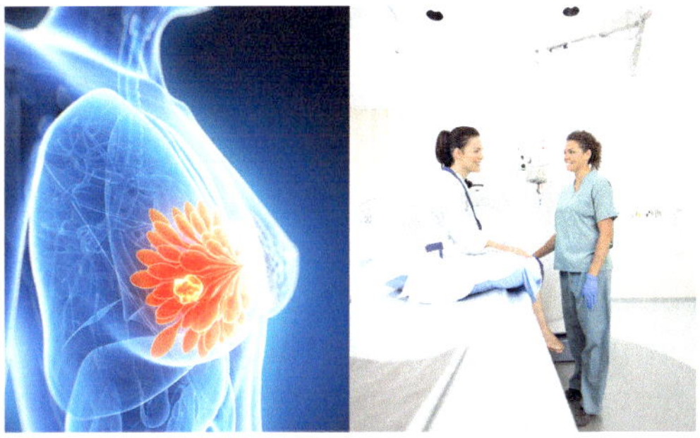

Figure 9.18. The advancement of nuclear medicine, particularly the widespread use of PET-CT imaging, has significantly improved diagnostic capabilities and patient outcomes.

Source: https://kiranpetct.com/wp-content/uploads/2024/05/breast-cancer.png.

9.4.6. Ethical Dilemmas in Radiopharmaceutical Use

Developments in nuclear medicine, such as PET-CT imaging and radiopharmaceuticals, have made it much easier to diagnose and treat cancer. Even so, such innovations raise difficult ethical questions that should be considered with care. Since radiation and unexpected problems can happen, it is difficult for patients to give their informed consent. Also, making sure that advanced radiopharmaceuticals are given fairly to all patients is a concern for healthcare systems. Ensuring the accuracy and clinical utility of emerging PET biomarkers remains critical, as misleading results can lead to inappropriate treatment decisions or unnecessary patient anxiety (Boers *et al.*, 2020). Apart from diagnosis, radiomolecular precision oncology points out that quality control, correct dosing, and ethical rules are required for theragnostic use. Dealing with these ethical issues helps ensure that patients are safe and that nuclear medicine is done ethically.

9.4.7. Training and Certification for Practitioners

Since these fields need a lot of skill and attention to detail, people working in nuclear medicine and PET-CT must be well-trained and certified. To ensure both the right diagnosis and patient safety, professionals must thoroughly understand radiopharmaceuticals, imaging methods, and safety rules. Standardized competencies for working with PET-CT are usually required by law, and these are taught during certification programs. They usually consist of classroom learning, hands-on experience in hospitals, and tough tests to test both theory and practice. Also, it is important to keep learning to stay up-to-date with new technology and updated best practices in this fast-changing field. More and more, training involves using simulations and teamwork to help people improve their decision-making skills. The integration of such comprehensive education frameworks ultimately improves diagnostic accuracy and patient outcomes, underscoring the importance of standardized certification pathways for practitioners in nuclear medicine and PET-CT (Kitsiou *et al.*, 2013) (Figure 9.19).

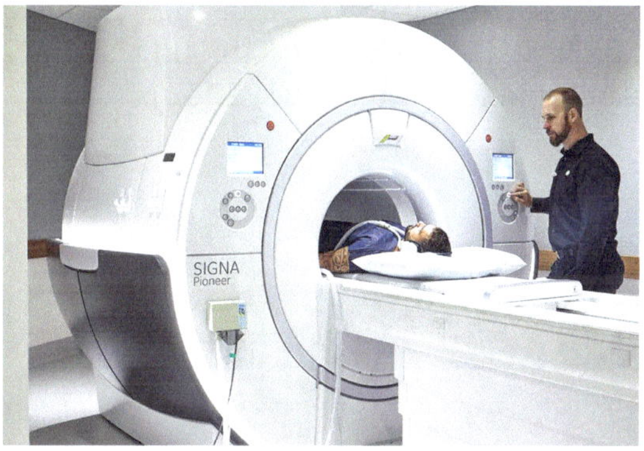

Figure 9.19. Professionals must acquire a deep understanding of radiopharmaceuticals, imaging techniques, and safety protocols to ensure accurate diagnosis and patient safety.

Source: https://www.prpimaging.com.au/wp-content/uploads/2021/04/PRP-4-11-195495.jpg.

9.4.8. Public Perception of Nuclear Medicine

New medical technology has greatly increased the public's understanding and acceptance of different ways to diagnose and treat diseases. Although PET-CT and other nuclear medicine techniques are very useful, the public is sometimes worried about their safety. These apprehensions are partially rooted in a general lack of understanding regarding the rigorous training and safety protocols that professionals in the field undergo, including those detailed in medical physics, which ensures patient and staff protection through precise radiation dosimetry and quality assurance measures (Newhauser *et al.*, 2022). Furthermore, many widespread myths and false information make people reluctant or afraid, which makes it harder for nuclear medicine to be entirely accepted. Giving clear information about the risks and benefits and using targeted education helps patients and the community feel more confident and informed. As nuclear medicine continues to evolve, addressing public perception challenges remains vital to maximize its clinical impact and acceptance (Lyon *et al.*, 2022).

9.4.9. Future Directions in Ethical Practices

Because of progress in nuclear medicine and PET-CT imaging, it is necessary to address ethical matters that involve patient safety, privacy of data, and the environment. Since AI is being used in healthcare to improve diagnosis and tailor treatments, ensuring AI decisions are open and responsible is very important. Using new types of imaging can help reduce radiation exposure, which is an ethical obligation to protect patients while maintaining accurate diagnoses. Ensuring that everyone, especially those from vulnerable populations, can use these advanced techniques is also important in future ethics. Also, using biodegradable contrast agents and more energy-efficient systems is necessary for reducing the environmental issues associated with imaging procedures. Embracing these multidimensional ethical imperatives will require interdisciplinary collaboration and continuous refinement of regulatory frameworks to harmonize innovation with moral responsibility in nuclear medicine (Abualigah *et al.*, 2024; Adadzi *et al.*, 2024).

Test Your Knowledge

1. What are the main problems that can happen from radiation exposure in nuclear medicine?
2. What safety measures are needed when using radiopharmaceuticals for PET scans?

SUMMARY

Thanks to new nuclear medicine techniques such as PET-CT, it is now much easier to accurately diagnose several clinical problems. The combined metabolic and anatomical information provided by PET-CT allows for more precise characterization of lesions, as evidenced by studies demonstrating high sensitivity and specificity in assessing solitary pulmonary nodules (Bobek-Billewicz *et al.*, 2012). Moreover, the collaboration between nuclear medicine specialists and radiologists, while beneficial, does not drastically alter overall diagnostic performance, though it may improve negative predictive value (Bobek-Billewicz *et al.*, 2012). Although PET-CT is very accurate, some diagnostic errors do occur; a few percent of PET-CT reports require addenda because of errors in perception or decision-making, and the type of imaging can affect the rate of these errors. They demonstrate that constant efforts to improve quality and teamwork between different specialists can help patients the most. Ultimately, PET-CT represents a valuable tool in modern medicine, balancing substantial diagnostic benefits with the need for cautious interpretation and ongoing evaluation (Bobek-Billewicz *et al.*, 2012).

Better imaging technologies have significantly improved the accuracy of nuclear medicine diagnoses. Scintigraphy and PET-CT help provide extra information on how organs function, which is not available from anatomical imaging. Scintigraphy gives two-dimensional pictures and is still important for checking the whole body, even as other methods improve. PET-CT offers a better resolution and three-dimensional view, which helps find pathological changes earlier and, in more detail, than CT or MRI. In human medicine, this is now more important, especially for difficult cases like fever of unknown origin, since it helps locate the infectious or inflammatory focal point after initial standard diagnostics. The integration of PET-CT into clinical guidelines underscores its growing role in personalized patient management, emphasizing the need for ongoing research to optimize its indications and applications across different medical fields (Palestro *et al.*, 2024; Spriet *et al.*, 2024).

KEY TERMS FROM THIS CHAPTER

- Prostate-specific membrane antigen (PSMA)
- Radiopharmaceuticals
- Receptor status
- Molecular biology
- Gamma rays
- Neurological disorders
- Radioactive materials
- Metabolic activity
- Tumor metabolism
- Clinical imaging
- Cardiovascular diseases
- Glucose uptake

CRITICAL THINKING QUESTIONS

1. **Which of the following most accurately states the idea behind Nuclear Medicine imaging?**
   a. Magnetic resonance of hydrogen nuclei
   b. Ionizing radiation emitted by radiopharmaceuticals within the body
   c. Reflection of sound waves from tissues
   d. X-ray transmission through body tissues
2. **What is the main role of a radiopharmaceutical in nuclear medicine?**
   a. To enhance contrast in CT scans
   b. To emit gamma radiation for imaging
   c. To produce an MRI image
   d. To detect calcium deposits in bones
3. **In which of these imaging devices is Nuclear Medicine most often applied?**
   a. Ultrasound scanner
   b. PET scanner
   c. Gamma camera (SPECT)
   d. MRI scanner
4. **What does PET stand for in Nuclear Medicine?**
   a. Positron Emission Tomography
   b. Proton Emission Tomography
   c. Photographic Emission Tomography
   d. Positron Energy Tomography
5. **Which of these is the most often used radiopharmaceutical in PET scans?**
   a. Technetium-99m
   b. Fluorodeoxyglucose (FDG)
   c. Iodine-131
   d. Barium sulfate

Short Answer Questions

1. In what way does a PET scan create images that show how tissues are active?
2. What part does PET-CT play in diagnosing neurological illnesses?
3. What is the main worry when using radiopharmaceuticals in Nuclear Medicine?
4. What are the recent advancements in PET-CT technology?
5. What is a potential future improvement in PET-CT imaging?

Answers to Critical Thinking Questions

1. (b); 2. (b); 3. (c); 4. (a); 5. (b)

REFERENCES

1. Aarntzen, E. H. J. G., Kneilling, M., La Fougere, C., Mulder, G., *et al.* (2022). A role for artificial intelligence in molecular imaging of infection and inflammation. https://core.ac.uk/download/534681230.pdf (accessed on 1st June 2025).
2. Abualigah, L., Banu, S. A., Dhama, K., Mamachan, R., *et al.* (2024). Unleashing the future: Exploring the transformative prospects of artificial intelligence in veterinary science. https://core.ac.uk/download/620832362.pdf (accessed on 1st June 2025).
3. Adadzi, J., Anderson, II. J., Azi, C. I., Carsrud, *et al.* (2024). Transformative advancements in diagnostic imaging: Reducing risks, enhancing accuracy, and promoting sustainability. https://core.ac.uk/download/621451782.pdf (accessed on 1st June 2025).
4. Adak, S., Bhalla, R., Luthra, S. K., Mandal, *et al.* (2012). *Radiotracers for SPECT Imaging: Current Scenario and Future Prospects.* https://core.ac.uk/download/43366298.pdf (accessed on 1st June 2025).
5. Ajani, J. A., D'Amico, T. A., Bentrem, D. J., Chao, J., Cooke, D. T., Corvera, C. U., Das, P., *et al.* (2022). Gastric cancer, version 2.2022, NCCN clinical practice guidelines in oncology. *Journal of the National Comprehensive Cancer Network, 20*, 167–192. https://doi.org/10.6004/jnccn.2022.0008 (accessed on 1st June 2025).
6. Albano, D., Altini, C., Baldari, S., Bartoli, *et al.* (2021). State of the art of 18F-FDG PET/CT application in inflammation and infection: A guide for image acquisition and interpretation. https://core.ac.uk/download/554203023.pdf (accessed on 1st June 2025).
7. Albert, N. L., Chang, S., Deroose, C. M., Fraioli, *et al.* (2024). Joint EANM/EANO/RANO/SNMMI practice guideline/procedure standards for diagnostics and therapy (theranostics) of meningiomas using radiolabeled somatostatin receptor ligands: Version 1.0. https://core.ac.uk/download/621201183.pdf (accessed on 1st June 2025).
8. Alotaibi, N. A., Glaudemans, A. W. J. M., Kwee, T. C., Yakar, *et al.* (2020). Diagnostic errors in clinical FDG-PET/CT. https://core.ac.uk/download/345435689.pdf (accessed on 1st June 2025).
9. AlSaadi, A., Jain, A., Al-Jabri, A., Delanerolle, G., Zabah, J., Shi, J. Q., Phiri, P., *et al.* (2024). *Technological Advances in SPECT and SPECT/CT Imaging.* https://core.ac.uk/download/613741130.pdf (accessed on 1st June 2025).
10. Aparici, C. M., Cheung, H., Lawhn-Heath, C., Lopez, *et al.* (2018). Metastatic cervical paravertebral solitary fibrous tumor detected by fluorodeoxyglucose positron emission tomography-computed tomography. https://core.ac.uk/download/323062391.pdf (accessed on 1st June 2025).
11. Auletta, S., Carideo, L., Galli, F., Lauri, *et al.* (2016). Immunoscintigraphy for therapy decision making and follow-up of biological therapies. *International Journal of Nuclear Medicine Research.* https://core.ac.uk/download/153364883.pdf (accessed on 1st June 2025).
12. Azad, G., Cook, G. J. R., & Padhani, A. R. (2016). *Bone Imaging in Prostate Cancer: The Evolving Roles of Nuclear Medicine and Radiology.* https://core.ac.uk/download/45323707.pdf (accessed on 1st June 2025).
13. Babicky, M. L., French, R. P., Hoh, C. K., Jaquish, *et al.* (2014). *Generation of Orthotopic Patient-Derived Xenografts from Gastrointestinal Stromal Tumor.* https://core.ac.uk/download/323066735.pdf (accessed on 1st June 2025).

14. Baianu, I. (2011). *Early Diagnosis of Alzheimer's Disease by NIRF Spectroscopy and Nuclear Medicine – v.4.0.* https://core.ac.uk/download/pdf/290232.pdf (accessed on 1st June 2025).

15. Bankstahl, J., Belcari, N., Krämer, S., Vandenberghe, *et al.* (2015). Accurate molecular imaging of small animals taking into account animal models, handling, anesthesia, quality control and imaging system performance. https://core.ac.uk/download/55743381.pdf (accessed on 1st June 2025).

16. Basu, S., & Kalshetty, A. (2017). Volumetric high-resolution computed tomography in evaluating pulmonary metastases from differentiated thyroid carcinoma: Considerations for evolving the optimal diagnostic pathway. *Nuclear Medicine Communications.* https://www.semanticscholar.org/paper/563f6c5a64fb0b730f73f92886f0583deb15cde0 (accessed on 1st June 2025).

17. Belal, S. L., Edenbrandt, L., Enqvist, O., Frantz, *et al.* (2023). *Applications of Artificial Intelligence in PSMA PET/CT for Prostate Cancer Imaging.* https://core.ac.uk/download/571662722.pdf (accessed on 1st June 2025).

18. Benjamens, S., Moers, C., Pol, R. A., Slart, *et al.* (2020). Kidney transplantation and diagnostic imaging: The early days and future advancements of transplant surgery. https://core.ac.uk/download/519039042.pdf (accessed on 1st June 2025).

19. Bobek-Billewicz, M., D'Amico, A., Gorczewski, K., Kużdżał, *et al.* (2012). PET-CT evaluation of solitary pulmonary nodules: With or without a radiologist? *Nuclear Med. Rev.* https://core.ac.uk/download/344354990.pdf (accessed on 1st June 2025).

20. Bochev, P., Kaprelyan, A., & Klissarova, A. (2014). *Use of 18F-FDG PET/CT in Patients with Acute Ischemic Stroke.* https://core.ac.uk/download/389005622.pdf (accessed on 1st June 2025).

21. Boers, J., De Vries, E. F. J., Glaudemans, A. W. J. M., Hospers, *et al.* (2020). *Application of PET Tracers in Molecular Imaging for Breast Cancer.* https://core.ac.uk/download/345432574.pdf (accessed on 1st June 2025).

22. Boussios, S., Carneiro, G., Evans, P. M., Mikropoulos, *et al.* (2024). *The Application of Radiomics and AI to Molecular Imaging for Prostate Cancer.* https://core.ac.uk/download/603232360.pdf (accessed on 1st June 2025).

23. Brunetti, A., Cuocolo, A., Ferro, A., Gargiulo, *et al.* (2012). *PET/CT Imaging in Mouse Models of Myocardial Ischemia.* https://core.ac.uk/download/pdf/8702226.pdf (accessed on 1st June 2025).

24. Calderoni, L., Giovanella, L., & Fanti, S. (2024). Endocrinology application of molecular imaging: Current role of PET/CT. *Journal of Endocrinological Investigation, 47*, 2383–2396. https://www.semanticscholar.org/paper/dc735ba8ff5f4af9f9763d13fd030b42131519ec (accessed on 1st June 2025).

25. Carsrud, N. D. V., Flores, J. V., Holets, H. M., Kadivi, *et al.* (2024). Transformative precision: Investigative summary of PET/CT-guided radiation therapy simulation in comprehensive cancer management. *European Journal of Theoretical and Applied Sciences.* https://core.ac.uk/download/603903713.pdf (accessed on 1st June 2025).

26. Ceci, F., Castellucci, P., Graziani, T., Farolfi, A., Fonti, C., Lodi, F., Bianchi, L., *et al.* (2019). MP09-15 68Ga-PSMA-11 PET/CT in recurrent prostate cancer: Efficacy in different clinical stages of PSA failure. *The Journal of Urology, 201*, e113, e114. https://www.semanticscholar.org/paper/cda76e95baad3720b6df477e56580bcf89d18308 (accessed on 1st June 2025).

27. Dhami, S. (2008). *Strategic Analysis of the Commercialization Potential of a Novel Algorithm.* https://core.ac.uk/download/638896345.pdf (accessed on 1st June 2025).

28. Drey, N., Husson, O., May, K. A., Murray, *et al.* (2020). Radiation exposure awareness from patients undergoing nuclear medicine diagnostic 99mTc-MDP bone scans and 2-deoxy-2-(18F) fluoro-D-glucose PET/computed tomography scans. *Nuclear Medicine.* https://core.ac.uk/download/305120002.pdf (accessed on 1st June 2025).

29. Drey, N., Husson, O., May, K., Murray, *et al.* (2019). *Ionizing Radiation Exposure from Medical Imaging – A Review of Patient's (un)awareness.* https://core.ac.uk/download/266989986.pdf (accessed on 1st June 2025).

30. Glaudemans, A. W., Rouzet, F., Galli, G., Signore, A., *et al.* (2015). *Imaging Infection and Inflammation.* https://core.ac.uk/download/54518572.pdf (accessed on 1st June 2025).

31. Hogg, P., Medvedec, H., Testanera, G., Waterstram-Rich, *et al.* (2011). *Euro-American Discussion Document on Entry and Advanced Level Practice in Nuclear Medicine.* https://core.ac.uk/download/1666480.pdf (accessed on 1st June 2025).

32. Islam, M. R., Zohra, F. T., & Watabe, H. (2025). Current applications and advancements of state-of-the-art technology of PET-CT. *Bangladesh Journal of Nuclear Medicine.* https://www.semanticscholar.org/paper/12b89e3a31b744c2b4276ce8f282580a3ccfeec4 (accessed on 1st June 2025).

33. Jain, A., Kheruka, S., Usmani, S., Al Riyami, K., Al Busaidi, A., Bichpuria, S., & Al Sukaiti, R. (2025). Exploring tumor heterogeneity: The role of PET/CT with various radiopharmaceuticals in diagnosis and treatment guidance. *Advances in Radiotherapy & Nuclear Medicine.* https://www.semanticscholar.org/paper/ca3aa00cec29ea3229f8aa8223aa5c7fe378f95e (accessed on 1st June 2025).

34. Jokerst, J. V., & Wang, J. (2016). *Stem Cell Imaging: Tools to Improve Cell Delivery and Viability.* https://core.ac.uk/download/323064235.pdf (accessed on 1st June 2025).

35. Jussing, E. (2022). *Development of Radiometal-Based Labelling Techniques and Tracers for Non-invasive Molecular Imaging.* https://core.ac.uk/download/516463870.pdf (accessed on 1st June 2025).

36. Kashyap, P., Kaur, C. D., Kumar, A., Mishra, *et al.* (2020). *Theranostics: New Era in Nuclear Medicine and Radiopharmaceuticals.* https://core.ac.uk/download/322580751.pdf (accessed on 1st June 2025).

37. Kerrie, T., Lokitz, S., Hawley, M., Sibley, C., *et al.* (2025). Ten poster presentations for the 56th Annual Meeting of the Southwestern Chapter of the Society of Nuclear Medicine. https://www.semanticscholar.org/paper/b80247f5266ba10d9568ca77224552524025d220 (accessed on 1st June 2025).

38. Kitsiou, A., Caforio, A. L. P., Porta-Sanchez, A., Vahanian, A., Iung, B., Carrera, C., Szymanski, C., *et al.* (2013). ESC core curriculum for the general cardiologist (2013). *European Heart Journal.* https://core.ac.uk/download/55756305.pdf (accessed on 1st June 2025).

39. Lambelle, A. (2017). *Moderated Posters Session – Ischemia Detection.* https://www.semanticscholar.org/paper/4b62299d0119454d301bc00096a0944a3fd1608c (accessed on 1st June 2025).

40. Law, I., Albert, N. L., Arbizu, J., Boellaard, R., Drzezga, A., Galldiks, N., La Fougère, C., *et al.* (2018). Joint EANM/EANO/RANO practice guidelines/SNMMI procedure standards for imaging of gliomas using PET with radiolabeled amino acids and [18F]FDG: Version 1.0. *European Journal of Nuclear Medicine and Molecular Imaging, 46*, 540–557. https://doi.org/10.1007/s00259-018-4207-9 (accessed on 1st June 2025).

41. Lowrance, W. T., Dreicer, R., Jarrard, D. F., Scarpato, K. R., Kim, S. K., Kirkby, E., Buckley, D., *et al.* (2023). Updates to advanced prostate cancer: AUA/SUO guideline (2023). *The Journal of Urology, 209*, 1082–1090. https://doi.org/10.1097/ju.0000000000003452 (accessed on 1st June 2025).

42. Lyon, A. R., López-Fernández, T., Couch, L. S., Asteggiano, R., Aznar, M. C., Bergler-Klein, J., Boriani, G., *et al.* (2022). 2022 ESC guidelines on cardio-oncology developed in collaboration with the European Hematology Association (EHA), the European Society for Therapeutic Radiology and Oncology (ESTRO) and the International Cardio-Oncology Society (IC-OS). *European Heart Journal, 43*, 4229–4361. https://doi.org/10.1093/eurheartj/ehac244 (accessed on 1st June 2025).

43. Nag, S. (2017). *Image Registration Techniques: A Survey*. http://arxiv.org/abs/1712.07540 (accessed on 1st June 2025).

44. Newhauser, W., Gress, D. A., Mills, M., Jordan, D. W., Sutlief, S. G., Martin, M., & Jackson, E. F. (2022). Medical physics workforce in the United States. *Journal of Applied Clinical Medical Physics, 23.* https://doi.org/10.1002/acm2.13762 (accessed on 1st June 2025).

45. Palestro, C., Abikhzer, G., Bar-Sever, Z., Bartel, T., Brady, R., Grady, E. E., Israel, O., *et al.* (2024). Summary: Appropriate use criteria for the use of nuclear medicine in fever of unknown origin. *Journal of Nuclear Medicine: Official Publication, Society of Nuclear Medicine.* https://www.semanticscholar.org/paper/373842207d1a50e4cb32813f8684e9e91c021387 (accessed on 1st June 2025).

46. Pawar, Y. P., Shimpi, H., Shrivastav, A., Awasare, S. U., Rakshit, S., Karpe, M., Damle, A. A., *et al.* (2024). Role of advance nuclear medicine imaging techniques in preclinical drug development and three R's in animal research. *Journal of Laboratory Animal Science.* https://www.semanticscholar.org/paper/872cfab68fb460e6cccc2938a232921c5865a79c (accessed on 1st June 2025).

47. Petisca, T. S. C. (2024). Internship report at a clinical research unit – CRU2C: The specifics of clinical research with radiopharmaceuticals. https://core.ac.uk/download/621577770.pdf (accessed on 1st June 2025).

48. Ramanathan, V., Gamage, S. P., Karunathilaka, U., Wickramasinghe, W., & Tudugala, R. (2024). Assessing radiation exposure of fingers of PET/CT technologists during 18F-FDG procedures using active extremity dosimeters: A single-center study. *Journal of Radiological Protection: Official Journal of the Society for Radiological Protection.* https://www.semanticscholar.org/paper/f5b3341385eed375a2204444b903496a60f2069d (accessed on 1st June 2025).

49. Roya, M., van Snick, J. H., Slart, R., Noordzij, W., Stormezand, G., Willemsen, A., Boellaard, R., *et al.* (2024). Clinical performance comparison of a long versus a short axial field-of-view PET/CT using EARL-compliant reconstructions. *Molecular Imaging and Biology, 26*, 780–789. https://www.semanticscholar.org/paper/b84774c18cef7ea8933cb4bb9d79d03694c0de60 (accessed on 1st June 2025).

50. Samim, A., Tytgat, G. A. M., Bleeker, G., Wenker, S. T. M., Chatalic, K. L. S., Poot, A. J., Tolboom, N., *et al.* (2021). Nuclear medicine imaging in neuroblastoma: Current status and new developments. *Journal of Personalized Medicine, 11*, 270. https://doi.org/10.3390/jpm11040270 (accessed on 1st June 2025).

51. Seibert, A. J., Baird, C. T., Clements, J. B., de Boer, *et al.* (2018). AAPM medical physics practice guideline 10.a.: Scope of practice for clinical medical physics. https://core.ac.uk/download/286729023.pdf (accessed on 1st June 2025).

52. Singh, S., & Gutta, A. (2022). A review of the role of nuclear medicine imaging in diagnostic dentistry. *South African Dental Journal.* https://www.semanticscholar.org/paper/8cdbe3fb65f0292e7b5a03d0a1c2c3d79f7c8643 (accessed on 1st June 2025).

53. Skovorodko, K., Komiagienė, R., Maciusovic, M., Gilys, L., Vajauskas, D., Grigonienė, V., Žiliukas, J., *et al.* (2022). Nationwide survey on radiation doses received by patients in nuclear medicine imaging procedures. *Journal of Radiological Protection, 42.* https://www.semanticscholar.org/paper/1f81c5d1d8aac89c436d5f6f1a537013cf35bca5 (accessed on 1st June 2025).

54. Soliman, K., Alenezi, A., Alrushoud, A., Altimyat, S., Albander, H., & Alruwaili, T. (2018). Applied radiation protection physics. *Nuclear Medicine Physics.* https://www.semanticscholar.org/paper/afdf9e30d79b14308200246168271 81ee82af1af (accessed on 1st June 2025).

55. Spriet, M., & Vandenberghe, F. (2024). Equine nuclear medicine in 2024: Use and value of scintigraphy and PET in equine lameness diagnosis. *Animals: An Open Access Journal from MDPI, 14.* https://www.semanticscholar.org/paper/2774334ddf6883c7c3debab676526ae9e47fc6de (accessed on 1st June 2025).

56. Tapper, W., Carneiro, G., Mikropoulos, C., Thomas, S. A., Evans, P. M., & Boussios, S. (2024). The application of radiomics and AI to molecular imaging for prostate cancer. *Journal of Personalized Medicine, 14.* https://www.semanticscholar.org/paper/0e3bafe8aa1895605ab9dc95a9dada411e11c81f (accessed on 1st June 2025).

INTERVENTIONAL RADIOLOGY

10

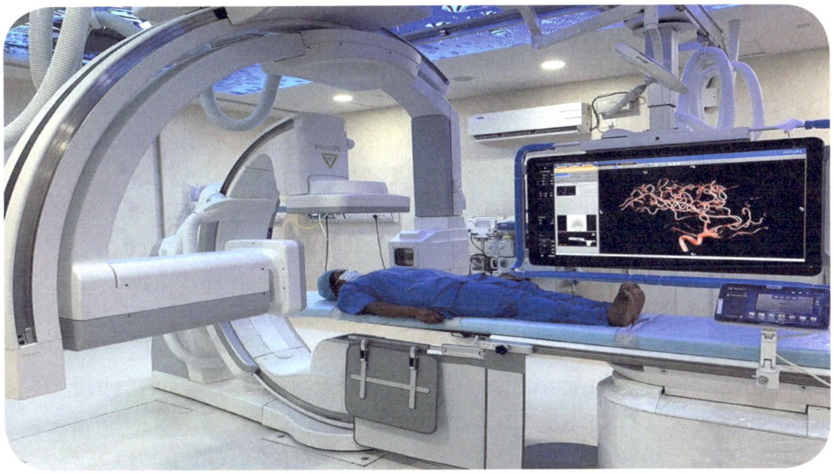

Introduction

With new medical technology, healthcare delivery has been changing, and these advances have improved how patients are treated. Among these, interventional radiology has become very important because it combines imaging with minimally invasive treatments to manage many conditions. Because of this approach, patients may not need traditional surgery, which helps them recover faster and with fewer risks. Interventional radiology is supported by using advanced imaging methods such as magnetic resonance imaging and computed tomography, which allow for precise work inside the body. Moreover, the recent surge in artificial intelligence applications within radiology enhances diagnostic accuracy and procedural efficiency, allowing radiologists to focus on complex decision-making and personalized patient care (Pesapane *et al.*, 2018). As a result, interventional radiology exemplifies the shift towards more objective and patient-centered medical practice, underscoring its growing importance in contemporary medicine (Mathijssen, 2020).

LEARNING OBJECTIVES

After studying this chapter, you will be able to:

1. Identify techniques in interventional radiology;
2. Explain imaging modalities in interventional radiology;
3. Learn patient care and safety in interventional radiology;
4. Describe applications and impact of interventional radiology.

Definition of Interventional Radiology

Because of medical imaging, it is now possible to diagnose and treat many conditions without the need for major surgery. Interventional radiology shows this progress by using advanced imaging to direct less invasive procedures that help diagnose and treat diseases in most organs. This area of medicine combines the accuracy of radiology with procedures, so that doctors can treat patients by inserting catheters, performing biopsies, or fixing blood vessels without the need for open surgery. Interventional radiology minimizes risks and speeds up recovery, which helps patients and allows doctors to treat conditions that are risky to operate on with traditional surgery. It links the process of diagnosing with the process of treating, putting the patient at the center, and using imaging technology. Though primarily recognized for its vascular interventions, the field directly supports advancements in managing diseases like pulmonary fibrosis and interstitial lung disease, where imaging-defining pathology and guiding treatment are crucial (Raghu *et al.*, 2018) (Figure 10.1).

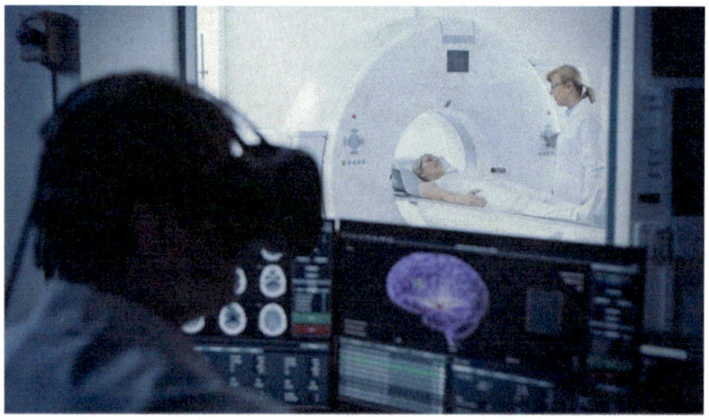

Figure 10.1. Interventional radiology exemplifies this evolution by utilizing advanced imaging techniques to guide minimally invasive procedures that diagnose and treat diseases in nearly every organ system.

Source: https://i0.wp.com/blog.medicai.io/wp-content/uploads/2024/09/iStock-1074166520.jpg.

Historical Background and Evolution

The progress of medical technology in the 20th and 21st centuries has played a key role in forming today's healthcare practices, such as interventional radiology. At the beginning, interventional radiology was based on the use of imaging in diagnosis, and it gradually became a way to treat diseases without major surgery. This evolution parallels broader trends in state and institutional interventions aimed at improving health outcomes through innovation and systematic regulation, as seen in economic and health system reforms during this period (Khurtovskyi, 2025). More investments and a focus on technology in health care show that the world is moving towards improved patient outcomes. Nonetheless, challenges remain in equitable resource distribution and integration within health systems, issues highlighted in recent analyses of development assistance for health, which underline the need for sustained investment in system strengthening alongside technological advances (Xie *et al.*, 2025). It is clear from this history that medical progress and policy changes have played a big role in shaping interventional radiology.

Importance in Modern Medicine

Improvements in medical technology have greatly changed how diseases are diagnosed and treated, and interventional radiology is now a key specialty. Interventional radiology, which makes use of imaging for minimally invasive procedures, helps patients recover more quickly and saves healthcare money. Even so, using radiologic equipment means it is very important to have strict rules to manage radiation levels. Ensuring patient safety involves addressing potential risks from high radiation doses during complex procedures, a challenge underscored by incidents of overexposure attributed to insufficient staff training and equipment misuse (Damilakis *et al.*, 2017). Using checklists, dose alerts, and having regulations has improved safety during procedures by blending new technology with careful attention. Moreover, the integration of interventional radiology continues to improve treatment precision and outcomes, reflecting its indispensable role in contemporary healthcare (Figure 10.2).

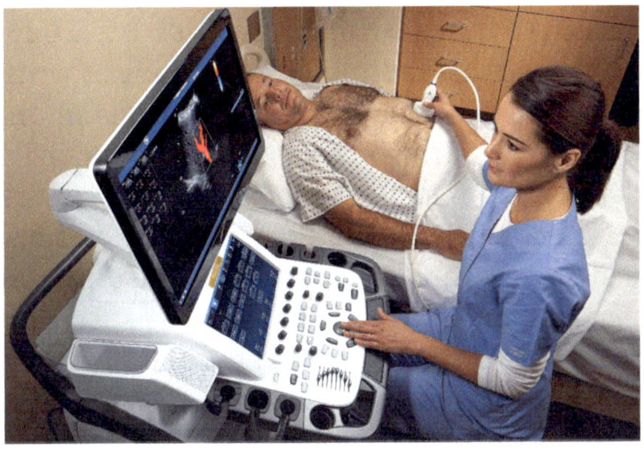

Figure 10.2. By enabling minimally invasive techniques guided by imaging, interventional radiology reduces the need for traditional surgeries, leading to decreased patient recovery times and lower healthcare costs.

Source: https://www.itnonline.com/sites/default/files/field/image/Ultrasound_Abdominal_GE_Vivid%20E95_PR.jpg.

Overview of Techniques Used

Because of advances in imaging, minimally invasive procedures in medicine have become more accurate and safer for patients. A number of image-guided methods are used in interventional radiology for both diagnosing and treating patients. For instance, arterial embolizations targeting critical vessels in the brain, viscera, and peripheral vasculature have become standard practices in trauma care, showcasing the successful integration of these methods in complex clinical scenarios (Sclafani, 2025). Additionally, image-guided liver biopsy exemplifies the meticulous approach of interventional radiology, with percutaneous and transjugular techniques tailored to specific hepatobiliary conditions, emphasizing the importance of procedural understanding and complication management (Ma *et al.*, 2024). They reveal how interventional radiology is flexible, showing its key role in today's healthcare by being precise, effective, and minimally invasive.

Comparison with Traditional Surgical Methods

New medical technology has made it possible to do surgery in less invasive ways, which often leads to shorter recovery times and fewer complications for patients.

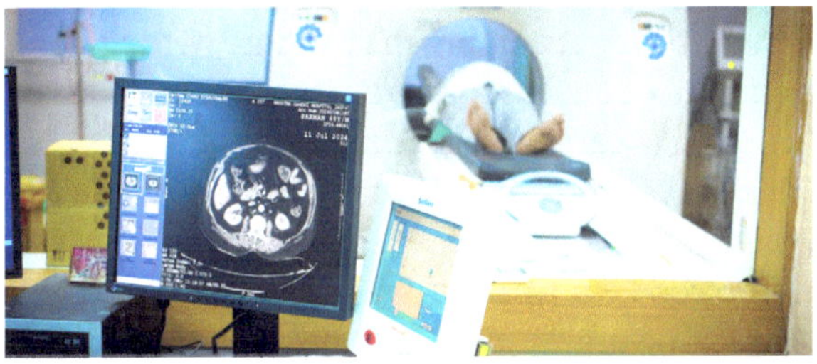

Figure 10.3. Advancements in medical technology have introduced less invasive techniques that significantly contrast with traditional surgical methods, particularly in terms of patient recovery and complication rates.

Source: https://www.mgmch.org/uploads/LargeImages/24pg_radio-diagnosis.jpg.

For example, minimally invasive lumbar procedures such as oblique lumbar interbody fusion combined with the Wiltse approach demonstrate reduced muscle damage and shorter hospital stays compared to conventional posterior-only surgeries, while still achieving effective clinical and radiological outcomes in patients with degenerative lumbar scoliosis (Zhang *et al.*, 2025). Likewise, modified autologous bone grafting techniques for maxillary alveolar defects have shown faster recovery times and lower complication rates than traditional methods, with complete bone regeneration occurring within a year and significantly improved bone density measures

(Eshiev & Eshiev, 2024). These comparisons underline the growing role of interventional radiology and minimally invasive procedures in reducing patient morbidity, optimizing clinical results, and enhancing postoperative quality of life, marking a clear advantage over more invasive, traditional surgical approaches (Figure 10.3).

Role of Imaging in Interventional Procedures

Thanks to advances in imaging, doctors can now see what they are doing in real time, which helps them succeed in interventional procedures. Clinicians can use fluoroscopy, ultrasound, CT, and MRI to guide tools inside the body, which helps reduce invasiveness and leads to better results. In particular, fluoroscopy plays a central role in guiding interventions while necessitating careful management of radiation exposure to protect both patients and medical staff, as highlighted by recent studies measuring radiation doses during procedures to optimize safety protocols (Baron, 2024). Additionally, in specialized fields like pediatric thoracic interventions, tailored imaging approaches are essential to address unique anatomical and physiological challenges, ensuring both diagnostic clarity and procedural efficacy (Beyoğlu, 2024). Advanced imaging improves the accuracy of diagnoses and helps doctors perform minimally invasive treatments, which improves patient care and helps interventional radiology progress.

Patient Demographics and Common Conditions Treated

Interventional radiology takes care of patients with a wide range of medical backgrounds and levels of risk. A lot of the time, patients who have had surgery before or who have chronic conditions are advised to use minimally invasive approaches to prevent issues caused by traditional surgery. Gastrointestinal disorders, including bowel obstructions and enterocutaneous fistulas, represent a significant portion of cases managed through image-guided interventions, which can reduce morbidity and improve quality of life where conservative treatments fail or surgery poses substantial risks (Holzwanger *et al.*, 2025). Interventional radiology techniques, which depend on advanced imaging, are commonly used for treating bone diseases such as osteoporosis and Paget's disease. Procedures like vertebroplasty and bone biopsies not only assist in accurate assessment but also provide therapeutic benefits, illustrating the specialty's critical role in managing conditions that affect a wide demographic spectrum (Donna *et al.*, 2024) (Figure 10.4).

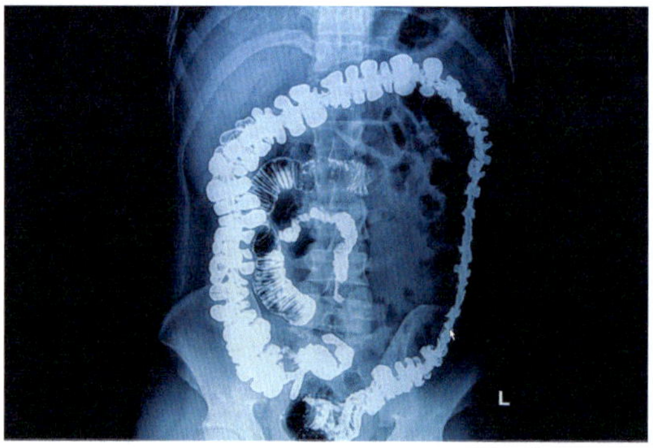

Figure 10.4. Gastrointestinal disorders, including bowel obstructions and enterocutaneous fistulas, represent a significant portion of cases managed through image-guided interventions.

Source: https://cdn-prod.medicalnewstoday.com/content/images/articles/322/322309/barium-swallow-image-highlighting-intestine.jpg.

Future Trends in Interventional Radiology

The field of interventional radiology is about to be transformed by new technologies, which will open up better options for patient treatment and more efficient procedures. Among these, artificial intelligence (AI) stands out as a transformative force, with its capacity to optimize risk assessment, procedural planning, and real-time decision-making, thereby improving outcomes and workflow within clinical settings. AI's integration spans pre-procedural imaging analysis, intra-procedural guidance, and post-procedural monitoring, highlighting a comprehensive influence throughout the patient care continuum (Nguyen *et al.*, 2024). Additionally, the evolution of digital imaging techniques, including advancements in X-ray technology and photon-counting computed tomography (CT), provides higher resolution images with reduced radiation doses, facilitating more precise interventions and expanded diagnostic capabilities (Rayyani *et al.*, 2024). Working together among various specialties and creating strong policies is important for using these innovations well. It is expected that in the future, treatments will be more personalized, data-based, and less invasive, which will greatly benefit and expand interventional radiology.

10.1. Techniques in Interventional Radiology

Learning Outcome

1. Understand angiography and its applications;
2. Explain biopsy procedures and techniques;
3. Focus on drainage procedures and catheter placements;
4. Describe endovenous laser therapy for varicose veins;
5. Learn radiofrequency ablation for tumors;
6. Define transjugular intrahepatic portosystemic shunt (TIPS);
7. Discuss uterine artery embolization for fibroids;
8. Learn vertebroplasty and kyphoplasty for spinal fractures;
9. Understand innovations in minimally invasive techniques.

Technological progress is always changing the way minimally invasive medical procedures are done. In interventional radiology, this progress is exemplified by the integration of small-scale robotic devices and augmented reality (AR) systems, both enhancing precision and expanding the scope of treatable vascular conditions. Small-scale robots have the potential to navigate intricate vascular anatomies autonomously, overcoming challenges such as accessing narrow or damaged vessels while reducing reliance on traditional tethered devices (Alwahdani Nsamn, 2024). Meanwhile, AR applications provide interventionalists with three-dimensional live overlays during image-guided procedures, improving spatial orientation and accuracy, particularly in complex puncture techniques that involve respiratory organ movement (Fehrenbach, 2023). Because these AR tools are available on common smartphones, they provide an inexpensive option to regular guidance systems, which may help reduce radiation and the time needed for the procedure. Still, using these new techniques in practice involves ongoing scientific checks to handle problems with technology and the wide range of cases seen in clinics, so they can truly improve patient care.

10.1.1. Angiography and its Applications

Better methods for diagnosis and treatment have made vascular interventions more accurate and safe. An important development is angiography, which involves injecting contrast material into blood vessels to help doctors both find and treat problems in the same session. By using angiography, doctors can spot stenosis, aneurysms, and occlusions in the blood vessels, enabling them to make informed treatment decisions and benefit the patient. Apart from diagnostics, it is used to plan angioplasty, stenting, and embolization, which shows its vital role in interventional radiology. Using angiography and small tools reduces the risk to patients and the time needed for recovery, which is a modern trend in medicine. Furthermore, ongoing advancements and clinical guidelines emphasize the importance of angiographic techniques within a multidisciplinary framework to optimize care and adapt to complex cases, reinforcing its foundational role in contemporary vascular management (Adler *et al.*, 2015; Baddour *et al.*, 2015) (Figure 10.5).

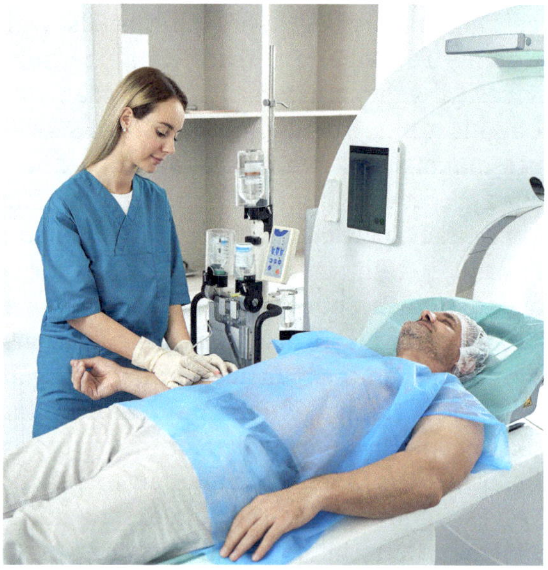

Figure 10.5. Angiography plays a crucial role in identifying vascular abnormalities such as stenosis, aneurysms, and occlusions, facilitating real-time decision-making that improves patient outcomes.

Source: https://www.elitenicosia.com/wp-content/uploads/2024/04/BT-anjiyografi.jpg.

10.1.2. Biopsy Procedures and Techniques

Because of progress in interventional radiology, biopsies are now more precise and safer for patients. The change from traditional surgical biopsies to image-guided percutaneous methods now allows doctors to take tissue samples with less invasiveness. An example is using CT-guided biopsies for lung lesions, which provide real-time guidance to help the needle reach the right spot, but these procedures may result in pneumothorax or bleeding. Risk factors like emphysema, lesion depth, and pleural puncture influence complication rates, emphasizing the need for meticulous procedural planning (Elshafee *et al.*, 2019). Moreover, combining biopsy with minimally invasive treatments, such as radiofrequency ablation in osteoid osteoma management, highlights the dual diagnostic and therapeutic potential within interventional radiology (Parmeggiani *et al.*, 2021). By using these integrated methods, doctors can analyze tissues more precisely, which also leads to better patient outcomes and safety, proving the importance of tailored biopsy approaches today.

10.1.3. Drainage Procedures and Catheter Placements

Managing fluid collections and vascular access is very important in interventional radiology, especially for cases in gynecology and obstetrics. By using imaging, it is possible to drain abscesses, seromas, lymphoceles, and malignant ascites without major surgery, which helps patients recover more quickly. Using central venous catheters and other catheters, chemotherapy, antibiotics, and parenteral nutrition can be given to patients for a longer period, which helps improve their treatment. Doctors use imaging to guide these techniques, which helps them be more accurate and reduces the risk of problems. Also, using catheters for embolization can manage severe bleeding, such as in cases of abnormally invasive placenta, and uterine artery embolization is more effective and better for preserving fertility than internal iliac artery occlusion. Collectively, these drainage and catheter-based interventions exemplify the vital role of interventional radiology in improving clinical outcomes through targeted, less invasive therapies (Soyer *et al.*, 2020; Yu *et al.*, 2013) (Figure 10.6).

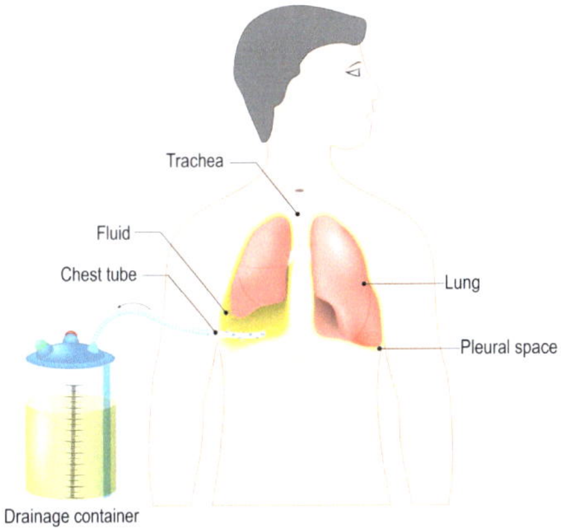

Figure 10.6. Chest tube insertion.

Source: https://cdn-prod.medicalnewstoday.com/content/images/articles/322/322161/diagram-of-plural-effusion-showing-chest-tube-insertion.jpg.

10.1.4. Endovenous Laser Therapy (EVLT) for Varicose Veins

Vascular conditions are now handled with minimally invasive surgery, which gives patients less pain and allows them to recover faster than with traditional surgery. Among these innovations, endovenous laser therapy (EVLT) has emerged as a prominent treatment for varicose veins, which are commonly caused by venous insufficiency. EVLT uses laser heat to damage the problem vein, which then closes and is absorbed by the body. This approach, which is guided by ultrasound, shows the main principle of interventional radiology: using images to target therapy. The growing evidence base highlights EVLT's efficacy, safety, and reduced complication rates compared to conventional approaches, contributing to its inclusion in updated clinical guidelines worldwide (Gianesini *et al.*, 2019). Furthermore, multidisciplinary care—emphasizing specialized vascular teams—enhances patient outcomes by integrating EVLT with comprehensive management plans tailored to individual risk profiles (Byers *et al.*, 2017). Because of technological progress, EVLT is now used more frequently for treating varicose veins in interventional radiology.

10.1.5. Radiofrequency Ablation for Tumors

Minimally invasive therapies have greatly improved the way tumors are handled, mainly by using interventional radiology to treat cancerous tissue with accuracy. Radiofrequency ablation (RFA) has emerged as a pivotal modality, leveraging localized thermal energy to induce tumor necrosis while preserving surrounding healthy structures. Its efficacy is particularly noteworthy in palliating metastatic bone disease, where RFA combined with vertebroplasty not only achieves rapid pain relief but also demonstrates durable local tumor control, enhancing patients' quality of life without significant adverse effects (Faiella *et al.*, 2024). Apart from skeletal tumors, RFA is helping to develop new treatments for pancreatic ductal adenocarcinoma by interfering with the tumor environment to overcome chemoresistance and immunosuppression.

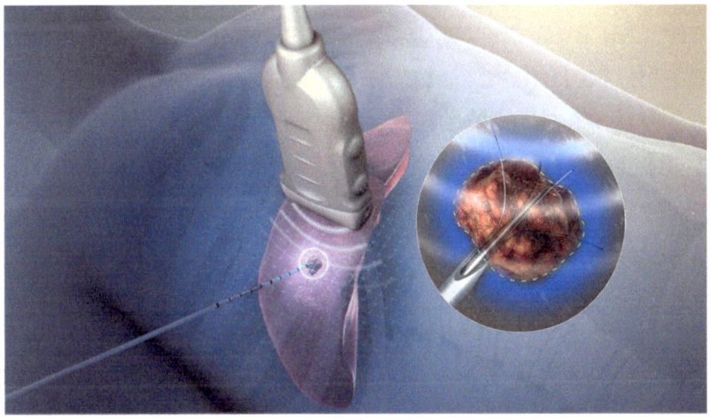

Figure 10.7. Radiofrequency ablation for tumors.

Source: https://upload.wikimedia.org/wikipedia/commons/thumb/e/e6/Radiofrequency_ablation.jpg/1200px-Radiofrequency_ablation.jpg.

By modifying the stroma and enhancing immune activation, RFA may potentiate the effects of systemic therapies, although it remains adjunctive rather than standard care (Grandis *et al.*, 2023). Together, these applications underscore the critical role of RFA in expanding interventional radiology's therapeutic arsenal against diverse tumor types (Figure 10.7).

10.1.6. Transjugular Intrahepatic Portosystemic Shunt (TIPS)

Managing complications due to portal hypertension has improved a lot because of new minimally invasive procedures. Among these, TIPS has become a pivotal therapeutic intervention. The method is to connect the portal and systemic veins inside the liver to help reduce portal pressure, which helps prevent variceal bleeding and ascites. To perform the procedure, advanced imaging and technical abilities are needed, mainly provided by interventional radiologists in a team with other specialists. New stent designs, for example, polytetrafluoroethylene stents, have made it easier for patients to maintain a clear bile duct and have lessened the risk of hepatic encephalopathy. Picking the right patients is very important, considering both the benefits and risks, especially for heart and liver health, to improve their chances of survival and quality of life. While more research is needed to standardize protocols, consensus among experts underscores TIPS as an indispensable endovascular therapy in portal hypertension management within interventional radiology (Boike *et al.*, 2021; Lee *et al.*, 2023).

10.1.7. Uterine Artery Embolization for Fibroids

New minimally invasive methods have made it much easier to treat a variety of gynecological problems, especially uterine fibroids. Among these developments, uterine artery embolization (UAE) has emerged as a pivotal interventional radiology procedure that offers a less invasive alternative to traditional surgical methods. The uterine arteries are selectively blocked using this method, which cuts off the blood supply to fibroids and makes them shrink without damaging the uterus. Recent evidence demonstrates that UAE not only alleviates symptoms such as abnormal bleeding and pelvic pain but also promotes substantial fibroid volume reduction, with studies reporting an average decrease of nearly 20% post-procedure and symptom resolution in 80% of patients (Mansour *et al.*, 2022). Before and after embolization, using multiparametric MRI helps improve the accuracy of treatment and the way results are measured. As interventional radiology continues to evolve, the UAE exemplifies the integration of targeted, organ-sparing therapies that improve patient quality of life with reduced recovery times (Tanaka *et al.*, 2023) (Figure 10.8).

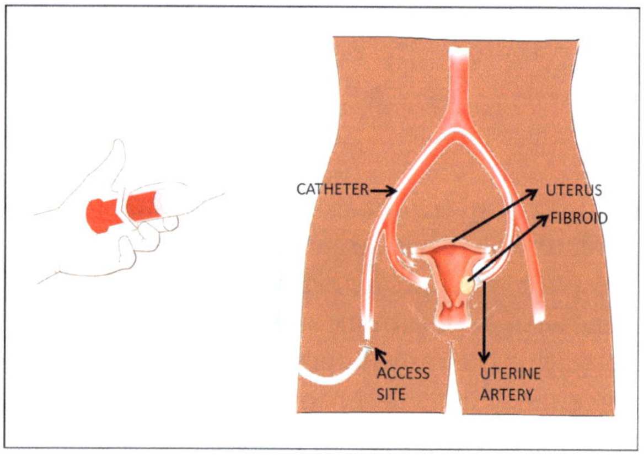

Figure 10.8. Advancements in minimally invasive techniques have significantly transformed the management of various gynecological conditions, particularly uterine fibroids.

Source: https://i0.wp.com/radiology.wales/wp-content/uploads/2018/10/UFE-procedure.png?fit=1382%2C940&ssl=1.

10.1.8. Vertebroplasty and Kyphoplasty for Spinal Fractures

A spinal fracture caused by osteoporosis or metastatic bone disease is a major problem in medicine because it can be painful and lead to deformity. Vertebroplasty and kyphoplasty, which are offered by interventional radiology, have greatly improved how these fractures are managed. In vertebroplasty, a percutaneous injection of bone cement is used to stabilize the fractured vertebra and reduce pain, and in kyphoplasty, a balloon is also inserted to restore the height of the vertebra before cement is injected. These procedures relieve pain quickly, improve movement, and help avoid more serious surgeries, which is very useful for patients with few other options. Their role complements pharmacologic strategies aimed at addressing underlying bone fragility, as highlighted by the importance of integrating bone-targeted therapies, including bisphosphonates, in managing skeletal complications of cancer and osteoporosis (Coleman *et al.*, 2020; LeBoff *et al.*, 2022). Having these interventions highlights the importance of using multiple disciplines in interventional radiology today.

10.1.9. Innovations in Minimally Invasive Techniques

Thanks to new medical technology, the number of traditional open surgeries has decreased greatly. Here, interventional radiology is remarkable for always finding new ways to perform minimally invasive treatments that improve outcomes for patients. Percutaneous biopsy and treatment can be done precisely with image-guided methods, which reduces damage to tissues and helps patients recover faster. Notably, the development of transarterial chemoembolization and radiofrequency ablation exemplifies the integration of innovative approaches to treat malignancies effectively while reducing systemic side effects (Maher *et al.*, 2011). Besides, using these techniques helps manage the problems that come with cancer more safely and effectively, proving that interventional radiology is playing a bigger role in cancer care. Despite regulatory challenges, ongoing research efforts aimed at improving molecular imaging and nanotechnology applications continue to drive progress, promising even more sophisticated and patient-friendly interventions in the near future (Bradley *et al.*, 2009) (Figure 10.9).

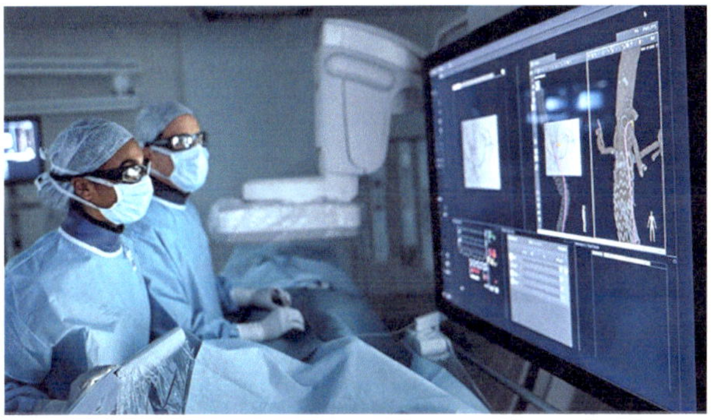

Figure 10.9. By utilizing image-guided methods, practitioners are able to perform precise percutaneous biopsies and targeted treatments, minimizing tissue damage and promoting faster recovery times.

Source: https://www.philips.com/c-dam/corporate/newscenter/global/standard/resources/healthcare/2024/lumiguide/teaser-igt2023-lumiguide-perform-fast.jpg.

Test Your Knowledge

1. How does interventional radiology differ from diagnostic radiology?
2. What imaging techniques are most often used in interventional radiology?

10.2. Imaging Modalities in Interventional Radiology

Learning Outcome

1. Understand X-ray fluoroscopy, and its role;
2. Explain computed tomography (CT) in guidance;
3. Learn magnetic resonance imaging (MRI) applications;
4. Focus on ultrasound as a real-time imaging tool;
5. Define contrast agents used in imaging;
6. Discuss safety considerations in imaging;
7. Know integration of imaging technologies;
8. Discuss advances in imaging techniques;
9. Identify challenges in imaging during procedures.

Better imaging tools have made interventional radiology procedures much more accurate and safer. Among various imaging modalities, Cone beam computed tomography (CBCT) has emerged as a significant tool, offering superior spatial resolution with reduced radiation exposure compared to conventional CT scans. This capability facilitates detailed visualization of complex anatomical structures, enabling refined assessment of fractures, cartilage lesions, and joint disorders, which is crucial for planning and guiding interventions (Desimpel *et al.*, 2018).

Fluoroscopy is still important for real-time guidance because it can show moving images, and ultrasound gives a safe option for examining soft tissues. Combining these modalities enables interventional radiologists to adjust their imaging methods to match the needs of each patient, which improves the success of procedures and patient outcomes. Also, the use of CBCT and other advanced imaging techniques provides more accurate diagnoses, and helps track progress during follow-up, making them essential in the field of interventional radiology.

10.2.1. X-ray Fluoroscopy and its Role

The use of advanced imaging has revolutionized interventional radiology by allowing doctors to see what they are doing in real time, which improves the accuracy of procedures and the outcomes for patients. X-ray fluoroscopy is especially important because it enables doctors to watch the procedure as it happens and guide the intervention. With fluoroscopy, doctors can view the movement of instruments and contrast agents inside the body, which helps them guide catheters and devices properly during difficult procedures. Even so, it is necessary to carefully control the amount of radiation, as using it too much or too often can cause tissue reactions, so strict rules for dose monitoring and patient safety are needed. Optimizing the use of fluoroscopy and managing doses safely is possible because of qualified medical physicists. The evolving landscape of imaging informatics and AI-driven analytics further promises to augment fluoroscopy's capabilities, optimizing procedural planning and enhancing diagnostic accuracy in interventional radiology (Fisher *et al.*, 2022; Panayides *et al.*, 2020) (Figure 10.10).

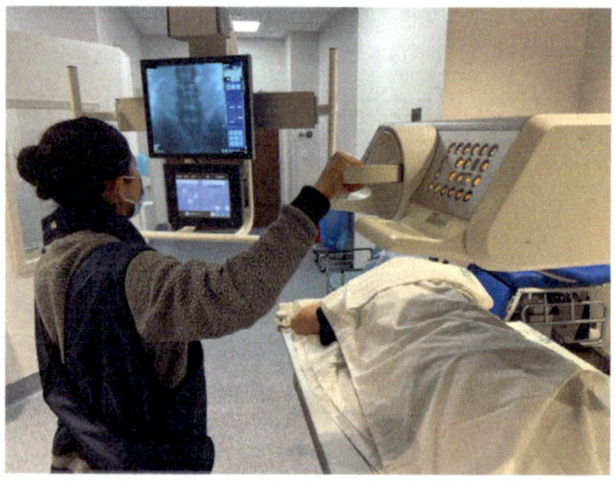

Figure 10.10. X-ray fluoroscopy.

Source: https://www.laiic.com/cdn/shop/articles/fluoroscopy_los_angeles_explained_2100x.webp?v=1682966034.

10.2.2. Computed Tomography (CT) in Guidance

Because of new imaging technologies, minimally invasive procedures are now safer and more accurate, and CT is a key tool in interventional radiology. CT guidance allows doctors to see the anatomy in real time, which helps them place needles and guide devices accurately during different interventions. It helps to perform the procedure well and reduces harm to nearby tissues. Still, since CT imaging uses ionizing radiation, it is very important to strictly follow safety rules to keep patients safe. Implementation of dose optimization strategies, including time-outs, checklists, and dose alerts, is crucial to prevent radiation overexposure and associated tissue reactions, especially in complex procedures such as perfusion studies (Damilakis *et al.*, 2017). Furthermore, the integration of medical physics expertise is essential in maintaining dose accuracy and ensuring compliance with practice guidelines that govern safe and effective CT use in intervention (Seibert *et al.*, 2018). All of these measures show that it is important to ensure both the effectiveness of CT-guided interventions and the safety of the patients during these procedures.

10.2.3. Magnetic Resonance Imaging (MRI) Applications

Because of new imaging technologies, interventional radiology can now perform more accurate and less invasive procedures. MRI is especially notable because it provides strong contrast between soft tissues and can be viewed from various angles, which makes it important for accurate diagnosis and treatment planning. MRI's detailed pictures and information, which do not use ionizing radiation, make it very useful for guiding surgeries in the brain, muscles, and abdomen. Also, recent progress in machine learning and deep learning has made MRI more useful by improving image analysis and interpretation, enabling instant decisions during procedures. These innovations support differentiation between pathological and treatment-related changes, thereby tailoring interventions more effectively (Shen *et al.*, 2017; Zhu *et al.*, 2022). For this reason, MRI is being used in interventional radiology, highlighting the strong connection between advanced imaging and computer-based techniques, which helps patients and allows for more treatment options.

10.2.4. Ultrasound as a Real-time Imaging Tool

New imaging tools have greatly improved both the precision and safety of procedures done in radiology. Ultrasound is unique because it offers real-time images, which improve how accurately procedures are done and how well patients recover.

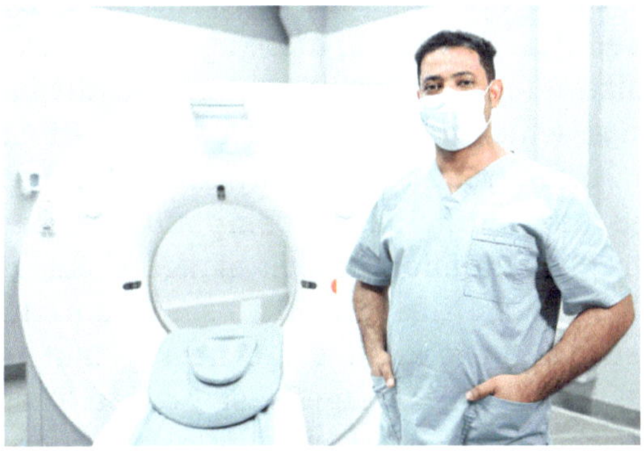

Figure 10.11. The evolution of imaging technologies has profoundly impacted the precision and safety of interventional procedures in radiology.

Source: https://www.ahu.edu/sites/default/files/styles/fc_800x533/public/media/1200314173859729.o1cflrytgf9gyxdvjl7n_height640.png?h=4c1fc98e&itok=i1ZKcqjM.

Because of its dynamic imaging, doctors can instantly check the position of the needle, blood flow, and tissue changes, which helps prevent complications. It is very important in vascular interventions because the detailed images and accurate information guide the treatment of diseases such as portal hypertension or access to the heart. Ultrasound is also safer than fluoroscopy because it does not use ionizing radiation, which is especially important for people at risk. Using Doppler and contrast-enhanced ultrasound improves vascular imaging, which helps doctors perform targeted treatments in difficult cases. These attributes exemplify ultrasound's expanding role as both a diagnostic and therapeutic tool within interventional radiology practice (Dhar *et al.*, 2023) (Figure 10.11).

10.2.5. Contrast Agents used in Imaging

Medical imaging has advanced mainly because of contrast agents, which help highlight internal structures during interventional radiology procedures. Because of these agents, it is easier to distinguish between normal and diseased tissues, which helps with accurate diagnostics and better treatments. X-ray and CT imaging often use iodine-based compounds because their high atomic number makes them very visible on the images. MRI uses gadolinium-based agents to change the nearby magnetic field, which makes images easier to see. Thanks to advances in digital imaging, these contrast agents can now be used for quick image capture and live viewing, which is very important during minimally invasive procedures. Furthermore, novel contrast agents continue to emerge, offering enhanced safety profiles and specificity, which are pivotal in reducing complications and improving outcomes in interventional radiology (Vassallo *et al.*, 2004).

10.2.6. Safety Considerations in Imaging

To manage patient safety in interventional radiology well, one must know the risks of radiation exposure and strictly follow the set protocols. Being exposed to too much radiation during procedures can cause serious harm to the skin, which is why it is very important to receive proper training and use equipment properly. Following checklists, pausing for time-outs before doing procedures, and using real-time dose alerts have helped a lot in avoiding accidental radiation doses. Having clear guidelines for each department's duties in prevention, investigation, and dose assessment is necessary to deal with incidents well and keep improving the quality of care. Similarly, it is important to use standard methods to report and assess radiation doses, putting more focus on describing risks qualitatively rather than using numbers to avoid misunderstanding a person's risk. These safety practices align closely with medical physics guidelines that advocate for specialized training and consistent protocol adherence to safeguard patient welfare throughout imaging procedures (Damilakis *et al.*, 2017; Seibert *et al.*, 2018).

10.2.7. Integration of Imaging Technologies

Improvements in technology have greatly changed interventional radiology by bringing together various imaging devices and advanced tools. AR and virtual reality (VR) are increasingly incorporated to enhance procedural accuracy through real-time visualization and detailed anatomical reconstructions, allowing clinicians to navigate complex vascular and soft tissue structures more effectively (Bhatti *et al.*, 2025). Concurrently, the integration of sensorless haptic feedback in robotic-assisted systems, particularly in image-guided interventions such as MRI, has improved the tactile perception during percutaneous procedures, bridging the gap between robotic precision and surgeon intuition (Vogt *et al.*, 2024). They help guide procedures, improve how doctors are trained, and make it easier to diagnose, which in turn reduces errors and improves patient outcomes. Continued development in AI and more accessible designs is essential to overcome current limitations, facilitating a comprehensive, multimodal imaging environment that supports personalized and minimally invasive radiologic interventions (Bhatti *et al.*, 2025; Vogt *et al.*, 2024) (Figure 10.12).

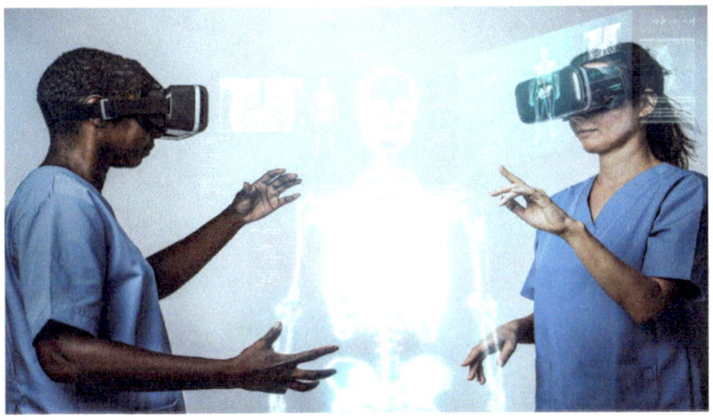

Figure 10.12. Augmented reality (AR) and virtual reality (VR) are increasingly incorporated to enhance procedural accuracy through real-time visualization and detailed anatomical reconstructions, allowing clinicians to navigate complex vascular and soft tissue structures more effectively.

Source: https://media.licdn.com/dms/image/v2/D4D12AQGEk0o1atlNKA/article-cover_image-shrink_720_1280/article-cover_image-shrink_720_1280/0/1710918503341?e=2147483647&v=beta&t=07k59izuYod3uoW2hie4HvKf_Yz4rNCgIpGfZ9VZ0SE.

10.2.8. Advances in Imaging Techniques

Because of advancements in medical imaging, interventional radiology can now perform procedures that are both more accurate and less invasive. The use of digital radiography, ultrasound, MRI, and CT has made it much easier for radiologists to perform interventions safely and correctly. Advanced imaging methods help doctors perform precise interventions in prenatal and musculoskeletal care, which lowers risks and speeds up recovery. For example, MRI-guided high-intensity focused ultrasound leverages thermal ablation to treat bone metastases with minimal collateral damage, highlighting how imaging advances refine both diagnosis and therapy (Sgalambro *et al.*, 2022). Additionally, the miniaturization of instruments combined with enhanced digital optics has made fetoscopic interventions feasible, expanding interventional radiology's applications in high-risk pregnancies by improving the identification and treatment of fetal conditions (Sharma *et al.*, 2022). All of these innovations together are a major reason why interventional radiology keeps growing and improving.

10.2.9. Challenges in Imaging During Procedures

Because of new technology, medical imaging is now a key element in both diagnosis and interventional treatments. Still, there are many difficulties in using imaging during interventions that influence both the safety and success of the procedure. Using contrast agents to see soft tissues is necessary, but it leads to issues with toxicity and the amount that can be used, which can make delicate vascular procedures more complicated. Due to the patient's changing blood flow, contrast agents can cause the images to be inconsistent and sometimes out of sync, which makes it hard to keep guiding the procedure. Also, the frequent use of CT and fluoroscopy, which are X-ray-based, means that patients are exposed to radiation, and this must be considered along with the need for the procedure. Addressing these issues is critical as interventional radiology continues to evolve, requiring innovations that enhance real-time visualization while minimizing risks and improving outcomes (Datta *et al.*, 2024; Lecomte *et al.*, 2023) (Figure 10.13).

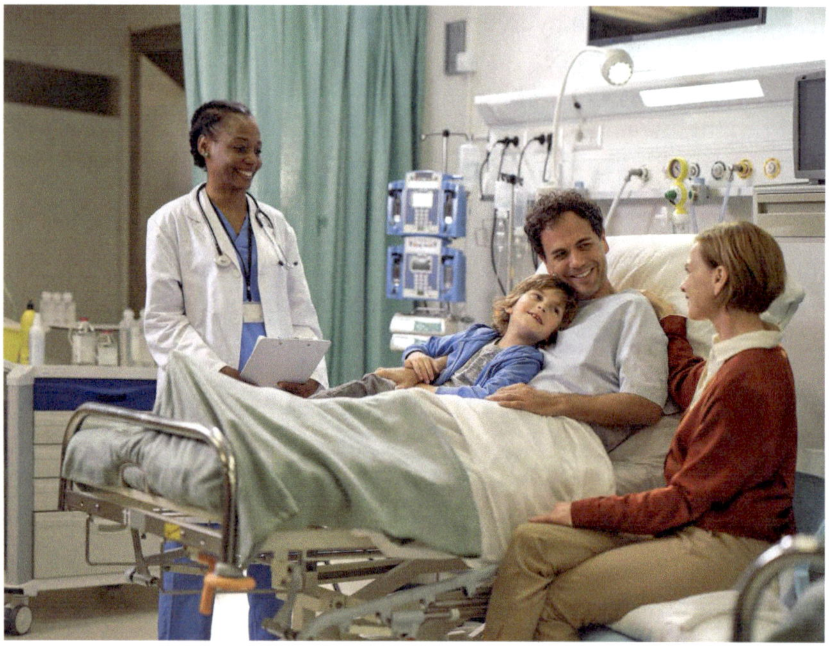

Figure 10.13. The reliance on contrast agents to visualize soft tissues, while essential, introduces concerns regarding toxicity and restricted allowable volumes, complicating their use in delicate vascular procedures.

Source: https://assets.isu.pub/document-structure/240304090334-d58a7bf76cace577f0c8f5ab233762af/v1/739d792df76e482fa930368f55203caf.jpeg.

Test Your Knowledge

1. What is the main idea behind doing a percutaneous biopsy in interventional radiology?
2. How is a catheter-based procedure performed in interventional radiology?
3. What is angioplasty, and how does it fit into interventional radiology?

10.3. Patient Care and Safety in Interventional Radiology

Learning Outcome

1. Understand pre-procedural assessment and preparation;
2. Explain the informed consent process;
3. Focus on sedation and anesthesia options;
4. Discuss monitoring during procedures;
5. Know post-procedural care and follow-up;
6. Identify complications and risk management;
7. Focus on patient education and communication;
8. Learn ethical considerations in patient care;
9. Describe quality assurance in interventional radiology.

Taking care of patients and keeping them safe in interventional radiology calls for a team effort, good communication, strict adherence to protocols, and ongoing training of medical staff. Complex therapies, such as PSMA-targeted radiopharmaceutical treatment for metastatic castration-resistant prostate cancer, highlight the necessity for vigilant monitoring of adverse events and strict radiation safety practices to optimize treatment outcomes while minimizing harm (Calais *et al.*, 2024).

Creating a strong safety culture in healthcare institutions is also very important, as evidenced by efforts that stress transparency, reporting errors, and improving quality to ensure better care for patients. When healthcare teams collaborate, they can better manage challenges, and provide more effective care to patients, which increases safety and satisfaction. Therefore, using proven safety methods and encouraging ongoing learning help raise the standards of patient care in interventional radiology.

10.3.1. Pre-procedural Assessment and Preparation

Good patient outcomes in interventional radiology are achieved by being very thorough before the procedure. At this step, the doctor reviews the patient's past health, the medicines they are on, and possible risks to design the best intervention for them. Reviewing imaging helps confirm the need for the procedure and find any anatomical difficulties that may affect the safety of the approach. In addition, laboratory tests are done to check blood clotting and organ health, which helps prevent problems during the operation.

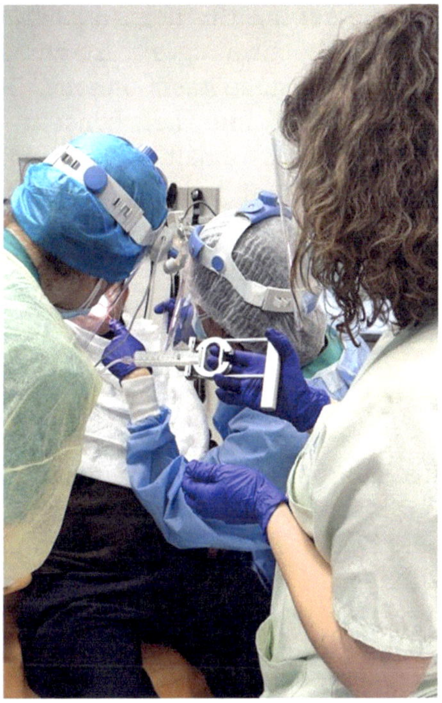

Figure 10.14. Effective patient outcomes in interventional radiology heavily depend on meticulous pre-procedural assessment and preparation.

Source: https://onlinelibrary.wiley.com/cms/asset/62760283-e30b-4175-87de-3a891e0c6fbe/cyt13375-toc-0001-m.jpg.

10.3.2. Informed Consent Process

Clearly communicating with patients is very important for both patient autonomy and ethical medical care in advanced fields such as interventional radiology. Because these procedures are minimally invasive yet may carry risks, patients in this specialty must be fully informed about what they involve. Since interventional radiology is highly technological and hands-off, it becomes important for clinicians to make sure patients can understand the details. Nurses play a pivotal role in this dialogue, supporting patient education and facilitating consent by bridging technical information and individual patient concerns (Boone *et al.*, 2012). Working together like this helps maintain legal and ethical rules, encourages trust, and allows patients to understand their options. Despite the prominence of informed consent, some procedural nuances remain under-explained, indicating a need for ongoing refinement in communication strategies within interventional radiology practice (Karabulut *et al.*, 2015).

10.3.3. Sedation and Anesthesia Options

Because of progress in interventional radiology, a detailed approach to sedation and anesthesia is now needed to ensure patient safety and the procedure's success. Using virtual evaluations and thorough testing has changed perioperative care by making it possible to select the right sedation for each patient and procedure. Those undergoing safe procedures might be given moderate sedation without thorough testing, but those who are at higher risk must be tested more carefully to help select the type of anesthesia, which could be general or monitored anesthesia care. The adoption of telehealth for preoperative evaluations facilitates patient optimization and reduces exposure risks, particularly vital in the context of infectious disease considerations such as COVID-19 (Lu *et al.*, 2020). Moreover, personalized sedation plans are designed to minimize complications while addressing specific procedural demands, reinforcing the critical role of anesthesia in advancing the precision and safety of interventional radiology practices (Wolf *et al.*, 2018) (Figure 10.15).

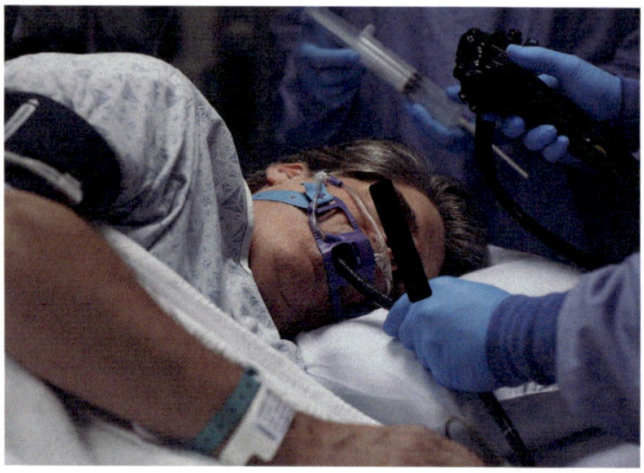

Figure 10.15. Advancements in interventional radiology have necessitated a nuanced approach to sedation and anesthesia to ensure patient safety and procedural efficacy.

Source: https://www.bjaed.org/cms/10.1016/j.bjae.2022.02.006/asset/728f4e92-5ef6-4041-9779-7e9d6aa1ce04/main.assets/gr1_lrg.jpg.

10.3.4. Monitoring During Procedures

Keeping patients safe during interventional radiology requires constant and thorough monitoring so that any problems can be spotted and managed right away. It means constantly monitoring vital signs, blood pressure, and the patient's brain activity so that any emergency can be handled promptly. Advanced imaging technologies, often integrated with artificial intelligence systems, enhance the precision and reliability of procedural monitoring by facilitating dynamic assessment of anatomical changes and catheter placements (Davenport *et al.*, 2019). Moreover, multidisciplinary teams utilize protocol-driven monitoring strategies to optimize outcomes, tailoring interventions based on diagnostic criteria and patient-specific risk factors (Raghu *et al.*, 2018). Careful observation during procedures lowers risks and helps doctors make the right decisions, crucial for patient safety and the success of the procedure. As a result, monitoring patients closely is still very important in interventional radiology, helping to advance less invasive treatments and keep patients safe.

10.3.5. Post-procedural Care and Follow-up

Good management after interventional radiology procedures is needed to help patients recover well and avoid complications. After the intervention, patients must be monitored to find out if they develop bleeding, infection, or device complications. After a procedure, patients are usually assessed for vital signs, pain is managed, and imaging is done to check if the treatment worked and to decide on any further actions. It is also important to have follow-up appointments to check how well the patient is recovering and if the treatment is still effective, which may involve teamwork from different experts. For instance, integrating individualized follow-up plans tailored to specific conditions, such as tumors managed with image-guided therapy, can enhance functional restoration and quality of life (Agrawal *et al.*, 2025). Additionally, in cases where psychological impacts arise, structured support and counseling interventions might be essential to address patient needs beyond the physical recovery (Davis *et al.*, 2024). In the end, good care after a procedure and careful follow-up are essential in the progress of interventional radiology.

10.3.6. Complications and Risk Management

Improvements in interventional radiology have made it possible to use less invasive treatments, which greatly reduce the chance of complications, but still, managing risks is very important. Certain procedures, such as lymphovenous anastomosis for refractory chylothorax in infants, highlight the delicate balance between innovative treatment and the susceptibility to life-threatening outcomes, including persistent lymphatic leaks that demand precise surgical intervention to restore lymphatic circulation effectively (Weissler *et al.*, 2018). Similarly, extracorporeal membrane oxygenation (ECMO), frequently utilized in critical care settings, exemplifies the complexity of managing invasive therapies where severe complications like intracranial hemorrhage impose high mortality risks and necessitate vigilant monitoring, prompt imaging, and tailored anticoagulation strategies to mitigate adverse events (Cavayas *et al.*, 2018). Consequently, interventional radiology demands a multidisciplinary approach integrating early diagnosis, patient-specific risk stratification, and adaptive procedural techniques to optimize safety and improve prognosis in complex clinical scenarios (Figure 10.16).

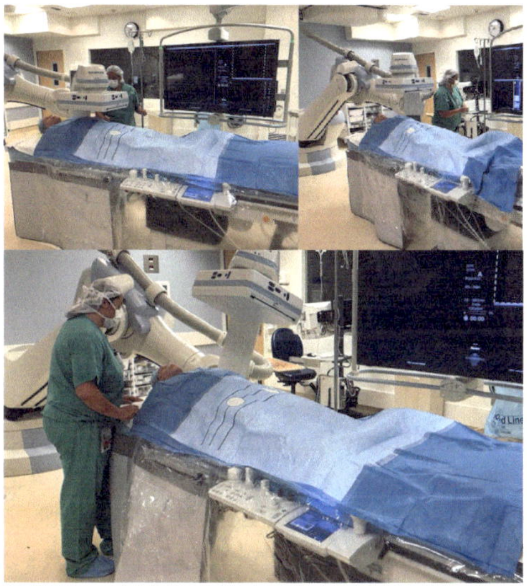

Figure 10.16. Advancements in interventional radiology have introduced minimally invasive therapies that significantly reduce patient morbidity, yet the potential for complications remains a critical concern requiring meticulous risk management.

Source: https://health.ucdavis.edu/radiology/images/MYEXAM/myir/IRprocedure.jpg.

10.3.7. Patient Education and Communication

Good management of interventional radiology procedures requires clear communication and proper education of patients to lower risks and help them recover well. Patients should be informed about the procedure as well as about the possibility of radiation exposure and the rare risks it may bring, such as reactions in tissues due to higher doses. Giving explanations that fit each patient's needs helps reduce anxiety and ensures that patients understand what is happening, which is necessary for ethical care. Making sure healthcare providers know how to communicate well in stressful situations helps them explain things like dose alerts and safety procedures to patients, which encourages openness and trust. Preventative strategies, including the use of checklists and time-outs, should be explained to patients as safeguards in the procedure, reinforcing safety culture in clinical settings (Damilakis *et al.*, 2017). Having visual aids and usable resources helps a lot, and this can be improved by using illustrations available in digital archives. All in all, this way of communicating supports patients in becoming more involved and safer during interventional radiology procedures.

10.3.8. Ethical Considerations in Patient Care

Advances in interventional radiology have made it possible to perform many procedures with less invasive methods, which benefits patients. But at the same time, these developments raise several ethical problems in how patients are cared for, such as gaining consent, revealing risks, and ensuring everyone has access to the latest technologies. Patients must be fully informed about potential complications, such as those observed in procedures like ultrasound-guided lung biopsies, where risks of pneumothorax and hemorrhage must be clearly communicated to ensure autonomous decision-making (Kayastha *et al.*, 2024). Additionally, healthcare systems face ethical challenges related to equipment maintenance and operations, as outdated or malfunctioning devices can jeopardize patient safety and treatment efficacy, underscoring the need for organizational resilience and proactive equipment management (O'Leary *et al.*, 2024). Balancing technological capabilities with patient-centered care demands vigilance in ethical standards to uphold trust, optimize safety, and provide justifiable interventions within interventional radiology practices (Figure 10.17).

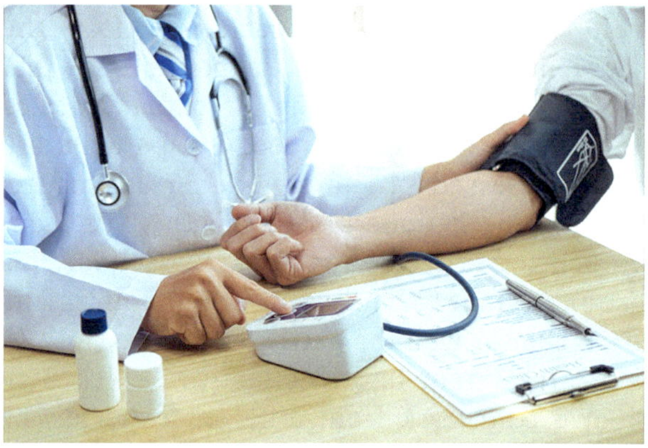

Figure 10.17. The advancement of interventional radiology has significantly transformed diagnostic and therapeutic procedures, offering minimally invasive options that improve patient outcomes.

Source: https://cdn.prod.website-files.com/64498fa255036a077feafca4/6536de2e70fd908c6954179a_pad.png.

10.3.9. Quality Assurance in Interventional Radiology

Because interventional radiology is advancing and seeing more patients, it is very important to maintain high standards. To ensure that quality is always maintained, equipment is checked and operators are assessed regularly to reduce dangers from radiation and mistakes during the procedure. Recent studies emphasize the necessity of precise measurement and calibration of X-ray parameters such as kilovoltage, dose, and exposure time, highlighting inherent uncertainties that must be factored into quality assessments to avoid inaccurate evaluations of equipment function (Senthilkumar *et al.*, 2024). Moreover, comprehensive assessments that include multidisciplinary input from radiologists, technologists, and medical physicists enhance adherence to evolving safety guidelines while identifying potential gaps in current protocols (Chaple *et al.*, 2024). By using such approaches, both patients and doctors are protected, and the field of interventional radiology continues to improve and advance.

Test Your Knowledge

1. What steps are taken to stop infection from happening during interventional radiology treatments?
2. What methods are used to keep an eye on patients before, during and following interventional radiology procedures?

10.4. Applications and Impact of Interventional Radiology

Learning Outcome

1. Explain the role in cancer treatment and management;
2. Know the treatment of vascular diseases;
3. Discuss management of gastrointestinal conditions;
4. Focus on interventional radiology in trauma care;
5. Describe pediatric applications and considerations;
6. Discuss cost-effectiveness compared to traditional surgery;
7. Define patient outcomes and quality of life improvements;
8. Know research and clinical trials in interventional radiology;
9. Understand global perspectives and access to care.

Better medical imaging methods have greatly improved both the diagnosis and treatment of patients. Interventional radiology shows this improvement by using small procedures and imaging to treat many conditions with high accuracy and less risk. Because of this approach, patients recover more quickly and have fewer complications than with traditional surgery, which benefits both healthcare quality and cost. Moreover, the integration of clinical decision support systems, aligned with evidence-based imaging referral guidelines, has streamlined the use of interventional radiology, ensuring appropriateness and optimizing resource allocation (Tay *et al.*, 2024). They make sure patients are safe, protect them from getting too much radiation, and help them reduce their wait time. Additionally, interdisciplinary collaboration and continuous training, as highlighted in broader patient safety strategies, cultivate a culture of safety essential for successful outcomes in interventional radiology (Falade *et al.*, 2024). All of these applications show that interventional radiology plays a major role in making healthcare more efficient, safe, and cost-effective.

10.4.1. Role in Cancer Treatment and Management

Minimally invasive techniques have made it possible for many cancer patients to get new kinds of treatment, especially with the help of interventional radiology. By employing targeted procedures such as celiac plexus blocks, interventional radiologists can effectively manage intractable abdominal pain associated with pancreatic cancer, reducing reliance on high-dose opioids and mitigating related adverse effects, thus improving patient quality of life (Ahmed *et al.*, 2023).

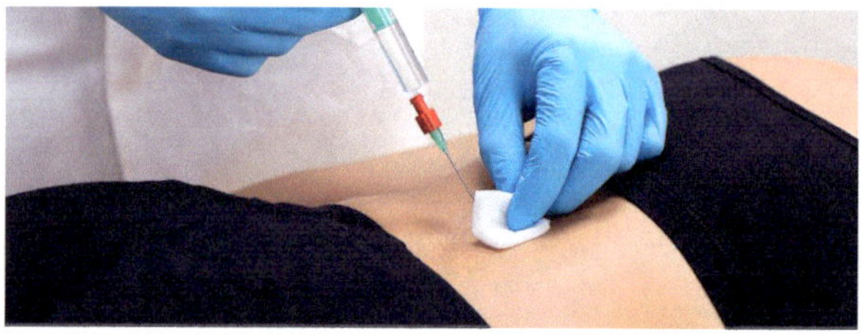

Figure 10.18. By employing targeted procedures such as celiac plexus blocks, interventional radiologists can effectively manage intractable abdominal pain associated with pancreatic cancer, reducing reliance on high-dose opioids and mitigating related adverse effects, thus improving patient quality of life.

Source: https://www.advancedpainmedical.com/wp-content/uploads/2023/08/celiac-plexus-block.jpg.

In addition, radiofrequency ablation and trans-arterial chemoembolization are now considered good ways to treat liver metastases from thyroid cancer that cannot be removed by surgery. These techniques enable localized tumor control, especially when hepatic tumor burden is limited, offering symptom relief and potential disease stabilization even in patients undergoing systemic therapies like tyrosine kinase inhibitors (Nervo *et al.*, 2021). Overall, interventional radiology plays a pivotal role in cancer treatment and management by providing tailored, less invasive options that complement systemic approaches, optimize symptom control, and extend therapeutic possibilities within multidisciplinary care frameworks (Figure 10.18).

10.4.2. Treatment of Vascular Diseases

With new developments in interventional radiology, patients with vascular diseases now have less invasive choices than before. In particular, thrombolysis and mechanical thrombectomy have emerged as vital techniques for treating acute thrombotic events, especially in pediatric populations where options were previously limited (Tarango *et al.*, 2017). The goal of these endovascular procedures is to quickly restore blood flow in the veins, which can ease acute symptoms and might help prevent post-thrombotic syndrome. However, such interventions require specialized expertise and carry risks including bleeding complications, emphasizing the necessity for careful patient selection and management (Tarango *et al.*, 2017). In addition, interventional radiology is involved in more than thrombotic disease; it offers both diagnostic and treatment options for complex vascular conditions by using different imaging techniques. Because the scope is growing, it is more important than ever to keep researching and training to make sure these advanced treatments are accessible and effective in different healthcare settings.

10.4.3. Management of Gastrointestinal Conditions

With new medical technology, the way complex gastrointestinal conditions are treated has undergone significant changes, especially with the use of interventional radiology. Newer techniques allow doctors to treat acute gastrointestinal bleeding, problems with enteral feeding, and luminal strictures with minimally invasive surgery instead of the usual open surgery. Interventional radiology helps to stop bleeding accurately with angiographic embolization and also supports endoscopic procedures, thereby enhancing patient care. The use of these procedures often means patients heal faster and have fewer complications, so they are preferred for high-risk patients. In addition, effective treatment of these conditions depends on the teamwork of interventional radiologists, gastroenterologists, and surgeons. This evolving paradigm shift highlights the importance of continued research and clinical collaboration to optimize procedural outcomes and expand the therapeutic arsenal available for gastrointestinal disease management (Alshalali *et al.*, 2023; McCowan *et al.*, 2017) (Figure 10.19).

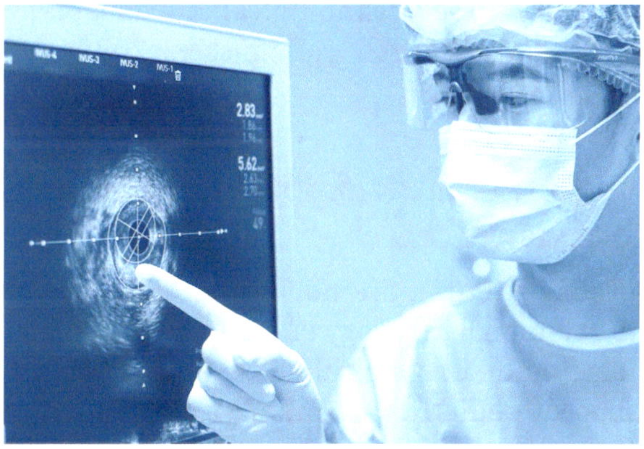

Figure 10.19. Interventional radiology not only facilitates precise localization and control of bleeding through angiographic embolization but also complements endoscopic procedures, thus enhancing overall patient care.

Source: https://drihealthgroup.com/sites/default/files/2024-12/DRI_Interventional-Radiology_12-16.jpg.

10.4.4. Interventional Radiology in Trauma Care

Modern medicine has significantly improved by using minimally invasive techniques to treat acute injuries, mainly in trauma care. Interventional radiology allows doctors to use images to guide procedures that quickly stop bleeding, secure damaged blood vessels, and make it possible to diagnose quickly without surgery. In trauma situations, these benefits matter a lot since fast actions can greatly affect whether a patient survives and recovers well. Also, performing embolization and angiographic stenting increases the accuracy of treatment and lowers the risk of serious complications from extensive surgery. Even though interventional radiology was mainly used for elective or chronic cases, it is now being used more often in emergency trauma, which improves patient care and resource management. This evolving role underscores the necessity of multidisciplinary collaboration and continuous guideline updates to incorporate technological advancements safely and effectively (Mathijssen, 2020; Schi Mødt *et al.*, 2019).

10.4.5. Pediatric Applications and Considerations

Because children are not like adults, the way interventional radiology is practiced in pediatric medicine differs from that for adults. The age range of pediatric patients is from premature infants to adolescents, almost as tall as adults, so they need special adjustments in equipment and procedures. Because of these differences, doctors must be extra attentive to the needs before, during, and after the procedure and use customized approaches for liver, chest, and musculoskeletal conditions. Also, it is important to think about how treatments might affect the growth and development of the patient. In some cases, doctors have treated refractory idiopathic intracranial hypertension in children using cerebrospinal fluid diversion, optic nerve sheath fenestration, and venous sinus stenting, which have shown mixed results and different complication risks. Optic nerve sheath fenestration is a promising treatment for pediatric visual symptoms, with few complications, and venous sinus stenting is a specialized, promising procedure in a few centers. These clinical nuances reinforce the complexity inherent in pediatric interventional radiology and underscore the necessity for expertise in this domain (Friso *et al.*, 2024; Young *et al.*, 2022) (Figure 10.20).

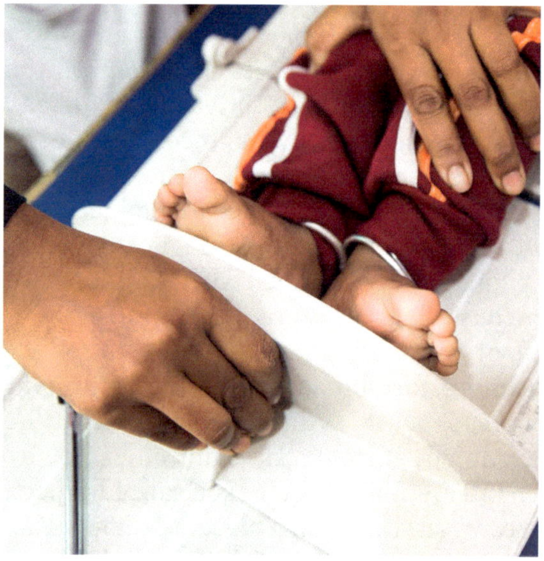

Figure 10.20. Pediatric patients range from premature infants to adolescents nearing adult size, requiring customized equipment adaptations and procedural modifications.

Source: https://images.gatesnotes.com/12514eb8-7b51-008e-41a9-512542cf683b/568c0fed-a24f-432f-b612-50b633afa25a/Exemplars-in-Global-Health_2020_vNext_1500x1500-01.jpg?w=1400&h=900&fit=clip&fm=jpg&q=75.

10.4.6. Cost-effectiveness Compared to Traditional Surgery

Medical technology has placed more importance on making sure treatments are effective and still affordable. Because of the minimally invasive nature of interventional radiology, patients usually spend less time in the hospital and recover more quickly, which helps reduce immediate medical expenses. However when we look at how much it costs over the years, things get more complicated. For example, a study comparing UAE with surgery for fibroid treatment found that, while UAE initially appeared more cost-effective due to reduced invasiveness and recovery time, the need for re-intervention in nearly one-third of patients diminished this benefit over five years (Dutton *et al.*, 2011). In the end, even though interventional radiology can save money and risks in the beginning, the savings may disappear once more procedures are required. This detailed knowledge of cost-effectiveness points out the need for decisions that fit each patient and for full economic assessments.

10.4.7. Patient Outcomes and Quality of Life Improvements

Because of new medical treatments, managing serious conditions is now much easier, resulting in better health and quality of life for patients. Especially, interventional radiology has become a useful way to quickly treat severe nosebleeds and sudden hearing loss in the inner ear. Interventional radiology helps avoid major surgeries by offering targeted arterial embolization and intratympanic steroid administration, which also speed up recovery and reduce the risk of problems. For example, management of severe epistaxis now involves stepwise procedures, from nasal packing to endovascular embolization, optimizing bleeding control while minimizing patient discomfort and hospitalization duration (Tunkel *et al.*, 2020). Similarly, early diagnosis and timely intratympanic steroid treatment for sudden hearing loss can substantially improve hearing restoration, thereby mitigating long-term auditory impairment and associated psychosocial impacts (Chandrasekhar *et al.*, 2019). These advancements collectively underscore interventional radiology's pivotal role in improving not only clinical outcomes but also overall patient well-being (Figure 10.21).

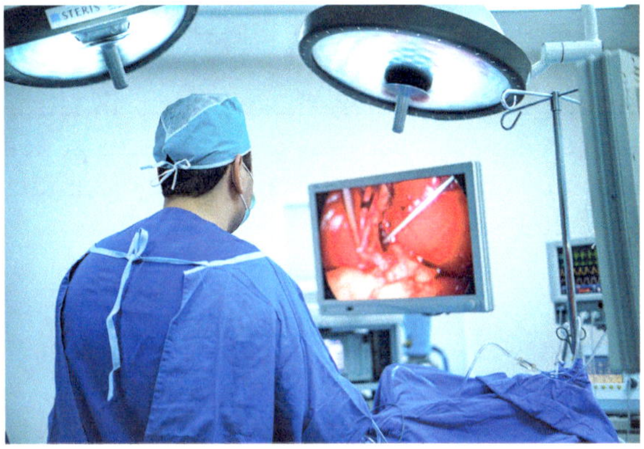

Figure 10.21. In particular, interventional radiology has emerged as a minimally invasive approach that effectively addresses acute problems such as severe nosebleeds and sudden sensorineural hearing loss.

Source: https://static.wixstatic.com/media/84da7d_490b1e8dda004a30a258a45852562896~mv2.png/v1/fill/w_980,h_654,al_c,q_90,usm_0.66_1.00_0.01,enc_avif,quality_auto/84da7d_490b1e8dda004a30a258a45852562896~mv2.png.

10.4.8. Research and Clinical Trials in Interventional Radiology

The progress in interventional radiology is largely due to strong research and well-designed clinical trials, which have made it an important part of modern medicine. One study protocol highlights the importance of patient involvement by comparing the usual way referring physicians give information to a more detailed approach by interventional radiologists with explanatory videos. This randomized controlled trial aims to evaluate improvements in patient knowledge, satisfaction, and anxiety, thereby underscoring the importance of proactive clinical involvement and innovative educational tools in procedural settings (García Jurado *et al.*, 2025). The MR CLEAN series and similar landmark trials in stroke intervention clearly show the major changes that research in interventional radiology brings to clinical care. Because of these studies, endovascular treatment was improved, and the timing of procedures and the use of drugs became more precise, highlighting the strong teamwork between radiologists and neurologists. Together, these efforts illustrate the evolving evidence base that enhances patient outcomes and advances the specialty (Samuels *et al.*, 2024).

10.4.9. Global Perspectives and Access to Care

Developments in technology have greatly changed healthcare worldwide, especially in interventional radiology, which uses minimally invasive techniques that call for expert tools and knowledge. Even so, there are still large differences in access, mainly in low- and middle-income countries, as a lack of resources and infrastructure makes it hard to provide for everyone. The pandemic brought attention to the challenges and benefits of using telemedicine and digital tools for remote consultations, training, and follow-up care, which supports equal access to interventional radiology services. However, these virtual solutions also introduced concerns related to digital fatigue and the need for sustainable, user-friendly technologies that accommodate diverse populations and clinical environments (Bashshur *et al.*, 2020; Wiederhold, 2020). Addressing global inequities necessitates collaborative international efforts that integrate telehealth innovations with investments in local infrastructure and workforce development, ensuring that interventional radiology can be both accessible and effective worldwide, ultimately improving patient outcomes on a global scale (Figure 10.22).

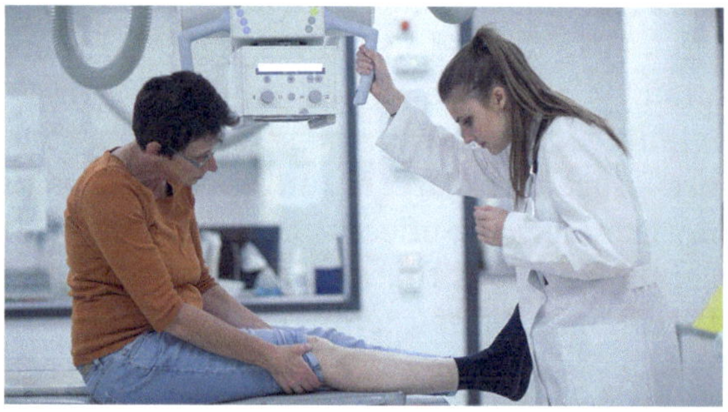

Figure 10.22. Advancements in technology have dramatically transformed healthcare delivery across the globe, particularly within interventional radiology, where minimally invasive procedures require specialized expertise and equipment.

Source: https://medicalbuyer.co.in/wp-content/uploads/2021/03/xray-story.jpg.

Test Your Knowledge

1. In what ways does interventional radiology help with cancer management?
2. In what ways is interventional radiology used to treat chronic pain?

SUMMARY

Thanks to new techniques in interventional radiology, patients can now receive treatment and diagnoses with less pain and a faster recovery. Still, introducing new technologies such as artificial intelligence means it is important to check regulatory and ethical aspects to make sure everything is safe and effective. The current challenges include establishing robust legal frameworks and quality standards that address the medico-legal implications inherent in AI-assisted procedures, particularly given the evolving nature of radiologist liability and autonomous diagnostic systems (Ungureanu *et al.*, 2025). Furthermore, clinical factors like perioperative medication management continue to influence procedural risks, as demonstrated by increased postoperative hemorrhage rates in patients on antiplatelet therapy, underscoring the need for comprehensive patient assessment and individualized care planning (Pinchuk *et al.*, 2024). To ensure a bright future, interventional radiology should bring together progress in technology, strict monitoring, and responsible clinical decisions.

With the improvements in interventional radiology, this field is now more important in medicine because it improves both diagnosis and treatment. Through technologies such as Biomechanical Computed Tomography analysis, clinicians can opportunistically assess bone strength and fracture risk without additional patient burden, highlighting its integration into broader diagnostic workflows (Bouxsein *et al.*, 2020). Furthermore, the role of specialized practitioner frameworks, as seen in consultant radiographer models, contributes significantly to service improvements by optimizing patient throughput, ensuring cost-effectiveness, and fostering multidisciplinary collaboration (Miller *et al.*, 2010). All these developments show that interventional radiology overcomes the limits of standard imaging, helping patients with less invasive treatments that improve their health and make healthcare easier. Because of new technologies and career advancements, interventional radiology helps detect diseases early and provides suitable treatment methods, making it a vital part of healthcare today.

KEY TERMS FROM THIS CHAPTER

- Interventional radiology
- Personalized patient care
- Pulmonary fibrosis
- Checklists
- Arterial embolizations
- Transjugular techniques
- Fluoroscopy
- Vertebroplasty
- Decision-making
- Open surgery
- Interstitial lung disease
- Dose alerts
- Image-guided liver biopsy
- Hepatobiliary conditions
- Paget's disease
- Patient care continuum

CRITICAL THINKING QUESTIONS

1. **What is the primary role of interventional radiology (IR)?**
   a. To visualize soft tissues using X-rays
   b. To treat diseases and conditions using imaging guidance
   c. To perform surgery without any imaging support
   d. To conduct physical therapy treatments
2. **What imaging method is most often used in interventional radiology?**
   a. X-ray
   b. CT scan
   c. MRI
   d. All of the above
3. **Which of the options below shows a typical minimally invasive interventional radiology procedure?**
   a. Open-heart surgery
   b. Percutaneous coronary intervention (PCI)
   c. Brain surgery
   d. Organ transplant
4. **In which procedure is a catheter inserted to remove or break up a blood clot?**
   a. Angioplasty
   b. Thrombolysis
   c. Embolization
   d. Biopsy
5. **What is the purpose of angioplasty in interventional radiology?**
   a. To remove a tumor
   b. To widen narrowed blood vessels
   c. To treat infections
   d. To inject contrast agents for imaging

Short Answer Questions

1. What is the primary goal of transarterial embolization (TAE) in cancer treatment?
2. Which risks are most common in interventional radiology procedures?
3. What part does robotic assistance play in performing interventional radiology procedures?
4. Why should patients keep to bed rest for several hours after a catheter-based procedure?
5. What is the most common problem that happens after a percutaneous biopsy done by interventional radiology?

Answers to Critical Thinking Questions

1. (b); 2. (d); 3. (b); 4. (b); 5. (b)

REFERENCES

1. Adler, Y., Charron, P., Imazio, M., Badano, L. P., Barón-Esquivias, G., Bogaert, J., Brucato, A., *et al.* (2015). 2015 ESC Guidelines for the diagnosis and management of pericardial diseases. *European Heart Journal, 36*, 2921–2964. https://doi.org/10.1093/eurheartj/ehv318 (accessed on 1st June 2025).
2. Agrawal, A., Sakale, H., Goyal, R., Mishra, A., Gaurav, P., & Inamdar, A. (2025). Comprehensive management of distal femur osteosarcoma in a 15-year-old male: A multidisciplinary approach and long-term follow-up. *Journal of Orthopedic Case Reports, 15*, 74–79. https://www.semanticscholar.org/paper/99237bfdf00015e06a9d474739a8db617961f354 (accessed on 1st June 2025).
3. Ahmed, K., Mahmoud, A., Mohammed, K. A., & Ibrahim, B. (2023). Role of interventional radiology in upper abdominal cancer pain management. *Egyptian Journal of Radiology and Nuclear Medicine, 54*, 1–7. https://www.semanticscholar.org/paper/dc1813e6ee5218e0b3b802bbbbf1e68c759b0149 (accessed on 1st June 2025).
4. Alshalali, A. A., Alharthi, A. A., Alzaidi, F. A., Alhasawi, I. M., Alshamrani, L. A., Almasoudi, M. A., Hussain, M. S., *et al.* (2023). *Role of Interventional Radiology in Management of Gastrointestinal Bleeding*. https://core.ac.uk/download/603897406.pdf (accessed on 1st June 2025).
5. Alshammary, N. S., & Alwahdani, M. N. (2024). The effectiveness of interventional radiology procedures in minimally invasive treatments: (Critical review). *The Medical Journal of Cairo University.* https://www.semanticscholar.org/paper/52ab4ba46159f2bb6ffbac2e68b73e57342dedad (accessed on 1st June 2025).
6. Baddour, L. M., Wilson, W. R., Bayer, A. S., Fowler, V. G., Tleyjeh, I. M., Rybak, M. J., Baršić, B., *et al.* (2015). Infective endocarditis in adults: Diagnosis, antimicrobial therapy, and management of complications. *Circulation, 132,* 1435–1486. https://doi.org/10.1161/cir.0000000000000296 (accessed on 1st June 2025).
7. Baron, K. (2024). Evaluating the radiation dose involved in interventional radiology procedures. *The Arab Journal of Interventional Radiology.* https://www.semanticscholar.org/paper/71215e72727e611e49ebbbb18e6a5226f8d81df0 (accessed on 1st June 2025).
8. Bashshur, R. L., Doarn, C. R., Frenk, J., Kvedar, J. C., & Woolliscroft, J. O. (2020). Telemedicine and the COVID-19 pandemic: Lessons for the future. *Telemedicine Journal and e-Health, 26,* 571–573. https://doi.org/10.1089/tmj.2020.29040.rb (accessed on 1st June 2025).
9. Beyoğlu, R. (2024). Radiological imaging and interventional procedures of the thorax in children. *Turkish Journal of Thoracic and Cardiovascular Surgery, 32*, S10–S20. https://www.semanticscholar.org/paper/6885b98e9276f2eefe8d37c450c47f4bf7574aab (accessed on 1st June 2025).
10. Bhatti, H., Moeed, M., Bhatti, A., Ali, M., Shahid, S., Javed, M., Ali, S., *et al.* (2025). Augmented and virtual reality in radiology: A comparative analysis of clinical applications and outcomes. *Journal of Medical & Health Sciences Review.* https://www.semanticscholar.org/paper/6970f5a361f418f10ab30bd58d61657b5337b988 (accessed on 1st June 2025).
11. Boike, J., Thornburg, B., Asrani, S. K., Fallon, M. B., Fortune, B. E., Izzy, M., Verna, E. C., *et al.* (2021). North American practice-based recommendations for transjugular intrahepatic portosystemic shunts in portal hypertension. *Clinical Gastroenterology and Hepatology, 20,*

1636–1662.e36. https://doi.org/10.1016/j.cgh.2021.07.018 (accessed on 1st June 2025).

12. Boone, N. B. (2012). *A Qualitative Descriptive Study of the Work of Nurses in Interventional Radiology.* https://core.ac.uk/download/477678860.pdf (accessed on 1st June 2025).

13. Bouxsein, M. L., Clarke, B. L., Cosman, F., Keaveny, *et al.* (2020). *Biomechanical Computed Tomography Analysis (BCT) for Clinical Assessment of Osteoporosis.* https://core.ac.uk/download/323308619.pdf (accessed on 1st June 2025).

14. Bradley, W. G., Glazer, G. M., Hricak, H., Krestin, *et al.* (2009). Advancing radiology through informed leadership: Summary of the proceedings of the Seventh Biannual Symposium of the International Society for Strategic Studies in Radiology (IS3R), 23–25 August 2007. https://core.ac.uk/download/pdf/8303029.pdf (accessed on 1st June 2025).

15. Byers, P. H., Belmont, J. W., Black, J. H., De Backer, J., Frank, M., Jeunemaître, X., Johnson, D., *et al.* (2017). Diagnosis, natural history, and management in vascular Ehlers–Danlos syndrome. *American Journal of Medical Genetics Part C: Seminars in Medical Genetics, 175,* 40–47. https://doi.org/10.1002/ajmg.c.31553 (accessed on 1st June 2025).

16. Calais, J., Morris, M. J., Kendi, A. T., Kalebasty, A. R., Tutrone, R., Anderson, M. J., Sartor, O. (2024). Best patient care practices for administering PSMA-targeted radiopharmaceutical therapy. *Journal of Nuclear Medicine, 65,* 1666–1671. https://www.semanticscholar.org/paper/f6e44ecc63d73d78bce41f8b1070083d3ca5a798 (accessed on 1st June 2025).

17. Cavayas, Y. A., Del Sorbo, L., & Fan, E. (2018). Intracranial hemorrhage in adults on ECMO. *Perfusion, 33,* 42–50. https://doi.org/10.1177/0267659118766435 (accessed on 1st June 2025).

18. Chandrasekhar, S. S., Tsai, S. B., Schwartz, S., Bontempo, L., Faucett, E. A., Finestone, S. A., Hollingsworth, D. B., *et al.* (2019). Clinical practice guideline: Sudden hearing loss (Update). *Otolaryngology, 161.* https://doi.org/10.1177/0194599819859885 (accessed on 1st June 2025).

19. Chaple, P., & Luhariya, A. (2024). A cross-sectional observational study on quality assurance and radiation safety in interventional radiology. *F1000Research.* https://www.semanticscholar.org/paper/58fecfe203b172681242887b181b4fa19dc10e4d (accessed on 1st June 2025).

20. Coleman, R. E., Hadji, P., Body, J. J., Santini, D., Chow, E., Terpos, E., Oudard, S., *et al.* (2020). Bone health in cancer: ESMO Clinical Practice Guidelines. *Annals of Oncology, 31,* 1650–1663. https://doi.org/10.1016/j.annonc.2020.07.019 (accessed on 1st June 2025).

21. Damilakis, J., Ebdon-Jackson, S., Frush, D. P., Loose, *et al.* (2017). Unintended and accidental medical radiation exposures in radiology: Guidelines on investigation and prevention. https://core.ac.uk/download/96883276.pdf (accessed on 1st June 2025).

22. Datta, A., Bhowmik, B., Alam, S. Z., Islam, M. T., & Sultana, S. N. (2024). Second International Conference and Workshop on Interventional Radiology 2023, Dhaka, Bangladesh: Advancements, achievements, and challenges. *Journal of Clinical Interventional Radiology ISVIR.* https://www.semanticscholar.org/paper/5b55c77cd86cd28735a9fcd6647b99444480b745 (accessed on 1st June 2025).

23. Davenport, T. H., & Kalakota, R. (2019). The potential for artificial intelligence in healthcare. *Future Healthcare Journal, 6,* 94–98. https://doi.org/10.7861/futurehosp.6-2-94 (accessed on 1st June 2025).

24. Davis, R. S., Devaney, J., Halligan, S. L., Meiser-Stedman, R., Oliveira, P., Smith, P., Stallard, P., *et al.* (2024). The feasibility and acceptability of delivering a group trauma-focused intervention to children in care. *The British Journal of Clinical Psychology, 64*, 86–109. https://www.semanticscholar.org/paper/03e82752a2ad310e796029a52f618997669b6cbd (accessed on 1st June 2025).

25. De Grandis, M. D., Ascenti, V., Lanza, C., Di Paolo, G., Galassi, B., Ierardi, A., Carrafiello, G., *et al.* (2023). Locoregional therapies and remodeling of tumor microenvironment in pancreatic cancer. *International Journal of Molecular Sciences, 24.* https://www.semanticscholar.org/paper/a1f54709ec31fb3c469c3506d712a5b06ea6ffb2 (accessed on 1st June 2025).

26. Desimpel, J., Posadzy, M., & Vanhoenacker, F. (2018). *Cone Beam CT of the Musculoskeletal System: Clinical Applications.* https://core.ac.uk/download/147045015.pdf (accessed on 1st June 2025).

27. Dhar, J., & Samanta, J. (2023). Endoscopic ultrasound-guided vascular interventions: An expanding paradigm. *World Journal of Gastrointestinal Endoscopy, 15,* 216–239. https://doi.org/10.4253/wjge.v15.i4.216 (accessed on 1st June 2025).

28. Di Donna, A., Masala, S., Muto, G., Marcia, S., Giordano, F., & Muto, M. (2024). Metabolic bone diseases: Recommendations for interventional radiology. *Seminars in Musculoskeletal Radiology, 28*(5), 641–650. https://www.semanticscholar.org/paper/d007a57991903651f0b1030f91cc0bf44c3747bc (accessed on 1st June 2025).

29. Dutton, G., Edwards, R., Goodwin, S., Hehenkamp, W., Homer, H., Katsumori, *et al.* (2011). Randomized comparison of uterine artery embolization (UAE) with surgical treatment in patients with symptomatic uterine fibroids (REST trial): 5-year results. https://core.ac.uk/download/9391452.pdf (accessed on 1st June 2025).

30. Elshafee, A. S., Karch, A., Ringe, K. I., Shin, H. O., Raatschen, H. J., Soliman, N., Wacker, F., *et al.* (2019). Complications of CT-guided lung biopsy with a non-coaxial semi-automated 18-gauge biopsy system: Frequency, severity and risk factors. *PLoS ONE, 14*, e0213990–e0213990. https://doi.org/10.1371/journal.pone.0213990 (accessed on 1st June 2025).

31. Eshiev, A. M., & Eshiev, D. A. (2024). Comparative evaluation of surgical treatment of congenital alveolar cleft in children. *Head and Neck. Russian Journal.* https://www.semanticscholar.org/paper/0ff75a6fb41e13cdd93bc5b61adb4ddbab5dcc3c (accessed on 1st June 2025).

32. Faiella, E., Vaccarino, F., Pacella, G., Santucci, D., Vergantino, E., Bruno, A., Ragone, R., *et al.* (2024). Exploring the efficacy of combining radiofrequency thermal ablation or microwave ablation with vertebroplasty for pain control and disease management in metastatic bone disease—A systematic review. *Current Oncology, 31,* 5422–5438. https://www.semanticscholar.org/paper/90a5963f2761456308ff3c39d75986e1ba049aee (accessed on 1st June 2025).

33. Falade, I., Gyampoh, G., Akpamgbo, E., Chika, O., Obodo, O. R., Okobi, O., Aguguo, J., *et al.* (2024). A comprehensive review of effective patient safety and quality improvement programs in healthcare facilities. *Medical Research Archives.* https://www.semanticscholar.org/paper/07eabf23f3cd7f447c92812d7e886a8af8d59414 (accessed on 1st June 2025).

34. Fehrenbach, U. (2023). Augmented reality applications in interventional radiology: Possibilities and challenges. *Cardiovascular and Interventional Radiology, 46*, 680, 681. https://www.semanticscholar.org/paper/a4f6d2244b642735f78b0a461fdb104f666a4998 (accessed on 1st June 2025).

35. Fisher, R., Applegate, K. E., Berkowitz, L. K., Christianson, O., Dave, J. K., DeWeese, L., Harris, N., *et al.* (2022). AAPM Medical Physics Practice Guideline 12.a: Fluoroscopy dose management. *Journal of Applied Clinical Medical Physics, 23.* https://doi.org/10.1002/acm2.13526 (accessed on 1st June 2025).

36. Friso, S., Giacobbo, V., Toscano, L. M., Baldo, B., Guariento, C., Lacarra, F., Pin, J. N., *et al.* (2024). A systematic review of surgical and interventional radiology procedures for pediatric idiopathic intracranial hypertension. *Frontiers in Pediatrics, 12.* https://www.semanticscholar.org/paper/e62aace55c94b26bfe848adf0170126acfd48cf8 (accessed on 1st June 2025).

37. García, J. P. B., Espejo, H. J. E., Lombardo, G. M. S., Pérez, M. M. E., Barranco, A. S., García-Revillo, J., Font Ugalde, P., *et al.* (2025). CLINTERVENTIONAL protocol: A randomized controlled trial to evaluate clinical consultations and audiovisual tools for interventional radiology. *European Radiology Experimental, 9.* https://www.semanticscholar.org/paper/d709d63853e9c981a83ddbcd40e71081664905e4 (accessed on 1st June 2025).

38. Gianesini, S., Obi, A., Onida, S., Baccellieri, D., Bissacco, D., Borsuk, D., Campisi, C., *et al.* (2019). Global guidelines trends and controversies in lower limb venous and lymphatic disease. *Phlebology: The Journal of Venous Disease, 34,* 4–66. https://doi.org/10.1177/0268355519870690 (accessed on 1st June 2025).

39. Glikson, M., Nielsen, J. C., Kronborg, M. B., Michowitz, Y., Auricchio, A., Barbash, I. M., Barrabés, J. A., *et al.* (2021a). 2021 ESC guidelines on cardiac pacing and cardiac resynchronization therapy. *European Heart Journal, 42,* 3427–3520. https://doi.org/10.1093/eurheartj/ehab364 (accessed on 1st June 2025).

40. Glikson, M., Nielsen, J. C., Kronborg, M. B., Michowitz, Y., Auricchio, A., Barbash, I. M., Barrabés, J. A., *et al.* (2021b). 2021 ESC guidelines on cardiac pacing and cardiac resynchronization therapy. *EP Europace, 24,* 71–164. https://doi.org/10.1093/europace/euab232 (accessed on 1st June 2025).

41. Heimbach, J. K., Kulik, L., Finn, R. S., Sirlin, C. B., Abécassis, M., Roberts, L. R., Zhu, A. X., *et al.* (2017). AASLD guidelines for the treatment of hepatocellular carcinoma. *Hepatology, 67,* 358–380. https://doi.org/10.1002/hep.29086 (accessed on 1st June 2025).

42. Holzwanger, D., Trikantzopolous, E., Nauheim, D., Chauhan, A. S., Milsom, J. W., & Pua, B. B. (2025). Fusion of interventional radiology with surgery and endoscopy to advance therapies in complex gastrointestinal disease. *Seminars in Interventional Radiology.* https://www.semanticscholar.org/paper/f7e30f7d809a4db4ebc374aac7e98b8237e9b6ad (accessed on 1st June 2025).

43. Karabulut, N. (2015). Requirements for manuscript submission: What every author needs to know and comply with to facilitate the review process. https://core.ac.uk/download/227065151.pdf (accessed on 1st June 2025).

44. Kayastha, P., Adhikari, B., Paudel, S., Suwal, S., Shingh, S. S., Chapagain, P., & Regmi, P. (2024). Ultrasound guided biopsy among patients with lung lesions undergoing procedures in interventional radiology of a tertiary care center. *JNMA: Journal of the Nepal Medical Association, 62,* 27–29. https://www.semanticscholar.org/paper/d11fedcc9fcf5e9d1b2ef5817a8ce25eeeb6e66a (accessed on 1st June 2025).

45. Khurtovskyi, V. (2025). The evolution of state economic regulation: Theoretical approaches and contemporary challenges. *Electronic Scientific Journal Intellectualization of Logistics*

and Supply Chain Management #1 2020. https://www.semanticscholar.org/paper/c57ce0f29b1cbd95754afa4b742ccbc5614e584f (accessed on 1st June 2025).

46. LeBoff, M. S., Greenspan, S. L., Insogna, K., Lewiecki, E. M., Saag, K. G., Singer, A., & Siris, E. S. (2022). The clinician's guide to prevention and treatment of osteoporosis. *Osteoporosis International, 33,* 2049–2102. https://doi.org/10.1007/s00198-021-05900-y (accessed on 1st June 2025).

47. Lecomte, F., Scarponi, V., Alvarez, P., Verde, J., Dillenseger, J., Vibert, E., & Cotin, S. (2023). Enhancing fluoroscopy-guided interventions: A neural network to predict vessel deformation without contrast agents. *Proceedings of the 15th Hamlyn Symposium on Medical Robotics 2023.* https://www.semanticscholar.org/paper/783183a7262980435fc870d7276a342d8fb25ff6 (accessed on 1st June 2025).

48. Lee, E., Eghtesad, B., García-Tsao, G., Haskal, Z. J., Hernández-Gea, V., Jalaeian, H., Kalva, S. P., *et al.* (2023). AASLD practice guidance on the use of TIPS, variceal embolization, and retrograde transvenous obliteration in the management of variceal hemorrhage. *Hepatology, 79,* 224–250. https://doi.org/10.1097/hep.0000000000000530 (accessed on 1st June 2025).

49. Lu, A. C., Schmiesing, C. A., Mahoney, M., Cianfichi, L., Semple, A., Watt, D., Fischer, S. P., *et al.* (2020). COVID-19 preoperative assessment and testing: From surge to recovery. *Annals of Surgery, 272,* e230–e235. https://doi.org/10.1097/sla.0000000000004124 (accessed on 1st June 2025).

50. Ma, J., Yu, Q., & Van Ha, T. V. (2024). Image-guided liver biopsy: Perspectives from interventional radiology. *Seminars in Interventional Radiology, 41*(5), 500–506. https://www.semanticscholar.org/paper/a2778c53603bd78d0f4374ca18e4a09615b26555 (accessed on 1st June 2025).

51. Maher, M. M., O'Connor, O. J., O'Neill, S. B., Ryan, *et al.* (2011). *Interventional Radiology and the Care of the Oncology Patient.* https://core.ac.uk/download/pdf/8631075.pdf (accessed on 1st June 2025).

52. Mansour, M. A., Raheem, M., & Ibrahim, W. (2022). Assessment of post therapeutic response of uterine artery embolization for treatment of uterine fibroids. *Journal of the Bahrain Medical Society.* https://www.semanticscholar.org/paper/6855d2177e963493e4e9e4a922907b43b5c10ad9 (accessed on 1st June 2025).

53. Mathijssen, I. M. J. (2020). Updated guideline on treatment and management of craniosynostosis. *Journal of Craniofacial Surgery, 32,* 371–450. https://doi.org/10.1097/scs.0000000000007035 (accessed on 1st June 2025).

54. McCowan, T. C., Patel, A. M., Ray, D. M., Srinivasan, *et al.* (2017). Complementary roles of interventional radiology and therapeutic endoscopy in gastroenterology. *World Journal of Radiology* https://core.ac.uk/download/269303742.pdf (accessed on 1st June 2025).

55. Miller, L., & Price, R. (2010). *An Evaluation of the Impact of Implementation of Consultant Practitioners in Clinical Imaging.* https://core.ac.uk/download/9840194.pdf (accessed on 1st June 2025).

56. Nervo, A., Ragni, A., Retta, F., Calandri, M., Gazzera, C., Gallo, M., Piovesan, A., *et al.* (2021). Interventional radiology approaches for liver metastases from thyroid cancer: A case series and overview of the literature. *Journal of Gastrointestinal Cancer, 52,* 823–832. https://www.semanticscholar.org/paper/a5a32f990bd0de26043f3298be481d4ae3e9073a (accessed on 1st June 2025).

57. Nguyen, R. (2024). *Interventional Radiology's Exploration into Artificial Intelligence.* https://core.ac.uk/download/619706208.pdf (accessed on 1st June 2025).

58. O'Leary, C., Mafeld, S., Hilario, K., Chan, T. Y., & Jaberi, A. (2024). Managing angiography unit failure in interventional radiology: Lessons in crisis management and considerations in prevention. *Canadian Association of Radiologists Journal = Journal l'Association Canadienne des Radiologistes.* https://www.semanticscholar.org/paper/0edf143ea4ef4129c9d1ab45a816d5ceaa449442 (accessed on 1st June 2025).

59. Panayides, A. S., Amini, A. A., Filipović, N., Sharma, A., Tsaftaris, S. A., Young, A. A., Foran, D. J., *et al.* (2020). AI in medical imaging informatics: Current challenges and future directions. *IEEE Journal of Biomedical and Health Informatics, 24,* 1837–1857. https://doi.org/10.1109/jbhi.2020.2991043 (accessed on 1st June 2025).

60. Parmeggiani, A., Martella, C., Ceccarelli, L., Miceli, M., Spinnato, P., & Facchini, G. (2021). Osteoid osteoma: Which is the best minimally invasive treatment option? *European Journal of Orthopedic Surgery & Traumatology, 31,* 1611–1624. https://doi.org/10.1007/s00590-021-02946-w (accessed on 1st June 2025).

61. Pascarella, G., Strumia, A., Piliego, C., Bruno, F., Del Buono, R., Costa, F., Scarlata, S., *et al.* (2020). COVID-19 diagnosis and management: A comprehensive review. *Journal of Internal Medicine, 288,* 192–206. https://doi.org/10.1111/joim.13091 (accessed on 1st June 2025).

62. Pesapane, F., Codari, M., & Sardanelli, F. (2018). Artificial intelligence in medical imaging: Threat or opportunity? Radiologists again at the forefront of innovation in medicine. *European Radiology Experimental, 2.* https://doi.org/10.1186/s41747-018-0061-6 (accessed on 1st June 2025).

63. Pinchuk, A., Tonchev, N., Stein, K. P., Swiatek, V. M., Dumitru, C. A., Neyazi, B., Sandalcioglu, I. E., *et al.* (2024). Impact of perioperative acetylsalicylic acid (ASA) administration on postoperative intracranial hemorrhage (pICH) and thromboembolic events in patients with intracranial meningiomas. *Journal of Clinical Medicine, 13.* https://www.semanticscholar.org/paper/e6d7daf60a727a6ef26183db54ac9f712b899935 (accessed on 1st June 2025).

64. Raghu, G., Rémy-Jardin, M., Myers, J. L., Richeldi, L., Ryerson, C. J., Lederer, D. J., Behr, J., *et al.* (2018). Diagnosis of idiopathic pulmonary fibrosis. An official ATS/ERS/JRS/ALAT clinical practice guideline. *American Journal of Respiratory and Critical Care Medicine, 198,* e44–e68. https://doi.org/10.1164/rccm.201807-1255st (accessed on 1st June 2025).

65. Rayyani, A. A., Shalalni, A. A., Radwan, A. H., Shibli, K. A., Jabin, J. Y., Mokli, M. A. Y., Mabuj, J. M., *et al.* (2024). Digital X-ray imaging: Emphasis can be placed on developments in digital X-ray technologies and their applications in diagnosis and treatment. https://core.ac.uk/download/616775625.pdf (accessed on 1st June 2025).

66. Samuels, N., Van De, G. R. A., Roos, Y., Dippel, D., & Van Der Lugt, A. (2024). Advancements in diagnostic and interventional radiology for stroke treatment: The path from trial to bedside through the pre-MR CLEAN, MR CLEAN, and MR CLEAN II eras. *Insights into Imaging, 15.* https://www.semanticscholar.org/paper/89d1a3e306d1608cf5504300942e9f40dd79a46c (accessed on 1st June 2025).

67. Schiødt, M., Otto, S., Fedele, S., Bedogni, A., Nicolatou-Galitis, O., Guggenberger, R., Herlofson, B. B., *et al.* (2019). Workshop of European task force on medication-related osteonecrosis of the jaw—Current challenges. *Oral Diseases, 25,* 1815–1821. https://doi.org/10.1111/odi.13160 (accessed on 1st June 2025).

68. Sclafani, S. J. A. (2025). The origins of interventional radiology as a treatment of the trauma patient: A personal perspective. *Seminars in Interventional Radiology.* https://www.semanticscholar.org/paper/5faadbbbdf5b5ca8e304c90ba531125a371adadc (accessed on 1st June 2025).

69. Seibert, A. J., Baird, C. T., Clements, J. B., De Boer, *et al.* (2018). *AAPM Medical Physics Practice Guideline 10.a.: Scope of Practice for Clinical Medical Physics.* https://core.ac.uk/download/286729023.pdf (accessed on 1st June 2025).

70. Senthilkumar, M., Senthil, K. C., Parmar, R., & Velmurugan, J. (2024). Uncertainty evaluation of non-invasive multi-parameter detector measurements in quality assurance of diagnostic radiology. *Journal of Cancer Research and Therapeutics.* https://www.semanticscholar.org/paper/af5bd292e4328455c507e45a3730cf016d89242a (accessed on 1st June 2025).

71. Sgalambro, F., Zugaro, L., Bruno, F., Palumbo, P., Salducca, N., Zoccali, C., Barile, A., *et al.* (2022). Interventional radiology in the management of metastases and bone tumors. *Journal of Clinical Medicine, 11.* https://www.semanticscholar.org/paper/297d8b28a84074a0575f2b8f0c1b573fecd23773 (accessed on 1st June 2025).

72. Sharma, R., Thakkar, H., Baisoya, R., & Tiwari, T. N. (2022). Fetal intervention: Less developed field of interventional radiology. *Enormous Journal of Medical Sciences and Current Research.* https://www.semanticscholar.org/paper/499c2b065296c7f177a42cc7a14d037e8b67bb36 (accessed on 1st June 2025).

73. Shen, D., Wu, G., & Suk, H. I. (2017). Deep learning in medical image analysis. *Annual Review of Biomedical Engineering, 19,* 221–248. https://doi.org/10.1146/annurev-bioeng-071516-044442 (accessed on 1st June 2025).

74. Soyer, P., Barat, M., Loffroy, R., Barral, M., Dautry, R., Vidal, V., Pellerin, O., *et al.* (2020). The role of interventional radiology in the management of abnormally invasive placenta: A systematic review of current evidences. *Quantitative Imaging in Medicine and Surgery, 10*(6), 1370–1391. https://www.semanticscholar.org/paper/eb64000480f9c6bd89c485fabb863168b08d33de (accessed on 1st June 2025).

75. Tanaka, M., Keefe, N. A., Caridi, T., Kohi, M., & Salazar, G. (2023). Interventional radiology in obstetrics and gynecology: Updates in women's health. *Radiographics: A Review Publication of the Radiological Society of North America, Inc., 43*(3), e220039. https://www.semanticscholar.org/paper/fc8e6cfd3985a6210c693e69cb5158498872b5ea (accessed on 1st June 2025).

76. Tarango, C., & Manco-Johnson, M. J. (2017). Pediatric thrombolysis: A practical approach. *Frontiers in Pediatrics, 5.* https://doi.org/10.3389/fped.2017.00260 (accessed on 1st June 2025).

77. Tay, Y. X., Foley, S. J., Killeen, R., Ong, M. E., Chen, R. C., Chan, L. P., Mak, M. S., *et al.* (2024). Impact and effect of imaging referral guidelines on patients and radiology services: A systematic review. *European Radiology, 35,* 532–541. https://www.semanticscholar.org/paper/f9fe67bad8838e51c50670dbbde12fee785c5941 (accessed on 1st June 2025).

78. Tunkel, D. E., Anne, S., Payne, S. C., Ishman, S. L., Rosenfeld, R. M., Abramson, P. J., Alikhaani, J. D., *et al.* (2020). Clinical practice guideline: Nosebleed (epistaxis). *Otolaryngology, 162.* https://doi.org/10.1177/0194599819890327 (accessed on 1st June 2025).

79. Ungureanu, A. M., Matei, S., & Malita, D. (2025). Controversies in the application of AI in radiology—Is there medico-legal support? Aspects from Romanian practice. *Diagnostics, 15.*

https://www.semanticscholar.org/paper/288ba342d57fc5ea98e9d4cf8fba85d8e01522d7 (accessed on 1st June 2025).

80. Vassallo, P. (2004). *Radiology.* https://core.ac.uk/download/46601887.pdf (accessed on 1st June 2025).

81. Vogt, I., Eisenmann, M., Schlünz, A., Kowal, R., Düx, D. M., Thormann, M., Glandorf, J., *et al.* (2024). MRI-compatible and sensorless haptic feedback for cable-driven medical robotics to perform teleoperated needle-based interventions. *International Journal of Computer Assisted Radiology and Surgery, 20,* 179–189. https://www.semanticscholar.org/paper/9d589d50d8004dd08d9d5afba1d8b30c420dbb4d (accessed on 1st June 2025).

82. Weissler, J. M., Cho, E. H., Koltz, P. F., Carney, M. J., Itkin, M., Laje, P., Levin, L. S., *et al.* (2018). Lymphovenous anastomosis for the treatment of chylothorax in infants: A novel microsurgical approach to a devastating problem. *Plastic & Reconstructive Surgery, 141,* 1502–1507. https://doi.org/10.1097/prs.0000000000004424 (accessed on 1st June 2025).

83. Wiederhold, B. K. (2020). Connecting through technology during the coronavirus disease 2019 pandemic: Avoiding "Zoom fatigue." *Cyberpsychology Behavior and Social Networking, 23,* 437, 438. https://doi.org/10.1089/cyber.2020.29188.bkw (accessed on 1st June 2025).

84. Wolf, A. M. D., Fontham, E. T. H., Church, T. R., Flowers, C. R., Guerra, C. E., LaMonte, S. J., Etzioni, R., *et al.* (2018). Colorectal cancer screening for average-risk adults: 2018 guideline update from the American Cancer Society. *CA A Cancer Journal for Clinicians, 68,* 250–281. https://doi.org/10.3322/caac.21457 (accessed on 1st June 2025).

85. Xie, S., Du, S., Huang, Y., Luo, Y., Chen, Y., Zheng, Z., Yuan, B., *et al.* (2025). Evolution and effectiveness of bilateral and multilateral development assistance for health: A mixed-methods review of trends and strategic shifts (1990–2022). *BMJ Global Health, 10.* https://www.semanticscholar.org/paper/57629859d00fd3cad8830f76bd7d5ea6cc5d2e38 (accessed on 1st June 2025).

86. Young, V. A., Thakor, A., & Josephs, S. (2022). Update on pediatric interventional radiology. *Radiographics: A Review Publication of the Radiological Society of North America, Inc., 42*(6), 1580–1597. https://www.semanticscholar.org/paper/4b0a4288b34f3a3100fedec0a2d436b471dfd5ab (accessed on 1st June 2025).

87. Yu, H., & Stavas, J. (2013). The role of interventional radiology in management of benign and malignant gynecologic diseases. *Obstetrical & Gynecological Survey, 68,* 691–701. https://www.semanticscholar.org/paper/c909b51f4cf23da1fd862d67305212450c668cc2 (accessed on 1st June 2025).

88. Zhang, X., Wang, Y., Lu, Y., Li, J., Sun, Z., Zeng, Y., Li, W., *et al.* (2025). Comparison of modified oblique lateral interbody fusion and posterior-only approach in the treatment of degenerative lumbar scoliosis. *Orthopedic Surgery.* https://www.semanticscholar.org/paper/4b723bcabaeba2f4b21b780c3147a1029f239b89 (accessed on 1st June 2025).

89. Zhu, M., Li, S., Kuang, Y., Hill, V., Heimberger, A. B., Zhai, L., & Zhai, S. (2022). Artificial intelligence in the radiomic analysis of glioblastomas: A review, taxonomy, and perspective. *Frontiers in Oncology, 12.* https://doi.org/10.3389/fonc.2022.924245 (accessed on 1st June 2025).

EMERGENCY AND TRAUMA RADIOLOGY

11

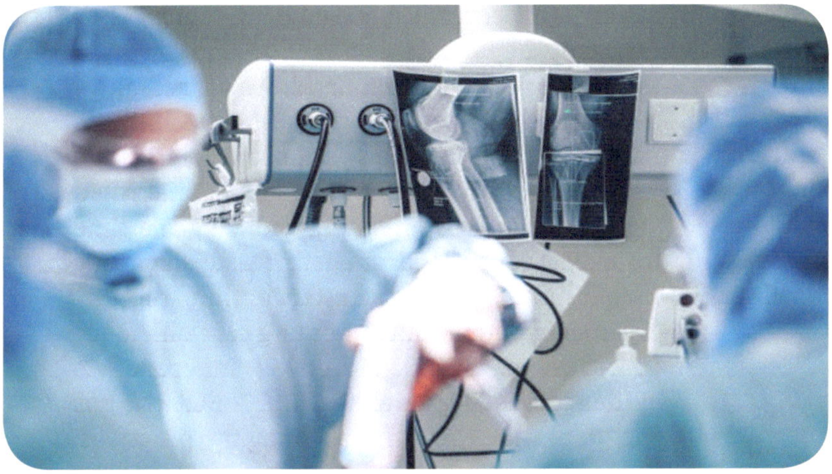

LEARNING OBJECTIVES

After studying this chapter, you will be able to:

1. Identify types of imaging modalities in emergency radiology;
2. Explain common trauma cases and their radiological assessment;
3. Know interpretation of radiological findings;
4. Focus on ethical and legal considerations in emergency radiology.

Introduction

In the critical context of emergency medicine, the rapid and accurate assessment of trauma patients is imperative for effective management and improved outcomes. Radiology plays a pivotal role in this process, offering detailed visualization that guides clinical decisions essential for addressing life-threatening injuries. The complexity of trauma cases necessitates advanced imaging techniques to identify subtle yet significant internal damage, such as that seen in severe traumatic brain injuries, which have been elucidated through innovative molecular profiling approaches like proximity extension assays, revealing dynamic biomarker patterns linked to inflammation and tissue repair (Dyhrfort *et al.*, 2023). Similarly, the comprehensive evaluation of pelvic and acetabular fractures relies heavily on high-resolution CT and MRI imaging, supplemented by a thorough understanding of anatomy and biomechanics, as detailed in specialized surgical texts that also emphasize interdisciplinary collaboration between radiologists and surgeons (Nagel, 2015). This integration of cutting-edge imaging and clinical expertise forms the foundation of emergency and trauma radiology, underscoring its essential role in optimizing patient care.

Definition of Emergency and Trauma Radiology

It is very important in medicine to make a quick and correct diagnosis of injuries, especially in situations where time matters a lot. Emergency and trauma radiology deals with the imaging of urgent injuries and serious health problems. This sub-discipline encompasses the use of various radiologic techniques, such as computed tomography (CT), X-ray, and ultrasound, aimed at identifying traumatic injuries efficiently to guide immediate clinical decision-making and intervention. Quickly interpreting imaging studies means critical injuries can be treated promptly and patients are not exposed to unnecessary procedures.

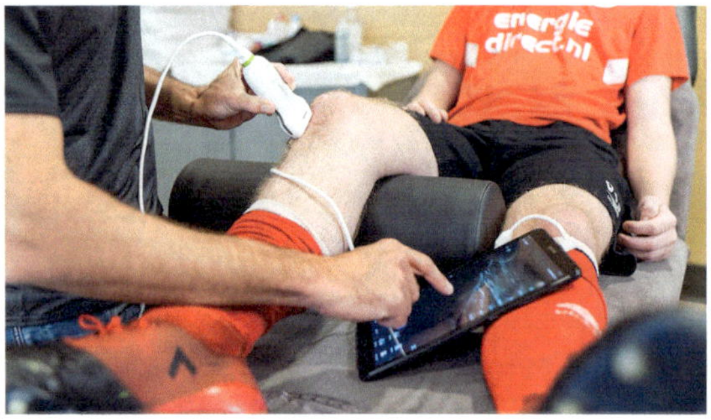

Figure 11.1. In medical practice, the rapid and accurate diagnosis of injuries is crucial, especially in high-stakes scenarios where time is of the essence.

Source: https://www.philips.com/c-dam/corporate/newscenter/global/standard/resources/healthcare/2024/treatment-for-top-athletes/header-philips-lumify-portable-ultrasound-with-psv-player.jpg.

Recent advancements and guidelines, including those for pediatric head trauma, underscore the importance of targeted imaging to balance diagnostic accuracy with patient safety, particularly in minimizing excessive radiation exposure and managing incidental findings effectively (Bingham *et al.*, 2020). The integration of technology and clinical protocols in emergency and trauma radiology reflects its dynamic role in acute healthcare settings (Figure 11.1).

Importance of Radiology in Emergency Medicine

Quick and correct judgment in emergency medicine depends a lot on fast and accurate imaging of traumatic injuries, which radiology provides. The integration of streamlined imaging protocols, such as those implemented in pediatric trauma centers, has demonstrated significant improvements in reducing the time from emergency department arrival to diagnostic imaging and operative intervention, thereby enhancing patient outcomes and care efficiency (Cross *et al.*, 2019). Moreover, adherence to evidence-based guidelines, like PECARN, has the potential to optimize imaging practices, balancing the immediate need for diagnostic clarity against the risks of unnecessary radiation exposure (Bingham *et al.*, 2020). Although the full adoption of such guidelines remains a challenge, their application helps to standardize care and minimize incidental findings that can complicate clinical management and increase patient anxiety (Bingham *et al.*, 2020). Due to these advancements, radiology plays a vital role in emergency and trauma situations by enabling rapid diagnosis and informing critical medical decisions.

Overview of Common Emergencies Requiring Radiology

In emergencies and trauma situations, it is very important to use imaging quickly and correctly to help manage patients and improve their outcomes. Many urgent problems, for example, vascular injuries, fractures, bleeding in the brain, and organ lacerations, require radiologic evaluation. Vascular emergencies, in particular, pose a significant threat due to the risk of hypovolemic shock or ischemia, demanding prompt detection primarily via computed tomography, which offers detailed multiphasic imaging superior to ultrasound in many cases (Lucio *et al.*, 2013). Additionally, advancements in telemedicine have expanded access to radiologic expertise, enabling remote consultations and facilitating faster diagnosis and intervention, which is vital in both urban and rural environments (Campus *et al.*, 2022). Because of these technologies, critical imaging reports can be shared and accessed no matter where the patient is located. Consequently, the integration of various imaging modalities tailored to specific emergencies remains essential in optimizing trauma care (Figure 11.2).

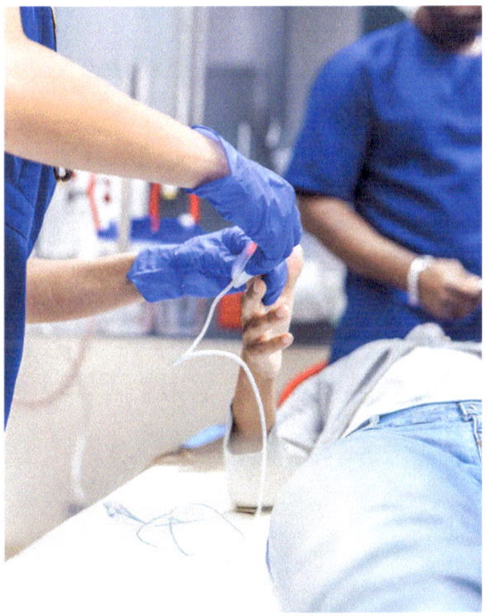

Figure 11.2. In emergency and trauma settings, timely and accurate imaging is critical to guide clinical management and improve patient outcomes.

Source: https://geimshospital.com/wp-content/uploads/2025/03/Emergency-and-trauma-img.jpg.

Role of Radiologists in Trauma Care

Because trauma care requires prompt attention, radiologists play a crucial role in ensuring proper diagnosis and swift action. Radiologists play a crucial role in analyzing CT scans, X-rays, and ultrasounds, which often show internal injuries that are not seen with a physical exam alone. Their skill in finding severe conditions such as internal bleeding, injuries to organs, or blood vessel damage helps decide what treatment to give and how to perform surgery. In addition, new imaging techniques have expanded the radiologist's duties, helping with accurate assessments and planning for less invasive treatments. Cooperation between emergency physicians and trauma surgeons allows for a multidisciplinary way of managing trauma. By being part of the trauma team, radiologists make sure patients are diagnosed quickly and continue to be monitored, which improves their chances of survival and reduces the risk of problems from missed or delayed injuries.

Technological Advances in Radiology

Thanks to advances in radiology over the years, handling emergency and trauma cases has become more accurate and faster. Advances such as the development of high-resolution computed tomography (CT) and digital radiography have significantly improved image clarity, enabling clinicians to detect subtle injuries that might otherwise be missed. New portable imaging tools have enabled doctors to quickly assess patients in critical care and take immediate action. In addition, electronic storage and telemedicine make it possible to share images quickly, which is very important in trauma cases because time is so important. Because of these advancements, doctors can be more certain about their findings, and patients are exposed to less radiation. Such progress underscores the pivotal role of continual innovation in radiologic technology to meet the pressing demands of emergency medicine, as exemplified in the historical trajectory and modern advancements documented in recent studies (Figure 11.3).

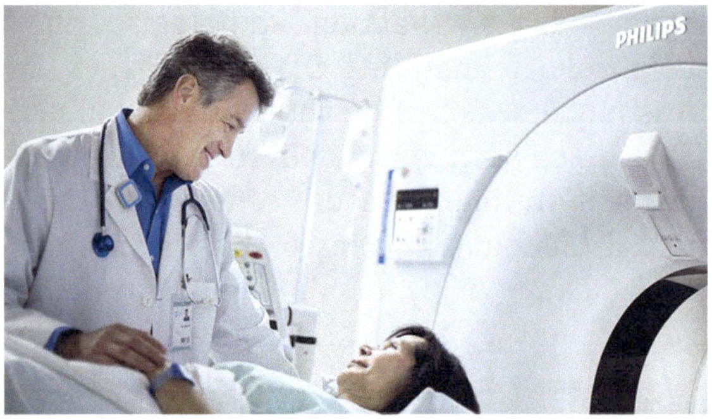

Figure 11.3. The evolution of radiology over the past decades has drastically transformed the management of emergency and trauma cases, enhancing diagnostic accuracy and expediting treatment decisions.

Source: https://www.philips.com/c-dam/corporate/innovation-and-you/global/jul-2020/radiology-tech-patient.jpg.

Challenges in Emergency and Trauma Radiology

When there is an emergency or trauma, radiology must handle various issues that can affect the fast and accurate identification of serious conditions. Lack of specialized imaging tools and trained radiologists in underserved areas makes it challenging to manage patients effectively. Pediatric radiology underscores this difficulty, as it demands specific precautions against ionizing radiation and tailored imaging protocols, which are often unavailable in developing regions burdened by high injury rates and infectious diseases (Brandt *et al.*, 2011). Besides, the requirement to interpret images quickly in emergencies is challenging because there are not enough expert staff, which results in the use of teleradiology, but this also needs strong infrastructure. Thanks to new technology, it is now easier to diagnose diseases, but looking after the equipment and ensuring its quality is still a challenge, mainly where money and support are not enough. Solving these issues requires working with other countries, better training, and advanced technology in radiology for trauma care, which is demonstrated in global radiology projects.

Significance of Timely Diagnosis

Rapidly spotting injuries and critical health problems in emergency and trauma care is very important for the patient's survival and recovery. Failing to diagnose a disease promptly can lead to more severe health issues due to missed dangerous complications, underscoring the importance of radiology in making timely clinical decisions. Advanced modalities, such as computed tomography and focused ultrasonography, enable clinicians to detect internal bleeding, organ ruptures, and other emergent pathologies that might not be apparent through physical examination alone (Muhmmed *et al.*, 2024). This is especially critical in cases like traumatic diaphragmatic rupture, where swift recognition and intervention are paramount to stabilize hemodynamics and prevent fatal outcomes (Artha *et al.*, 2024). Consequently, the integration of timely radiologic assessment into trauma protocols enhances the accuracy and speed of diagnosis, facilitating prompt treatment and ultimately improving prognoses in emergency settings (Figure 11.4).

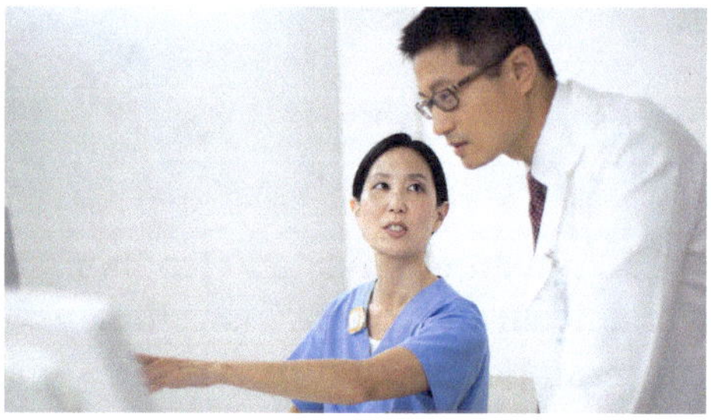

Figure 11.4. Delays in diagnosis can exacerbate morbidity due to missed or overlooked life-threatening complications, underscoring the indispensable role of radiologic imaging in expediting clinical decision-making.

Source: https://www.philips.com/c-dam/corporate/innovation-and-you/global/jul-2020/hero-radiologists.jpg.

11.1. Types of Imaging Modalities in Emergency Radiology

Learning Outcome

1. Explain the basics and applications of X-rays;
2. Discuss computed tomography (CT) scans in trauma;
3. Perform magnetic resonance imaging (MRI) in emergencies;
4. Focus on ultrasound in emergency settings;
5. Explain the uses of fluoroscopy in trauma;
6. Know contrast agents and their importance;
7. Learn radiation safety considerations;
8. List the limitations of each modality;
9. Discuss future trends in imaging technologies.

Many different imaging methods are used in emergency and trauma radiology to quickly and accurately diagnose patients for good management. The main reason conventional radiography is used first is that it is quick, easy to use, and can rapidly show fractures, dislocations, and injuries of the chest. Computed tomography (CT) offers superior sensitivity for complex trauma, especially in detecting intracranial hemorrhages, vascular injuries, and abdominal organ damage, facilitating prompt surgical decisions. Ultrasound, particularly focused assessment with sonography in trauma (FAST), is invaluable for its bedside applicability and lack of ionizing radiation, allowing for quick evaluation of internal bleeding. Magnetic resonance imaging (MRI) is less commonly used emergently but is critical for soft tissue, spinal cord, and subtle brain injury assessment when time and patient stability permit. The integration of these modalities, enhanced by advanced clinical roles such as consultant radiographers, improves service efficiency and patient throughput in emergency departments (Miller *et al.*, 2010). Meanwhile, the visual representation of these techniques forms an essential educational foundation for practitioners.

11.1.1. X-rays: Basics and Applications

The use of modern imaging has greatly improved how emergency and trauma situations are handled and managed. X-rays are still important because they are easy to use, quick and show the skeleton as well as some abnormalities in soft tissue. They play a key part in early trauma evaluations by finding fractures, dislocations, and foreign objects which can guide the choice of treatment. While emerging technologies like point-of-care ultrasound show promise in complementing traditional imaging, X-rays continue to serve as a baseline tool, often guiding further diagnostic steps or interventions (Joseph Österwalder *et al.*, 2023).

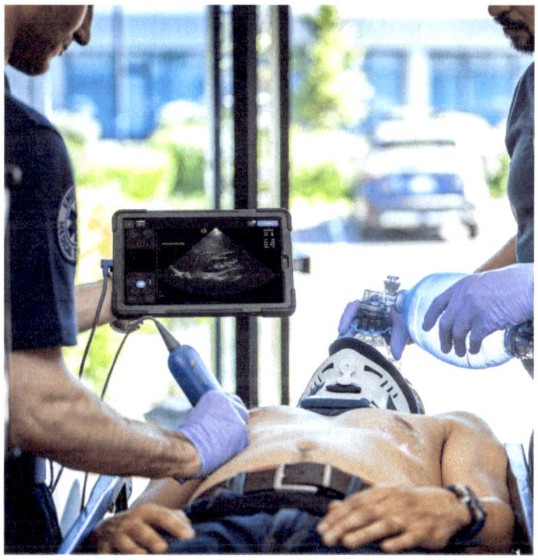

Figure 11.5. X-rays remain foundational due to their accessibility, speed, and ability to provide clear visualization of skeletal structures and certain soft tissue abnormalities.

Source: https://echonous.com/wp-content/uploads/2024/05/Emergency-Medicine.png.

Additionally, the potential incorporation of artificial intelligence within radiologic interpretation may enhance accuracy and efficiency, particularly under the high-pressure circumstances of emergency care, though challenges related to validation and standardization persist (Taciuc *et al.*, 2024). Thus, X-rays remain indispensable in trauma radiology, bridging time-sensitive diagnostic needs with established clinical protocols (Figure 11.5).

11.1.2. Computed Tomography (CT) Scans in Trauma

In emergency trauma care, fast and correct diagnosis is essential for improving patient outcomes, especially when there is major bleeding or internal injuries. Because of advanced imaging, clinicians can quickly evaluate patients and decide on the best course of action. In many cases, CT scans are important because they provide detailed images of the inside, which is useful when physical examination and ultrasound are not enough to detect all the damage. Using CT imaging helps doctors plan treatments that fit each person's needs, which is crucial for managing bleeding and coagulopathy after trauma. CT scans are often used in conjunction with bedside ultrasound, such as e-FAST, a quick method for detecting free fluid and pneumothorax. The integration of CT scans into clinical algorithms ensures a more thorough evaluation process, ultimately contributing to uniform care standards and improved survival rates among severely injured patients (Samuel *et al.*, 2018; Spahn *et al.*, 2019).

11.1.3. Magnetic Resonance Imaging (MRI) in Emergencies

Fast and accurate imaging is very important in emergency and trauma care for managing patients and achieving better outcomes. MRI is able to find soft tissue injuries, damage to the spinal cord, and brain problems that other imaging tests might miss. Because MRI was traditionally hard to use quickly and in emergencies, improvements in technology and automation have made it much more practical for urgent cases. The integration of AI-driven protocols and digital innovations, as part of the broader healthcare digitalization trend, is facilitating faster image processing and interpretation, thereby expanding MRI's role in acute care scenarios (Chengoden *et al.*, 2023). Also, it is important to use advanced imaging technologies according to ethical and legal guidelines in emergencies. Consequently, MRI is becoming an indispensable tool in trauma radiology, complementing traditional methods to provide comprehensive diagnostic insights in critical situations (Figure 11.6).

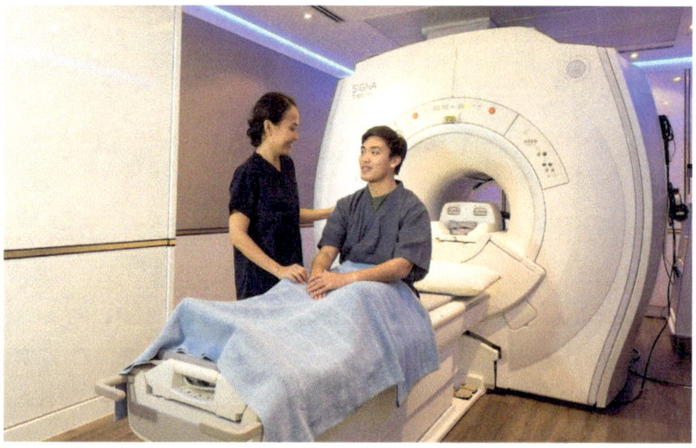

Figure 11.6. Magnetic Resonance Imaging (MRI) offers distinct advantages in identifying soft tissue injuries, spinal cord trauma, and subtle brain pathologies that may go undetected with other imaging modalities.

Source: https://radlink.com.sg/wp-content/uploads/2025/03/MRI-machine-from-Radlink-with-patient-HD-landscape.jpg.

11.1.4. Ultrasound in Emergency Settings

Thanks to the fast progress and easy use of portable ultrasound, emergency and trauma care can now do quick assessments right at the patient's bedside. Point-of-care ultrasound (POCUS) has proven especially valuable in resource-limited settings, offering a focused approach to detect critical conditions such as internal bleeding, cardiac abnormalities, or pneumothorax without the delay of transport to imaging suites. This technology bridges gaps in healthcare delivery, particularly in underserved regions where conventional imaging is scarce, by facilitating early diagnosis of infectious diseases and trauma injuries through protocols like FASH and FASE (Abdalla *et al.*, 2015). Also, new developments in teleultrasound may help experienced doctors guide nonmedical staff in obtaining images that can be used for diagnosis. Preliminary studies indicate that remote examinations can be rapidly performed with high image accuracy for cardiac, pulmonary, and abdominal assessments, enhancing the utility of ultrasound in emergency scenarios (Austin *et al.*, 2019). Because of this, ultrasound helps to improve patient care by speeding up the process of diagnosis and treatment in emergency and trauma cases.

11.1.5. Fluoroscopy: Uses in Trauma

It is very important to quickly and accurately assess injuries in emergency and trauma situations to manage patients well. Fluoroscopy offers dynamic images that let doctors see inside the body and guide procedures, which is especially helpful for treating complex trauma cases. It makes it possible for clinicians to find fractures, track joint reductions, and help in removing foreign bodies, improving the accuracy of diagnosis more than with static X-rays. The integration of advanced technologies, such as artificial intelligence, has further improved fracture detection accuracy, reducing diagnostic errors significantly and supporting clinical decision-making in traumatology (Beikmane *et al.*, 2023). Additionally, the combination of fluoroscopy with adjunctive imaging, like ultrasound, aids in the localization and extraction of radiolucent soft tissue foreign bodies, a frequent challenge in urgent care environments (Merritt *et al.*, 2013). Thus, fluoroscopy's role in trauma radiology extends beyond diagnosis to actively guiding therapeutic interventions, emphasizing its essential utility in emergency medical practice (Figure 11.7).

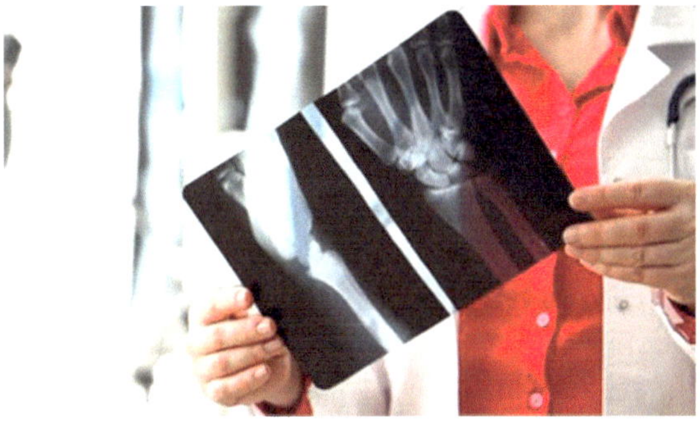

Figure 11.7. Fluoroscopy serves as a dynamic imaging modality that provides real-time visualization of anatomical structures and guides interventional procedures, particularly useful in complex trauma cases.

Source: https://www.hopkinsmedicine.org/-/media/images/health/2_-treatment/radiology/xray-for-extremities-teaser.jpg?h=217&iar=0&mh=260&mw=380&w=380&hash=966038D0E7221FCF5AFF75443D905F68.

11.1.6. Contrast Agents and Their Importance

Quick and accurate diagnosis is very important in emergency and trauma radiology for treating patients well. Contrast agents make it much easier to see blood vessels, organs, and any abnormalities, which speeds up the process of making choices. For example, contrast-enhanced ultrasound (CEUS) has demonstrated substantial utility in acute trauma settings, offering real-time assessment without the risks associated with ionizing radiation or iodinated contrast media. This is particularly advantageous in vulnerable populations such as children, where minimizing exposure to harmful substances is critical (Cantisani *et al.*, 2016). Also, contrast agents used with CT and MRI give detailed images of the body's structure and function, which help find hemorrhages, damage to blood vessels, or reduced blood supply to organs. They help doctors make more accurate diagnoses and choose the best interventions, which positively influence patient outcomes.

11.1.7. Radiation Safety Considerations

In emergency and trauma radiology, it is crucial to minimize the amount of radiation patients receive. Many times, a quick diagnosis relies on using more than one imaging method, but it is important to weigh the benefits against the possible risks of radiation. One significant advancement to reduce radiation exposure is the increasing utilization of contrast-enhanced ultrasound, especially in pediatric populations, which offers a radiation-free alternative for evaluating certain conditions traditionally assessed with CT scans (Cantisani *et al.*, 2016).

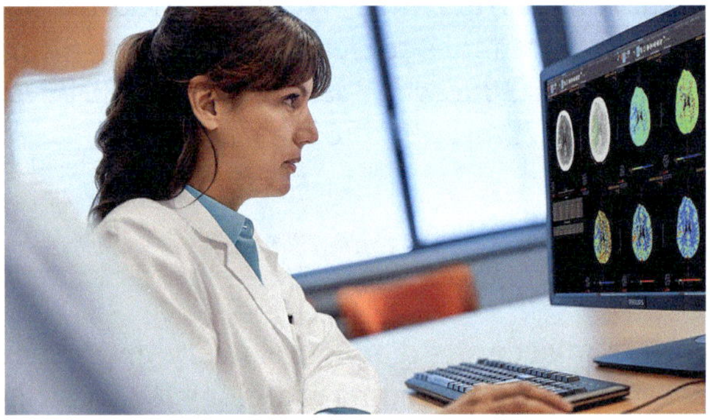

Figure 11.8. Rapid diagnosis often necessitates multiple imaging modalities; however, careful consideration must be given to balancing diagnostic benefits with potential radiation risks.

Source: https://www.philips.com/c-dam/corporate/newscenter/global/standard/resources/healthcare/2024/ai-driven-enterprise-informatics/header-female-doctor-looking-at-images-mr-perfusion.jpg.

Additionally, optimization of imaging parameters, adherence to the ALARA (As Low As Reasonably Achievable) principle, and the use of shielding can further mitigate unnecessary exposure. Picking the right protocol for the patient's symptoms can ensure imaging is not performed twice and that the procedure is safe. These measures collectively contribute to the responsible use of radiologic resources in trauma settings, ensuring patient well-being while maintaining the efficacy of emergency care (Figure 11.8).

11.1.8. Limitations of Each Modality

In emergency and trauma radiology, it is important to pick an imaging method that is both fast, accurate, and available, but each one has its own limits. Even though chest X-rays can be done fast and are available in most places, they have an uneven ability to detect thoracic injuries and may overlook important signs that need immediate attention. Ultrasound is very useful for detecting soft tissue foreign bodies and guiding surgery, since it shows images live and does not use radiation, but it is only as good as the person operating it, and can have trouble with some injuries hidden by gas or bone. Abdominal X-rays and ultrasounds, frequently used in penetrating trauma assessment, can be inaccurate when used in isolation, necessitating confirmatory computed tomography or surgical exploration to avoid missed diagnoses (Lieshout *et al.*, 2009). Furthermore, reliance solely on X-rays for foreign body localization is limited due to their inability to detect radiolucent objects such as wood, whereas adjunctive ultrasound improves detection rates but still demands technical expertise for effective application (Merritt *et al.*, 2013).

11.1.9. Future Trends in Imaging Technologies

Healthcare is being improved through the use of advanced technologies that enhance the detection of diseases and the care provided to patients. With the use of AI, virtual reality, augmented reality, and the Internet of Medical Things, emergency and trauma radiology can make imaging more accurate and instant. The concept of the Metaverse, encompassing these technologies, offers immersive and personalized diagnostic experiences that could transform emergency interventions and streamline workflow efficiencies (Chengoden *et al.*, 2023). Additionally, the emergence of Digital Twins—virtual replicas of patients—holds significant potential to tailor imaging protocols and anticipate complications, thereby improving clinical outcomes through precision medicine (Armeni *et al.*, 2022). Despite some issues, these innovations are set to improve and speed up the way trauma is diagnosed, which will help doctors decide quickly and lower costs. Consequently, the future of imaging technologies in trauma care is characterized by increasingly intelligent, connected, and patient-centered systems (Figure 11.9).

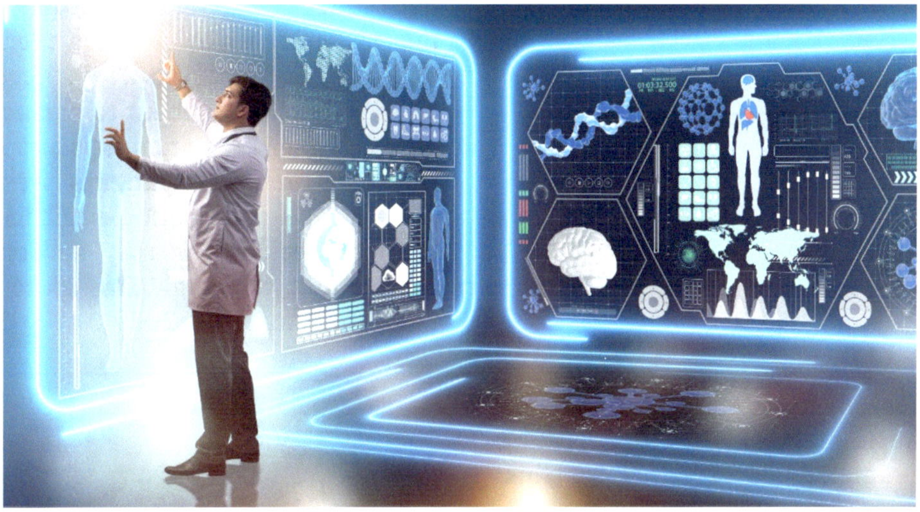

Figure 11.9. In emergency and trauma radiology, the convergence of artificial intelligence, virtual and augmented reality, and the Internet of Medical Things promises to revolutionize imaging modalities by enabling more precise, real-time assessments.

Source: https://images-cdn.welcomesoftware.com/Zz0wYzg1MmMwYTQ4NDgxMWVjODg1NjhlZTgwMDg2MWNiNw==/Advantages%20of%20AI%20for%20radiology.jpeg.

Test Your Knowledge

1. Which imaging method is usually used for suspected acute head injury?
2. What radiological signs suggest a skull fracture?

11.2. Common Trauma Cases and Their Radiological Assessment

Learning Outcome

1. Know imaging protocols in head injuries;
2. Understand radiological findings of chest trauma;
3. Explain abdominal trauma;
4. Discuss imaging techniques in pelvic fractures;
5. Know x-ray protocols in extremity injuries;
6. Focus on spinal injuries;
7. Understand special considerations in pediatric trauma;
8. Identify imaging challenges in geriatric trauma;
9. Perform a comprehensive assessment of multi-system trauma.

When there is an emergency, a quick and correct diagnosis matters a lot for treating trauma, and radiology is essential for this. When patients have blunt abdominal injuries, fractures, or traumatic brain injuries, imaging is used to find any serious problems that may be life-threatening. Because CT scans are highly sensitive and specific, they are preferred to show clear images of the internal organs, bones, and blood vessels. For example, abdominal trauma cases may benefit from CT imaging with oral intestinal opacification, which enhances diagnostic accuracy, especially in post-surgical patients where complications could arise (Abu-Zidan *et al.*, 2020). Plain radiographs remain essential for initial assessment of bone injuries, while advanced imaging aids surgeons in preparing for and monitoring treatment. Radiological findings and clinical examination together allow for quick action, which helps lower the number of deaths and serious injuries in trauma patients. So, radiology is crucial for deciding how to treat emergency and trauma cases.

11.2.1. Head Injuries: Imaging Protocols

Advancements in imaging technology have significantly influenced the management of trauma patients, particularly in assessing head injuries, where rapid and accurate diagnosis is critical. CT remains the cornerstone for head trauma imaging due to its accessibility and speed, enabling detection of intracranial hemorrhages, skull fractures, and other critical injuries. However, the decision to employ whole-body or head-specific CT protocols requires careful clinical judgment to balance diagnostic benefits against radiation exposure risks. Studies highlight that even patients presenting with good clinical status but experiencing high-risk trauma mechanisms may harbor significant injuries detectable only through comprehensive imaging (Blaz *et al.*, 2009).

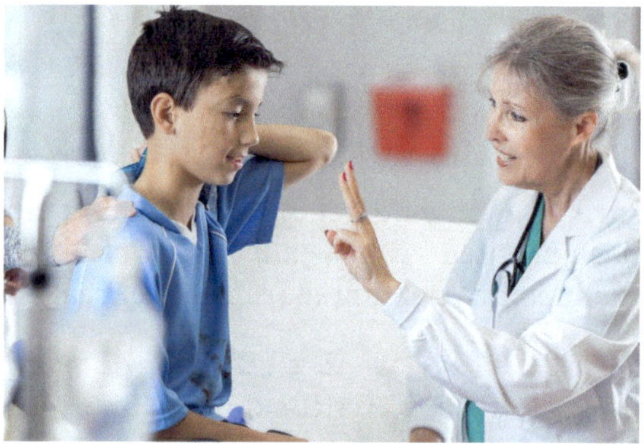

Figure 11.10. Advancements in imaging technology have significantly influenced the management of trauma patients, particularly in assessing head injuries, where rapid and accurate diagnosis is critical.

Source: https://cdn-prod.medicalnewstoday.com/content/images/articles/179/179837/head-injury.jpg.

In pediatric populations, adherence to evidence-based guidelines like PECARN aims to optimize CT use by reducing unnecessary scans while ensuring high-risk cases are not missed; nevertheless, real-world implementation remains inconsistent, leading to frequent incidental findings that may cause unwarranted anxiety and further tests (Bingham *et al.*, 2020). Thus, refining imaging protocols to align with clinical criteria is essential for improving patient outcomes in emergency and trauma radiology (Figure 11.10).

11.2.2. Chest Trauma: Radiological Findings

It is very important to identify chest trauma quickly in an emergency to guide the proper care and avoid deadly complications. To diagnose rib fractures, pulmonary contusions, pneumothorax, hemothorax, and cardiac tamponade, radiological imaging is crucial. Because chest X-rays are easy to acquire and are available everywhere, they are the first imaging test used to detect rib fractures and large pneumothoraces. CT is better at detecting minor injuries such as small pneumothoraces, lung lacerations, and vascular injuries, which helps doctors decide between surgery and non-surgical methods. Being skilled in interpreting these results helps radiologists improve patient care after a trauma. Additionally, integration of advanced imaging protocols contributes to improved diagnostic accuracy in diverse patient populations, including pediatric cases, who require specialized radiological approaches to minimize radiation exposure while ensuring comprehensive evaluation (Brandt *et al.*, 2011). This points out the crucial place of imaging in diagnosing chest injuries in emergency and trauma radiology.

11.2.3. Abdominal Trauma: Computed Tomography (CT) Versus. Ultrasound

It is very important to make a fast and correct diagnosis in trauma cases, especially when looking for abdominal injuries. CT is generally seen as the best method for assessing abdominal trauma since it is very sensitive and can spot small injuries, but ultrasound is now considered important because it is fast, non-invasive, and does not use radiation. CEUS has shown promise, particularly in pediatric patients, offering detailed imaging without the risks associated with ionizing radiation and iodinated contrast agents, aligning with evolving preferences for safer, patient-friendly diagnostics (Cantisani *et al.*, 2016). Moreover, streamlined trauma protocols that incorporate both FAST and CT have demonstrated improved efficiency, reducing time to imaging and definitive care, which is crucial for favorable outcomes in blunt abdominal trauma (Cross *et al.*, 2019). Thus, ultrasound complements CT in emergency radiology by enhancing rapid triage and minimizing radiation exposure, while CT remains indispensable for comprehensive injury evaluation (Figure 11.11).

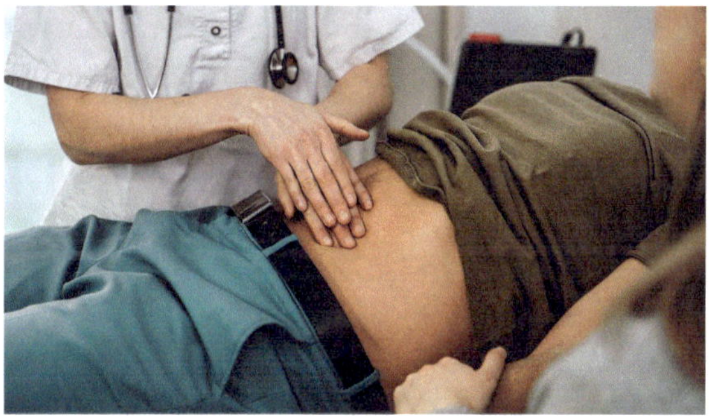

Figure 11.11. Rapid and accurate diagnosis in trauma settings is critical for effective patient management, especially in assessing abdominal injuries.

Source: https://media.post.rvohealth.io/wp-content/uploads/2024/04/doctor-examining-patient-stomach-abdomen-area-for-pain-1296x728-header.jpg.

11.2.4. Pelvic Fractures: Imaging Techniques

Because pelvic fractures are complicated, quick and accurate imaging is needed to manage them well in emergencies. In most cases, the first assessment is done with plain radiographs, which quickly show the overall situation but can miss serious injuries. CT is now widely used because it clearly shows both the bones and surrounding soft tissue damage, which makes it easier for trauma surgeons and interventional radiologists to work together. Moreover, advancements in imaging aim to identify active bleeding sources amenable to angioembolization, a critical intervention in life-threatening hemorrhages triggered by pelvic trauma (Battisti *et al.*, 2021). At the same time, using artificial intelligence and machine learning in trauma radiology may help improve how accurately injuries are found and how smoothly the process runs. However, these tools are still in early developmental stages with limited FDA-approved applications, and the scarcity of robust datasets for pelvic trauma remains a challenge for broad clinical adoption (Beckmann *et al.*, 2023). These imaging tools and advancements are essential for improving patient outcomes after pelvic fractures.

11.2.5. Extremity Injuries: X-ray Protocols

When a trauma patient is being treated urgently, accurate and prompt imaging is very important for deciding on treatment. While advanced imaging modalities like CT are pivotal for assessing complex polytrauma cases, conventional radiography remains the cornerstone for initial evaluation of extremity injuries due to its accessibility and speed (Mauro *et al.*, 2012). Usually, standard X-ray protocols involve anteroposterior, lateral, and oblique views to make sure all the bones and joints are well seen. They are meant to prevent missed fractures and dislocations, which are frequently seen in emergency care. In addition, radiologists can use systematic imaging methods to focus on urgent cases, which helps speed up treatment. Despite technological advances, X-rays continue to offer an optimal balance between diagnostic efficacy and resource management, especially in emergency departments where rapid assessment is essential (Smith *et al.*, 2017). Consequently, detailed X-ray protocols for extremity injuries remain fundamental in the practice of emergency and trauma radiology (Figure 11.12).

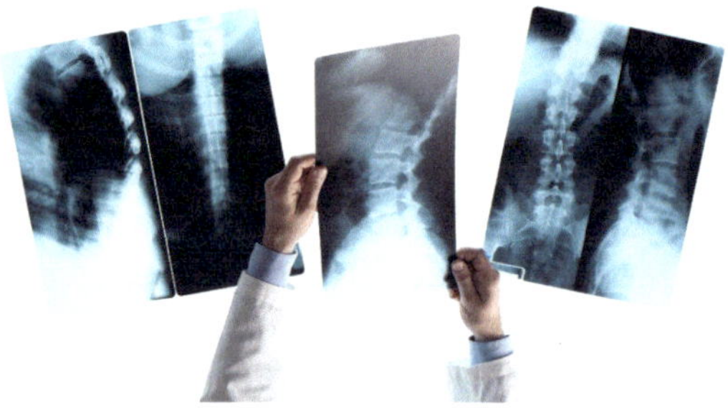

Figure 11.12. X-ray protocols in extremity injuries.

Source: https://www.envrad.com/content/uploads/2021/02/doctor-holding-x-rays.jpg.

11.2.6. Spinal Injuries: Magnetic Resonance Imaging (MRI) Versus Computed Tomography (CT)

The selection of an imaging test in emergency and trauma radiology can strongly affect the accuracy of diagnosis and the care given to the patient. Studies conducted lately show that CT is still the main imaging option because it is quick and widely accessible, but MRI is better at finding soft tissue and ligament injuries that CT might miss. For instance, MRI can reveal injuries that not only alter therapeutic decisions but also identify cases requiring surgical intervention that might be underestimated by CT alone (Alkadhi *et al.*, 2018). Moreover, in pediatric populations, MRI demonstrates high safety and feasibility, reducing the need for follow-up imaging without compromising diagnostic confidence, although logistical challenges such as longer scan times and sedation requirements persist (Sirén *et al.*, 2024). Because of this, using MRI in spinal trauma protocols improves the way spinal injuries are classified and managed, but more research is needed to confirm its cost-effectiveness and to find the best way to use it together with CT in urgent situations.

11.2.7. Pediatric Trauma: Special Considerations

The special needs of children in trauma management are due to their unique anatomy and physiology, so emergency and trauma radiology must be adapted for them. Unlike adults, children have flexible bones, a bigger head, and a smaller body, which makes them more likely to have different injuries and makes it harder to interpret imaging. Besides, some patients may not show obvious signs of injury, which is why doctors must use clinical assessment and prompt radiologic studies to find serious injuries. Treatment without surgery is usually chosen for hepatic and renal injuries to reduce the risks from surgery and anesthesia.

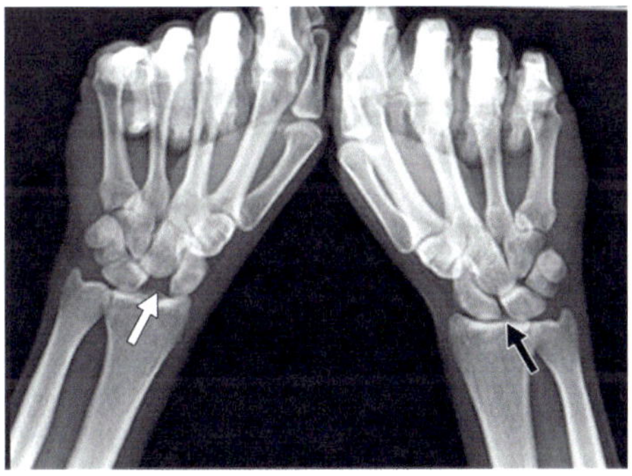

Figure 11.13. Children present unique challenges in trauma management due to their distinct anatomical and physiological characteristics, which necessitate specialized consideration in emergency and trauma radiology.

Source: https://www.ajronline.org/cms/10.2214/AJR.14.12589/asset/images/large/09_14_12589_11a.jpeg.

This method relies on close observation of images to determine the extent of damage and the appropriate treatment. Multidisciplinary collaboration among trauma surgeons, interventional radiologists, and critical care teams is vital to restore homeostasis and optimize outcomes in pediatric trauma patients (Coccolini *et al.*, 2019; Coccolini *et al.*, 2020) (Figure 11.13).

11.2.8. Geriatric Trauma: Imaging Challenges

More elderly trauma patients are now being treated, which requires changes to the usual imaging protocols in emergency and trauma radiology. Older people usually have unusual symptoms and other medical conditions that can make it harder to see injuries on scans, which may result in missed or delayed diagnoses. In addition, changes in the body of older adults, such as lower bone density and different tissue contrast, mean radiologists must be extra cautious and use suitable imaging methods to judge the extent of injuries. Radiologic criteria for this group are being considered in updated triage systems, which stresses the importance of quick and accurate imaging to improve patient care. Advances in telemedicine may provide promising avenues for remote expert consultation, though widespread integration remains limited (AlDossary *et al.*, 2017). National guidelines continue to evolve, highlighting the necessity of ongoing research to refine imaging approaches that address the intricate needs of geriatric trauma care (Adams *et al.*, 2024).

11.2.9. Multi-system Trauma: Comprehensive Assessment

Care for patients with serious injuries should focus on quickly spotting and treating any life-threatening problems. In multi-system trauma, a careful evaluation depends on using advanced imaging that clearly reveals the extent of injuries to the muscles, organs, and blood vessels to help with quick intervention. When there are many injuries or overlapping fractures, radiologists play a key role in finding the correct diagnosis, since missing or late diagnosis can increase the risk of complications. For example, operative strategies for complex femoral fractures rely heavily on precise imaging to tailor fixation techniques, optimizing outcomes in urgent surgical scenarios (von Rüden *et al.*, 2015). Additionally, understanding the biomechanics of injury and employing appropriate imaging protocols enhances diagnostic accuracy in spinal and pelvic trauma, areas frequently complicated by associated soft tissue and neurovascular compromise (Guglielmi *et al.*, 2017). Thus, a comprehensive radiologic assessment that integrates clinical context and advanced imaging findings is essential for improving patient prognosis in emergency and trauma settings (Figure 11.14).

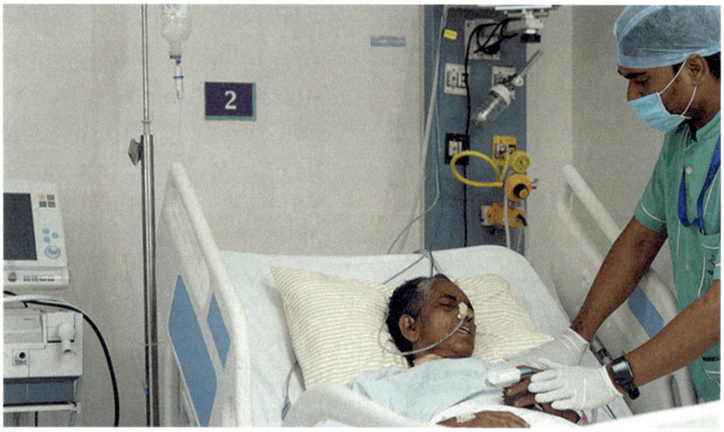

Figure 11.14. Effective management of patients with complex injuries demands an integrated approach that prioritizes rapid identification and stabilization of life-threatening conditions.

Source: https://www.apexhospitals.com/_next/image?url=https%3A%2F%2Fbed.apexhospitals.com%2Fuploads%2Ficu_13fed0a1c8.png&w=1920&q=75.

Test Your Knowledge

1. What imaging should be performed for suspected cervical spine injury in trauma?
2. How can imaging identify rib fractures, and why are they clinically important?

11.3. Interpretation of Radiological Findings

Learning Outcome

1. Identify key indicators of trauma on x-rays;
2. Explain common pitfalls in CT scan interpretation;
3. Focus on MRI findings in soft tissue injuries;
4. Know the ultrasound signs of internal bleeding;
5. Describe the importance of clinical correlation;
6. Explain the role of radiologists in emergency departments;
7. Discuss communication of findings to clinicians;
8. Know the use of radiology in surgical decision-making;
9. Learn case studies: successful diagnoses.

Reading radiological images correctly is very important in managing emergency and trauma cases, as it affects both the decisions made and the results for patients. The ability of radiologists to discern subtle yet critical indicators of injury can significantly outperform predictive scoring systems designed to identify serious blunt bowel and mesenteric injuries, underscoring the indispensability of expert analysis in acute settings (O'Toole *et al.*, 2024). Despite the availability of advanced imaging modalities, reliance on non-radiologist interpretation, such as emergency medicine trainees assessing cervical spine CTs, has demonstrated limited concordance with definitive radiological reports, even when structured reporting templates are introduced (Malhotra *et al.*, 2024). It shows that having a radiologist involved quickly and skillfully is necessary to make correct diagnoses and prevent complications. Including radiologist knowledge in emergency radiology enables the proper interpretation of challenging trauma images and provides efficient and effective care for patients.

11.3.1. Key Indicators of Trauma on X-rays

It is very important to correctly identify trauma using imaging in emergency and trauma radiology, because delays or errors can seriously harm patients. Trauma to the bones can be seen on X-rays as fractures, dislocations, and abnormal joint positions, which point to structural damage. Also, soft tissue swelling, gas in the soft tissues, or joint effusions can give an indirect idea of how severe the trauma is. Analyzing the pelvis, spine, and ribs for subtle fractures is difficult because many structures are close together, and some injuries may be overlooked. The early radiographic recognition of these indicators guides prompt intervention, essential in managing major bleeding or coagulopathy often associated with severe injuries (Spahn *et al.*, 2019).

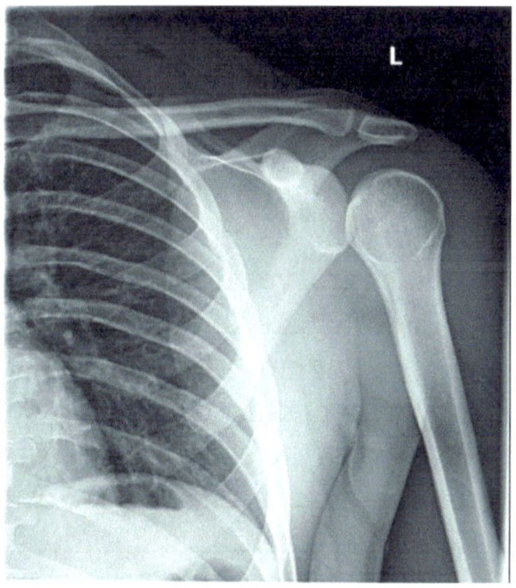

Figure 11.15. Key indicators of trauma on X-rays include fractures, dislocations, and abnormal joint alignments, which signal underlying structural compromise.

Source: https://static.cambridge.org/binary/version/id/urn:cambridge.org:id:binary:78448:20160617100819578-0248:44988fig1_29.png?pub-status=live.

Given the global scarcity of diagnostic resources, as highlighted by the diagnostic gap in many low-income settings, optimizing the interpretation of available X-rays remains pivotal in trauma care (Fleming *et al.*, 2021). Consequently, training and standardized protocols enhance diagnostic accuracy and improve patient prognosis after traumatic events (Figure 11.15).

11.3.2. Computer Tomography (CT) Scan Interpretation: Common Pitfalls

Because CT scans are used in emergencies and trauma, their quick and reliable interpretation is very important for patient care, but there are many things that can affect the accuracy of the diagnosis. One common error involves underappreciation of subtle fractures or soft tissue injuries, which can be overlooked amid the urgency following major trauma incidents, as seen in disaster-related mass casualties where rapid assessment is necessary (Ilgar *et al.*, 2024). Additionally, CT's limited sensitivity in detecting non-hemorrhagic brain injuries or lesions within the posterior fossa necessitates cautious evaluation, as misinterpretation can delay critical intervention (Almamoori *et al.*, 2024). Radiologists should watch out for artifacts and patient movements that may mask pathology, which means they should always review the case with the clinician and sometimes use MRI for more detailed images. Utilizing a range of medical specialties and understanding the limitations and pitfalls of CT scans enhances the accuracy and speed of decisions in trauma care. It is very important to address and reduce these challenges to make CT scans more useful in emergency situations.

11.3.3. Magnetic Resonance Imaging (MRI) Findings in Soft Tissue Injuries

In emergency and trauma radiology, proper imaging is very important for guiding the management of patients, especially those with soft tissue injuries. Because MRI is very sensitive to soft tissue changes, it is now considered the best modality for detecting them. An example is that MRI is better at identifying ligament damage, bruised muscles, and hematomas, which are often present in trauma but not easily seen on CT scans. This is most noticeable when a person has complex injuries, and the degree of soft tissue damage helps decide the treatment plan. Based on studies, in trauma situations such as non-self-inflicted strangulation, MRI is much better at detecting injuries and is more accurate, which can help prevent misjudging the severity of the injuries and improve patient outcomes. While MRI requires greater resources and expertise, its ability to provide detailed soft tissue characterization underscores its critical value in trauma assessments (Arneberg *et al.*, 2023). Moreover, its application in pediatric spinal trauma emphasizes safety and feasibility, offering comprehensive evaluation without radiation exposure and minimizing the need for repeated imaging (Sirén *et al.*, 2024) (Figure 11.16).

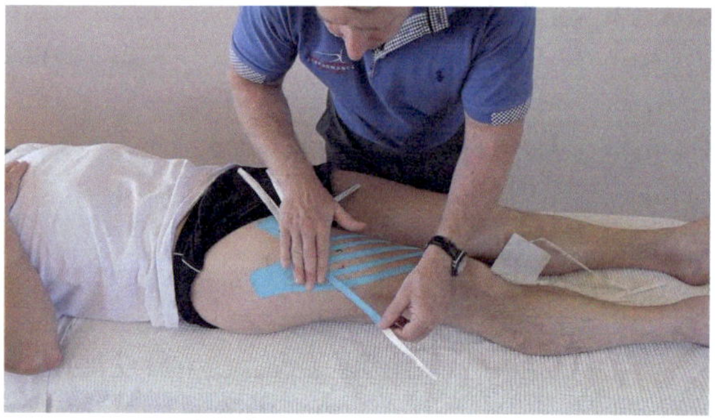

Figure 11.16. MRI demonstrates enhanced capability in identifying ligamentous damage, muscle contusions, and hematomas, which often accompany trauma but are not readily apparent on CT scans.

Source: https://i.ytimg.com/vi/VIGIgEHN-wA/maxresdefault.jpg.

11.3.4. Ultrasound Signs of Internal Bleeding

It is very important in emergency and trauma radiology to quickly and accurately spot internal bleeding for the sake of the patient's treatment and outcome. Ultrasound is very important in diagnosis, especially through the FAST exam, which helps find free fluid in the peritoneal, pericardial, or pleural spaces, which can indicate bleeding. In sonography, the signs of internal bleeding are fluid collections that are anechoic or hypoechoic, unusual shapes of organs, and breaks in the normal tissue borders. Ultrasound can detect blood more easily because it can spot changes in fluid echogenicity, which helps tell apart fresh blood from clotted or organized hematomas. Additionally, in specialized settings such as postpartum hemorrhage, ultrasound aids procedural guidance for interventions like pelvic artery embolization, illustrating its expanding role in bleeding control (Renzo *et al.*, 2015). As ultrasound technology continues to evolve, its portability and diagnostic utility in diverse clinical contexts, including resource-limited areas, further underscore its value in trauma care (Abdalla *et al.*, 2015).

11.3.5. Importance of Clinical Correlation

In emergency and trauma cases, accurate diagnosis and effective treatment rely on linking radiologic images to what is happening clinically. Even with radiologic images, it is sometimes hard to see the whole picture of the injury, so a doctor needs to consider the patient's condition when interpreting the images. For example, post-traumatic bleeding and coagulopathy require timely recognition and management, which is guided not only by imaging but also by patient presentation, laboratory findings, and physical examination (Spahn *et al.*, 2019). By noticing these connections, doctors can design treatments that are better suited to each patient, which can improve results and reduce unnecessary deaths. Moreover, understanding the dynamic physiological changes after trauma ensures that radiologic evaluations are not viewed in isolation but as components of a broader clinical pathway (Rossaint *et al.*, 2016). This multidisciplinary approach emphasizes the need for radiologists to collaborate closely with trauma teams, thereby strengthening the accuracy of diagnosis and the efficacy of therapeutic strategies in emergency care (Figure 11.17).

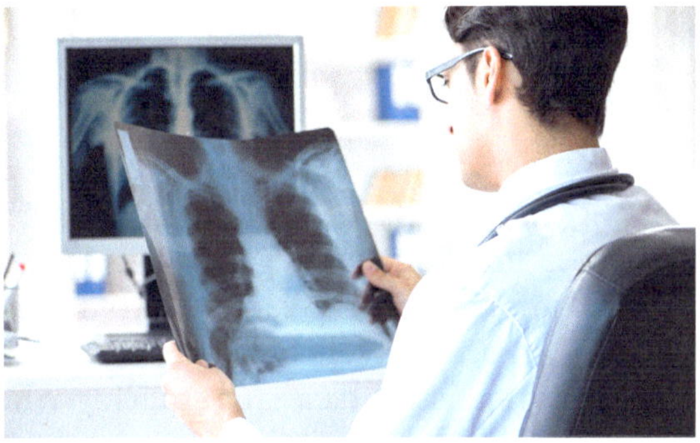

Figure 11.17. Radiologic images alone cannot always reveal the full extent or severity of injury, making clinical correlation essential to interpret imaging results appropriately.

Source: https://blog.powerliens.com/wp-content/uploads/04-15-2025-April-Blog-2-Featured-Image.png.

11.3.6. Role of Radiologists in Emergency Departments

Working together in the emergency department is very important for managing trauma patients, and radiologists are key members of the team. Over time, disagreements about territory in clinical roles have made it difficult for emergency physicians and radiologists to give seamless care, mainly related to imaging. Still, progress in clinical protocols and the use of specialized radiographers under frameworks like the Career Progression Framework has helped improve teamwork among different professions. These developments have not only optimized radiologists' time but also enhanced departmental efficiency and patient throughput by allowing consultant radiographers to support diagnostic services (Miller *et al.*, 2010). Although emergency physicians now use imaging in the clinic, radiologists are needed for proper interpretation, consultations on challenging cases, and decision-making. This dynamic relationship within the ED underscores the ongoing importance of radiologists in delivering timely and accurate diagnostics vital to trauma care (Edwards *et al.*, 2018).

11.3.7. Communication of Findings to Clinicians

Reporting the results of radiological tests to clinicians is crucial in emergency and trauma care, as it informs patient care and treatment. Fast and correct delivery of imaging results allows doctors to start treatment quickly when a patient is bleeding heavily or has coagulation problems. Having multidisciplinary teams involved improves this process, so radiologists can give focused, useful information that helps doctors decide on care for patients. Additionally, clarity in reporting helps mitigate misunderstandings that could delay critical treatment, underscoring the need for standardized protocols within institutions to ensure consistency and reliability (Geldsetzer, 2020).

Because emergency situations are always changing, communication between radiologists and clinicians must be flexible and address both new technologies and human aspects. Moreover, addressing misconceptions and ensuring accurate understanding among healthcare providers, as highlighted by public perception challenges in medical communication, further exemplifies the importance of clear, evidence-based messaging (Geldsetzer, 2020) (Figure 11.18).

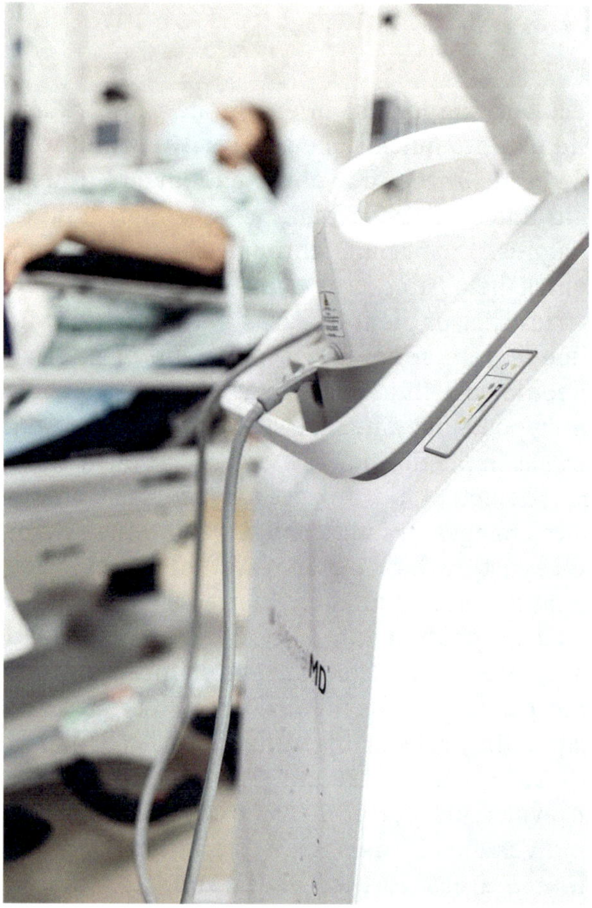

Figure 11.18. Rapid and accurate transmission of imaging results facilitates timely intervention, particularly in cases of major bleeding and coagulopathy where prompt management is essential.

Source: https://www.spectral-ai.com/wp-content/uploads/2024/04/diagnostic-tests-fo-burns.jpg.

11.3.8. Use of Radiology in Surgical Decision-Making

When dealing with emergencies and trauma, using imaging quickly and correctly guides the surgeon, leading to better outcomes for patients. Radiology gives surgeons important details to judge the severity of an injury, decide if surgery is necessary, and select the best surgical procedure. For instance, MRI has been shown to reliably detect pediatric spinal injuries that require surgical treatment, while also minimizing unnecessary follow-up imaging, highlighting both its diagnostic value and safety profile in emergent scenarios (Sirén *et al.*, 2024). Moreover, interventional radiology techniques such as pelvic artery embolization serve as minimally invasive alternatives or adjuncts to surgery in controlling life-threatening hemorrhage, exemplified by their effectiveness in preventing hysterectomy during abnormal placental implantation complications (Renzo *et al.*, 2015). So, using advanced radiologic techniques leads to better diagnoses and helps surgeons decide on treatment, which results in less illness and better clinical outcomes for patients with trauma.

11.3.9. Case Studies: Successful Diagnoses

Emergency and trauma radiology advancements have made it much easier to diagnose patients quickly and accurately, which has improved patient outcomes. A hybrid emergency room system allowed for quick computed tomography, surgery, and interventional radiology, so there was no need to move the patient, which was important in managing a difficult case of blunt traumatic injury with blocked blood vessels and organ damage. The integration of imaging and immediate therapeutic intervention allowed for timely damage control surgery and successful resuscitation, highlighting the system's life-saving potential in severe blunt trauma cases (Omoto *et al.*, 2024). Also, a rare example of bilateral intertrochanteric hip fractures in an elderly trauma patient showed that working together and using precise imaging helped with successful surgical repair and recovery. This coordinated approach underscored how detailed imaging can inform optimal treatment strategies, even in multifaceted injury patterns, leading to positive recovery outcomes (Tang *et al.*, 2024). All these case studies highlight the crucial role that emergency radiology plays in helping doctors diagnose and treat trauma patients.

Test Your Knowledge

1. What are the limitations of ultrasound in blunt abdominal trauma?
2. What are common CT findings in renal trauma?

11.4. Ethical and Legal Considerations in Emergency Radiology

Learning Outcome

1. Discuss informed consent in emergency situations;
2. Explain patient privacy and confidentiality;
3. Know the legal implications of misdiagnosis;
4. Focus on ethical dilemmas in imaging decisions;
5. Describe a radiologist's responsibility in emergencies;
6. Learn documentation and reporting standards;
7. Describe interdisciplinary collaboration and ethics;
8 Explain the impact of technology on ethical practices;
9. Understand future ethical challenges in radiology.

Emergency radiology requires fast imaging and also following ethical and legal guidelines. Because there are not enough radiologists in many healthcare places, interpretation of images is delayed, which leads radiographers and others to take on tasks that are not part of their job descriptions. This practice, although often essential to expedite trauma patient management, carries significant legal risks because it conflicts with established professional scopes of practice, potentially exposing practitioners and institutions to litigation (Van der Venter *et al.*, 2016). Also, during emergency department overcrowding, safety for patients requires that teams from different fields work together to avoid errors and ensure the quality of care. Ethics require that findings are openly shared and patient confidentiality is respected, no matter how busy the department gets. So, it is still very important for emergency radiology to balance urgent patient care with following regulations and ethics, which call for regular updates to policies and teamwork among professionals to look after both patients and providers.

11.4.1. Informed Consent in Emergency Situations

When doctors are under pressure in the clinic, they must make decisions quickly and with uncertainty, which can change the usual process of getting patient consent. Emergency and trauma radiology illustrate this problem, as urgent testing can be very important for the patient's health, but often does not give time for detailed consent discussions. Shared decision making (SDM) offers a promising framework to navigate these complexities, enabling clinicians to balance the urgency of care with patient autonomy by transparently discussing risks, benefits, and alternatives when feasible (Arterburn *et al.*, 2016).

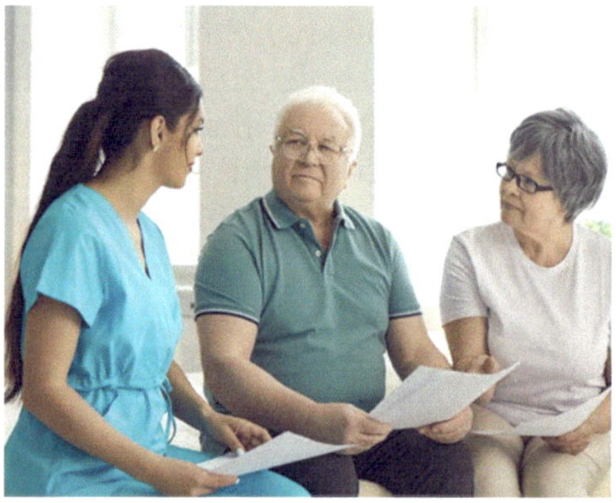

Figure 11.19. Emergency and trauma radiology exemplify this dilemma, as timely diagnostic testing can decisively influence patient outcomes but may not allow for extensive informed consent discussions.

Source: https://www.medical-professionals.com/wp-content/uploads/2022/02/Informed-Consent3.webp.

But when patients are unable to communicate or when quick action is necessary, doctors rely on set guidelines to make decisions that are best for the patient, which stresses the importance of ethical safeguards. Advances such as point-of-care devices providing rapid diagnostic results may further facilitate timely interventions, but they also emphasize the importance of clear communication to uphold consent principles even in exigent circumstances (Carden *et al.*, 2016) (Figure 11.19).

11.4.2. Patient Privacy and Confidentiality

In emergency and trauma radiology, since care is urgent and complicated, exchanging information quickly among different teams is important, but keeping patient privacy and confidentiality is still essential. It is important to protect sensitive health information follow rules, and keep patients comfortable when they are at their most vulnerable. Digital health technologies now make it easier to share data securely, but they also open up new opportunities for attacks, so strong protection is needed. The integration of innovative tools such as digital twins could revolutionize individualized care while requiring stringent safeguards to prevent unauthorized access and misuse of patient information (Armeni *et al.*, 2022). Furthermore, the growing reliance on diagnostic imaging underscores the need for robust data governance frameworks that address disparities in access and confidentiality, particularly in resource-limited settings where data infrastructure may be less developed (Fleming *et al.*, 2021). Protecting patient privacy in emergency situations is necessary to go along with effective care and fairness in healthcare.

11.4.3. Legal Implications of Misdiagnosis

In emergency and trauma radiology, making quick and correct diagnoses is key for the patient's health, but challenges and cognitive biases can sometimes cause mistakes, which can be very concerning for doctors. When someone is misdiagnosed, especially in emergency departments, healthcare providers may be sued for malpractice if they are accused of not meeting the proper standard of care. The complexity increases with the integration of advanced technologies such as artificial intelligence, which, while offering potential to reduce human error, introduces new legal and ethical questions regarding liability and accountability for diagnostic decisions (Brown *et al.*, 2023). Additionally, the evolving use of digital twins in healthcare may transform diagnostic processes, but regulatory uncertainties further complicate the legal landscape surrounding errors and patient safety (Armeni *et al.*, 2022). Understanding these implications is essential for clinicians to navigate medico-legal risks effectively while fostering trust and justice in emergency radiology practice (Figure 11.20).

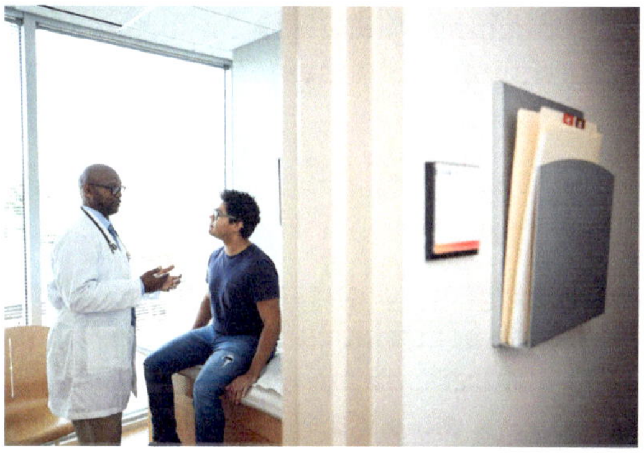

Figure 11.20. When a diagnostic error occurs, especially in high-stakes settings like emergency departments, healthcare providers may face malpractice claims stemming from alleged negligence or failure to meet the standard of care.

Source: https://garmeylaw.com/wp-content/uploads/AdobeStock_236127587-1.jpeg.

11.4.4. Ethical Dilemmas in Imaging Decisions

During emergency and trauma radiology, those working in the field must often decide what is most important: getting a quick diagnosis or considering ethics. When doctors overimage because of defensive medicine or self-referrals, patients may get exposed to radiation without need, healthcare costs may rise, and patients could face possible harm. These consequences underscore the ethical imperative to justify every imaging examination carefully, ensuring patient safety while optimizing care effectiveness (Cantone *et al.*, 2019). Also, the rise of artificial intelligence in imaging creates new ethical issues, for example, who is responsible for errors in diagnosis, how AI works, and how much say doctors still have in their decisions. Addressing these concerns requires multidisciplinary collaboration and education, integrating digital health competencies to uphold patient-centric values and fairness in emergent care settings (Angelos *et al.*, 2022). All in all, dealing with these situations calls for using new technologies while remaining guided by important ethical rules in trauma and emergency radiology.

11.4.5. Radiologist's Responsibility in Emergencies

During emergency care, the radiologist assumes additional responsibilities, collaborating with the team to ensure accurate and timely diagnoses, which in turn affects the patient's response to treatment. Quick decisions and choosing which imaging to do first are crucial, since delays might increase the effects of trauma or hide new changes. Radiologists should be able to use new technologies such as artificial intelligence and advanced imaging tools to help with diagnosis and make the process more efficient in stressful situations. They are also required to keep in touch with emergency physicians and trauma surgeons, so intervention can begin right away if serious findings are discovered. This duty underscores the need to address global disparities in diagnostic accessibility, especially in low-resource environments where diagnostic gaps markedly affect mortality and morbidity rates (Fleming *et al.*, 2021). Embracing innovations like digital platforms and immersive technologies within the Metaverse could further empower radiologists to deliver enhanced, adaptive care during emergencies (Chengoden *et al.*, 2023) (Figure 11.21).

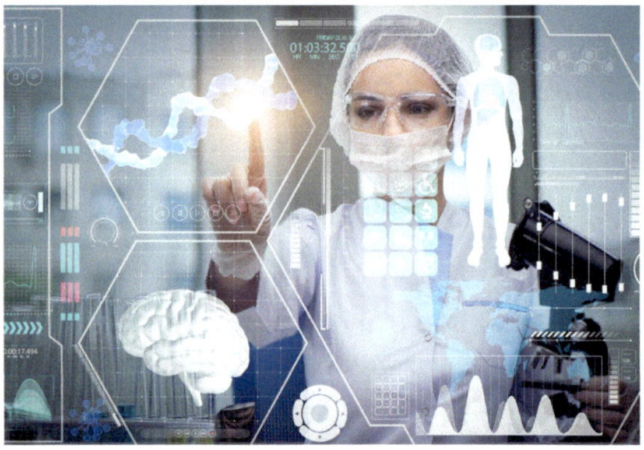

Figure 11.21. Radiologists must be adept at leveraging emerging technologies, such as artificial intelligence and enhanced imaging modalities, to improve diagnostic precision and efficiency in chaotic settings.

Source: https://www.gehealthcare.com/-/jssmedia/gehc/us/images/articles/leveraging-the-power-of-advanced-technologies-and-ai-to-improve-efficiencies-across-radiology.jfif?h=5677&iar=0&w=8503&rev=-1&hash=0ED2BF70B4E846B446692D532A5D469A.

11.4.6. Documentation and Reporting Standards

Good and prompt communication in emergency and trauma radiology helps improve patient results and allows different teams to cooperate well. It is important that the standards for documentation and reporting allow for the fast and accurate creation of provisional reports from emergency imaging, which helps with quick clinical decisions. Studies have highlighted discrepancies between initial and addendum reports, particularly when off-site radiologists are involved, underscoring the necessity for on-site expert review to minimize errors and potential harm to patients (Ball *et al.*, 2017). Additionally, following established guidelines for reporting ensures consistency, reduces the likelihood of misinterpretation, and supports both legal and quality assurance in emergency situations. Additionally, integrating documentation protocols that capture critical findings efficiently aids in the swift identification of life-threatening conditions such as traumatic injuries or acute cardiac events (Bandeeri *et al.*, 2004). So, following strict rules for recording and reporting is necessary in emergency and trauma radiology to improve how accurate the diagnosis is, decrease the number of errors, and keep patients safe.

11.4.7. Interdisciplinary Collaboration and Ethics

The best patient care in emergency and trauma radiology comes from health professionals uniting and each using their own knowledge and skills. In situations where the pace and risks are high, working together across different fields is important for quick and accurate care, but it also leads to ethical issues about how people communicate, who is responsible, and the rights of patients. When multiple disciplines converge, such as neurologists, internal specialists, anesthesiologists, and trauma surgeons coordinating through structured protocols, the collective goal remains optimizing patient outcomes while navigating the nuances of professional boundaries and moral accountability (Braun *et al.*, 2016). Problems can occur when professionals disagree, which may affect decisions and put patients at risk. So, making sure the multidisciplinary team has clear standards and shared values protects both the trust of patients and the quality of care provided. The focus on dynamic collaboration supported by evolving governance structures underscores the ethical imperative to reduce adverse events and enhance treatment efficacy in emergency settings (Almathal *et al.*, 2024) (Figure 11.22).

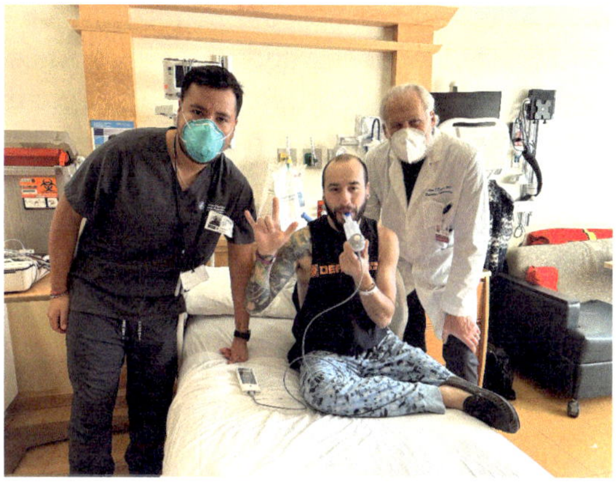

Figure 11.22. When multiple disciplines converge, such as neurologists, internal specialists, anesthesiologists, and trauma surgeons coordinating through structured protocols, the collective goal remains optimizing patient outcomes while navigating the nuances of professional boundaries and moral accountability.

Source: https://www.nymc.edu/media/schools-and-colleges/nymc/images/intouch-photos/2020-2023-intouch-photos/NicholasBrandner.jpg.

11.4.8. Impact of Technology on Ethical Practices

Improvements in technology have greatly changed how emergency and trauma radiology services are delivered, but they have also brought new ethical issues. Because of digital imaging and tele-radiology, critical radiographic examinations can be accessed and interpreted quickly from a distance, which can lead to better and faster decisions for patients. At the same time, depending more on technology can make people worry about data security, patient privacy, and the correctness of diagnoses made without seeing the patient. In addition, because there are not enough radiologists in several places, radiographers often take on tasks that are not part of their usual job to handle urgent cases. While this shift can improve service delivery, it also challenges existing regulatory frameworks and exposes practitioners to potential legal risks, as seen in South Africa's struggle to formalize radiographer reporting despite recognized needs (Van der Venter *et al.*, 2016). Ethical issues should also cover how technology is used to ensure that trauma unit staff remain responsible and protect their patients.

11.4.9. Future Ethical Challenges in Radiology

As technology advances and demand for rapid diagnostic imaging increases, emergency and trauma radiology must address significant ethical issues. The evolving roles within radiographic practice, such as the implementation of consultant radiographer positions, have demonstrated improvements in patient throughput and service efficiency, yet they also raise questions about maintaining professional standards and ensuring adequate training (Miller *et al.*, 2010). Additionally, the shortage of radiologists worldwide has led to informal collaborations between radiographers and medical practitioners, which—although beneficial for timely patient management—occupy a legal gray area and pose liability risks (Van der Venter *et et al.*, 2016). Balancing the lack of workers with the need for clear rules that safeguard both patients and practitioners will be a future ethical issue. In addition, providing equal use of advanced imaging equipment and protecting patient privacy and informed consent are very important. Due to these challenges, it is crucial for emergency and trauma radiology to continue discussing and developing policies to uphold ethical standards.

Test Your Knowledge

1. What are examples of breaches of patient confidentiality?
2. Why is protecting patient information important in medical practice?

SUMMARY

While emergency and trauma radiology has improved the early care of seriously injured patients, it remains challenging to ensure uniform and optimal care and results. Treatment of major bleeding and coagulopathy in complex trauma cases depends on teamwork and the use of evidence-based guidelines. Using structured clinical guidelines that fit the resources available at each institution has shown good results in saving patients' lives and lowering their risk of illness. Besides, learning new things and using advanced imaging methods help make the radiologic evaluation fast and accurate, which allows for quick treatment. Continuously improving trauma radiology practices based on strong research and agreement among experts will greatly help advance trauma care. Adaptation of these principles within diverse clinical environments holds the potential to harmonize treatment standards and improve outcomes universally (Rossaint *et al.*, 2016; Spahn *et al.*, 2019).

To provide good trauma care, medical staff need to use diagnostics quickly and correctly to avoid missing any injuries and help patients recover better. The implementation of structured protocols, such as the formalized trauma tertiary survey (TTS), has shown potential in enhancing early injury detection and reducing delayed diagnoses, although existing evidence emphasizes the need for more rigorous, controlled studies to confirm these benefits (Beller *et al.*, 2015). Concurrently, advancements in radiology practice through the adoption of career progression frameworks, particularly the introduction of consultant radiographer roles, have contributed to increased service capacity, improved interprofessional collaboration, and better utilization of medical staff time (Miller *et al.*, 2010). All these efforts combined support efficient patient management in emergency and trauma cases by making imaging quicker, helping with diagnosis, and improving care routes. While challenges remain in quantifying cost-benefit outcomes, the integration of formalized protocols and expanded professional roles signifies a promising direction for enhancing trauma radiology services and ultimately improving patient safety and quality of care (Beller *et al.*, 2015; Miller *et al.*, 2010).

KEY TERMS FROM THIS CHAPTER

- Traumatic brain injuries
- Proximity extension assays
- Tissue repair
- Emergency
- Patient safety
- Ischemia
- Physical exam
- Assessments
- Molecular profiling
- Biomarker
- Acetabular fractures
- Trauma radiology
- Hypovolemic shock
- Consultations
- Internal bleeding
- Planning

CRITICAL THINKING QUESTIONS

1. **What is the most commonly used initial imaging modality in trauma cases?**
   a. MRI
   b. CT scan
   c. Ultrasound
   d. X-ray
2. **Which of the following is part of the standard trauma imaging protocol for a polytrauma patient?**
   a. Whole-body MRI
   b. Focused Assessment with Sonography in Trauma (FAST)
   c. Electrocardiography (ECG)
   d. Nuclear scintigraphy
3. **The primary imaging modality for detecting intracranial hemorrhage in the emergency setting is:**
   a. MRI
   b. CT without contrast
   c. CT with contrast
   d. Skull X-ray
4. **In a patient with suspected spinal trauma, the initial imaging of choice is usually:**
   a. Whole-spine MRI
   b. CT of the spine
   c. Bone scintigraphy
   d. PET-CT
5. **Which imaging finding is most concerning for an epidural hematoma?**
   a. Crescent-shaped hyperdensity
   b. Biconvex (lens-shaped) hyperdensity
   c. Ring-enhancing lesion
   d. Hypodense area in the frontal lobe

Short Answer Questions

1. Which sign on a CT scan suggests a basilar skull fracture?
2. What is the best initial imaging modality to evaluate a pneumothorax in an unstable patient?
3. What is the primary purpose of a FAST scan in abdominal trauma?
4. What is the main advantage of CT in trauma over plain radiography?
5. What is the primary concern with giving IV contrast in trauma patients?

Answers to Critical Thinking Questions

1. (d); 2. (b); 3. (b); 4. (b); 5. (b)

REFERENCES

1. Abdalla, A. B., Adler, B., Balasubramanian, B., Belard, S., Reddy, B. K., Bonnard, P., *et al.* (2015). Point-of-care ultrasound assessment of tropical infectious diseases—A review of applications and perspectives. *Am. J. Trop. Med. Hyg.* https://core.ac.uk/download/286716207.pdf (accessed on 1st June 2025).
2. Abu-Zidan, F. M., Ansaloni, L., Baiocchi, G. L., Biffl, W., *et al.* (2020). The Operative management in Bariatric Acute abdomen (OBA) Survey: Long-term complications of bariatric surgery and the emergency surgeon's point of view. *World Journal of Emergency Surgery*. https://core.ac.uk/download/286570102.pdf (accessed on 1st June 2025).
3. Adams, S. D., Ahmed, N., Behbahaninia, M., Bongiovanni, T., *et al.* (2024). Geriatric trauma triage: Optimizing systems for older adults—A publication of the American Association for the Surgery of Trauma Geriatric Trauma Committee. *Trauma Surg. Acute Care Open*. https://core.ac.uk/download/619411519.pdf (accessed on 1st June 2025).
4. AlDossary, S., Bradford, N. K., Martin-Khan, M. G., Smith, A. C., *et al.* (2017). A systematic review of the methodologies used to evaluate telemedicine service initiatives in hospital facilities. *International Journal of Medical Informatics.* https://core.ac.uk/download/83972862.pdf (accessed on 1st June 2025).
5. Alkadhi, H., Andreisek, G., Hodler, J., Rufibach, K., *et al.* (2018). Magnetic resonance imaging frequently changes classification of acute traumatic thoracolumbar spine injuries. *Skeletal Radio*. https://core.ac.uk/download/159146667.pdf (accessed on 1st June 2025).
6. Almamoori, H. Z. K., Changizi, V., Zeinalkhani, F., & Nasser, A. F. (2024). Evaluation of brain injury classifications accuracy by using CT scan and T2-star weighted image MRI in the emergency department. *International Journal of Innovative Research in Medical Science*. https://www.semanticscholar.org/paper/79b4582ace5ee0d0f8e170796c1faf7c04d81267 (accessed on 1st June 2025).
7. Almathal, B. F. F., Alrashdi, S. T. M., Alrashidi, T. M. A., Al Rashidi, W. H. M., Al-Rashidi, A. F. D., Alrasheedi, N. H., Alzabni, I. M. A., *et al.* (2024). *Multidisciplinary Collaboration in Emergency Medical Services*. https://core.ac.uk/download/616775692.pdf (accessed on 1st June 2025).
8. Angelos, P., Ansaloni, L., Cobianchi, L., Dal Mas, F., *et al.* (2022). *Artificial Intelligence and Surgery: Ethical Dilemmas and Open Issues.* https://core.ac.uk/download/535109030.pdf (accessed on 1st June 2025).
9. Armeni, P., Polat, I., De Rossi, L. M., Diaferia, L., Meregalli, S., & Gatti, A. (2022). Digital twins in healthcare: Is it the beginning of a new era of evidence-based medicine? A critical review. *Journal of Personalized Medicine, 12*, 1255. https://doi.org/10.3390/jpm12081255 (accessed on 1st June 2025).
10. Arneberg, L., Blunier, S., Exadaktylos, A. K., Gonzenbach, M., *et al.* (2023). Imaging of alert patients after non-self-inflicted strangulation: MRI is superior to CT. *European Radiology*. https://core.ac.uk/download/592040306.pdf (accessed on 1st June 2025).
11. Arterburn, D. E., Barton, M., Berkman, N. D., Charles, C., Edmonds, S. W., Elwyn, G., *et al.* (2016). The 2016 Academic Emergency Medicine Consensus Conference, shared decision making in the emergency department: Development of a policy-relevant patient-centered research agenda—Diagnostic testing breakout session report. https://core.ac.uk/download/155271748.

pdf (accessed on 1st June 2025).

12. Artha, P. A. K., & Sudiasa, I. K. (2024). 028. Traumatic diaphragmatic rupture with unstable hemodynamic: A case report of a rare surgical trauma emergency. *JBN (Jurnal Bedah Nasional)*. https://www.semanticscholar.org/paper/e6657754be9fff029f5fec8db4158d075ef64dd8 (accessed on 1st June 2025).

13. Austin, B., Davis, W., Le, D. Q., Ma, M., *et al.* (2019). Feasibility evaluation of commercially available video conferencing devices to technically direct untrained nonmedical personnel to perform a rapid trauma ultrasound examination. *Diagnostics*. https://core.ac.uk/download/323310769.pdf (accessed on 1st June 2025).

14. Ball, C., Drinkwater, K., Frost, C., Higginson, I., *et al.* (2017). The accuracy of interpretation of emergency abdominal CT in adult patients who present with non-traumatic abdominal pain: Results of a UK national audit. *Clinical Radiology*. https://core.ac.uk/download/74229438.pdf (accessed on 1st June 2025).

15. Bandeeri, N., Henry, J. A., Meredith, C., Treacy, M., *et al.* (2004). The prevalence of cocaine-Associated chest pain in a London hospital. *Emergency Medicine Journal*. https://core.ac.uk/download/5230488.pdf (accessed on 1st June 2025).

16. Battisti, S., Brandi, N., Carrafiello, G., Catena, F., Di Saverio, S., Giampalma, E., Golfieri, R., *et al.* (2021). Proposal of standardization of every step of angiographic procedure in bleeding patients from pelvic trauma. *Eur. J. Med. Res*. https://core.ac.uk/download/483510083.pdf (accessed on 1st June 2025).

17. Beckmann, N. M., Delproposto, Z. S., Dreizin, D., Feng, A., *et al.* (2023). Artificial intelligence CAD tools in trauma imaging: A scoping review from the American Society of Emergency Radiology (ASER) AI/ML expert panel. *Emerg. Radiol.* https://core.ac.uk/download/619410994.pdf (accessed on 1st June 2025).

18. Beikmane, D., Boginskis, V., Cernavska, I., Sauka, A., *et al.* (2023). *Artificial Intelligence Effectivity in Fracture Detection*. https://core.ac.uk/download/591338260.pdf (accessed on 1st June 2025).

19. Beller, E. M., Byrnes, J., Del Mar, C., Geeraedts, L., *et al.* (2015). What is the effect of a formalized trauma tertiary survey procedure on missed injury rates in multi-trauma patients? Study protocol for a randomized controlled trial. *Trials*. https://core.ac.uk/download/196601000.pdf (accessed on 1st June 2025).

20. Bingham, P., Hook, M., Shah, P., Tsao, K., *et al.* (2020). Implementation of Pediatric Emergency Care Applied Research Network (PECARN) guidelines for traumatic brain injury in a rural tertiary care center. https://core.ac.uk/download/289036100.pdf (accessed on 1st June 2025).

21. Blaz, M., Golebiowski, M., Palczewski, P., Swiatkowski, M., *et al.* (2009). Is whole-body trauma MDCT justified in patients in good clinical condition but with dangerous trauma mechanism? *Pol. J. Radiol.* https://core.ac.uk/download/161629231.pdf (accessed on 1st June 2025).

22. Brandt, A., Malkin, A. A., Zanoni, B., Khoury, B., Stuckler, D., Krupinski, E. A., Patton, G. C., *et al.* (2011). Pediatric radiology seen from Africa. Part I: Providing diagnostic imaging to a young population. *Pediatr Radiol*. https://core.ac.uk/download/pdf/10674304.pdf (accessed on 1st June 2025).

23. Braun, M., Lindner, T., Moeckel, M., Ploner, M., *et al.* (2016). *Implementation of an In-House*

Management Routine. https://core.ac.uk/download/199426895.pdf (accessed on 1st June 2025).

24. Brown, C., Nazeer, R., Gibbs, A., Pagé, P., & Mitchell, A. R. J. (2023). Breaking bias: The role of artificial intelligence in improving clinical decision-making. *Cureus*. https://doi.org/10.7759/cureus.36415 (accessed on 1st June 2025).
25. Cagini, L., Carrafiello, G., Floridi, C., Fonio, P., Genovese, E. A., Ianora, A. A. S., *et al.* (2013). *Abdominal Vascular Emergencies: US and CT Assessment*. https://core.ac.uk/download/54579828.pdf (accessed on 1st June 2025).
26. Campus, G., Ramos-Gomez, F., Schulze, R. K. W., Wolf, T. G., *et al.* (2022). *Effectiveness of Telemedicine and Teledentistry After the COVID-19 Pandemic*. https://core.ac.uk/download/543781825.pdf (accessed on 1st June 2025).
27. Cantisani, V., Deganello, A., Dietrich, C. F., Duran, C., *et al.* (2016). *Role of Contrast-Enhanced Ultrasound (CEUS) in Pediatric Practice: An EFSUMB Position Statement*. https://core.ac.uk/download/74320188.pdf (accessed on 1st June 2025).
28. Carden, A. J., Galante, J. M., Gross, E., Mattice, C., *et al.* (2016). *Prospective Observational Study of Point-of-Care Creatinine in Trauma*. https://core.ac.uk/download/323070373.pdf (accessed on 1st June 2025).
29. Chengoden, R., Victor, N., Huynh-The, T., Yenduri, G., Jhaveri, R. H., Alazab, M., Bhattacharya, S., *et al.* (2023). Metaverse for healthcare: A survey on potential applications, challenges and future directions. *IEEE Access, 11*, 12765–12795. https://doi.org/10.1109/access.2023.3241628 (accessed on 1st June 2025).
30. Coccolini, F., Moore, E. E., Kluger, Y., Biffl, W., Leppäniemi, A., Matsumura, Y., Kim, F., *et al.* (2019). Kidney and Uro-trauma: WSES-AAST guidelines. *World Journal of Emergency Surgery, 14*. https://doi.org/10.1186/s13017-019-0274-x (accessed on 1st June 2025).
31. Cross, K., Fallat, M. E., Laniewicz, M., Nti, M., *et al.* (2019). A novel streamlined trauma response team training improves imaging efficiency for pediatric blunt abdominal trauma patients. *Journal of Pediatric Surgery*. https://core.ac.uk/download/187423820.pdf (accessed on 1st June 2025).
32. Di Renzo, G. C., Epicoco, G., Fischer, M., Gerli, S., *et al.* (2015). Endovascular management of massive post-partum hemorrhage in abnormal placental implantation deliveries. *Eur. Radiol.* https://core.ac.uk/download/141695765.pdf (accessed on 1st June 2025).
33. Dyhrfort, P., Svedung, W. T., Clausen, F., Enblad, P., Hillered, L., & Lewén, A. (2023). A dedicated 21-plex proximity extension assay panel for high-sensitivity protein biomarker detection using microdialysis in severe traumatic brain injury: The next step in precision medicine? *Neurotrauma Reports, 4*, 25–40. https://www.semanticscholar.org/paper/13fe8b389f1b3773878a14d5af80ab8d0c7323e5 (accessed on 1st June 2025).
34. Edwards, F. J. (2018). *Good Interdepartmental Relationships: The Foundations of a Solid Emergency Department*. https://core.ac.uk/download/pdf/327264117.pdf (accessed on 1st June 2025).
35. Fleming, K. A., Horton, S., Wilson, M. L., Atun, R., DeStigter, K., Flanigan, J., Sayed, S., *et al.* (2021). The Lancet Commission on diagnostics: Transforming access to diagnostics. *The Lancet, 398*, 1997–2050. https://doi.org/10.1016/s0140-6736(21)00673-5 (accessed on 1st June 2025).

36. Geldsetzer, P. (2020). Knowledge and perceptions of COVID-19 among the general public in the United States and the United Kingdom: A cross-sectional online survey. *Annals of Internal Medicine, 173*, 157–160. https://doi.org/10.7326/m20-0912 (accessed on 1st June 2025).
37. Guglielmi, G., & Nasuto, M. (2017). Emergency and trauma in MSK radiology. *Seminars in Musculoskeletal Radiology, 21*, 165, 166. https://www.semanticscholar.org/paper/b2f351fba12ac3b6df6d8275991b24d4f7c66176 (accessed on 1st June 2025).
38. Ilgar, M., & Dağ, N. (2024). Emergency radiology in the first 24 h of two major earthquakes on the same day and radiologic evaluation of trauma cases. *Tomography, 10*, 1320–1330. https://www.semanticscholar.org/paper/8344ffdc9d823e4ef1974ace7b6495af3bfe4b1f (accessed on 1st June 2025).
39. Malhotra, G., Varma, D., & Mitra, B. (2024). Evaluating accuracy of cervical spine computed tomography interpretation by emergency trainees with the use of a structured protocol. *Emergency Medicine Australasia: EMA*. https://www.semanticscholar.org/paper/4f92c1c08b78a3eb808b0805e13da3da85ae71a8 (accessed on 1st June 2025).
40. Mauro, E. (2012). *Computed Tomography in Polytrauma: Experience in a Radiology Emergency First Level*. https://core.ac.uk/download/14705636.pdf (accessed on 1st June 2025).
41. Merritt, S. L. (2013). The use of ultrasound as an adjunct to X-ray for the localization and removal of soft tissue foreign bodies in an urgent care setting. https://core.ac.uk/download/217670466.pdf (accessed on 1st June 2025).
42. Miller, L., & Price, R. (2010). *An Evaluation of the Impact of Implementation of Consultant Practitioners in Clinical Imaging*. https://core.ac.uk/download/9840194.pdf (accessed on 1st June 2025).
43. Muhmmed, B., Muhmmed, A., Mohammed, D., Alsaeedi, S., Salem, A., Mohammed, Y., Alotibi, F. O., *et al.* (2024). *Radiology in Emergency Medicine: Life-Saving Imaging*. Power System Technology. https://www.semanticscholar.org/paper/64f1ceaad160e745a4b22e0bb715d7cee391faa6 (accessed on 1st June 2025).
44. Nagel, L. L. (2015). Fractures of the pelvis and acetabulum by Tile *et al. Acta Radiologica, 56*(12), NP52. https://www.semanticscholar.org/paper/72978eb6fb51a4aa9a92028a96bf2285e98a5b9a (accessed on 1st June 2025).
45. O'Toole, D. M., Warrington, N. V., Matthees, N. G., Kupanoff, K. M., Bogert, J. N., Jones, M. D., Soe-Lin, H., *et al.* (2024). Abdominal computed tomography scoring systems and experienced radiologists in the radiological diagnosis of small bowel and mesenteric injury. *Emergency Radiology, 31*, 193–201. https://www.semanticscholar.org/paper/8b8f809cf2b18b050a876d91028557ac29780fd9 (accessed on 1st June 2025).
46. Omoto, R., Umemura, Y., Kato, M., Nakahori, Y., & Fujimi, S. (2024). A case of multiple organ injury resuscitated by collaboration of damage control surgery and interventional radiology in hybrid emergency room. *Acute Medicine & Surgery, 11*. https://www.semanticscholar.org/paper/393578d64245d78bf320d216255f08af9be77173 (accessed on 1st June 2025).
47. Österwalder, J., Polyzogopoulou, E., & Hoffmann, B. (2023). Point-of-care ultrasound—History, current and evolving clinical concepts in emergency medicine. *Medicina, 59*, 2179. https://doi.org/10.3390/medicina59122179 (accessed on 1st June 2025).
48. Rossaint, R., Bouillon, B., Černý, V., Coats, T., Duranteau, J., Fernández-Mondejar, E., Filipescu,

D., *et al.* (2016). The European guideline on management of major bleeding and coagulopathy following trauma. *Critical Care* (4th edn., Vol. 20). https://doi.org/10.1186/s13054-016-1265-x (accessed on 1st June 2025).

49. Samuel, A. E., Chakrapani, A. T., & Moideen, F. (2018). Accuracy of extended focused assessment with sonography in trauma (e-FAST) performed by emergency medicine residents in a level one tertiary center of India. *DOAJ (Directory of Open Access Journals), 2*, e15–e15. https://doi.org/10.22114/ajem.v0i0.69 (accessed on 1st June 2025).

50. Sirén, A. (2024). Magnetic resonance imaging in pediatric spinal trauma – Retrospective analysis of feasibility, safety, and diagnostic value in the emergency department. https://core.ac.uk/download/619888893.pdf (accessed on 1st June 2025).

51. Smith, J. H. (2017). *The Orthopedic Athletic Trainer's Handbook.* https://core.ac.uk/download/211328807.pdf (accessed on 1st June 2025).

52. Spahn, D. R., Bouillon, B., Černý, V., Duranteau, J., Filipescu, D., Hunt, B. J., Komadina, R., *et al.* (2019). The European guideline on management of major bleeding and coagulopathy following trauma: Fifth edition. *Critical Care, 23.* https://doi.org/10.1186/s13054-019-2347-3 (accessed on 1st June 2025).

53. Taciuc, I. A., Dumitru, M., Vrînceanu, D., Gherghe, M., Manole, F., Marinescu, A., Şerboiu, C., *et al.* (2024). Applications and challenges of neural networks in otolaryngology (Review). *Biomedical Reports, 20.* https://doi.org/10.3892/br.2024.1781 (accessed on 1st June 2025).

54. Tang, Z., Wu, Q., Li, P., & Wei, X. (2024). Bilateral intertrochanteric fractures in an elderly patient following high-energy trauma: A case report. *BMC Musculoskeletal Disorders, 25.* https://www.semanticscholar.org/paper/579071509589913bb66a4d6c83f6ffda0358045c (accessed on 1st June 2025).

55. Van der Venter, R. (2016). Reporting on radiographic images in after-hours trauma units: Experiences of radiographers and medical practitioners. https://core.ac.uk/download/188177818.pdf (accessed on 1st June 2025).

56. Lieshout Van , E. M. M., Patka, P., Ringburg, A. N., Schipper, I. B., *et al.* (2009). Accuracy of conventional imaging of penetrating torso injuries in the trauma resuscitation room. *Eur. J. Emerg. Med.* https://core.ac.uk/download/19184956.pdf (accessed on 1st June 2025).

57. Von Rüden, C., Tauber, M., Woltmann, A., Friederichs, J., Hackl, S., Bühren, V., Hierholzer, C. (2015). Surgical treatment of ipsilateral multi-level femoral fractures. *Journal of Orthopedic Surgery and Research, 10.* https://www.semanticscholar.org/paper/0435338373239ecd1efc6d757dc9c61dcf02c68a (accessed on 1st June 2025).

RADIOLOGY INFORMATICS AND AI

12

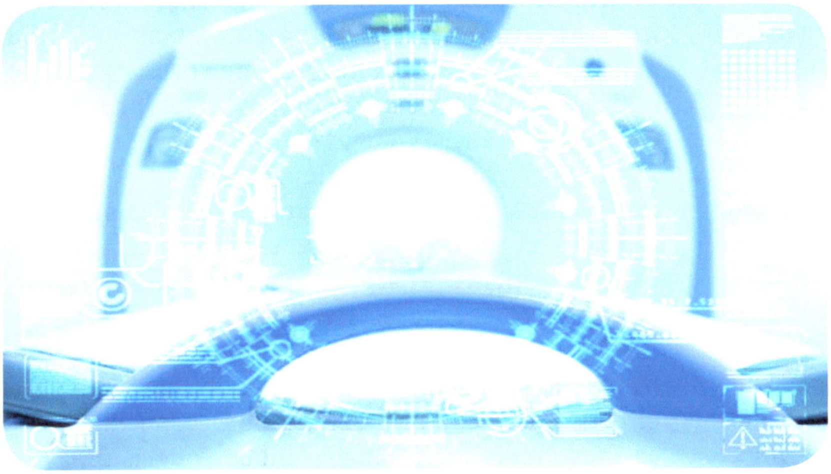

LEARNING OBJECTIVES

After studying this chapter, you will be able to:

1. Know the fundamentals of radiology informatics;
2. Explain the role of AI in radiology;
3. Discuss the benefits of integrating AI with radiology informatics;
4. Find out what challenges and restrictions radiology informatics and AI are facing.

Introduction

Improvements in technology have kept changing healthcare by using data analysis and computational tools. The emergence of artificial intelligence (AI) and machine learning (ML) has significantly enhanced the ability to interpret vast and varied medical datasets, offering substantial promise in fields such as radiology informatics. They make it possible for machines to automatically find important patterns in medical images and other clinical information, which helps doctors make better diagnoses and choose the proper treatment for each patient. Because radiology depends on studying images, AI-powered tools can greatly help it by improving both accuracy and the way it operates. Also, the challenges related to data privacy and algorithm transparency highlight why AI should be developed with strict validation and patient privacy in mind. As a result, the synergy between radiology informatics and AI heralds a transformative shift toward precision medicine and improved clinical outcomes (Dagi *et al.*, 2021; Warnat-Herresthal *et al.*, 2021).

Definition of Radiology Informatics

The use of technology in medical imaging has revolutionized traditional methods, enabling faster and more accurate diagnoses. Radiology informatics is about using information technology to handle the collection, storage, and study of radiological information. It brings together tools and strategies that make the job of radiologists more efficient, help with image reading, and allow for easy storage and access of images. This discipline plays a critical role in utilizing quantitative imaging biomarkers and artificial intelligence to refine diagnostic accuracy and prognostication, particularly in complex diseases such as interstitial lung disease, where quantitative CT and AI-driven methods offer objective assessments (Fanni *et al.*, 2021). Moreover, radiology informatics supports collaborative and decentralized data sharing efforts, which are essential in developing comprehensive machine learning models while adhering to privacy regulations, thereby advancing precision medicine (Warnat-Herresthal *et al.*, 2021). Through these innovations, radiology informatics represents the convergence of imaging science and computational intelligence (Figure 12.1).

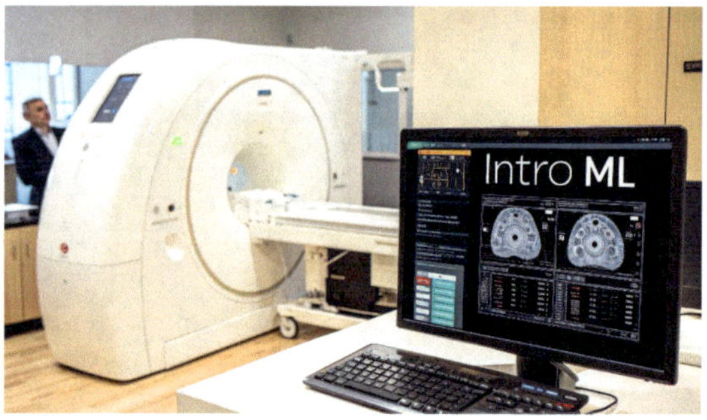

Figure 12.1. Radiology informatics refers to the specialized field that focuses on the acquisition, management, and analysis of radiological data through advanced information systems.

Source: https://cdn.outrank.so/c0c46267-c6c4-4083-a08c-9f225f163943/a84d11a5-7a24-4702-8c71-61d337cd02da.jpg.

Overview of Artificial Intelligence (AI) in Healthcare

Recently, the use of AI in healthcare has shown great promise for changing different medical fields, for example, radiology. Using machine learning and deep learning, AI is able to study large blood transcriptome and imaging datasets, which helps in early diagnosis of diseases such as leukemia and problems in the lungs. Innovative decentralized approaches, such as Swarm Learning, facilitate data sharing across institutions while preserving patient privacy and adhering to regulatory frameworks, thus addressing a critical barrier to widespread AI deployment (Warnat-Herresthal *et al.*, 2021). Even with great improvements in AI for nephrology and other specialties, it is still difficult to prove that these technologies are helping patients. The growing adoption of AI underscores the necessity for comprehensive digital strategies and ethical governance frameworks to ensure safe, equitable, and effective clinical implementation, especially as these tools increasingly influence decision-making in precision medicine (Ho *et al.*, 2021).

Importance of Radiology Informatics in Modern Medicine

Artificial intelligence being used in radiology greatly changes how medical care is delivered, so radiologists now need to learn new skills. Because they understand both medicine and technology, radiologists are able to choose and use AI-powered tools that improve how and what they diagnose. However, many of these new techniques are developed by people other than radiologists, which creates important ethical, legal, and workforce issues that need to be resolved before they can be used safely and effectively. Radiology informatics provides the framework through which these challenges can be managed, emphasizing the importance of roles such as the Chief Radiologist Information Officer to oversee AI integration and maintain professional standards (Ratnayake, 2021). Additionally, understanding technical factors—such as the impact of image resolution on AI performance—is essential for optimizing diagnostic outcomes and guiding future research (Lakhani, 2020). Thus, radiology informatics is indispensable for harnessing AI's potential while safeguarding patient care in modern medicine (Figure 12.2).

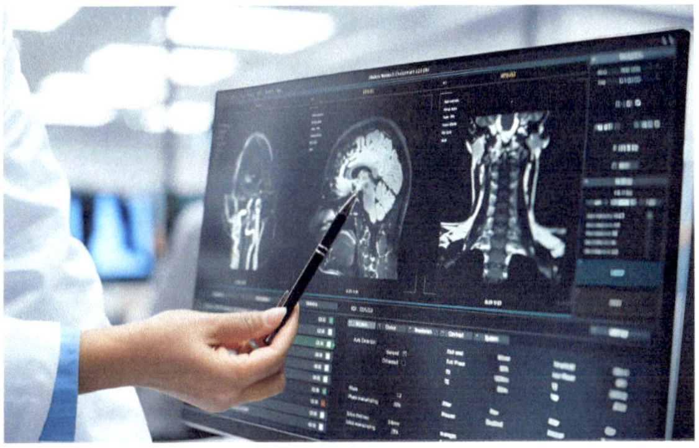

Figure 12.2. As experts at the intersection of clinical medicine and technology, radiologists are uniquely positioned to evaluate and implement AI-driven tools that enhance diagnostic accuracy and workflow efficiency.

Source: https://lakezurichopenmri.com/wp-content/uploads/2024/06/MRI-and-Artificial-Intelligence-The-Future-of-Diagnostics.jpg.

Historical Context of Radiology Informatics

Radiology informatics has changed over time due to wider changes in healthcare technology and data management, mainly because more is expected from medical imaging in terms of accuracy, efficiency, and accessibility. The early goal was to create digital versions of images instead of using film, which allowed for better storage and easier sharing needed for today's diagnostics. At the same time, the increase in complex radiological procedures required healthcare providers to have systems that made it easy for them to communicate. The history of informatics highlights how organizations and technological problems were handled by new informatics solutions, which made it possible for artificial intelligence to develop. Also, adopting informatics in radiology was complicated by the fact that healthcare systems and resources vary widely, which pointed out the differences in healthcare access and utilization. Studies on unmet healthcare needs indicate that systemic limitations in availability and accessibility shaped how radiology informatics evolved, reinforcing the importance of adaptable, scalable technologies to meet diverse clinical demands (Chen *et al.*, 2023).

The Role of Artificial Intelligence (AI) in Enhancing Radiology

AI in radiology has made it possible to analyze images more accurately and consistently, which has helped solve past problems with accuracy and efficiency. AI-based tools, which are sometimes called the Bionic Radiologist, support decision-making by using both algorithms and human experience to improve the accuracy of disease assessments and treatment advice. Because of this, radiologists face fewer opportunities to miss care and are able to keep learning, which helps them spend more time with patients and discuss cases with other specialists.

Even with all these benefits, introducing AI in healthcare can be challenging because of worries about assigning diagnoses to machines and guaranteeing patient safety, which requires cultural and leadership changes. Furthermore, collaboration across cancer informatics centers facilitates sharing innovations that improve AI applications in oncology and radiology, highlighting the importance of national forums and consortia in advancing these technologies for personalized patient care (Barnholtz-Sloan *et al.*, 2020; Dewey *et al.*, 2019) (Figure 12.3).

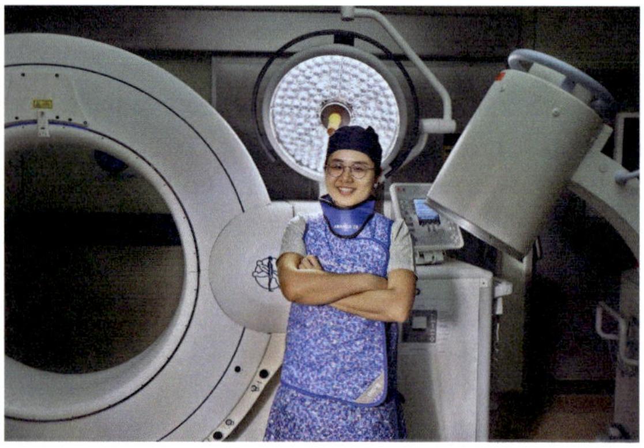

Figure 12.3. Bionic radiologist.

Source: https://www.healthcarescholarships.sg/ScholarStories/PublishingImages/2023/amanda-er-operating-theatre.JPG.

Scope of Radiology Informatics and Artificial Intelligence (AI)

Thanks to new technology, medical imaging has changed a lot, and this has made radiology informatics a key area that combines managing data with advanced analysis. In this situation, AI helps radiology informatics by improving image acquisition, interpretation, and decision-making in clinical care. AI's application in modalities such as computed tomography, magnetic resonance imaging, and echocardiography has enabled more accurate, efficient, and personalized diagnostics, thereby improving patient outcomes and management strategies (Martins *et al.*, 2024).

However, the adoption of AI also introduces challenges related to the interpretability of complex machine learning models, often described as black boxes, which raise important ethical and legal concerns regarding transparency and accountability (Marey *et al.*, 2024). It is important to handle these issues by using explainable AI and having clear regulations to make sure AI technologies are used properly in radiology informatics.

12.1. The Fundamentals of Radiology Informatics

Learning Outcome

1. Identify components of radiology informatics;
2. Explain data management in radiology;
3. Define picture archiving and communication systems (PACS);
4. Focus on electronic health records (EHR) integration;
5. Discuss workflow optimization in radiology departments;
6. Describe standards and protocols in radiology informatics;
7. Know security and privacy concerns;
8. Learn interoperability challenges;
9. Understand future trends in radiology informatics.

Using the latest technology in medical education helps healthcare professionals get ready for the challenges they will face in the future. Therefore, radiologists must be familiar with radiology informatics, which deals with organizing, examining, and using imaging data through computer tools. This knowledge helps improve how work is done, how images are understood, and how AI systems are added. New frameworks for teaching AI in radiology residencies stress the value of using a planned and multidisciplinary strategy. By fostering collaboration between AI experts and radiologists, educational initiatives have successfully increased residents' confidence and competence in AI applications, illustrating the practicality and impact of such curricula (Hofmeijer *et al.*, 2024). In addition, using visualization tools and digital platforms has made it much easier to explain complex informatics topics, as illustrated by tools that show how data is exchanged in radiology departments. All these actions demonstrate how important informatics basics are for the progress of radiology in the age of AI.

12.1.1. Components of Radiology Informatics

Because advanced technologies are now part of healthcare, managing medical data in radiology requires a variety of approaches. Several important parts of radiology informatics make it easier to obtain, store, and review imaging data. Key elements include Picture Archiving and Communication Systems (PACS), Radiology Information Systems (RIS), and teleradiology platforms, which together enable efficient workflow management and remote access to imaging studies. Also, using standard data formats such as DICOM helps various systems share data without issues. AI is integrated into these systems to assist with image analysis and decision-making, enhancing the accuracy of diagnoses and the overall efficiency of the hospital. Robust data security protocols and ethical governance frameworks are also vital, addressing concerns related to patient privacy and consent while fostering trust in AI-powered radiology applications (Kuwaiti *et al.*, 2023; Liu *et al.*, 2023). These components collectively form the backbone of modern radiology informatics, positioning it as a crucial enabler in transforming healthcare delivery (Figure 12.4).

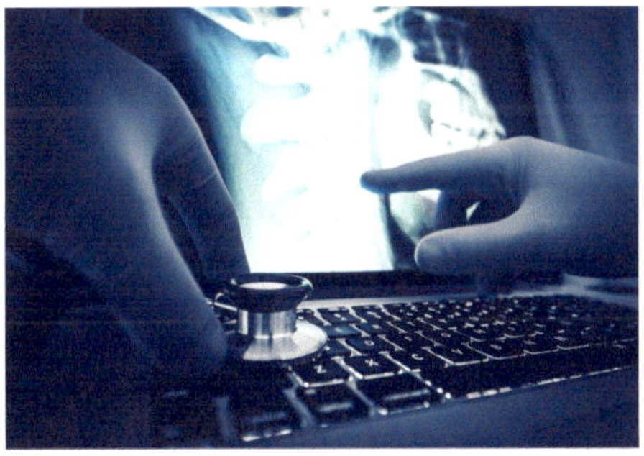

Figure 12.4. Radiology informatics encompasses several critical components that streamline the acquisition, storage, and analysis of imaging information.

Source: https://demigos.com/media/cache/a2/26/a226ac1b1488933f1bc75b1d78d1121e.jpg.

12.1.2. Data Management in Radiology

Efficient handling of vast amounts of imaging data is critical for advancing radiology practices, especially as artificial intelligence (AI) becomes increasingly integrated into diagnostic workflows. Well-organized data systems make it easy to keep, access, and review complicated radiological images, which helps doctors make better diagnoses and write reports more efficiently. Also, to implement machine learning, there needs to be strong datasets, which means paying close attention to data quality and organization. AI can be used to its best if issues such as data privacy, interoperability, and understanding algorithms are dealt with, so that patient information remains safe and everyone receives fair care. It is important to add informatics and data sciences to radiology education to help future doctors and scientists meet these new challenges. As AI-driven tools evolve, collaborative efforts to refine data management practices will be pivotal in maximizing their benefits in clinical radiology settings (Mbata *et al.*, 2024; Sharma *et al.*, 2024).

12.1.3. Picture Archiving and Communication Systems (PACS)

Radiology informatics has advanced a lot thanks to digital technology, which improves how quickly and accurately diagnoses are made. A major factor in this progress is the use of PACS, which made it possible to handle, access, and share medical images digitally and more easily. This shift from traditional film-based methods to integrated PACS facilitated faster diagnostic processes, improved accessibility for radiologists, and supported multidisciplinary collaboration within healthcare settings, ultimately contributing to better patient care outcomes (Canguit *et al.*, 2025). Lately, using artificial intelligence in PACS platforms has greatly increased these improvements. AI-powered tools, such as convolutional neural networks for image segmentation and natural language processing for report generation, have enhanced diagnostic precision and reduced interpretation times dramatically (Pérez-Sanpablo *et al.*, 2025). Despite these advances, challenges related to data security and interoperability must be addressed to fully realize the potential of AI-integrated PACS in transforming radiology informatics (Figure 12.5).

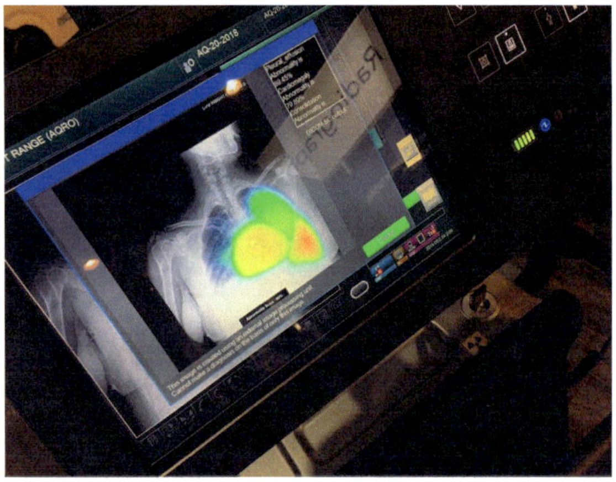

Figure 12.5. The evolution of radiology informatics has been markedly influenced by advancements in digital technologies that enhance both efficiency and diagnostic accuracy.

Source: https://www.itnonline.com/sites/default/files/field/image/Fujifilm_Reili_Artificial_intelligence_pneumothorax_X-ray_RSNA19_2.jpeg.

12.1.4. Electronic Health Records (EHR) Integration

For AI to make a big difference in radiology informatics, EHR integration must be done successfully. When healthcare systems can easily share data, doctors can see a complete patient record, which helps with accurate diagnoses and better treatment. Because AI-driven tools need a lot of data, which is often split and subject to strict privacy rules, it becomes very difficult to include them in new systems. Innovative approaches such as Swarm Learning address these issues by combining decentralized machine learning with blockchain technologies, ensuring data confidentiality while enhancing collaborative model training across multiple institutions (Warnat-Herresthal *et al.*, 2021). In addition, well-managed EHR can reduce paperwork, make patients more involved, and improve the way staff work, which helps doctors make better decisions. However, ethical and regulatory concerns remain, necessitating careful governance to safeguard patient rights and maintain trust in these advanced systems (Kuwaiti *et al.*, 2023). Therefore, utilizing EHRs effectively is crucial for enhancing radiology informatics that rely on AI.

12.1.5. Workflow Optimization in Radiology Departments

AI integration in radiology departments could improve how work is done by making things more efficient and accurate. Because AI can quickly review imaging information, radiologists can focus on urgent cases and cut down on delays in diagnosis, which benefits the patients. For example, recent studies demonstrate AI's high sensitivity and specificity in detecting bone fractures and other abnormalities, showing performance comparable to radiology residents while also minimizing missed diagnoses (Alejandro Díaz Moreno *et al.*, 2025). AI can also help automate tasks like organizing images and making reports which takes some of the administrative workload off radiology staff. However, optimizing workflow through AI also demands addressing concerns related to sustainability and operational costs, given the significant computational resources required for deep learning models (Koçak *et al.*, 2025). Balancing these challenges with the clinical benefits necessitates a holistic approach to AI integration that fosters productivity while maintaining environmental and economic viability within radiology departments (Figure 12.6).

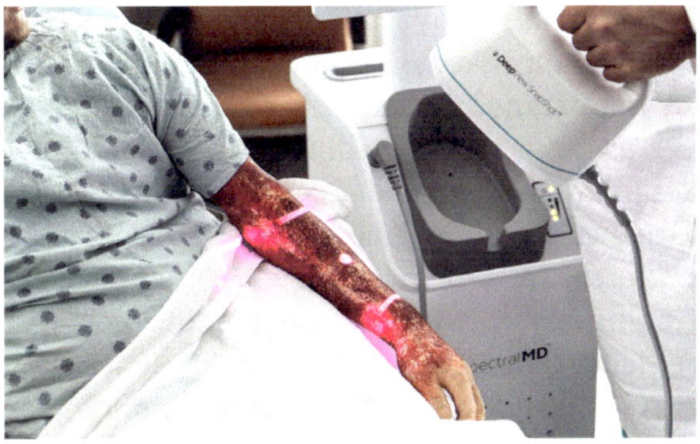

Figure 12.6. The integration of artificial intelligence (AI) within radiology departments has the potential to transform traditional workflows by enhancing efficiency and accuracy.

Source: https://www.spectral-ai.com/wp-content/uploads/2024/04/ai-and-medical-imaging.jpg.

12.1.6. Standards and Protocols in Radiology Informatics

Advancements in radiology informatics depend a lot on having and following strict standards and protocols that guarantee the accuracy, compatibility, and repeatability of the data. Using the same approaches is necessary for AI tools that need high-quality, well-labeled data to be effective in different medical settings. However, current research highlights significant gaps in reporting practices, with many studies lacking transparency in dataset descriptions, validation processes, and code availability, thereby hindering reproducibility and comparison of AI models in radiology (Alex *et al.*, 2021). To address these limitations, frameworks such as FUTURE-AI emphasize comprehensive guidelines encompassing fairness, traceability, robustness, and explainability throughout AI development and deployment phases (Lekadir *et al.*, n.d.). When these standards are included, radiology informatics supports AI applications that are reliable, efficient, and follow important ethical, legal, and operational rules needed for wide use in healthcare.

12.1.7. Security and Privacy Concerns

AI use in radiology informatics has greatly improved how accurate and efficient diagnoses are, but it has also raised major issues related to security and privacy that need to be handled properly. Since AI needs access to a lot of sensitive patient information, it is now very important to prevent unauthorized access and breaches. Because AI is complicated and healthcare networks are closely linked, the risk of data breaches and cyberattacks increases, which may threaten patient confidentiality. Ensuring that AI models follow the regulations for data privacy is necessary to keep patients and clinicians trusting the system. Dealing with these issues needs strong encryption, safe data storage, and clear rules for using AI in healthcare. Failure to mitigate these security and privacy risks could undermine the benefits of AI integration in radiology, hindering its widespread adoption and trustworthiness (Alhazime, 2024; Reshma, 2025) (Figure 12.7).

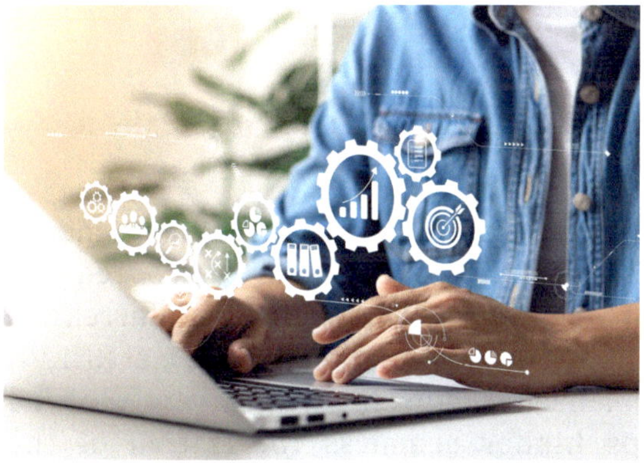

Figure 12.7. The integration of AI into radiology informatics has led to unprecedented advances in diagnostic accuracy and efficiency; however, it has also introduced substantial security and privacy challenges that must be carefully managed.

Source: https://www.icadmed.com/wp-content/uploads/2024/02/Common-Questions-Operations-1024x768.jpg.

12.1.8. Interoperability Challenges

A major issue in using artificial intelligence in radiology informatics is making different systems and datasets work together. Because medical imaging formats, clinical data structures, and standards are not the same everywhere, it becomes difficult to share and integrate data. Because there are no standardized frameworks, AI models have difficulties proving and repeating their results in various healthcare settings. Efforts like the OMOP Common Data Model and the Medical Imaging Common Data Model aim to tackle these issues by providing syntactic and semantic harmonization of imaging and clinical information, enabling large-scale collaboration and privacy-preserving data exchange (Jeon *et al.*, 2024). Furthermore, emerging technologies such as the Metaverse, integrating AI with virtual and augmented reality, underscore the necessity for adaptive interoperability solutions to bridge digital environments and healthcare systems effectively (Chengoden *et al.*, 2023). Dealing with these interoperability issues is necessary for AI-based radiology tools to be used reliably in hospitals.

12.1.9. Future Trends in Radiology Informatics

The quick development of AI and machine learning is helping to improve and speed up the way radiology informatics is used. Increasingly, radiologists are recognizing the necessity for formalized training in AI, as current knowledge gaps hinder seamless integration of these tools into clinical practice (Antolín *et al.*, 2022). Collaborative efforts led by prominent organizations like RSNA and MICCAI underscore the importance of addressing key challenges such as trust, reproducibility, and explainability to facilitate widespread acceptance of AI systems in medical imaging (Aboian *et al.*, 2024). Trends in the future will bring together clinical and imaging data, which supports personalized medicine and better results for patients. Also, changes in cultural values among radiologists are necessary to ensure that new innovations are used safely and ethically. Overall, the trajectory of radiology informatics hinges on interdisciplinary cooperation and enhanced educational frameworks to equip radiologists for an AI-augmented professional environment (Figure 12.8).

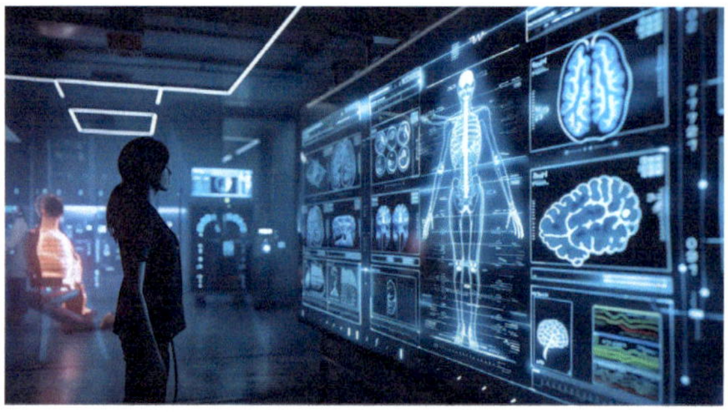

Figure 12.8. Rapid advancements in artificial intelligence (AI) and machine learning technologies are reshaping the landscape of radiology informatics, promising more efficient and accurate diagnostic processes.

Source: https://images.ctfassets.net/wt9spzbmicfl/7xha0jCBWVYr8NsahiXeJX/2f3e2bf5bee3fcc79be76b7a661ad457/AI_is_transforming_healthcare.webp.

Test Your Knowledge

1. In what ways does radiology informatics help radiologists communicate with other healthcare workers?
2. Which security steps are important for keeping patient data safe in radiology systems?

12.2. The Role of Artificial Intelligence (AI) in Radiology

Learning Outcome

1. Understand the definition and types of AI technologies;
2. Learn machine learning applications in radiology;
3. Explain deep learning and image analysis;
4. AI in diagnostic imaging;
5. Focus on predictive analytics in radiology;
6. Describe AI-assisted decision support systems;
7. List limitations of AI in radiology;
8. Know ethical considerations of AI use;
9. Learn case studies of AI implementation in radiology.

Artificial intelligence is now making a big difference in many medical areas, and radiology is leading the way. Thanks to machine learning and neural networks, AI can handle complex imaging data with great skill, which supports earlier and more accurate diagnoses. Notably, the development of intuitive interfaces that facilitate human-in-the-loop strategies has addressed key challenges related to training and annotating whole slide images, thereby improving model performance iteratively across various applications, including renal and prostate tissue segmentation (Ginley *et al.*, 2018).

Still, although AI has helped with accurate diagnoses in radiology, it has to deal with variations in reporting and the quality of studies. Nonetheless, recent research underscores the potential of sophisticated AI models to uncover hidden patterns by combining diverse data sources, ultimately enhancing reproducibility, interpretability, and patient outcomes within radiological practice (Baumgartner *et al.*, 2019).

12.2.1. Definition and Types of Artificial Intelligence (AI) Technologies

Thanks to the advancements in computer technology and the increasing availability of data, AI is now being utilized in various fields, including healthcare. Basically, AI is about systems that can do things that normally require human thinking such as learning, reasoning and solving problems. AI is mainly used in radiology informatics as machine learning, deep learning and natural language processing and each method helps in analyzing and interpreting medical images. Machine learning helps spot patterns in medical images and deep learning, with the help of neural networks, makes it possible to find more complex features in a lot of data which improves both accuracy and speed. Radiology reports can be understood more easily and workflow can be improved with natural language processing. All of these AI types together make it easier to diagnose and run daily operations in radiology, helping with issues like the amount of work and differences in how cases are interpreted. Understanding these foundational AI categories is crucial in leveraging their potential for advancing radiological practices (Kuwaiti *et al.*, 2023; Liu *et al.*, 2023) (Figure 12.9).

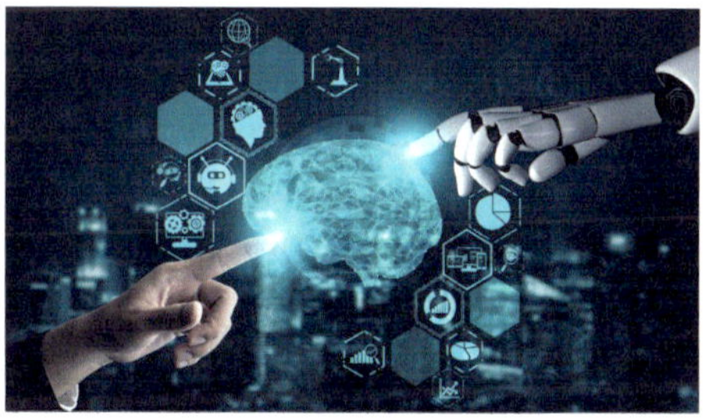

Figure 12.9. Artificial intelligence (AI) refers to systems designed to perform tasks that typically require human intelligence, encompassing learning, reasoning, and problem-solving.

Source: https://elm.umaryland.edu/elm-stories/2023/ArtIntell.jpg.

12.2.2. Machine Learning (ML) Applications in Radiology

Because of fast technological changes in healthcare, radiology has seen major improvements in its diagnostic procedures. Machine learning, which belongs to artificial intelligence, is now widely used to analyze complex imaging data more accurately and efficiently. Learning from large amounts of data allows them to spot patterns and issues that humans might not notice, which improves early disease detection and prediction. Also, machine learning helps automate everyday tasks, so radiologists can give more attention to complex decisions, which improves their workflow and lowers the risk of errors. Using these new technologies means medical education should focus on digital skills and ethics to make sure AI is used wisely with clinical knowledge. While much of the AI application focus has been on human medicine, parallels can be drawn to veterinary radiology, where machine learning similarly informs diagnostics and personalized treatment strategies, underscoring the broad transformative potential of these approaches (Abualigah *et al.*, 2024).

12.2.3. Deep Learning and Image Analysis

Improvements in artificial intelligence have made a significant impact on radiology, mainly by using deep learning models to improve medical image analysis. They have shown great potential in handling tasks such as identifying diseases and separating tissues, which are important for correct diagnosis and proper treatment planning. But it is still challenging to make these algorithms work well in different datasets and clinical settings. Studies reveal that many deep learning algorithms exhibit a noticeable decrease in performance when tested on external datasets compared to internal validation, highlighting issues related to overfitting and variability in imaging protocols (Yu *et al.*, 2022). Still, by using deep learning together with advanced imaging and data systems, it has become possible to create solutions that can scale for precision medicine. Furthermore, emerging methods combining three-dimensional reconstruction with in-silico modeling reinforce the potential of deep learning frameworks to revolutionize radiology informatics by facilitating more accurate and timely clinical decision-making (Panayides *et al.*, 2020) (Figure 12.10).

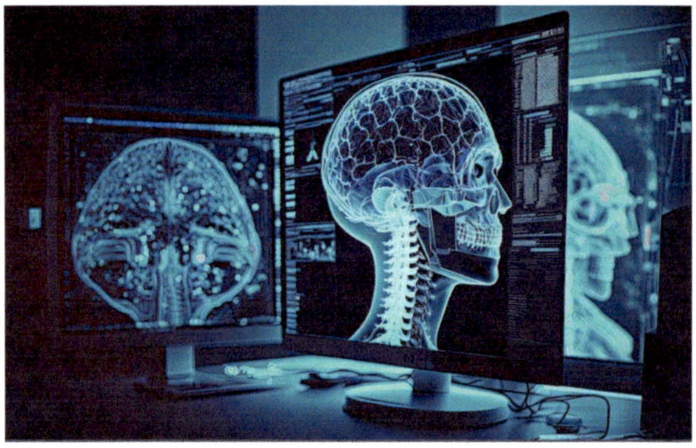

Figure 12.10. Advancements in artificial intelligence (AI) have significantly influenced the field of radiology, particularly through deep learning models that enhance medical image analysis.

Source: https://journal.medtigo.com/wp-content/uploads/2024/09/image-25.png.

12.2.4. Artificial Intelligence (AI) in Diagnostic Imaging

Thanks to progress in medical informatics, it is now easier and more accurate to interpret complex results from diagnostic imaging. New technologies use artificial intelligence to spot small changes and irregularities in imaging tests that might not be seen by people, which helps doctors make better diagnoses and care for their patients. With machine learning, it is possible to combine many types of data, which supports more detailed analysis and better grouping of diseases and their risks. Also, advanced training tools for radiologists, such as neuroradiology tutors, rely on AI to provide organized cases and interactive methods to help with education and decision-making. They rely on image description languages and statistical models of similarity and typicality to make learning environments that fit each learner's requirements. Even with these technologies, it is still challenging to make a reporting standard and make sure models are easy to understand, which helps maintain reproducibility and trust among doctors. Overall, AI's role in diagnostic imaging epitomizes the intersection of technological innovation with clinical informatics, advancing radiological practice markedly (Azevedo *et al.*, 2000; Baumgartner *et al.*, 2019).

12.2.5. Predictive Analytics in Radiology

Advances in technology have greatly improved healthcare services, especially by including advanced data analysis methods. Predictive analytics in radiology, which utilizes AI, is now considered a major breakthrough because it can analyze extensive imaging data and predict what will happen to patients. Combining machine learning and deep learning allows predictive models to detect patterns that are not obvious to the human eye, which improves diagnosis and makes it possible to intervene early.

They help doctors customize care for patients and also improve the way hospitals use their resources. However, the efficacy of predictive analytics hinges on the quality and transparency of the underlying datasets, as well as the ability to mitigate inherent biases in AI applications (Garg *et al.*, 2023). As a subset of AI's broader role in healthcare, predictive analytics exemplifies how computational intelligence approximates complex clinical conclusions from input data, thereby supporting radiologists in decision-making processes and ultimately improving patient care (Sridhar *et al.*, 2021) (Figure 12.11).

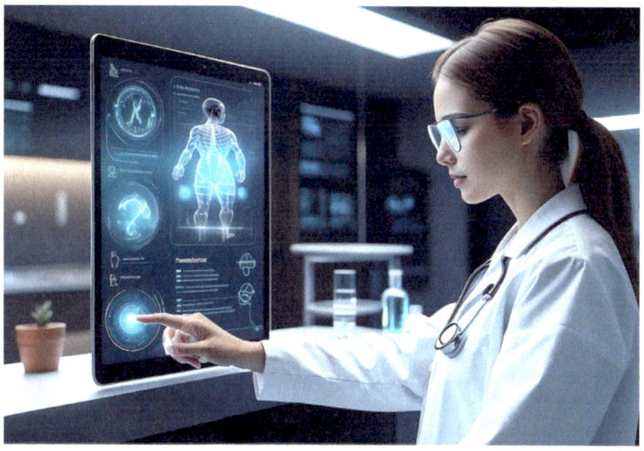

Figure 12.11. Predictive analytics in radiology has emerged as a transformative approach, leveraging artificial intelligence to interpret vast amounts of imaging data and forecast patient outcomes.

Source: https://www.buzzybrains.com/blog/wp-content/uploads/2024/07/Bigdata-in-healthcare.jpg.

12.2.6. Artificial Intelligence (AI)-Assisted Decision Support Systems

With AI in medical imaging, clinicians now have better support for making decisions due to the help provided by AI-based systems. They study large amounts of data to discover patterns that might be difficult for even experienced radiologists to spot, which improves how accurately and efficiently diagnoses are made. AI tools that use machine learning and predictive analytics assist in understanding complicated imaging scans and identifying diseases like cancer and neurological problems earlier. Still, the risk of technology disrupting the usual relationship between doctors and patients points to the need for a careful balance, so technology helps rather than replaces human decisions. It is also important to ensure that clinicians understand AI results and maintain patient trust in the system. As medical education evolves to include digital literacy and ethical reasoning, AI-assisted decision support stands as a pivotal component in radiology informatics, advancing both clinical outcomes and healthcare delivery (Ade *et al.*, 2023).

12.2.7. Limitations of Artificial Intelligence (AI) in Radiology

Even with the fast progress in AI in radiology, there are still some obstacles that stop it from being widely used. One major problem is that training neural networks can be very complex, and this often needs large amounts of annotated data that take a lot of effort to prepare. Although innovative human-in-the-loop strategies have been proposed to alleviate this burden by iteratively refining network performance through expert feedback, these methods still depend heavily on domain-specific expertise for accurate annotation (Ginley *et al.*, 2018).

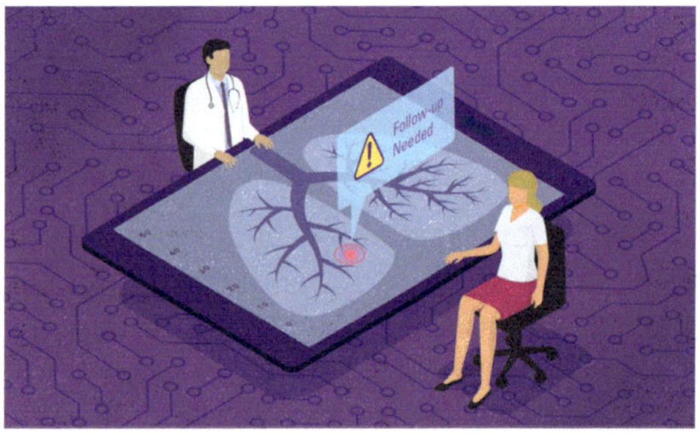

Figure 12.12. The limitations in data annotation, interpretability, and generalizability continue to impede the full potential of AI in radiology.

Source: https://catalyst.nejm.org/cms/10.1056/CAT.21.0469/asset/4ad02d2f-6252-4172-97a5-6fe1b34a0641/assets/graphic/cat.21.0469-hero.jpg.

Also, using regular natural language processing methods cannot fully grasp the meaning in radiology reports, which affects how accurate AI-based analysis is. Recent efforts employing large language models have shown promise in enhancing semantic similarity assessments, yet their applications remain largely experimental and require further validation before integration into clinical workflows (Li *et al.*, 2024). Consequently, the limitations in data annotation, interpretability, and generalizability continue to impede the full potential of AI in radiology (Figure 12.12).

12.2.8. Ethical Considerations of Artificial Intelligence (AI) Use

Because artificial intelligence is changing radiology informatics, its ethical impact should be examined closely. The use of AI to improve diagnosis is very beneficial, but it also brings up issues about privacy, biased algorithms, and transparency. Because AI systems rely on a lot of sensitive data, it is becoming more difficult to keep patient information private, so healthcare organizations must be more careful with data security. Also, if biases in the training data are not handled, they might continue to cause healthcare disparities and result in unequal treatment. When AI decisions are transparent, clinicians and patients can trust the system, agree to treatment, and hold the system accountable. Balancing the immense potential of AI-enhanced medical diagnostics with these ethical challenges is critical for developing responsible applications that prioritize patient welfare and uphold professional standards within radiology informatics (Ali *et al.*, 2023; Liu *et al.*, 2023).

12.2.9. Case Studies of Artificial Intelligence (AI) Implementation in Radiology

The use of AI in radiology has created a new era, and this is shown by case studies that carefully assess how AI affects practice. One such investigation implemented a Radiology AI lab employing advanced biometric techniques—including eye-tracking, heart rate monitoring, and facial expression analysis—to objectively measure radiologists' interactions with AI-assisted imaging methods (Paalvast *et al.*, 2025).

The study that used ultra-low-dose CT scans showed that having AI annotations improved the way doctors searched for information and made their decisions, suggesting better efficiency and accuracy. Heart rate variability on its own did not show a link to experience, but combining different biometric data gave a clearer picture of how radiologists behave, revealing the difficulties of combining humans and AI. They point out that AI in clinical settings has both advantages and difficulties, and stress that having objective monitoring systems in real time is very important. Such case studies form a critical foundation for the continued optimization and adoption of AI tools in radiological practice (Olivieri *et al.*, 2024).

Test Your Knowledge

1. In what ways does machine learning assist with understanding images in radiology?
2. What kinds of artificial intelligence are most often used in the field of radiology?

12.3. Benefits of Integrating Artificial Intelligence (AI) with Radiology Informatics

Learning Outcome

1. Understand improved diagnostic accuracy;
2. Learn enhanced workflow efficiency;
3. Discuss reduction in radiologist burnout;
4. Focus on the cost-effectiveness of AI solutions;
5. Describe personalized patient care;
6. Define real-time data analysis;
7. Discuss increased access to radiology services;
8. Focus on collaboration between radiologists and AI;
9. Know the future potential of AI in radiology.

AI and radiology informatics, when combined, can greatly improve how accurate and efficient healthcare systems are. Using advanced machine learning, radiologists can examine data more efficiently and precisely, which allows them to detect cancers and lung diseases sooner. This synergy not only enhances the capability of computer-aided diagnosis but also facilitates the handling of large, heterogeneous datasets from multiple sources without compromising patient privacy, as demonstrated by decentralized learning frameworks that maintain confidentiality while improving predictive power across distributed datasets (Warnat-Herresthal *et al.*, 2021). Furthermore, AI integration addresses critical challenges related to data security and robustness in clinical environments, offering methods to safeguard against adversarial threats while preserving privacy (Qayyum *et al.*, 2020). All of these benefits demonstrate that AI is important for improving radiology informatics, which leads to better care for patients.

12.3.1. Improved Diagnostic Accuracy

Using artificial intelligence in radiology informatics has greatly improved how accurately doctors interpret medical images. With AI, images can be segmented and analyzed in detail, which reduces mistakes and makes assessments more consistent among different doctors. For instance, iterative human-in-the-loop strategies utilize neural networks to refine diagnostic accuracy in pathology and radiology by incorporating expert feedback during training, which improves performance over time and adapts to diverse tissue types and imaging modalities (Ginley *et al.*, 2018). Moreover, the concept of the Bionic Radiologist exemplifies how AI-driven, consistent image analysis and scientifically grounded testing decisions improve disease probability assessments and treatment planning, fostering reliable and reproducible diagnostic outcomes (Dewey *et al.*, 2019). These advancements empower radiologists to deliver more personalized patient care, enhance early detection capabilities, and ultimately contribute to better clinical decision-making, exemplifying the transformative potential of AI in radiology informatics (Figure 12.13).

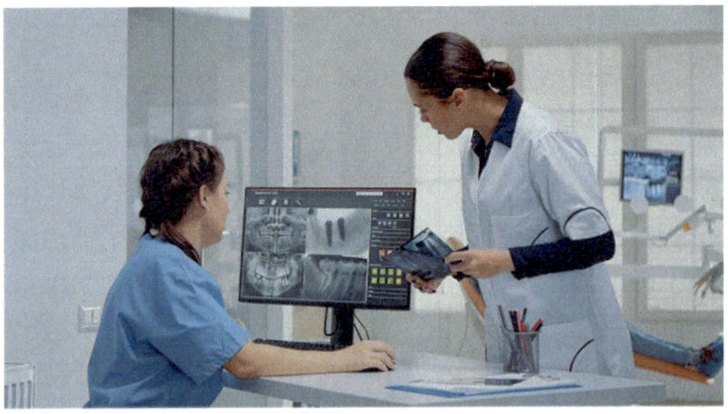

Figure 12.13. Advancements in radiology informatics, particularly through the integration of artificial intelligence, have significantly enhanced the precision of diagnostic interpretations.

Source: https://www.osplabs.com/wp-content/uploads/2021/12/810x435-5-5.jpg.

12.3.2. Enhanced Workflow Efficiency

Many parts of healthcare have been transformed by technology, and radiology informatics is leading the way. AI adoption in medical imaging has made it possible to complete diagnostics more quickly and improve how things are done. For instance, AI-enhanced PACS have demonstrated the ability to reduce diagnostic times by up to 90% for critical conditions by automating complex image analysis tasks such as early tumor detection and motion artifact correction (Pérez-Sanpablo *et al.*, 2025). Additionally, the incorporation of natural language processing tools has streamlined the generation and consistency of radiology reports, reducing reporting time by 30%–50% and thereby allowing radiologists to focus more on interpretation and patient care (Pérez-Sanpablo *et al.*, 2025). AI chatbots are now important helpers in medical decisions, as studies have found that people like their accuracy and ease of operation, which helps improve the way work is done and reduces mistakes. All of these developments highlight the crucial role AI plays in enhancing radiology and supporting patient care.

12.3.3. Reduction in Radiologist Burnout

The rising pressures on radiologists caused by more images to read and complicated cases have led to a lot of burnout. By adopting artificial intelligence, radiology workflows can address these issues by enhancing efficiency and reducing repetitive tasks. For instance, AI-assisted reporting can significantly decrease the time required to generate radiology reports without compromising diagnostic accuracy, thereby alleviating workload intensity and cognitive fatigue among practitioners (Acosta *et al.*, 2024). Moreover, the acceptance of AI and teleradiology in pediatric radiology, despite currently low routine utilization, reflects a growing recognition of their potential to support radiologists and improve care delivery (Sturm *et al.*, 2025). By streamlining report generation and facilitating remote consultations, AI-driven solutions pave the way for more manageable workloads and improved work-life balance, ultimately contributing to a reduction in radiologist burnout and fostering sustainable clinical practice environments (Figure 12.14).

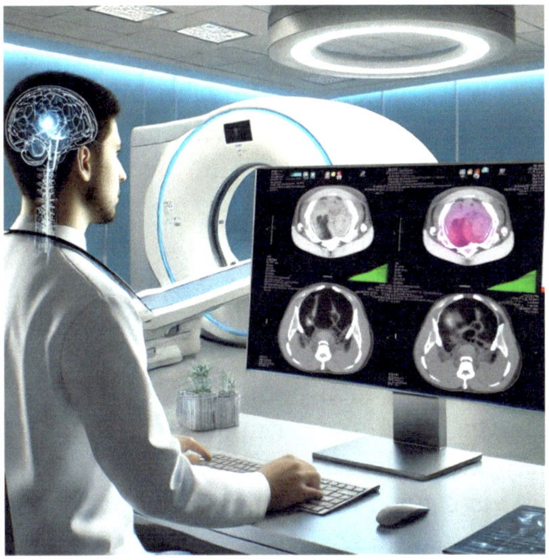

Figure 12.14. Integrating artificial intelligence into radiology workflows offers a promising avenue to mitigate these pressures by enhancing efficiency and reducing repetitive tasks.

Source: https://castlehilldx.com.au/wp-content/uploads/2025/01/Artifical-Intelligence-in-Radiology.webp.

12.3.4. Cost-Effectiveness of Artificial Intelligence (AI) Solutions

Because healthcare systems are under more pressure, new ways are needed to use resources wisely without sacrificing patient care. AI is helping radiology informatics by making operations more efficient and less costly. Radiologists have their workload reduced by AI, which also helps them make more accurate and speedy diagnoses. Because of this efficiency, healthcare institutions can save a lot of money, particularly when the change affects many patients. In addition, AI helps by sorting cases by their urgency and possible outcomes, which leads to more efficient use of resources. While it may cost a lot to start using AI in healthcare, the advantages over time, such as fewer misdiagnoses, quicker patient care, and improved planning, are worth it. These advantages reinforce AI's role as a cost-effective intervention in clinical workflows, an impact that is increasingly evident in developing nations that are adapting such technologies (Krishnan *et al.*, 2023; Liu *et al.*, 2023).

12.3.5. Personalized Patient Care

Thanks to improvements in radiology informatics and artificial intelligence, it has become easier to provide each patient with personalized care through accurate diagnosis and treatment. AI tools improve the analysis of medical images, making it possible to find clinical conditions earlier and more accurately, which helps doctors design the best treatment plans for each patient.

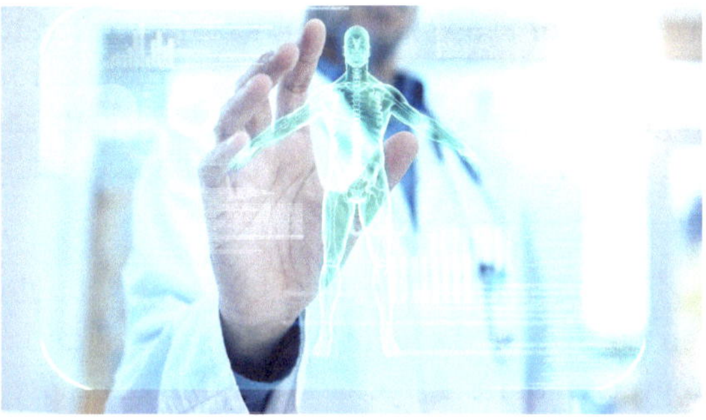

Figure 12.15. AI-powered tools enhance medical imaging analysis, enabling more accurate and timely detection of clinical conditions, which optimizes treatment plans specific to each patient's pathology and clinical history.

Source: https://www.technologyally.com/wp-content/uploads/2024/02/ai-medical-diagnosis-apps.jpg.

Also, the use of virtual and augmented reality in the Metaverse helps patients by offering interactive and flexible healthcare settings that improve communication between providers and patients. They not only give more accurate diagnoses but also help patients stay involved and follow treatment plans with personalized learning and rehab content. Still, it is important to govern these systems well to deal with ethical, privacy, and safety matters, so that patients receive fair and effective care. Thus, the synthesis of AI and informatics technologies holds great promise for revolutionizing personalized care in radiology (Chengoden *et al.*, 2023; Kuwaiti *et al.*, 2023) (Figure 12.15).

12.3.6. Real-Time Data Analysis

Because there is more and more medical imaging data, it is necessary to interpret it quickly and accurately, which can be achieved by using real-time data analysis in radiology informatics. Using AI in imaging makes it possible to analyze results quickly and make quick decisions, which benefits patients. The versatility of these algorithms is demonstrated by their ability to generalize across various imaging tasks and pathologies, a trait that underscores their robustness and clinical utility (Antonelli *et al.*, 2022).

Furthermore, decentralized approaches such as Swarm Learning enable the seamless integration of heterogeneous data sources from multiple institutions while preserving privacy and compliance with regulations (Warnat-Herresthal *et al.*, 2021). Because of this, AI models can be updated and improved in real time with new data while still protecting confidentiality. For this reason, real-time data analysis helps precision medicine and also leads to the development of adaptable and scalable radiology informatics systems for fast and personalized diagnostics.

12.3.7. Increased Access to Radiology Services

Thanks to progress in radiology informatics and artificial intelligence, it is now easier and more efficient for many people to receive radiology services. Because of PACS and other digital tools, storing and retrieving medical images is now much simpler and faster for clinicians from any location. This digital infrastructure not only enhances workflow efficiency but also contributes to shorter reporting times and reduced patient waiting periods, factors that improve satisfaction among both patients and healthcare providers (Alhur *et al.*, 2024). Additionally, AI-driven tools support consistent and accurate image analysis, mitigating disparities in diagnostic quality across different settings by providing uniform expertise and decision-making support (Dewey *et al.*, 2019). Because of these advances, learning and teamwork increase, which leads to better care for each patient and fewer missed diagnoses. So, making radiology services more widely available with the help of informatics and AI is crucial for reaching fair, prompt, and excellent healthcare outcomes.

12.3.8. Collaboration Between Radiologists and Artificial Intelligence (AI)

AI has made it possible to diagnose more accurately and handle workflow more efficiently in healthcare, mainly in radiology. AI systems use machine learning and predictive analytics to quickly look at medical images, notice faint changes, and help in making clinical choices. But the best outcome is reached when radiologists and AI work together, with human understanding adding to the accuracy of algorithms. Radiologists help by understanding a patient's background and symptoms, while AI is efficient and reliable in analyzing a lot of data and spotting patterns. With this collaboration, there are better test results, more efficient operations, less paperwork, and more individualized care. Even so, dealing with issues such as algorithmic bias and ethics requires people from various areas to team up and follow strong regulations. As the integration of AI in radiology continues to evolve, these cooperative dynamic holds promise for transforming patient care and advancing radiology informatics (Ghozali, 2024; Mbata *et al.*, 2024) (Figure 12.16).

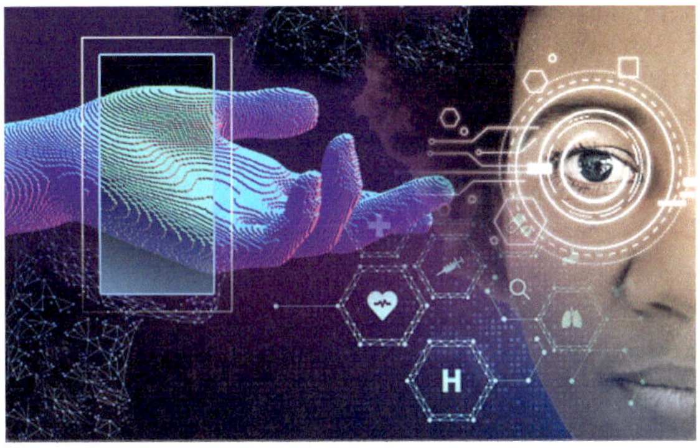

Figure 12.16. By leveraging machine learning algorithms and predictive analytics, AI systems can swiftly analyze medical images, identify subtle abnormalities, and support clinical decision-making processes.

Source: https://www.aha.org/sites/default/files/2023-05/How-AI-Is-Improving-Diagnostics-Decision-Making-and-Care.png.

12.3.9. Future Potential of Artificial Intelligence (AI) in Radiology

Radiology will be transformed by artificial intelligence, leading to more accurate diagnoses and better workflow, which will greatly benefit patients. Radiologists can make more accurate interpretations of complex images by using AI's ability to process information fast and recognize patterns, which helps them detect diseases earlier and reduces the risk of human mistakes. Innovations such as large language models have demonstrated potential in enhancing the semantic analysis of radiology reports, which improves the alignment of textual data with clinical truths, thus facilitating better communication and decision-making (Li *et al.*, 2024). Furthermore, AI's predictive capabilities extend beyond human capacity, allowing for personalized treatment plans and real-time monitoring, contributing to proactive healthcare management (Abualigah *et al.*, 2024). It is still very important to focus on data privacy and how AI can be properly combined with the knowledge of experts for AI to be used sustainably. As AI keeps advancing, it will likely play a bigger part in radiology and bring major benefits to both doctors and patients within radiology informatics and AI.

Test Your Knowledge

1. How do AI and MRI or CT scan interpretation interact?
2. What are the applications of AI in emergency radiology?

12.4. Challenges and Limitations of Radiology Informatics and Artificial Intelligence (AI)

Learning Outcome

1. Understand data quality and standardization issues;
2. Know resistance to change in clinical settings;
3. Focus on training and education for radiologists;
4. Identify regulatory and compliance challenges;
5. Consider ethical dilemmas in AI decision-making;
6. Know dependence on technology;
7. Describe financial barriers to implementation;
8. Address bias in AI algorithms;
9. Explain future research directions.

Bringing AI into radiology informatics is difficult mainly because there is not enough diverse data, and AI models are not always general enough. Even with new algorithm updates, many AI systems fail to perform the same way in different groups of patients and hospitals since there is not enough complete and representative data. This scarcity hinders rigorous evaluation and regulatory approval, as well as site-specific fine-tuning necessary to adapt models to local clinical nuances (Saenz *et al.*, 2023). Additionally, while challenges like the Medical Segmentation Decathlon have demonstrated that well-designed algorithms can generalize across multiple tasks, the training and deployment of such systems remain complex and resource-intensive (Antonelli *et al.*, 2022). Medical practices change from one place to another; there are differences in how data is labeled, and privacy issues make it more difficult to share and verify data. All of these challenges make it difficult for AI tools to be used more widely in radiology, which is why having strong, common ways to handle data and test models is important.

12.4.1. Data Quality and Standardization Issues

Although artificial intelligence has great potential in radiology, it is facing major obstacles because of problems with data quality and standardization. If data is not formatted the same way, images are not complete, and annotation methods differ, AI algorithms cannot be trusted and may not work in different situations. Besides, because there are no standard ways to store medical imaging data, it is hard for different healthcare institutions to share and use the data for AI model development and testing. The problem is made worse by separate health information systems that do not work well together, which results in data that is divided and may be biased. To deal with these issues, we must work together to build strong data governance systems and standardization guidelines for producing good-quality, compatible data. Without these foundational improvements, the full potential of AI-enhanced radiology in improving diagnostic accuracy and patient outcomes remains unattainable (Debnath *et al.*, 2023; Eymann *et al.*, 2024) (Figure 12.17).

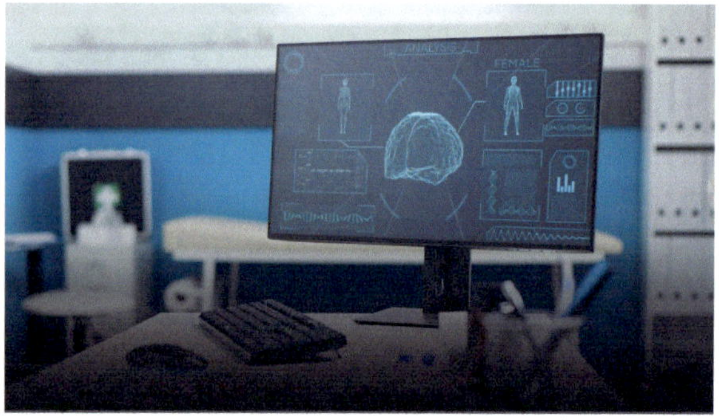

Figure 12.17. The integration of artificial intelligence (AI) into radiology holds immense promise, yet it is critically impeded by challenges related to data quality and standardization.

Source: https://d33xmv9j3wn8v0.cloudfront.net/uploads/2025/04/3-21_1.jpg.

12.4.2. Resistance to Change in Clinical Settings

Many healthcare experts are resistant to new technologies, which causes significant issues when implementing them in clinical settings. The reason for this resistance is that operating rooms are complex and unpredictable, and any inefficiency or inconsistent way of working adds a lot of stress to staff. If informatics and AI are not well-integrated, they can make these problems worse by disturbing how teams from nursing, anesthesia, and radiology usually communicate and work together. Also, worries about privacy, ethics, and how AI algorithms work cause some to be cautious about using them. To solve these challenges, technology should be introduced with a plan that ensures it fits well, is explained clearly, and that employees are trained to work together. As research highlights, advancing radiology informatics with AI demands balancing innovation with ethical considerations and user acceptance to overcome resistance and achieve meaningful improvements in patient care and operational efficiency (Bogari *et al.*, 2024; Esteves *et al.*, 2024).

12.4.3. Training and Education for Radiologists

As AI is being used more in radiology, the training of radiologists should also change to help them use these new technologies well. Studies today show that many radiologists lack knowledge of AI, and many believe that proper training can help close this gap. Surveys conducted among radiologists reveal a strong consensus that comprehensive academic programs incorporating medical informatics and AI should be embedded within radiology residency curricula, emphasizing the critical nature of understanding algorithmic processes and patient safety concerns (Antolín *et al.*, 2022). Furthermore, innovative computer-based training systems, such as case-based tutors utilizing structured image description languages and statistical models, offer promising avenues to enhance diagnostic skills through interactive and personalized learning experiences (Azevedo *et al.*, 2000). Such pedagogical advancements are essential to equip radiologists with the necessary knowledge and tools to effectively collaborate with AI technologies, ultimately improving diagnostic accuracy and patient outcomes in clinical practice (Figure 12.18).

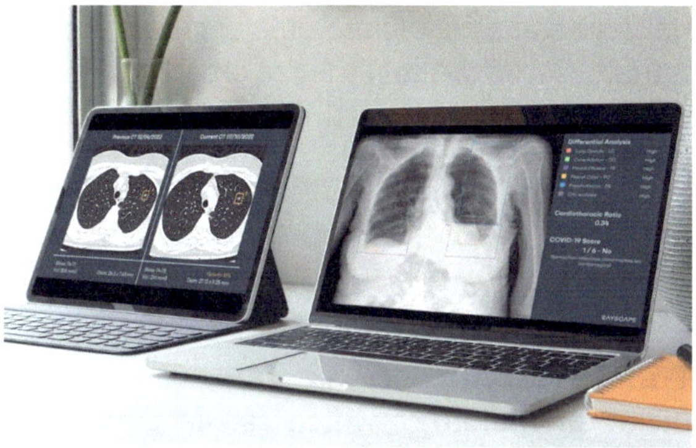

Figure 12.18. As the integration of artificial intelligence (AI) within radiology advances rapidly, the educational framework for radiologists must evolve accordingly to ensure competence in these emerging technologies.

Source: https://images.prismic.io/rayscape/87a4e503-ea68-4285-8044-960080bb1f27_smartmockups_lj3z7kx0%281%29.webp?auto=compress,format.

12.4.4. Regulatory and Compliance Challenges

Artificial intelligence is being introduced into radiology informatics, and this leads to many regulatory and compliance challenges that require careful handling. As AI technologies become increasingly sophisticated, issues related to trust, reproducibility, explainability, and accountability emerge as critical barriers to widespread clinical adoption (Aboian *et al.*, 2024). Policies must be updated to handle these issues and guarantee the safety of patients and their data, but the speed of innovation is usually faster than the speed of policy creation. Also, dealing with sensitive medical data creates serious privacy issues, so strict adherence to health information laws is required. The challenge extends to ensuring fairness and mitigating bias in AI algorithms, which require transparent and interpretable models to maintain ethical standards (Esteves *et al.*, 2024). Because of these various difficulties, it is important for technologists, clinicians, and regulators to work together to create guidelines that blend technology, ethics, and legal rules in radiology informatics.

12.4.5. Ethical Dilemmas in Artificial Intelligence (AI) Decision-Making

Artificial intelligence is being used more quickly in radiology, which can lead to major improvements, but it also raises important ethical concerns that should be closely examined. Because AI-based Clinical Decision Support Systems are playing a bigger role in diagnostic and treatment steps, more people are worried about bias, transparency, and accountability. If AI algorithms use biased data, they can harm equal access to healthcare, which means they should be closely watched and validated. Because some AI models are not fully transparent, clinicians have a hard time understanding and trusting the advice they get from machines, which makes it harder for them to make final decisions. It is important for developers, clinicians and regulators to team up to build strong systems that guarantee AI tools are safe and ethical at all stages. By systematically addressing these ethical considerations, the promise of AI can be harnessed without compromising patient welfare, aligning technological innovation with moral imperatives in radiology practice (Brady *et al.*, 2024; Elhaddad *et al.*, 2024) (Figure 12.19).

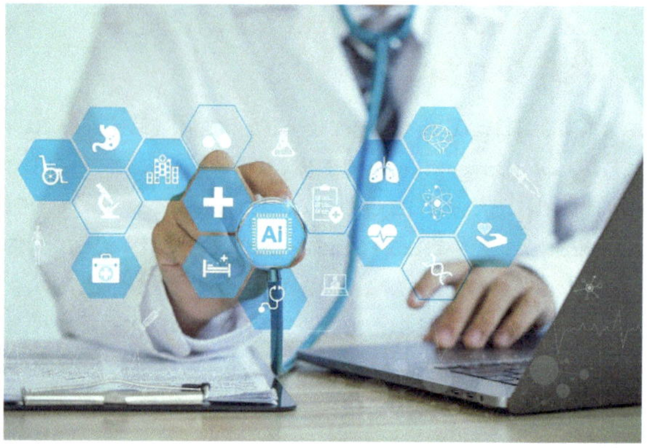

Figure 12.19. As artificial intelligence (AI)-driven Clinical Decision Support Systems become increasingly influential in diagnostic and treatment processes, concerns regarding bias, transparency, and accountability intensify.

Source: https://d2jx2rerrg6sh3.cloudfront.net/images/Article_Images/ImageForArticle_23905_16992787609573557.jpg.

12.4.6. Dependence on Technology

Advanced technologies are now essential in radiology, which demonstrates a major change in healthcare toward using digital tools and artificial intelligence. The reason for this dependence is that the huge amount of patient data and images must be analyzed quickly and precisely, which older approaches find hard to do. Electronic health records, combined with natural language processing, illustrate efforts to reduce clinician workload by automating the extraction and structuring of complex medical information, although challenges in commercial adoption remain (Braun *et al.*, 2023). Furthermore, generative AI technologies, such as large language models and adversarial networks, offer transformative potential in diagnostics and personalized treatment, yet their integration necessitates addressing concerns related to transparency, bias, and ethical standards (Esteves *et al.*, 2024). At the same time, while technology improves how things are done in radiology, being too dependent on it requires us to watch over its use to avoid it complicating the work of radiologists.

12.4.7. Financial Barriers to Implementation

Bringing advanced technologies into healthcare usually meets many challenges, and financial problems are the most significant. Because of the initial costs needed to purchase advanced imaging devices, design AI algorithms, and build a solid data system, radiology informatics and AI are often too expensive for under-resourced institutions. Also, the constant need to update software, train workers, and secure systems adds more expenses to the company.

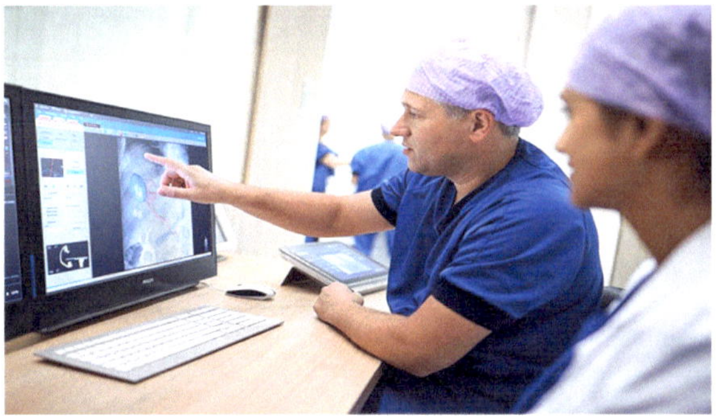

Figure 12.20. In the context of radiology informatics and AI, the initial investment required for acquiring sophisticated imaging hardware, developing AI algorithms, and maintaining robust data infrastructure can be prohibitive, particularly for under-resourced institutions.

Source: https://www.philips.com/c-dam/corporate/newscenter/global/standard/resources/healthcare/2024/fhi-informatics-data-cut/teaser-global-future-health-index-data-cut.jpg.

This economic strain is especially pronounced in developing countries, where healthcare budgets are already stretched thin by competing priorities and infrastructural deficits (Soyege *et al.*, 2025). Even in healthcare systems with a lot of resources, the effectiveness of using AI tools is still questioned because there are uncertainties about what the future will bring and how AI will be reimbursed. Hence, without sustainable funding models and strategic financial planning, the promise of AI-enhanced radiology may remain unrealized, limiting improvements in diagnostic accuracy and patient care (Adamchic, 2025) (Figure 12.20).

12.4.8. Addressing Bias in Artificial Intelligence (AI) Algorithms

Although AI in radiology can improve how accurate diagnoses are, the presence of bias in these algorithms causes serious ethical and practical issues. If the training data is not diverse enough, the model might give different results for patients from different groups. A solution to this should include improving fairness and also consider the specific needs and knowledge of the healthcare domain. Current efforts often emphasize group fairness, focusing on demographic equality at the macro level, yet individual fairness remains overlooked, which can undermine patient-specific care quality (Celi *et al.*, 2024). Trust and use of these systems by physicians are influenced by their being designed with transparency and to avoid bias. By leveraging socio-technical design principles, developers can create more robust systems that encourage clinician engagement and improve patient outcomes (Behrens *et al.*, 2022). Therefore, ensuring that AI algorithms are fair is crucial for both ethical and effective radiology informatics.

12.4.9. Future Research Directions

Because of progress in radiology informatics and artificial intelligence, it is necessary to keep exploring to handle existing issues and make use of new possibilities. Future research must prioritize enhancing model interpretability and transparency, particularly through the integration of explainable AI techniques such as SHAP and LIME, to foster clinician trust and ensure accountability in diagnostic processes (Alkhanbouli *et al.*, 2025). Also, it is important to create multi-modal data integration methods so that AI-based disease prediction models can be more accurate and reliable by using imaging, clinical, and genomic data together. Additionally, ethical considerations surrounding AI-generated medical images and their influence on diagnostic decisions warrant thorough investigation, paralleling discussions on image generation in other domains, as highlighted in related fields (Yu *et al.*, 2025). Customizing radiological studies using AI can boost the success of treatments and help fix differences in healthcare. All these directives will help to ensure that AI in radiology is more dependable, open, and focused on patients.

Test Your Knowledge

1. What are the potential ethical concerns regarding the use of AI in radiology?
2. How can bias in AI algorithms affect radiology outcomes and patient care?

SUMMARY

The use of artificial intelligence in radiology informatics is a major step forward in healthcare, helping to overcome problems such as a high workload and inaccurate diagnosis. AI improves image analysis, takes over routine duties, and helps radiologists detect diseases more accurately, without taking over their work. Even though AI has much potential, it is still difficult to use because of technical issues, privacy problems, and the lack of strong infrastructure in many healthcare settings. Even so, the ongoing development of AI in radiology is expected to enhance patient care and simplify how things are done in clinics, helping the healthcare system run more efficiently. The successful integration of AI will require ongoing collaboration between technologists and clinicians to optimize its benefits while mitigating risks, underscoring its essential role in the future of medical imaging and healthcare delivery (Krishnan *et al.*, 2023; Olawade *et al.*, 2023).

Thanks to new developments in artificial intelligence, there are now many possibilities in healthcare, and radiology informatics is leading this progress. Large language models (LLMs) exemplify these developments, demonstrating significant potential in enhancing diagnostic accuracy, streamlining workflow, and supporting clinical decision-making when integrated with human expertise. By handling a lot of data, such as patient information and research papers, they are able to improve patient treatment and speed up research. At the same time, there are still some difficulties, for example, biased data, the risk of sharing misleading information, and concerns about ethics, laws, and privacy. Additionally, there are few standardized methods for evaluating the usefulness and effectiveness of AI tools in medicine. Recognizing these limitations is very important when using and improving AI in radiology informatics. Continued research aimed at addressing these barriers will be essential to fully harness the capabilities of AI in medical contexts, ultimately improving healthcare outcomes and system efficiency (Nassiri *et al.*, 2024; Ye-Park *et al.*, 2024).

KEY TERMS FROM THIS CHAPTER

- Data analysis
- Machine learning (ML)
- Clinical information
- Privacy
- Transcriptome
- Leukemia
- Data sharing
- Teleradiology
- Computational tools
- Medical datasets
- Transparency
- Biomarkers
- Imaging datasets
- Swarm Learning
- Radiology Information Systems (RIS)

CRITICAL THINKING QUESTIONS

1. **What is the main purpose of a PACS in radiology?**
   a. Scheduling patients
   b. Storing and retrieving imaging data
   c. Performing image-guided surgery
   d. Managing billing information
2. **Which of the following standards is used for medical imaging data storage and transmission?**
   a. HL7
   b. JPEG
   c. DICOM
   d. PDF
3. **RIS (Radiology Information System) is primarily used to:**
   a. Reconstruct 3D images
   b. Manage patient records and workflows in radiology
   c. Conduct MRI scans
   d. Encrypt radiology data
4. **AI in radiology is commonly used for:**
   a. Performing surgeries
   b. Interpreting blood tests
   c. Assisting in image interpretation and anomaly detection
   d. Administering anesthesia
5. **What type of machine learning is most often used for image classification tasks in radiology?**
   a. Supervised learning
   b. Unsupervised learning
   c. Reinforcement learning
   d. Genetic algorithms

Short Answer Questions

1. What is Radiology Informatics, and why is it important in modern healthcare?
2. What are the key components of a Radiology Information System (RIS)?
3. How does a Picture Archiving and Communication System (PACS) facilitate radiology workflow?
4. What is the role of DICOM in radiology data management?
5. How does PACS improve patient care in radiology departments?

Answers to Critical Thinking Questions

1. (b); 2. (c); 3. (b); 4. (c); 5. (a)

REFERENCES

1. Aboian, M., Adewole, M., Bakas, S., Chang, K., *et al.* (2024). Clinical, cultural, computational, and regulatory considerations to deploy AI in radiology: Perspectives of RSNA and MICCAI experts. *Radiology: Artificial Intelligence.* https://core.ac.uk/download/614875585.pdf (accessed on 1st June 2025).
2. Abualigah, L., Banu, S. A., Dhama, K., Mamachan, T. J., *et al.* (2024). Unleashing the future: Exploring the transformative prospects of artificial intelligence in veterinary science. *Journal of Experimental Biology and Agricultural Sciences.* https://core.ac.uk/download/620832362.pdf (accessed on 1st June 2025).
3. Acosta, J. N., Dogra, S., Adithan, S., Wu, K., Moritz, M., Kwak, S., Rajpurkar, P. (2024). *The Impact of AI Assistance on Radiology Reporting: A Pilot Study Using Simulated AI.* https://www.semanticscholar.org/paper/d437b5b947118490e91efa1931917ffc1646384a (accessed on 1st June 2025).
4. Adamchic, I. (2025). Enhancing intracranial aneurysm detection with artificial intelligence in radiology. *Journal of Neurology & Neuromedicine.* https://www.semanticscholar.org/paper/b2988d4ab8688ece638881f72692ca1dbd4da8c2 (accessed on 1st June 2025).
5. Ade, R. P., Kumar, R., Nirala, R. K., Sonaji, P. G., *et al.* (2023). Uses of AI in field of radiology—What is state of doctor & patients communication in different disease for diagnosis purpose. *Journal for Research in Applied Sciences and Biotechnology.* https://core.ac.uk/download/597862415.pdf (accessed on 1st June 2025).
6. Al Hayek, A. H., Charara, J., & Geryes, M. (2025). Extent of artificial intelligence chatbots' integration into routine medical imaging: Exploring the boundaries of AI advancements. In *2025 International Conference on Control, Automation, and Instrumentation (IC2AI).* https://www.semanticscholar.org/paper/dff04bb64d6a5805b3e97f410af635664396917f (accessed on 1st June 2025).
7. Kuwaiti Al , A., Nazer, K., Alreedy, A. H., AlShehri, S. D., Almuhanna, A., Subbarayalu, A. V., Al Muhanna, D., *et al.* (2023). A review of the role of artificial intelligence in healthcare. *Journal of Personalized Medicine, 13,* 951. https://doi.org/10.3390/jpm13060951 (accessed on 1st June 2025).
8. Alex, B., Casey, A., Davidson, E., Dong, F., *et al.* (2021). The reporting quality of natural language processing studies – Systematic review of studies of radiology reports. *BMC Medical Imaging.* https://core.ac.uk/download/483871007.pdf (accessed on 1st June 2025).
9. Alhazime, Y. Y. (2024). Artificial intelligence transforming healthcare: Insights from a systematic review on nursing, midwifery, radiology, pharmacy, health administration, and social work applications. *Power System Technology.* https://www.semanticscholar.org/paper/ad998b12e11b7c6484e97d10af36f4d598a3ea1d (accessed on 1st June 2025).
10. Alhur, A. (2024). Clinician acceptance and adoption of PACS in radiology services: An exploratory study. *Indonesian Journal of Information Systems (IJIS).* https://core.ac.uk/download/617102161.pdf (accessed on 1st June 2025).
11. Ali, O., Abdelbaki, W., Shrestha, A., Elbaşi, E., Alryalat, M. A. A., & Dwivedi, Y. K. (2023). A systematic literature review of artificial intelligence in the healthcare sector: Benefits, challenges, methodologies, and functionalities. *Journal of Innovation & Knowledge, 8,* 100333. https://doi.org/10.1016/j.jik.2023.100333 (accessed on 1st June 2025).

12. Alkhanbouli, R., Almadhaani, H. M. A., Alhosani, F., & Simsekler, M. (2025). The role of explainable artificial intelligence in disease prediction: A systematic literature review and future research directions. *BMC Medical Informatics and Decision Making, 25.* https://www.semanticscholar.org/paper/a1b5e4b4a430058e33498e4d842734344d1fb7f9 (accessed on 1st June 2025).

13. Antolín, A., Eiroa, G. D., Escobar, A. M., Fernández Del, C. A. J., *et al.* (2022). The current state of knowledge on imaging informatics: A survey among Spanish radiologists. *Insights into Imaging.* https://core.ac.uk/download/534957993.pdf (accessed on 1st June 2025).

14. Antonelli, M., Reinke, A., Bakas, S., Farahani, K., Kopp-Schneider, A., Landman, B. A., Litjens, G., *et al.* (2022). The medical segmentation decathlon. *Nature Communications, 13.* https://doi.org/10.1038/s41467-022-30695-9 (accessed on 1st June 2025).

15. Azevedo, B., Du Boulay, B. A., Teather, D., Boshuizen, H., Brown, J., Collins, J., Teather, D., *et al.* (2000). *Structured Computer-Based Training in the Interpretation of Neuroradiological Images.* https://core.ac.uk/download/2709128.pdf (accessed on 1st June 2025).

16. Barnholtz-Sloan, J. S., Basu, A., Borowsky, A. D., Bui, A., *et al.* (2020). Cancer Informatics for Cancer Centers (CI4CC): Building a community focused on sharing ideas and best practices to improve cancer care and patient outcomes. https://core.ac.uk/download/288432567.pdf (accessed on 1st June 2025).

17. Baumgartner, C., Deserno, T., Hsu, W., *et al.* (2019). *Advancing Artificial Intelligence in Sensors, Signals, and Imaging Informatics.* https://core.ac.uk/download/323076975.pdf (accessed on 1st June 2025).

18. Behrens, A. J., Liu, J., & Noteboom, C. B. (2022). *A Design Theory for Intelligent Clinical Decision Support.* https://core.ac.uk/download/529573462.pdf (accessed on 1st June 2025).

19. Bogari, A. F., Alzahrani, F. A. A., Alzahrani, S. A. S., Hakami, A. A. M., Almotairi, A. D. J., Zamzami, S. A., *et al.* (2024). *Efficacy of Digital Operating Room Technology, Role of Nursing, Anesthesia and Radiology Team in OR Safety.* https://core.ac.uk/download/616775627.pdf (accessed on 1st June 2025).

20. Brady, A. P., Allen, B., Chong, J., Kotter, E., Kottler, N., Mongan, J., Oakden-Rayner, L., *et al.* (2024). Developing, purchasing, implementing and monitoring AI tools in radiology: Practical considerations. A multi-society statement from the ACR, CAR, ESR, RANZCR & RSNA. *Insights into Imaging, 15.* https://doi.org/10.1186/s13244-023-01541-3 (accessed on 1st June 2025).

21. Braun, M., Kolbe, L., & Neumann, C. (2023). *Natural Language Processing for Medical Texts – A Taxonomy to Inform Integration Decisions into Clinical Practice.* https://core.ac.uk/download/590878989.pdf (accessed on 1st June 2025).

22. Canguit, J. A., & Sison, M. O. (2025). Diagnostic efficiency, challenges and job satisfaction of radiologic technologists in picture archiving and communication system (PACS). *International Journal of Academic Research in Progressive Education and Development.* https://www.semanticscholar.org/paper/6e8773ca0a4c414bb361eb60203a62a8a09a1723 (accessed on 1st June 2025).

23. Celi, L. A., Cheng, L. T. E., Li, X., Liu, C., *et al.* (2024). *Towards Clinical AI Fairness: Filling Gaps in the Puzzle.* http://arxiv.org/abs/2405.17921 (accessed on 1st June 2025).

24. Chen, J., & Hou, F. (2023). Unmet needs for healthcare. *Health at a Glance.* https://doi.org/10.1787/c122a43b-en (accessed on 1st June 2025).

25. Chengoden, R., Victor, N., Huynh-The, T., Yenduri, G., Jhaveri, R. H., Alazab, M., Bhattacharya, S., *et al.* (2023). Metaverse for healthcare: A survey on potential applications, challenges and future directions. *IEEE Access, 11*, 12765–12795. https://doi.org/10.1109/access.2023.3241628 (accessed on 1st June 2025).

26. Dagi, T. F., Barker, F. G., & Glass, J. (2021). Machine learning and artificial intelligence in neurosurgery: Status, prospects, and challenges. *Neurosurgery, 89*, 133–142. https://doi.org/10.1093/neuros/nyab170 (accessed on 1st June 2025).

27. Debnath, S. (2023). Integrating information technology in healthcare: Recent developments, challenges, and future prospects for urban and regional health. *World Journal of Advanced Research and Reviews*. http://arxiv.org/abs/2307.16296 (accessed on 1st June 2025).

28. Dewey, M., & Wilkens, U. (2019). *The Bionic Radiologist: Avoiding Blurry Pictures and Providing Greater Insights*. https://core.ac.uk/download/228064788.pdf (accessed on 1st June 2025).

29. Díaz, M. A., Cano, A. R., Fernández, A. A., Álvarez, V. A., Carrascoso, A. J., López, A. J., García, C. D., *et al.* (2025). Diagnostic performance of an artificial intelligence software for the evaluation of bone X-ray examinations referred from the emergency department. *Diagnostics, 15*. https://www.semanticscholar.org/paper/2004b5268d521d8a1879485452944dadb4dd5cee (accessed on 1st June 2025).

30. Elhaddad, M., & Hamam, S. (2024). AI-driven clinical decision support systems: An ongoing pursuit of potential. *Cureus*. https://doi.org/10.7759/cureus.57728 (accessed on 1st June 2025).

31. Esteves, R. M. A. (2024). *Applications, Challenges, and Ethical Implications of Generative AI: A Systematic Review*. https://core.ac.uk/download/639216461.pdf (accessed on 1st June 2025).

32. Eymann, T., Fuhrmann, H., & Hennrich, J. (2024). Accelerating the adoption of artificial intelligence technologies in radiology: A comprehensive overview on current obstacles. https://core.ac.uk/download/616566150.pdf (accessed on 1st June 2025).

33. Fanni, S. C., D'Amore, C. A., Milazzo, A., De Liperi, A., Calandriello, L., Cicchetti, G., Baratella, E., *et al.* (2021). Role of quantitative imaging and deep learning in interstitial lung diseases. *Journal of Radiological Review, 8*. https://doi.org/10.23736/s2723-9284.21.00127-9 (accessed on 1st June 2025).

34. Garg, R., Gopichandran, L., Hote, P., Kahol, P., Venkatesan, A., *et al.* (2023). Artificial intelligence for smart patient care: Transforming future of nursing practice. *Int. J. Res. Med. Sci.* https://core.ac.uk/download/588568210.pdf (accessed on 1st June 2025).

35. Ghozali, M. T. (2024). How AI is changing healthcare: A review of innovations and challenges in health informatics. *Ranah Research: Journal of Multidisciplinary Research and Development*. https://www.semanticscholar.org/paper/63c0f388a311bb771d5127053eece954c2645cf6 (accessed on 1st June 2025).

36. Ginley, B., Govind, D., Jain, S., Jen, D., *et al.* (2018). Iterative annotation to ease neural network training: Specialized machine learning in medical image analysis. https://core.ac.uk/download/573411151.pdf (accessed on 1st June 2025).

37. Ho, C. W. L., & Caals, K. (2021). A call for an ethics and governance action plan to harness the power of artificial intelligence and digitalization in nephrology. *Seminars in Nephrology, 41*, 282–293. https://doi.org/10.1016/j.semnephrol.2021.05.009 (accessed on 1st June 2025).

38. Hofmeijer, E. I. S., Kwee, T., Lamers, M., Noordzij, W., *et al.* (2024). A framework to integrate artificial intelligence training into radiology residency programs: Preparing the future radiologist. https://core.ac.uk/download/620143327.pdf (accessed on 1st June 2025).

39. Jeon, K., Park, W. Y., Kahn, C. E., Nagy, P., You, S. C., & Yoon, S. H. (2024). Advancing medical imaging research through standardization. *Investigative Radiology*. https://doi.org/10.1097/rli.0000000000001106 (accessed on 1st June 2025).

40. Koçak, B., Ponsiglione, A., Romeo, V., Ugga, L., Huisman, M., Cuocolo, R., *et al.* (2025). Radiology AI and sustainability paradox: Environmental, economic, and social dimensions. *Insights into Imaging, 16*. https://www.semanticscholar.org/paper/23fc2744112849ad14874d6a309e931c4b936655 (accessed on 1st June 2025).

41. Krishnan, G., Singh, S., Pathania, M., Gosavi, S., Abhishek, S., Parchani, A., Dhar, M. (2023). Artificial intelligence in clinical medicine: Catalyzing a sustainable global healthcare paradigm. *Frontiers in Artificial Intelligence, 6*. https://doi.org/10.3389/frai.2023.1227091 (accessed on 1st June 2025).

42. Lakhani, P. (2020). The importance of image resolution in building deep learning models for medical imaging. *Radiology: Artificial Intelligence, 2*(1), e190177. https://www.semanticscholar.org/paper/7ec02c7837f863e7e66be8f1c7262362e4350139 (accessed on 1st June 2025).

43. Lekadir, K., & Petersen, S. (n.d.). FUTURE AI: International consensus guideline for trustworthy and deployable artificial intelligence in healthcare. *BMJ*. https://core.ac.uk/download/644556379.docx (accessed on 1st June 2025).

44. Li, S., Li, X., Liao, W., Liu, Q., *et al.* (2024). Reasoning before comparison: LLM-enhanced semantic similarity metrics for domain specialized text analysis. http://arxiv.org/abs/2402.11398 (accessed on 1st June 2025).

45. Liu, Y., Han, T., Ma, S., Zhang, J., Yang, Y., Tian, J., He, H., *et al.* (2023). Summary of ChatGPT-related research and perspective towards the future of large language models. *Meta-Radiology, 1*, 100017. https://doi.org/10.1016/j.metrad.2023.100017 (accessed on 1st June 2025).

46. Marey, A., Arjmand, P., Alerab, A. D. S., Eslami, M. J., Saad, A. M., Sanchez, N., Umair, M. (2024). Explainability, transparency and black box challenges of AI in radiology: Impact on patient care in cardiovascular radiology. *Egyptian Journal of Radiology and Nuclear Medicine*. https://www.semanticscholar.org/paper/a592922d239289cef17f539266c05c6e3019593c (accessed on 1st June 2025).

47. Martins, V. B. L., Viduedo, P. H. Z., Teixeira, T. A., Destefani, A. C., & Destefani, V. C. (2024). Advancing cardiovascular radiology with artificial intelligence: A comprehensive review of applications, challenges, and future directions. *Revista Ibero-Americana de Humanidades, Ciências e Educação*. https://www.semanticscholar.org/paper/850d73b76e11a3f05d7033f2f302fb574ee92144 (accessed on 1st June 2025).

48. Mbata, A. O., Soyege, O. S., Nwokedi, C. N., Tomoh, B. O., Mustapha, A. Y., Balogun, O. D., Forkuo, A. Y., *et al.* (2024). Machine learning for health informatics: An overview. *Journal of Frontiers in Multidisciplinary Research*. https://www.semanticscholar.org/paper/71612ca76b4e3848ae0d255139e5106e802b46bb (accessed on 1st June 2025).

49. Nassiri, K., & Akhloufi, M. A. (2024). Recent advances in large language models for healthcare. *BioMedInformatics, 4*, 1097–1143. https://doi.org/10.3390/biomedinformatics4020062 (accessed on 1st June 2025).

50. Olawade, D. B., Wada, O. J., David-Olawade, A. C., Kunonga, E., Abaire, O. J., Ling, J., *et al.* (2023). Using artificial intelligence to improve public health: A narrative review. *Frontiers in Public Health, 11*. https://doi.org/10.3389/fpubh.2023.1196397 (accessed on 1st June 2025).

51. Olivieri, F., Caputo, A., Leonetti, D., Castaldo, R., Avolio, R., Cocca, M., Errico, M., *et al.* (2024). Compositional analysis and mechanical recycling of polymer fractions recovered via the industrial sorting of post-consumer plastic waste: A case study toward the implementation of artificial intelligence databases. *Polymers, 16*. https://www.semanticscholar.org/paper/15f160d802dba7c4140b4b856a23fb20dba21bd9 (accessed on 1st June 2025).

52. Paalvast, O., Sevenster, M., Hertgers, O., De Bliek, H., Wijn, V., Buil, V., Knoester, J., *et al.* (2025). Radiology AI lab: Evaluation of radiology applications with clinical end-users. *Journal of Imaging Informatics in Medicine*. https://www.semanticscholar.org/paper/17a8da45b4fa024abc0ae790bf95546f2bb881b8 (accessed on 1st June 2025).

53. Panayides, A. S., Amini, A. A., Filipović, N., Sharma, A., Tsaftaris, S. A., Young, A. A., Foran, D. J., *et al.* (2020). AI in medical imaging informatics: Current challenges and future directions. *IEEE Journal of Biomedical and Health Informatics, 24*, 1837–1857. https://doi.org/10.1109/jbhi.2020.2991043 (accessed on 1st June 2025).

54. Park, Y. J., Pillai, A., Deng, J., Guo, E., Gupta, M., Paget, M., Naugler, C. (2024). Assessing the research landscape and clinical utility of large language models: A scoping review. *BMC Medical Informatics and Decision Making, 24*. https://doi.org/10.1186/s12911-024-02459-6 (accessed on 1st June 2025).

55. Pérez-Sanpablo, A., Quinzaños-Fresnedo, J., Gutiérrez-Martínez, J., Lozano-Rodríguez, I. G., & Roldán-Valadez, E. (2025). Transforming medical imaging: The role of artificial intelligence integration in PACS for enhanced diagnostic accuracy and workflow efficiency. *Current Medical Imaging*. https://www.semanticscholar.org/paper/07234831990987bd706bc40f023eabd193a1d8a2 (accessed on 1st June 2025).

56. Qayyum, A., Qadir, J., Bilal, M., & Al-Fuqaha, A. (2020). Secure and robust machine learning for healthcare: A survey. *IEEE Reviews in Biomedical Engineering, 14*, 156–180. https://doi.org/10.1109/rbme.2020.3013489 (accessed on 1st June 2025).

57. Ratnayake, M. (2021). Artificial intelligence and the radiologist's role. *Journal of Medical Imaging and Radiation Oncology, 65*. https://www.semanticscholar.org/paper/65a280c3efbf99fe88b50bf958603bcbff9cfc93 (accessed on 1st June 2025).

58. Reshma, R. (2025). Artificial intelligence in medical diagnostics and healthcare. *International Scientific Journal of Engineering and Management*. https://www.semanticscholar.org/paper/2d6517d405b412c0002e61bcba00cf665103a4da (accessed on 1st June 2025).

59. Saenz, A., Chen, E., Marklund, H., & Rajpurkar, P. (2023). The MAIDA initiative: Establishing a framework for global medical-imaging data sharing. *The Lancet Digital Health, 6*, e6–e8. https://doi.org/10.1016/s2589-7500(23)00222-4 (accessed on 1st June 2025).

60. Sharma, A., Al-Haidose, A., Al-Asmakh, M., & Abdallah, A. M. (2024). Integrating artificial intelligence into biomedical science curricula: Advancing healthcare education. *Clinics and Practice, 14*, 1391–1403. https://www.semanticscholar.org/paper/e85e52abfb24f6f4d50b428f3235e7aab1dccff1 (accessed on 1st June 2025).

61. Soyege, O. S., Nwokedi, C. N., Tomoh, B. O., Mustapha, A. Y., Mbata, A. O., Balogun, O. D., Forkuo, A. Y., *et al.* (2025). Health informatics in developing countries: Challenges and opportunities.

International Journal of Applied Research in Social Sciences. https://www.semanticscholar.org/paper/3328bddca58c52018fc7ed42fe0804ba9c6f1ff8 (accessed on 1st June 2025).

62. Sridhar, S., & Sridhar, S. (2021). *A Review Study on Role of AI in Healthcare*. https://core.ac.uk/download/478208454.pdf (accessed on 1st June 2025).

63. Sturm, M. J., von Kalle, T., Renz, D. M., Klee, D., Patsch, J., Spieth, S., Toso, S., *et al.* (2025). Artificial intelligence and teleradiology in pediatric radiology: A survey by the Society for German-speaking Pediatric Radiologists (GPR) and the Swiss Society for Pediatric Radiology (SGPR). *RoFo: Fortschritte auf dem Gebiete der Rontgenstrahlen und der Nuklearmedizin*. https://www.semanticscholar.org/paper/11d766bcabefff065e6d89e23cadbfda6dc2f978 (accessed on 1st June 2025).

64. Warnat-Herresthal, S., Schultze, H., Shastry, K. L., Manamohan, S., Mukherjee, S., Garg, V., Sarveswara, R., *et al.* (2021). Swarm learning for decentralized and confidential clinical machine learning. *Nature, 594*, 265–270. https://doi.org/10.1038/s41586-021-03583-3 (accessed on 1st June 2025).

65. Yu, A., Mohajer, B., & Eng, J. (2022). External validation of deep learning algorithms for radiologic diagnosis: A systematic review. *Radiology: Artificial Intelligence, 4*. https://doi.org/10.1148/ryai.210064 (accessed on 1st June 2025).

66. Yu, J., & Meng, T. (2025). EXPRESS: Image generative AI in tourism: Trends, impacts, and future research directions. *Journal of Hospitality & Tourism Research*. https://www.semanticscholar.org/paper/9bbe61f14ff70638b84a5c037c3ceb4d34dfc3b4 (accessed on 1st June 2025).

INDEX

E

F

G

H

I

J

K

L

M

N

U

V

X